CANCER PAIN:
Assessment, Diagnosis, and Management

CANCER PAIN: Assessment, Diagnosis, and Management

Dermot R. Fitzgibbon, MB, BCh
Associate Professor of Anesthesiology
Adjunct Associate Professor of Medicine
University of Washington School of Medicine
Seattle, Washington

John D. Loeser, MD
Professor Emeritus of Neurological Surgery and Anesthesiology
University of Washington School of Medicine
Seattle, Washington

Wolters Kluwer | Lippincott Williams & Wilkins
Health
Philadelphia · Baltimore · New York · London
Buenos Aires · Hong Kong · Sydney · Tokyo

Acquisitions Editor: Frances DeStefano
Product Manager: Nicole Dernoski
Project Manager: Bridgett Dougherty
Senior Manufacturing Manager: Ben Rivera
Marketing Manager: Angela Panetta
Cover Designer: Teresa Mallon
Production Service: Spearhead Global, Inc.

© 2010 by LIPPINCOTT WILLIAMS & WILKINS, a WOLTERS KLUWER business
530 Walnut Street
Philadelphia, PA 19106 USA
LWW.com

All rights reserved. This book is protected by copyright. No part of this book may be reproduced in any form by any means, including photocopying, or utilized by any information storage and retrieval system without written permission from the copyright owner, except for brief quotations embodied in critical articles and reviews. Materials appearing in this book prepared by individuals as part of their official duties as U.S. government employees are not covered by the above-mentioned copyright.

Printed in China

Library of Congress Cataloging-in-Publication Data
Fitzgibbon, Dermot R.
  Cancer pain : assessment, diagnosis, and management / Dermot R. Fitzgibbon, John D. Loeser.
      p. ; cm.
  Includes bibliographical references and index.
  ISBN-13: 978-1-60831-089-0
  ISBN-10: 1-60831-089-2
  1. Cancer pain. I. Loeser, John D. (John David), 1935- II. Title.
  [DNLM: 1. Neoplasms—drug therapy. 2. Pain—drug therapy. 3. Neoplasms—diagnosis. 4. Pain Measurement. QZ 267 F554c 2009]
  RC262.F58 2009
  616.99′4—dc22
                                                                    2009042385

Care has been taken to confirm the accuracy of the information presented and to describe generally accepted practices. However, the authors, editors, and publisher are not responsible for errors or omissions or for any consequences from application of the information in this book and make no warranty, expressed or implied, with respect to the currency, completeness, or accuracy of the contents of the publication. Application of the information in a particular situation remains the professional responsibility of the practitioner.

The authors, editors, and publisher have exerted every effort to ensure that drug selection and dosage set forth in this text are in accordance with current recommendations and practice at the time of publication. However, in view of ongoing research, changes in government regulations, and the constant flow of information relating to drug therapy and drug reactions, the reader is urged to check the package insert for each drug for any change in indications and dosage and for added warnings and precautions. This is particularly important when the recommended agent is a new or infrequently employed drug.

Some drugs and medical devices presented in the publication have Food and Drug Administration (FDA) clearance for limited use in restricted research settings. It is the responsibility of the health care provider to ascertain the FDA status of each drug or device planned for use in their clinical practice.

To purchase additional copies of this book, call our customer service department at (800) 638-3030 or fax orders to (301) 223-2320. International customers should call (301) 223-2300.

Visit Lippincott Williams & Wilkins on the Internet: at LWW.com. Lippincott Williams & Wilkins customer service representatives are available from 8:30 am to 6 pm, EST.

10 9 8 7 6 5 4 3 2 1

FOREWORD

Public recognition of the importance of the successful management of pain is reflected by increasing governmental and lay public consideration of pain as an important aspect of health care. The 106th U. S. Congress designated the calendar decade beginning January 1, 2001 as the "Decade of Pain Control and Research." In 2004, the International Association for the Study of Pain (IASP) as one of the activities in its Global Year Against Pain stated: "Relief of pain should be a human right." In 2008, IASP also declared a Global Year Against Cancer Pain and encouraged its chapters throughout the world to work within their countries to develop cancer pain management activities. Cancer pain can lead to intractable suffering; interdisciplinary care is often a prerequisite for successful management.

It is thus with perfect timing that Dr. Dermot Fitzgibbon, director of the Inpatient Cancer Pain Program at the University of Washington Medical Center and the Outpatient Cancer Pain Clinic at the Seattle Cancer Care Alliance, with the collaboration of Dr. John D. Loeser, professor emeritus and the previous director of the legendary Multidisciplinary Pain Center founded at the University of Washington by John J. Bonica in 1960, have provided us with a comprehensive interdisciplinary, patient-centered, guide to the assessment, diagnosis, and management of cancer pain.

With a combined experience of over 50 years in pain management and in the exacting spirit of Dr. John Bonica, both Drs. Fitzgibbon and Loeser have composed a detailed treatise that covers not only pain (with a lower case p) as a symptom, but also Pain (with a capital P), as a disease, with all its physiologic, pathologic, emotional, social, and existential dimensions. The readers of this book will understand the characteristics both of cancer pain in general and specific tumor processes and their effects on pain. They will also find guidance on assessment and diagnostic dilemmas, on symptom-directed management, on issues related to home infusion therapy, and on clinical approaches to the diagnosis, assessment, and treatment of depression, anxiety, sleep disturbances, substance abuse, and even future trends in diagnosis and treatment of cancer pain including the role of nanotechnology.

This book provides practical advice, hints, and pearls from the *praxis* of specialists but more importantly, allows us to glimpse the complexities of the management of the cancer patient with pain from a medical, systemwide, and humanistic perspective. Treating Pain in individuals with cancer does not only pose diagnostic enigmas, but requires that providers utilize managerial skills and exhibit personal tenacity in the attempt to manage symptoms including pain. The providers of care for patients with cancer and for cancer survivors with chronic pain must envision themselves as having a long-term relationship with and a commitment to their patient. Treating patients with terminal illness who may be on the verge of death mirrors brightly on one's own mortality and *that*, the courageous act of companionship and care, is the true success of the authors. This book is not a theoretical journey into the myriad of systematic reviews on cancer pain. It is a story of the authors' constant desire to comfort the uncomfortable and care for those for whom, sometimes, we have difficulty caring. As Jamie Mayerfeld wrote in his book *Suffering and Moral Responsibility*, "… treating Pain is like looking at the Sun, it is blinding, so we look away and thus many times by doing nothing wrong, we do something wrong…."[1]

I would like to thank Drs. Fitzgibbon and Loeser for this book, their friendship, and the privilege of writing the foreword.

Alex Cahana, MD, DPhil, DAAPM, FIPP
Hughes M. and Katherine Blake Endowed Professor
Professor and Chief, Division of Pain Medicine
Professor Bioethics and Humanities (adj.)
Professor Radiology (adj.)
Department of Anesthesiology and Pain Medicine
University of Washington
Seattle, Washington
July 2009

---
[1] Jamie Mayerfeld, *Suffering and Moral Responsibility*. Oxford University Press, 1999

PREFACE

Care of the cancer patient with pain is a complex, dynamic endeavor requiring both a long-term commitment and the ability to work with an interdisciplinary team. The diagnosis of cancer and its subsequent treatment mandates the need to respond in a timely fashion to multiple issues. In our experience, the types of care are dictated primarily by the patient, and the uniqueness and individuality of each complaint must be recognized. It is important that a treating clinician recognize the many different factors that influence a patient's perception of pain. Algorithmic approaches to care frequently do not work and may, in fact, encourage rigidity in patient management. We wish to provide clinicians involved in the care of cancer patients with an up-to-date and thorough description of all of these factors and to describe successful management strategies. It is our belief that comprehensive pain management requires the presence of an "overseeing" or managing physician who can coordinate all aspects of symptom management in cancer pain patients. In each chapter, we comprehensively review the many different publications available on the diagnosis and management of cancer pain and then present our approaches both to diagnosis and to care.

As tumor-directed treatments improve, more patients are surviving for longer periods but often have lingering pain and other symptoms that negatively impact their quality of life. This mandates a change in treatment strategy from simply using medications to palliate symptoms to a more comprehensive approach that focuses on outcome issues such as quality of life and functional improvement. Essential to this strategic change is the recognition of the complex roles that medications and other interventions may have in such situations. For example, high doses of psychoactive medications (such as opioids or benzodiazepines) can impair quality of life as well as alleviate pain. Inappropriate use of such medications can be detrimental and potentially life threatening. The goal in pain management must always be to improve and not impair quality of life.

A consistent approach is required in the management of patients with cancer and pain and a book on this subject should reflect this consistency. This is why we have chosen to write this book without contributing authors. We have relied on many of our colleagues' suggestion of references, for discussions and review of portions of the book, and for years of informal input. We particularly wish to thank Drs. Debra Schwinn, Jason Rockhill, Dan Silbergeld, and Trent Tredway for reviewing sections of our manuscript and providing expert advice.

We are especially grateful to the patients who have provided us with the experiences upon which this book is based. The mutual trust between patient and doctor has been the cornerstone of our endeavors. We would also like to recognize the faculty and staff at the University of Washington for their excellence in teaching, research, and clinical care. We have encountered many excellent health care providers who have worked unselfishly every day to provide compassionate and professional care to patients with cancer and pain. In particular, we thank the many oncologists who have collaborated with us for care. Cancer pain management requires a team approach and, in our institution, we witness this daily.

We all stand on the shoulders of those who have gone before us. Dr. Fitzgibbon would especially like to acknowledge Dr. Peter Freund for his foresight in career development. He would also like to recognize his late father for his insight and guidance. Both Drs. Fitzgibbon and Loeser thank their wives and children for their understanding and support. They also acknowledge the role that Dr. John J. Bonica played in their careers, in developing the Pain Center at the University of Washington, and in putting pain management onto the medical map throughout the world. We are privileged to continue the journey that he started.

Dr. John D. Loeser
Dr. Dermot R. Fitzgibbon
Seattle, Washington

CONTENTS

Foreword   *v*
Preface   *vii*

SECTION I — ASSESSMENT AND DIAGNOSIS

Chapter 1	Introduction and Epidemiology	2
Chapter 2	Cancer Pain Assessment and Diagnostic Issues	7
Chapter 3	The Perception of Pain	10
Chapter 4	The Process of Pain in the Cancer Patient	17
Chapter 5	Issues Affecting Well-Being in Cancer Patients	24
Chapter 6	Characteristics of Cancer Pain	32
Chapter 7	Tumor Processes and Pain	42
Chapter 8	Bone Metastases	76
Chapter 9	Visceral Pain	86
Chapter 10	Neuropathic Pain	89
Chapter 11	Metastatic Epidural Spinal Cord Compression	114
Chapter 12	Systematic Pain Assessment	120

SECTION II — MANAGEMENT

Chapter 13	Overview of Management	130
Chapter 14	Comprehensive Care of the Cancer Patient with Pain	135
Chapter 15	Primary Anticancer Treatments	138
Chapter 16	Symptom-Directed Pain Management: Medication	153
Chapter 17	Nonopioid Analgesics	159
Chapter 18	Adjuvant Drugs	171
Chapter 19	Opioid Analgesics	190
Chapter 20	Medication Misuse and Substance Abuse	231
Chapter 21	Symptom-Directed Pain Management Interventions	246
Chapter 22	Neuraxial Analgesia	270

Chapter 23	Spine and Bone Pain	303
Chapter 24	Depression, Anxiety, and Sleep	314
Chapter 25	Related Issues	323
Chapter 26	Specialized Pain Management	327
	Summary: Pain and Cancer	332

APPENDICES

Appendix A	Pain Disability Index (PDI)	333
Appendix B	Functional Assessment Cancer Therapy – General (FACT-G)	335
Appendix C	Structured Opioid Assessment for Patients with Pain (SOAPP)	337
Appendix D	Current Opioid Misuse Measure (COMM)	339
Appendix E	Driving Instructions for Patients Taking Opioids	341
Appendix F	Opioid Agreement	342
Appendix G	Consent to Assume Risks for Medical Marijuana	343
Appendix H	Physician Authorization for Medical Marijuana	345
Appendix I	Pittsburgh Sleep Quality Index (PSQI)	347
Appendix J	Patient Health Questionnaire-9 (PHQ-9)	352
Appendix K	1. Template for Initial Outpatient Pain Evaluation	353
	2. Template for Outpatient Pain Clinic Follow-up Visits	358
Appendix L	Patient Disability Questionnaire (PDQ)	363
Appendix M	Neuropathic Pain Scale (NPS)	365
Appendix N	CAGE Questionnaire	367
Index		369

SECTION I ■ ASSESSMENT AND DIAGNOSIS

CHAPTER 1 ■ INTRODUCTION AND EPIDEMIOLOGY

This section is designed to provide perspectives on the incidence and prevalence of cancer and related pain syndromes. Cancer is a significant public health problem in the United States, as well as in other developed countries. The incidence of cancer has increased worldwide by 19% in the past decade, most of which has been attributed to cases in developing countries.[1] By 2020, it has been estimated, up to 70% of the 20 million new cases of cancer predicted to occur yearly will be in the developing world.[2] Survival rates in developing countries are often less than one third of those for site-specific cancers in the developing world.[3] Cancers observed in developed countries tend to reflect hormonal and dietary profiles of their populations, with a high incidence of breast, colorectal, and prostate cancers. By contrast, populations in developing countries are susceptible to cancers stemming from infectious disease or nonmalignant disease associated with chronic infections; there is a greater incidence of cervical, liver, stomach, oropharyngeal, and esophageal cancers.

Men have a higher (45%) lifetime probability of developing cancer than women (38%); however, because of the relatively early age of breast cancer onset, women have a slightly higher probability of developing cancer before 60 years of age. Cancer is a major cause of death (22.8% of total deaths) in the United States and is second only to heart diseases (26.6% of total deaths). A total of 1,437,180 new cancer cases and 565,650 deaths from cancers were expected to occur in the United States in 2008.[4] One in four deaths that year in the United States was expected to be due to cancer. In 2008, approximately 560,000 Americans died from cancer: more than 1,500 deaths per day. Significant trends in the incidence and mortality rates of cancer include stabilization of the age-standardized, delay-adjusted incidence rates for all cancers combined, in men, from 1990 through 2004; a continuing increase in the incidence rate for women by 0.3% per year; and a 13.6% total decrease in age-standardized cancer death rates among men and women, combined, between 1991 and 2004. Overall cancer death rates in 2004 decreased by 18.4% and 10.5%, respectively, for men since 1990 and for women since 1991. The 5-year relative survival rate from cancer is 68% for whites and 57% for African Americans. For many sites, survival rates in African Americans are 10% to more than 20% lower than in whites. This is due, in part, to African Americans being less likely to receive a cancer diagnosis at an early, localized stage, when treatment can improve chances of survival. Additional factors that contribute to the survival differential include unequal access to medical care and tumor characteristics (Table 1.1). Survival rates for all cancers combined and for certain site-specific cancers have improved significantly since the 1970s, due, in part, to both earlier detection and advances in treatment. Survival rates markedly increased for cancers of the prostate, breast, colon, and rectum and for leukemia (Table 1.2).

Cancers of the prostate, lung and bronchus, and colon and rectum account for about 50% of all newly diagnosed cancers in men. Prostate cancer accounts for about 25% of incident cases in men. Approximately 91% of the new cases of prostate cancer will be diagnosed at local or regional stages, for which 5-year relative survival approaches 100%. For women in 2008, the three most commonly diagnosed types of cancer are cancers of the breast, lung and bronchus, and colon and rectum; these accounted for half of estimated cancer cases. Among all new cancer diagnoses in women, breast cancer alone accounts for 26% or 182,460 cases. Cancers of the lung and bronchus, prostate, and colon and rectum in men, and cancers of the breast, lung and bronchus, and colon and rectum in women continue to be the most common fatal cancers. These four cancers account for half of the total cancer deaths among men and women. Lung cancer surpassed breast cancer as the leading cause of cancer death in women in 1987 and accounted for 26% of all female cancer deaths in 2008. Death rates in the U.S. for all cancer sites combined

TABLE 1.1

FIVE-YEAR CANCER SURVIVAL (%), BY SITE AND RACE, 1996–2002, BASED ON CANCER PATIENTS DIAGNOSED 1996–2002 AND FOLLOWED-UP THROUGH 2003

Site	White	African American	% Difference
All sites	66	57	11
Breast (female)	90	77	13
Colon	66	54	12
Esophagus	17	15	5
Leukemia	50	39	11
Non-Hodgkin lymphoma	64	56	8
Oral cavity	62	40	22
Prostate	100	98	2
Rectum	66	59	7
Urinary bladder	83	65	18
Uterine cervix	75	66	9
Uterine corpus	86	61	25

(From Surveillance, Epidemiology, and End Results Program, 1975–2003, Division of Cancer Control and Population Sciences, National Cancer Institute, 2006)

TABLE 1.2

FIVE-YEAR RELATIVE SURVIVAL (%) DURING THREE TIME PERIODS, BY CANCER SITE, BASED ON CANCER PATIENTS FOLLOWED-UP THROUGH 2003

Site	1975–1977	1984–1986	1996–2002
All sites	50	53	66
Breast (female)	75	79	89
Colon	51	59	65
Leukemia	35	42	49
Lung and bronchus	13	13	16
Melanoma	82	86	92
Non-Hodgkin lymphoma	48	53	63
Ovary	37	40	45
Pancreas	2	3	5
Prostate	69	76	100
Rectum	49	57	66
Urinary bladder	73	78	82

(From Surveillance, Epidemiology, and End Results Program, 1975–2003, Division of Cancer Control and Population Sciences, National Cancer Institute, 2006)

decreased by 2.6% per year from 2002 to 2004 in men and by 1.8% per year in women during the same period. Mortality rates have continued to decrease across all four major cancer sites in men and in women, except for lung cancer in women, where rates continued to increase by 0.2% per year from 1995 to 2004.[4]

Lung cancer incidence rates declined in men and have plateaued in women after increasing for many decades. In both men and women, colorectal cancer incidence rates decreased from 1998 through 2004. Female breast cancer incidence rates decreased by 3.5% per year from 2001 to 2004 after increasing since 1980, likely reflecting both delays in diagnosis due to a decrease in mammography utilization and declines in hormone replacement therapy use among postmenopausal women. Prostate cancer incidence rates have stabilized from 1995 through 2004, following a short-term rapid increase and subsequent decrease between 1988 and 1995; these trends are thought to reflect changes in utilization of prostate-specific antigen testing.

Figures 1.1 and 1.2 reveal the estimated new cancer cases for the ten leading sites and estimated cancer deaths,

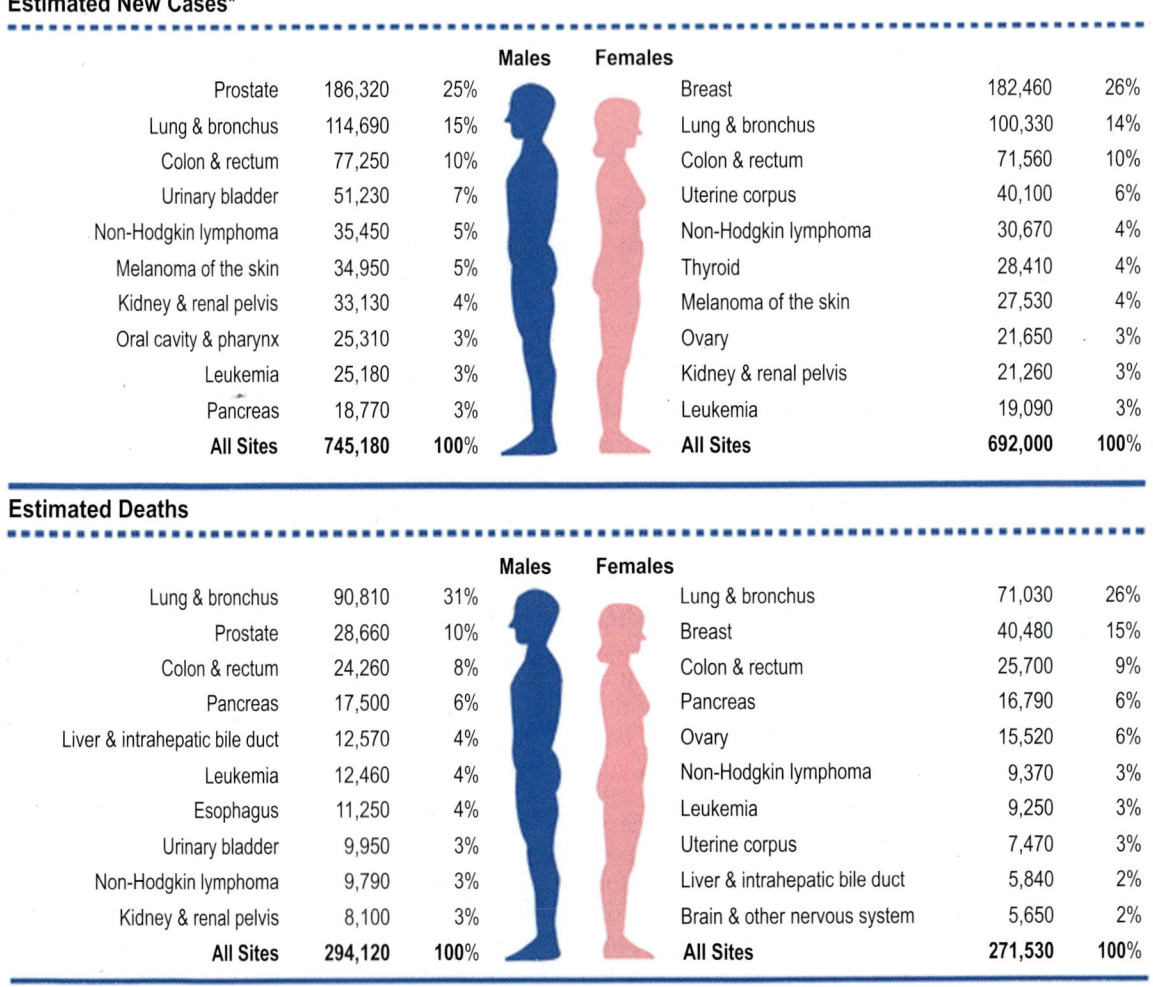

FIGURE 1.1 Ten leading cancer types for estimated new cancer cases and deaths, by sex, United States, 2008.

*Excludes basal and squamous cell skin cancers and in situ carcinomas except urinary bladder. Estimates were rounded to the nearest ten. (From Jemal A, et al. Cancer statistics, 2008. *CA Cancer J Clin*. 2008;58(2):71–96. Copyright 2008, American Cancer Society, Reprinted with permission of John Wiley & Sons, Inc.)

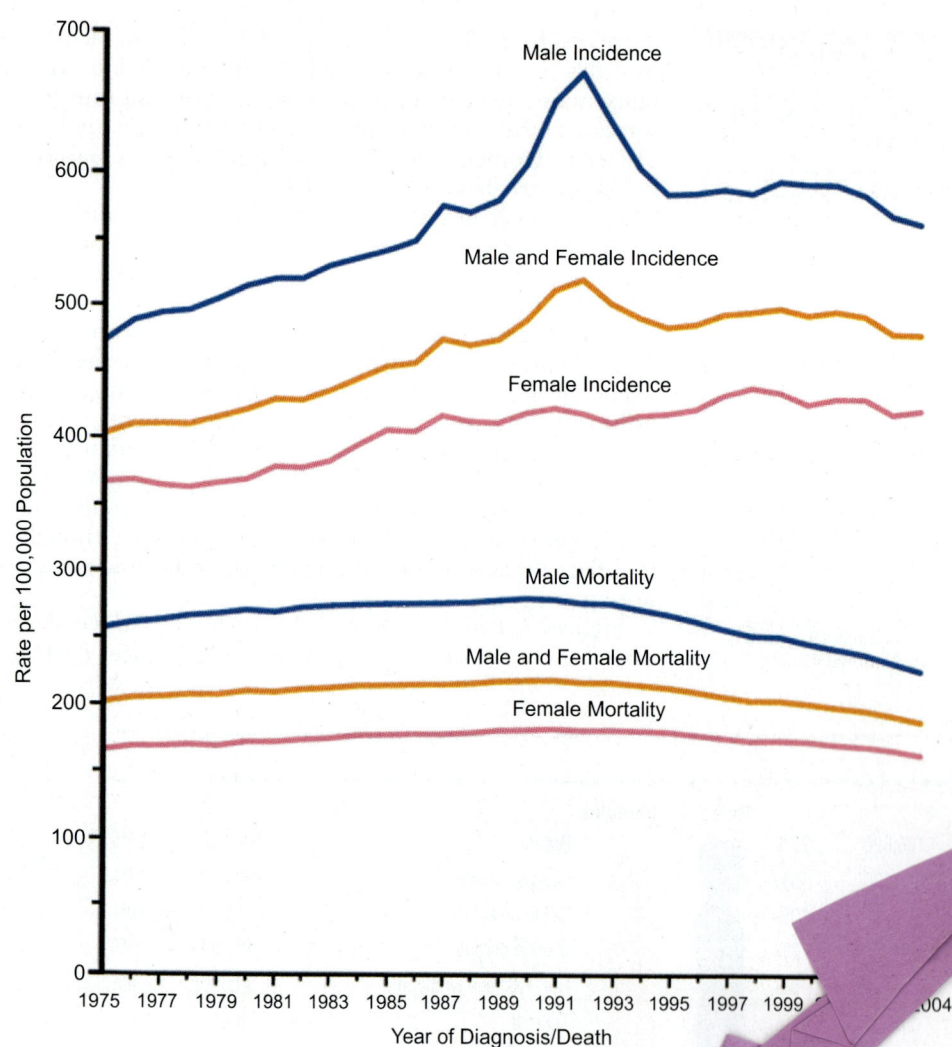

FIGURE 1.2 Annual age-adjusted cancer incidence and death rates* for all sites, by sex, United States, 1975 to 2004.
*Rates were age-adjusted to the 2000 U.S. standard population. Incidence rates were adjusted for delays in reporting.

by sex in the United States for 2008 and annual age-adjusted cancer incidence for all sites, from 1975 to 2004.

Among men under 40 years of age, leukemia is the most common fatal cancer, whereas cancer of the lung and bronchus predominates in men aged 40 years and older. Among women, leukemia is the leading cause of cancer death before age 20 years, breast cancer ranks first at age 20 to 59 years, and lung cancer ranks first at age 60 years and older. Five-year survival rates for many cancer sites and all cancers combined in both white and African Americans have notably improved. Survival has not improved significantly in the past 25 years for cancers of the lung, larynx, uterine corpus, cervix, and pancreas. Between 1996 and 2002, the relative survival rate of all cancers was 66% (excluding basal and squamous cell skin cancers and in situ carcinomas except of the urinary bladder).[5] Predicting the economic benefit of reduced cancer mortality may provide important information for resource allocation to cancer interventions that provide the greatest benefit. Bradley et al.[6] estimated that the annual productivity costs of cancer were approximately $115.8 billion in 2000 and projected a value of $147.6 billion for 2020. Death from lung cancer accounted for more than 27% of productivity costs. A 1% annual reduction in lung, colorectal, breast, leukemia, pancreatic, and brain cancer mortality lowered productivity costs by million per year. Investments in programs that target cancers with high incidence and/or cancers that occur younger, working-age individuals may yield the greatest reductions in productivity losses to society.

The prevalence of cancer-related pain has been estimated to be 30% to 50% in patients under chronic treatment and more than 70% in patients with advanced disease.[7] Thirty-three percent of patients receiving active treatment for metastatic disease have significant cancer-related pain, and this percentage increases to 60% to 90% in those with advanced disease[8–10] with the management of pain ultimately becoming the main focus of treatment.

Cancer is one of the medical conditions patients fear most.[11] The diagnosis of cancer initiates a cascade of complex decisions at a time when patients feel vulnerable and distressed. In the past, clinical decisions previously followed a single physician-generated standard; guidelines now include several options and the explicit recognition of the need to incorporate patients' preferences to determine the most appropriate treatment strategies. Consequently, the demands and stresses imposed on patients during treatment may be considerable. In addition to anxiety about cancer as a potentially lethal disease, patient and family anticipation that pain is inevitable and untreatable adds to patient and family distress.[11] Cancer pain has been shown to elevate psychological distress,[12–14]

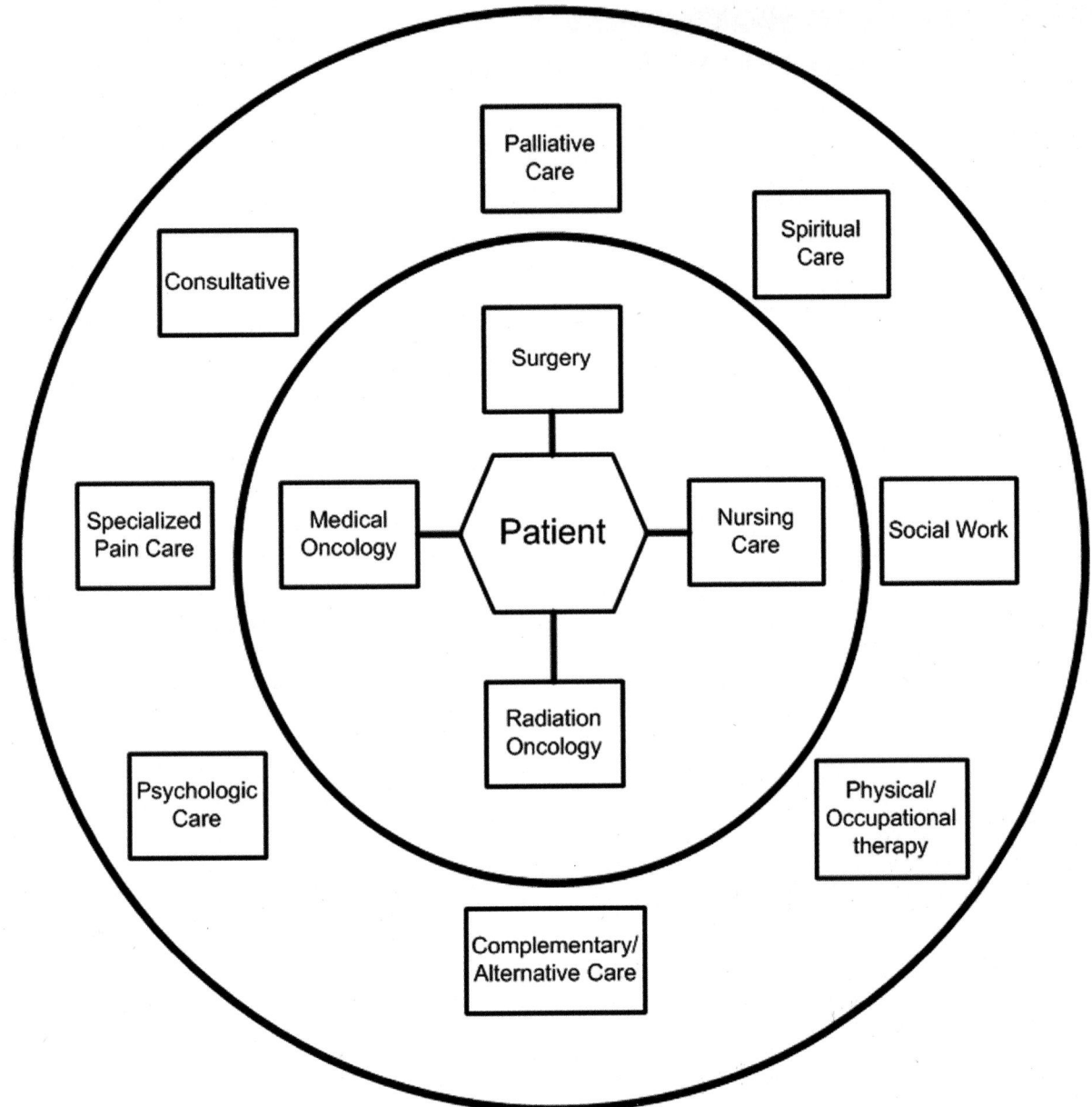

FIGURE 1.3 Interdisciplinary care teams of the cancer patient with pain.

alter social life,[15] disturb sleep,[16] and compromise enjoyment of life.[8]

There are many differences between cancer pain patients and those who experience acute pain and/or chronic nonmalignant pain. End-of-life considerations and palliative care are rarely major issues for acute and chronic nonmalignant pain conditions, but these concerns are extremely important for cancer pain patients, especially those with advanced disease. The complex medical and psychosocial aspects of comprehensive cancer care mandate a multi- and/or interdisciplinary approach. The changing nature of cancer pain, either in response to treatments directed at the tumor and/or progression of the tumor, requires vigilance. It is common that treatment strategies for pain must be altered as the patient progresses through his or her disease. Furthermore, cancer survivors require ongoing surveillance for symptoms and signs of recurrent disease. New pain complaints in cancer patients produce great anxiety and require careful assessment. Aggressive treatments of cancer will continue to improve survival; oncology patients will have even more long-term pain management issues. In this situation, different treatment strategies will be required over time. Comprehensive cancer care usually requires the simultaneous services of various health care providers (Fig. 1.3). Successful pain management requires that the person or persons responsible for pain management adopt, or at least become familiar with, an interdisciplinary framework. In addition, the humanitarian nature of cancer pain management, the focus on suffering and comfort, and the associated effects on patients' relatives all contribute to the uniqueness of the management of pain associated with cancer.

The prevalence of pain varies with the stage of cancer and its treatment (Table 1.3). It has been reported that the

TABLE 1.3

PREVALENCE OF PAIN WITH STAGES OF CANCER AND ITS TREATMENT

Stage of Disease	Prevalence of Pain
Active anticancer treatment	24% to 73%
Advanced cancer	58% to 86%
Cured of cancer (in remission)	21% to 46%

(From van den Beuken-van Everdingen MH, et al. Prevalence of pain in patients with cancer: A systematic review of the past 40 years. *Ann Oncol.* 2007; 18(9):1437–1449. By permission of the European Society for Medical Oncology.)

prevalence of pain ranged from 24% to 60% in patients on active anticancer treatment[17–18] and 62% to 86% in patients with advanced cancer.[19–21] Van den Beuken-van Everdingen et al.[22] estimated that the pain prevalence in patients with cancer was high and was influenced by disease stage, treatment, and survival: 64% (confidence interval [CI] 58% to 69%) in patients with metastatic, advanced, or terminal disease, 59% (CI 44% to 73%) in patients on anticancer treatment, and 33% (CI 21% to 46%) in patients whose cancer had been cured. However, there are problems associated with published prevalence data. Few data are available on the severity of the pain in different phases of cancer, and the available data has been inconclusive. Similarly, the relation between the prevalence of cancer pain and the type of cancer, phase of disease, age, gender, marital status, and education level has not been well studied.[23] Additional studies with well-designed methodology are needed to gain greater insight into the real extent of the pain and suffering experienced by cancer patients.

Controlling the pain associated with cancer is a major health care problem.[24–25] The presence of severe pain and other symptoms dramatically affects the quality of life of cancer patients and their families.[26] Pain and its treatment interact with other common cancer symptoms such as fatigue, weakness, dyspnea, nausea, constipation, and impaired cognition and magnify the negative impact of cancer pain.[27–28] It has been shown that cancer patients treated on an outpatient basis frequently (67%) have pain that is inadequately controlled, whereas 36% had pain severe enough to reduce their functional status.[24] This was particularly true at pain centers that predominantly treated minority patients, who were three times more likely than those treated elsewhere to have inadequate pain management[29] due to inadequate pain assessment, patient reluctance to report pain, and lack of staff time for pain management.[30]

We aim in this book to provide the basis for effective pain management at all stages of the cancer patient's clinical course, reviewing the published literature and documenting our strategies that are, as much as possible, based upon published evidence. Central to this theme, we believe that successful cancer pain management requires an accurate understanding of the factors that contribute to the patient's pain complaint. We also believe that there is a moral imperative to attempt to alleviate pain and suffering in our patients and their families.

References

1. Yach D, et al. The global burden of chronic diseases: Overcoming impediments to prevention and control. *JAMA.* 2004;291(21): 2616–2622.
2. Jones SB. Cancer in the developing world: A call to action. *BMJ.* 1999;319(7208):505–508.
3. Sener SF, Grey N. The global burden of cancer. *J Surg Oncol.* 2005;92(1):1–3.
4. Jemal A, et al. Cancer statistics, 2008. *CA Cancer J Clin.* 2008; 58(2):71–96.
5. Jemal A, et al. Cancer statistics, 2007. *CA Cancer J Clin.* 2007;57(1):43–66.
6. Bradley CJ, et al. Productivity costs of cancer mortality in the United States: 2000–2020. *J Natl Cancer Inst.* 2008;100(24):1763–1770.
7. Portenoy RK, Lesage P. Management of cancer pain. *Lancet.* 1999; 353(9165):1695–700.
8. Daut RL, Cleeland CS. The prevalence and severity of pain in cancer. *Cancer.* 1982;50(9):1913–1918.
9. Foley KM. The treatment of cancer pain. *N Engl J Med.* 1985;313(2):84–95.
10. Twycross R. *Pain relief in advanced cancer.* London: Churchill Livingstone, 1994.
11. Levin DN, Cleeland CS, Dar R. Public attitudes toward cancer pain. *Cancer.* 1985;56(9):2337–2339.
12. Ahles TA, Blanchard EB, Ruckdeschel JC. The multidimensional nature of cancer-related pain. *Pain.* 1983;17(3):277–288.
13. Carroll BT, et al. Screening for depression and anxiety in cancer patients using the Hospital Anxiety and Depression Scale. *Gen Hosp Psychiatry.* 1993;15(2):69–74.
14. Glover J, et al. Mood states of oncology outpatients: Does pain make a difference? *J Pain Symptom Manage.* 1995;10(2):120–128.
15. Strang P. Emotional and social aspects of cancer pain. *Acta Oncol.* 1992;31(3):323–326.
16. Hu DS, Silberfarb PM. Management of sleep problems in cancer patients. *Oncology (Huntingt).* 1991;5(9):23–27.
17. Pignon JP, et al. Adjusting for patient selection suggests the addition of docetaxel to 5-fluorouracil–cisplatin induction therapy may offer survival benefit in squamous cell cancer of the head and neck. *Anticancer Drugs.* 2004;15(4):331–340.
18. Rietman JS, et al. Impairments, disabilities and health related quality of life after treatment for breast cancer: A follow-up study 2.7 years after surgery. *Disabil Rehabil.* 2004;26(2):78–84.
19. Bradley N, Davis L, Chow E. Symptom distress in patients attending an outpatient palliative radiotherapy clinic. *J Pain Symptom Manage.* 2005;30(2):123–131.
20. Hwang SS, et al. Prediction of survival for advanced cancer patients by recursive partitioning analysis: role of Karnofsky performance status, quality of life, and symptom distress. *Cancer Invest.* 2004;22(5):678–687.
21. Wilson KG, et al. Structured interview assessment of symptoms and concerns in palliative care. *Can J Psychiatry.* 2004;49(6):350–358.
22. van den Beuken-van Everdingen MH, et al. Prevalence of pain in patients with cancer: A systematic review of the past 40 years. *Ann Oncol.* 2007;18(9):1437–1449.
23. van den Beuken-van Everdingen MH, et al. High prevalence of pain in patients with cancer in a large population-based study in The Netherlands. *Pain.* 2007;132(3):312–320.
24. Cleeland CS, et al. Pain and its treatment in outpatients with metastatic cancer. *N Engl J Med.* 1994;330(9):592–596.
25. Zhukovsky DS, et al. Unmet analgesic needs in cancer patients. *J Pain Symptom Manage.* 1995;10(2):113–119.
26. Cleeland CS. Cancer-related symptoms. *Semin Radiat Oncol.* 2000;10(3):175–190.
27. Coyle N, et al. Character of terminal illness in the advanced cancer patient: Pain and other symptoms during the last four weeks of life. *J Pain Symptom Manage.* 1990;5(2):83–93.
28. Grond S, et al. Prevalence and pattern of symptoms in patients with cancer pain: A prospective evaluation of 1635 cancer patients referred to a pain clinic. *J Pain Symptom Manage.* 1994;9(6):372–382.
29. Cleeland CS, et al. Pain and treatment of pain in minority patients with cancer: The Eastern Cooperative Oncology Group Minority Outpatient Pain Study. *Ann Intern Med.* 1997;127(9):813–816.
30. Anderson KO, et al. Minority cancer patients and their providers: Pain management attitudes and practice. *Cancer.* 2000;88(8): 1929–1938.

CHAPTER 2 ■ CANCER PAIN ASSESSMENT AND DIAGNOSTIC ISSUES

Multiple studies during the 1990s revealed less-than-optimal treatment of pain in patients with cancer.[1-4] Even with the subsequent availability of more-effective pain treatments and the publication of pain management guidelines, similar patient care deficiencies continue in the United States and in other countries.[5-9] The most frequently identified barriers to appropriate pain management in multiple studies have been physician underestimation of the patient's pain, inadequate pain assessment, and patient reluctance to report pain. A growing body of literature attests to the need for significant improvement in cancer pain assessment and treatment in their practice.[10-11] Poor pain control has been ascribed to lack of expertise by clinicians in assessing and managing cancer pain.[12] Knowledge deficits in the basic principles of cancer pain management have been revealed by interviews of practicing physicians.[13] Nurses and nursing students are also commonly deficient in their understanding of basic principles of cancer pain management.[1,14-15] Studies and expert opinion reveal that contemporary American medical education does not prepare medical students or residents to provide adequate care for the cancer patient with pain.[16-17] Educational interventions can successfully improve cancer pain knowledge and attitudes of health care professionals.[18]

A variety of assessment skills are required to integrate knowledge about pharmacology, pharmacokinetics, and pharmacodynamics, as well as patient characteristics such as individual variability and compliance with medications, side effects and quality-of-life determinants, and disease specifics in the diagnosis and management of the cancer patient with pain. These skills contribute to clinical judgment and decision-making, and require substantial individual experience. Studies of pain education in undergraduate medical students have generally focused on knowledge, and little is known about interviewing skills and pain evaluation. Leila et al.[19] suggested that formative assessment of both knowledge and communication skills is required for the development of a functional pain curriculum to train medical students in chronic pain management. Daylong cancer pain education workshops were as effective as hands-on experience in improving cancer pain knowledge and changing attitudes for postgraduate nurses, as observed by Lasch et al.[20]

Computer simulation software can be used to create tools that include the principles and ideals of cancer pain assessment and management as has been presented at professional society meetings, in published clinical guidelines, journal articles, and editorials. Such tools offer the opportunity to include platforms to move learning into the working environment of the student, health care provider, and institution. In addition, modern interactive software may provide the ability to efficiently assist in the identification of specific errors in knowledge, judgment, and practice patterns of the individual provider.[21] Because formal education and training in cancer pain management has not routinely been a part of medical education, efforts are needed to update both undergraduate curricula for those in training and continuing education for practicing providers. Continuing education is needed across many disciplines but, in order to ensure the provision of high-quality pain management care, it is especially important that continuing education reach providers such as oncologists, hematologists, urologists, surgeons, and radiation therapists who initially treat cancer patients, as well as primary care physicians, nurses, and social workers and other providers of psychosocial services. All members of the healthcare team need continuous updating of the skills, attitudes, and knowledge that can lead to superior management of the cancer patient with pain.

Patient training may help to reduce barriers to pain relief, improve appropriate medication use, and improve communication of pain-related needs. Effective strategies should have a sustained impact while requiring only reasonable amounts of professional time. Print materials reinforce face-to-face training, which may also include caregivers in the training session. Videos or DVDs help both providers and patients by presenting information in a standardized yet engaging manner, allowing face-to-face time to be individualized. The challenge, however, is to optimize professional time while achieving sustained, effective cancer pain control. Syrjala et al.[22] reported on patient training using integrated print and video material. Patients watched a video followed by about 20 min of manual-standardized training with an oncology nurse; training was focused on reviewing the printed material and adapted to individual patient concerns. A follow-up phone call at 72 hr post-training addressed individualized treatment content and pain communication. Assessments at baseline, 1, 3, and 6 months included barriers, the Brief Pain Inventory, opioid use, and physician and nurse ratings of their patients' pain. Trained versus control patients reported reduced barriers to pain relief ($P < .001$), lower usual pain ($P = .03$), and greater opioid use ($P < .001$). No pain training patients reported severe pain (>6 on a 0–10 scale) at 1 month ($P = .03$). The authors concluded that this method of brief individualized training effectively improved pain management over a 6-month period for cancer patients of varying diagnostic and demographic groups.

Clinicians have traditionally held clinical judgment and decision making in high regard. Technological developments and the growth of biomedical knowledge have vastly expanded the range of investigative and therapeutic possibilities. The goal of diagnosis is to place a nosologic label on a process that manifests itself in a patient over time. The nosologic labels used in diagnosis reflect the current level of scientific understanding of pathophysiology and disease. The utility of making specific diagnoses lies in selection of effective therapies, in making accurate prognoses, and in providing detailed explanations. In some situations, it is not necessary to arrive at an exact diagnosis in order to fulfill one or more of these objectives. Treatment is often initiated before an exact diagnosis is made. In medical diagnostic reasoning, there are also cases where recognition from compiled knowledge does not pertain. Some cases present an overwhelming array of seemingly contradictory information; others present with common conditions in unexpected or unusual manners; some patients manifest rare findings or disorders. Physicians are capable of reasoning with incomplete and imprecise information; and often make clinical judgments at times when they have unfulfilled information needs.

The tasks involved with medical management of a particular patient are complex. Clinicians typically define a disease, make a diagnosis, select a procedure, observe outcomes, assess possibilities, and assign preferences. In addition, there are wide variations in clinical judgments and decision making. Clinical judgments and decisions are not isolated cognitive events. Political, economic, ethical, legal, and sociological factors influence decisions. Individual physicians tend to follow what is considered standard and accepted in the community. A community standard evolves from statements published in national journals and textbooks, from the opinions of established physicians, and from new ideas brought to the community by new physicians.

Diagnosis begins with perception. Clinicians typically use methods of solving a medical problem for which no well-defined formula exists, but base decisions on informal methods or experience, and employ a form of trial-and-error iteration. A diagnostician, when he or she arrives at a diagnosis or diagnoses, has invoked certain concepts. These can be diseases, causes of diseases, or other notions that are relevant to the diagnosis and form a hierarchical structure. Clinicians frequently arrive at a diagnosis despite limited time or data.

Diagnostic errors are associated with a proportionately higher morbidity than is the case with other types of medical errors.[23-25] Common issues in diagnostic errors include errors or delay in diagnosis, failure to employ indicated tests, use of outmoded tests or therapy, and failure to act on results of monitoring or testing. Graber et al.[26] consider three major categories of diagnostic errors in medicine: no-fault errors, systems errors, and cognitive errors.

No-fault errors include cases where the illness is silent, masked, or presents in such an atypical fashion that making the correct diagnosis with the current state of medical knowledge would not be expected. Other examples would include the rare condition misdiagnosed as something more common, and the diagnosis missed because the patient does not present his or her symptoms clearly. A diagnosis missed or delayed because of patient noncompliance might also be viewed as a no-fault error.

System errors reflect flaws in the administrative structure of the health care system. Cognitive errors occur from inadequate knowledge or faulty data gathering, inaccurate reasoning, or faulty verification. In one study of adverse events associated with iatrogenic patient injury, cognitive failure was a factor in 57% of all events.[25] Compared with error-improvement strategies that focus on individual providers, system-level changes have the advantages of potentially decreasing error rates for all involved providers. Unfortunately, system improvements are not sustained over time. New policies tend to become forgotten and enthusiasm for improvement wanes. Clinicians, from their first days of training, are encouraged to search for unifying explanations of a patient's multiple symptoms. Overconfidence can also result in a clinician stopping the search for additional possibilities.

Setting and enforcing explicit performance standards for patient safety through regulatory and related mechanisms, such as licensing, certification, and accreditation, can define minimum performance levels for health professionals, the organizations in which they work, and the tools (drugs and devices) they use to care for patients.[27] The process of developing and adopting standards also helps to form expectations for safety among providers and consumers. The values and norms set by the health professions influence the practice, training, and education for providers. Thus, professional societies should become leaders in encouraging and demanding improvements in patient safety, by such actions as setting their own performance standards, convening and communicating with members about safety, incorporating attention to patient safety in training programs, and collaborating across disciplines. The medication process provides an example where implementing better systems will yield better human performance. Patients themselves also could provide a major safety check in most hospitals, clinics, and practice. They should know which medications they are taking, their appearance, and their side effects, and they should notify their doctors of medication discrepancies and the occurrence of side effects.

Good decision making involves sufficient search for possibilities, evidence, and goals, and fairness in the search for evidence and in the use of evidence. Teaching discriminative skills and providing more examples and repetition may improve clinical decision-making skills. Problem-based learning attempts to improve diagnostic skills through a process that emphasizes clinical reasoning. It may also be possible to improve diagnostic accuracy indirectly by a system-level approach. The development of clinical guidelines and treatment algorithms is an example of this. Guidelines standardize the approaches to clinical problems and minimize the variability in response patterns. However, when guidelines for a particular problem are available, clinicians may not follow the guidelines appropriately. Improvements in clinical skills and diagnostic procedures can have dramatic consequences in health care. Studies comparing the accuracy of clinical diagnosis in unselected patients who died in hospital in different medical eras have shown no decline of errors in the main diagnosis.[28-29] Sonderegger-Iseli et al.[30] assessed changes in diagnostic accuracy over 20 years using necropsy as the gold standard for diagnosis. Necropsy has the double role of a method by which to detect diagnostic errors and as a source of knowledge to be applied to future cases, which influences learning and adds to data on local epidemiology of diseases and quality control for technical investigations. The authors showed that the frequency of major diagnostic errors in unselected patients who died in hospital was halved over 20 years because of improved clinical skills and new diagnostic procedures.

References

1. Clarke EB, French B, Bilodeau ML, et al. Pain management knowledge, attitudes and clinical practice: The impact of nurses' characteristics and education. *J Pain Symptom Manage.* 1996;11:18–31.
2. Cleeland CS, Gonin R, Hatfield AK, et al. Pain and its treatment in outpatients with metastatic cancer. *N Engl J Med.* 1994;330:592–596.
3. Larue F, Colleau SM, Brasseur L, et al. Multicentre study of cancer pain and its treatment in France. *Br Med J* 1995;310:1034–1037.
4. Cleeland CS, Gonin R, Baez L, et al. Pain and treatment of pain in minority patients with cancer. The Eastern Cooperative Oncology Group Minority Outpatient Pain Study. *Ann Intern Med.* 1997;127:813–816.
5. Cascinu S, Giordani P, Agostinelli R, et al. Pain and its treatment in hospitalized patients with metastatic cancer. *Support Care Cancer.* 2003;11:587–592.
6. Dahl JL. Pain: impediments and suggestions for solutions. *J Natl Cancer Inst Monogr* 2004:124–126.
7. Enting RH, Oldenmenger WH, Van Gool AR, et al. The effects of analgesic prescription and patient adherence on pain in a Dutch outpatient cancer population. *J Pain Symptom Manage.* 2007;34:523–531.
8. Gallagher R, Hawley P, Yeomans W. A survey of cancer pain management knowledge and attitudes of British Columbian physicians. *Pain Res Manag.* 2004;9:188–194.
9. Jeon YS, Kim HK, Cleeland CS, et al. Clinicians' practice and attitudes toward cancer pain management in Korea. *Support Care Cancer.* 2007;15:463–469.
10. Payne R. Chronic pain: Challenges in the assessment and management of cancer pain. *J Pain Symptom Manage.* 2000;19:S12–S15.
11. Von Roenn JH, Cleeland CS, Gonin R, et al. Physician attitudes and practice in cancer pain management. A survey from the Eastern Cooperative Oncology Group. *Ann Int Med.* 1993;119:121–126.
12. Cleeland C. Research in cancer pain: What we know and what we need to know. *Cancer.* 1991;67:823–827.
13. Elliott TE, Murray DM, Elliott BA, et al. Physician knowledge and attitudes about cancer pain management: a survey from the Minnesota cancer pain project. *J Pain Symptom Manage.* 1995;10:494–504.
14. McCaffery M, Ferrell BR. Nurses' knowledge about cancer pain: A survey of five countries. *J Pain Symptom Manage.* 1995;10:356–369.
15. Sheehan DK, Webb A, Bower D, et al. Level of cancer pain knowledge among baccalaureate student nurses. *J Pain Symptom Manage.* 1992;7:478–484.
16. Sloan PA, Donnelly MB, Schwartz RW, et al. Cancer pain assessment and management by housestaff. *Pain.* 1996;67:475–481.
17. Sloan PA, Montgomery C, Musick D. Medical student knowledge of morphine for the management of cancer pain. *J Pain Symptom Manage.* 1998;15:359–364.
18. Ferrell BR, Winn R. Medical and nursing education and training opportunities to improve survivorship care. *J Clin Oncol.* 2006;24:5142–5148.
19. Leila NM, Pirkko H, Eeva P, et al. Training medical students to manage a chronic pain patient: Both knowledge and communication skills are needed. *Eur J Pain.* 2006;10:167–170.
20. Lasch KE, Wilkes G, Lee J, et al. Is hands-on experience more effective than didactic workshops in postgraduate cancer pain education? *J Cancer Educ.* 2000;15:218–222.
21. Sloan PA, LaFountain P, Plymale M, et al. Cancer pain education for medical students: The development of a short course on CD-ROM. *Pain Med.* 2002;3:66–72.
22. Syrjala KL, Abrams JR, Polissar NL, et al. Patient training in cancer pain management using integrated print and video materials: A multisite randomized controlled trial. *Pain.* 2008;135:175–186.
23. Brennan TA, Leape LL, Laird NM, et al. Incidence of adverse events and negligence in hospitalized patients. Results of the Harvard Medical Practice Study I. *N Engl J Med.* 1991;324:370–376.
24. Thomas EJ, Studdert DM, Burstin HR, et al. Incidence and types of adverse events and negligent care in Utah and Colorado. *Med Care.* 2000;38:261–271.
25. Wilson RM, Runciman WB, Gibberd RW, et al. The Quality in Australian Health Care Study. *Med J Aust.* 1995;163:458–471.
26. Graber M, Gordon R, Franklin N. Reducing diagnostic errors in medicine: What's the goal? *Acad Med.* 2002;77:981–992.
27. Institute of Medicine. To Err is Human; Building a Safer Health System. Washington, DC: National Academy Press, 1999.
28. Goldman L, Sayson R, Robbins S, et al. The value of the autopsy in three medical eras. *N Engl J Med.* 1983;308:1000–1005.
29. Kirch W, Schafii C. Misdiagnosis at a university hospital in 4 medical eras. *Medicine (Baltimore).* 1996;75:29–40.
30. Sonderegger-Iseli K, Burger S, Muntwyler J, et al. Diagnostic errors in three medical eras: A necropsy study. *Lancet.* 2000;355:2027–2031.

CHAPTER 3 ■ THE PERCEPTION OF PAIN

This section is designed to provide a background for the understanding of the anatomy, physiology, and psychology of pain. According to the classical Cartesian model, pain is a hard-wired sensory system in which noxious input is passively transmitted along sensory pathways to the brain. This is an inadequate model for nociceptive information processing. Pain perception is subject to substantial pro- and antinociceptive modulation at multiple levels in the central nervous system (CNS). Pain is a conscious experience, an interpretation of the nociceptive input that is influenced by memories, emotions, pathology, and genetic and cognitive factors.[1] Pain is not necessarily related directly to nociceptive drive or input; neither is it solely for vital protective functions. Contrary to previously held beliefs that pain resulted from a central summation in response to excessive sensory stimulation, it is now clear that many factors influencing pain perception are centrally mediated.[1] The astute clinician must ascertain the balance between peripheral and central influences and identify those that are caused by pathological as opposed to emotional or cognitive influences. Treatments must be targeted at the relevant causative factors.

NOCICEPTIVE TRANSMISSION

Nociceptive transmission represents the synaptic transfer of information about the intensity, duration, and location of peripheral noxious stimuli from nociceptive afferent axons to dorsal horn neurons. Nociceptors detect noxious stimuli and initiate the peripheral pathway to nociceptive pain. The nociceptor is highly modifiable in response to injury of its axon and to exposure to inflammation.[2] Some nociceptors are thinly myelinated (Aδ-fibers) but most are unmyelinated (C fibers), and these slowly conducting afferents represent the majority of sensory neurons in the peripheral nervous system. The nociceptor has four major functional components: the peripheral terminal that transduces external stimuli and initiates action potentials, the axon that conducts action potentials, the cell body that controls the identity and integrity of the neuron and is its metabolic factory, and the central terminal that forms the presynaptic element of the first synapse in the sensory pathway in the CNS (Fig. 3.1). Nociceptive neuron sensitivity is modulated by a large variety of mediators in the extracellular space. These mediators activate a large number of receptor classes, which in turn activate a plethora of signaling cascades (Fig. 3.2).[3] A variety of ion channels implicated in nociception are expressed in sensory neurons (Fig. 3.3). In disease states, various ion channels are activated by inflammatory signals and these signals sensitize sensory neuron channels, causing primary hyperalgesia. K^+ channels are main ion channels that stabilize the membrane potential by hyperpolarization. The role of the K^+ receptor in nociception is not well understood, but it is implicated because of its modulating potential.

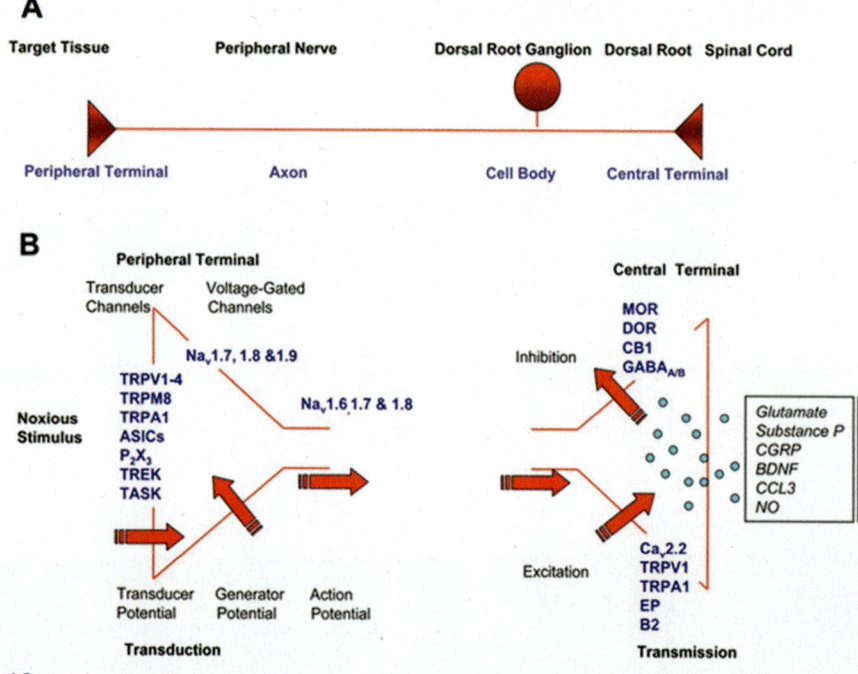

FIGURE 3.1 The nociceptor. A: Operational components of the nociceptor. B: Transduction is mediated by high-threshold transducer ion channels, which depolarize the peripheral terminal activating voltage-dependent sodium channels. Transmission occurs in response to calcium influx at the central terminal, releasing glutamate as well as multiple synaptic modulators and signaling molecules, and is subject to both excitatory and inhibitory influences. (From Woolf CJ, Ma Q. Nociceptors—noxious stimulus detectors. *Neuron*. 2007;55(3):353–364. Copyright 2007, with permission from Elsevier.)

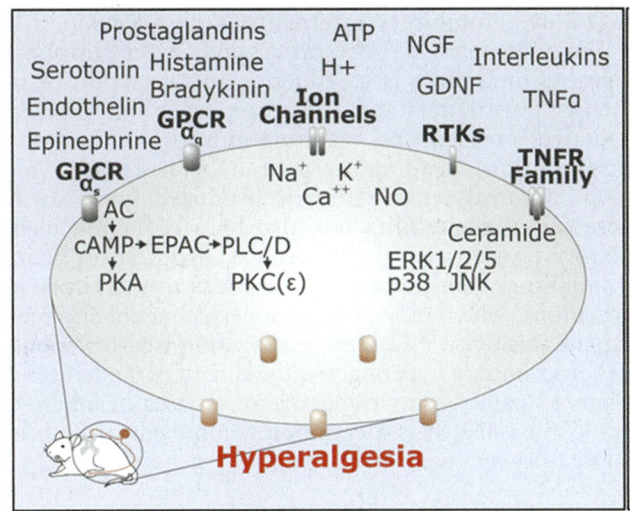

FIGURE 3.2 Signaling components in nociceptors. (From Hucho T, Levine JD. Signaling pathways in sensitization: toward a nociceptor cell biology. *Neuron.* 2007; 55(3):366. Copyright 2007, with permission from Elsevier.)

Voltage gated ion channels include Na^+, and Ca^{2+} channels. Na^+ channels are classified as tetrodotoxin-sensitive or -resistant. There are ten Na^+ channel genes, and these channels are responsible for rapid depolarization. Some voltage-gated Na^+ (Na_v) channels are involved in neuropathic pain.[4] Experiments with transgenic mice lines have clearly implicated Nav1.7, Nav1.8, and Nav1.9 in inflammatory pain, and possibly in neuropathic pain.[5]

There are several different types of voltage-dependent Ca^{2+} channels (L, N, P/Q, and R). Voltage-dependent calcium channels are formed as a complex of several different subunits (α_1, $\alpha_2\delta$, β_{1-4}, and γ). Gabapentin is known to interact with the $\alpha_2\delta$ subunit.[6] Nociceptive neurotransmitters such as substance-P and CGRP are released upon activation of L-, N-, and P/Q-type Ca^{2+} channels.

Transient receptor potential (TRP) ion channels are nonselective cation channels with variable permeability to Ca^{2+}; they are grouped into six families.[7] These families are classical (TRPC), vanilloid receptor–related (TRPV), melastatin-related (TRPM), mucolipins (TRPML), polycystins (TRPP), and ankyrin transmembrane protein–related (TRPA). TRP channels play important roles in sensation, because they detect a variety of stimuli, including vision, taste, smell, hearing, mechanosensation, thermosensation, and pain. For example, TRPV1 is activated by capsaicin, noxious heat (>43°C), and acid (a frequent stimulus in inflamed and ischemic tissues). Clones of TRPV[1–4] respond to noxious stimuli. The acid-sensing ion channel (ASIC) is activated by extracellular acid, like TRPV1. Currently, five ASIC genes are known in mammals (ASIC1–ASIC5). ASIC subtypes are modulated by NSAIDs.[8] Purinergic receptor subtype X channels (P2X) are adenosine triphosphate (ATP)-gated and have seven subtypes. P2X levels increase with inflammation[9] and may play a role in neuropathic pain.[10] Serotonin (5-HT) has several G protein–coupled metabotropic receptor subtypes and one ionotropic receptor (5-HT$_3$R). 5-HT$_3$R is involved in activation of nociceptor neurons by serotonin.[11]

Peripheral sensitization involves a lowering of the threshold of the nociceptor in response to inflammatory sensitizers. These activate the trafficking of sodium channels via diverse signal transduction pathways in the peripheral terminal, largely as a result of phosphorylation.[2] Phenotypic switches occur in nociceptors in response to inflammation and axonal injury, by virtue of exposure to retrograde transported signal molecules or the absence of target derived signals. The nociceptor neuron is highly specialized to respond only to noxious stimuli and to communicate this information accurately to the CNS. It is, however, not a static detector; the functional and chemical plasticity of the receptor ensures that its threshold and responsiveness, as well as the efficacy of its synaptic contacts, are regulated to reflect changes produced by activity, inflammation, and axonal injury. Heightened pain sensitivity can contribute to healing by helping avoid contact with the damaged body part until repair has occurred. Persistent alterations in nociceptors that drive pain in the absence of noxious stimuli or inflamed or damaged tissue represent, by contrast, a pathological change in the nociceptive system. Successful treatment of such pain requires restoring the nociceptor to its normal function.

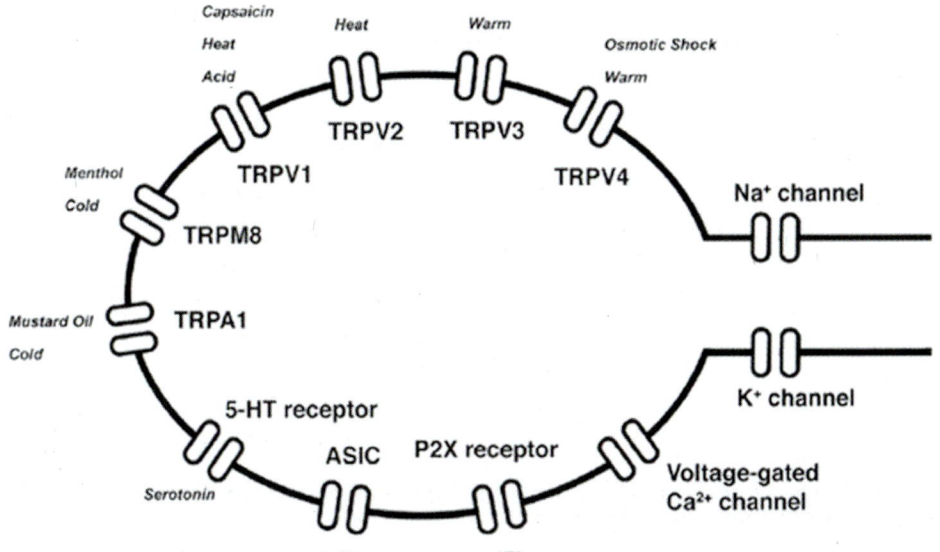

FIGURE 3.3 Ion channels expressed in sensory neurons. (From Lee Y, Lee CH, Oh U. Painful channels in sensory neurons. *Mol Cells.* 2005;20:315–324.)

With repeated peripheral noxious stimulation, the trigger for the change in receptive field properties is recruitment of receptive fields outside of this region, resulting in changes within the CNS and not an increased sensitivity of the peripheral terminals of sensory fibers innervating injured tissue.[2] Increased excitability triggered within the spinal cord by peripheral noxious inputs represents *central sensitization,* a state in which the response to normal inputs is greatly enhanced (Fig. 3.4). As such, pain does not simply reflect the presence, intensity, or duration of specific nociceptive stimuli in the periphery, but also changes in the function of the CNS.

The early phase of central sensitization is a form of activity-dependent synaptic plasticity driven by high levels of nociceptor input that, via transmitter release and action on the multiple receptors expressed on dorsal horn neurons, results in activation of intracellular kinases that phosphorylate ion channels and receptors, altering their distribution and function and increasing excitability and thereby pain sensitivity (Fig. 3.4B). The delayed or late phase of central sensitization involves changes in transcription in dorsal horn neurons. Some alterations in gene expression are activity driven, and restricted others are widespread, like the induction of cyclooxygenase 2 (COX-2) in central neurons after peripheral inflammation (Fig. 3.4C). Inhibitory interneurons play a major role in damping down sensory processing. After peripheral nerve lesions, there is a reduction in the action of inhibitory transmitters and a loss of γ-aminobutyric acid–mediated interneurons, resulting in a loss of inhibition (disinhibition), leading to pain hypersensitivity (Fig. 3.4D). Central sensitization is produced not only by increases in excitability but also by a reduction in inhibitory transmission due to reduced synthesis or action of inhibitory transmitters and to a loss of inhibitory interneurons, which may produce a persistent enhancement of pain sensitivity.[12] Central sensitization is also responsible for secondary hyperalgesia, the spread of tenderness or enhanced pain sensitivity outside of an area of injury, or tactile allodynia. It is a common component of both inflammatory and neuropathic pain.[2]

NEUROANATOMY OF CENTRAL PAIN PROCESSING

Nociceptive information ascends to the thalamus in the contralateral spinothalamic tract (STT) and to the medulla and brainstem via a spinoreticular (spinoparabrachial) and spinomesencephalic tracts. Spinal projections to the brain-

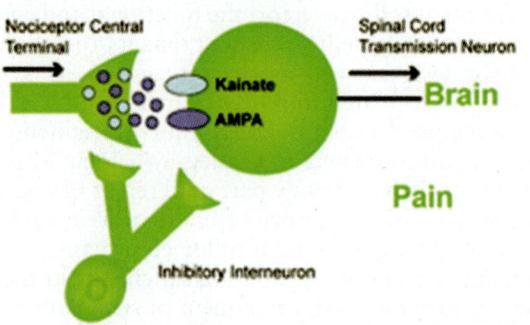

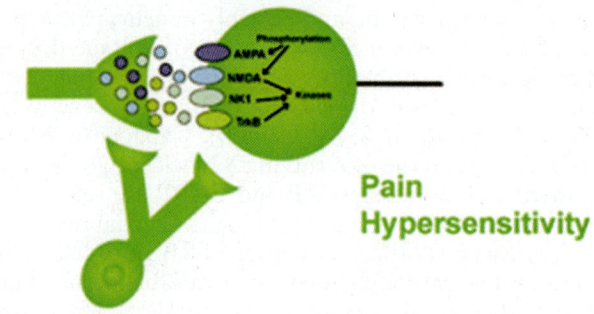

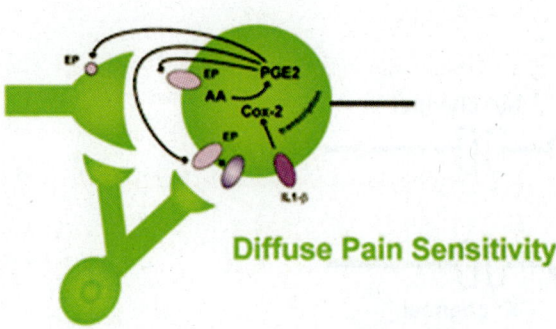

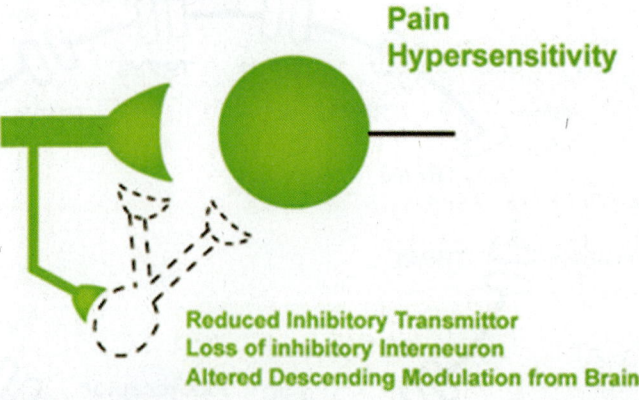

FIGURE 3.4 Normal and enhanced transmission in the spinal cord. (From Woolf CJ, Ma Q. Nociceptors—noxious stimulus detectors. *Neuron.* 2007;55:353–364.) AA, Arachidonic acid; AMPA, α-amino-3-hydroxy-5-methyl-4-isoxazole propionate; EP, prostaglandin receptor; IL1β, interleukin 1β; NK1, neurokinin 1; NMDA, N-methyl-D-aspartic acid; PGE2, prostaglandin E2; TrkB, tyrosine kinase B.

stem are important for integrating nociceptive activity with homeostatic, arousal, and autonomic processes, as well as providing a means to indirectly convey nociceptive information to forebrain regions after brainstem processing. Functional and anatomical divisions of the thalamus, the main relay site for nociceptive inputs to cortical and subcortical structures, have been made on the basis of their connections to specific spinal cord laminae in various animal species and in humans.[13]

Neuroimaging studies have uncovered a network of brain structures, sometimes referred to as the *pain matrix*, that process pain-related information.[14-15] This network for pain consistently includes the insular cortex, anterior cingulate cortex, somatosensory cortices, and thalamic nuclei, prefrontal cortical areas, and the amygdala (Fig. 3.5). The insula appears to receive information via a direct thalamo-insular connection[16] and can be considered a site for sensory and affective integration. It is a prominent structure in pain processing, as demonstrated by its rank as the most frequently activated structure in functional magnetic resonance imaging (fMRI) studies of pain.[14] Electrical stimulation of the posterior insula produces pain and/or thermal sensations in distinct sites on the contralateral hemibody[17] and damage in this region may produce pain asymbolia (pain is perceived, but does not cause suffering).[18] An increasing body of evidence links prefrontal cortical areas to the brain network for pain.[14,19] The role of the prefrontal cortex in cognitive functions, such as planning, decision making and detection of unfavorable outcomes, avoidance of emotion-based risky choices, and goal-directed behaviors, is well established.[20] An interface between ascending and descending systems, this brain area may also be important for the reciprocal interaction between cognitive and affective aspects of pain.

In addition to the contralateral thalamus, at least several cortical areas, including the contralateral SI, bilateral SII, anterior cingulate cortex, and insular cortices are involved in pain perception.[21] Pain perception is unique, because these cortical structures seem to be activated in parallel at nearly the same latency after the stimulus presentation. SI seems to play a role in basic pain processing, whereas SII and insula are involved in higher functions of pain perception. Emotional aspects of pain perception are mediated by anterior cingulate cortex and posterior insula/parietal operculum. The neuroanatomy of pain processing is shown in Figure 3.6.

In an acute pain experience, the most active areas are primary and secondary somatosensory, insular, anterior cingulate, and prefrontal cortices as well as the thalamus. Other regions such as basal ganglia, cerebellum, amygdala, hippocampus, and areas within the parietal and temporal cortices can also be active, dependent upon the particular set of circumstances for that individual. A reciprocal relationship exists between persistent pain and negative affective states such as fear, anxiety, and depression. Accumulating evidence points to the amygdala as an important site of such interaction.[22]

The anterior cingulate cortex has a pivotal role in human pain processing by integrating sensory, executive, attentional, emotional, and motivational components of pain.[23] Some evidence suggests that the amygdala is an important neural substrate of the reciprocal relationship between pain and negative affect.[24] The amygdala comprises several anatomically and functionally distinct nuclei. The central nucleus of the amygdala provides the output for major amygdala functions and modulates pain behavior through projections to descending pain control centers in the brainstem. The central nucleus receives purely nociceptive inputs from the dorsal horn via the parabrachial area and affect-related information from the circuitry of the lateral-basolateral amygdala.[24] In life-threatening situations, when survival demands immediate decisions, the amygdala acts to suppress attention to pain as a less important but possibly distracting factor to guarantee survival. As such, the amygdala assumes a pain-facilitating role when pain is the primary concern and deserves attention in conditions that activate or disturb the pain system.

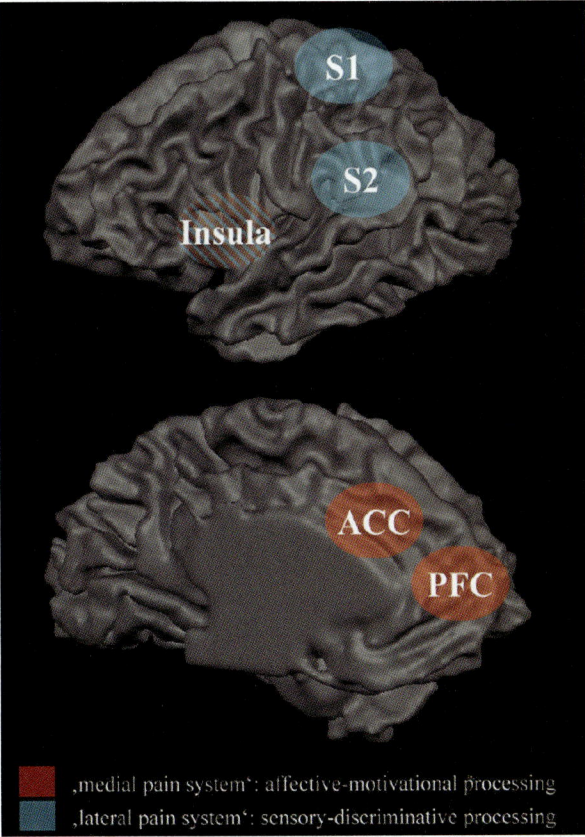

FIGURE 3.5 The pain neuromatrix. The lateral aspect (**top**) and mesial aspect (**bottom**) of the left hemisphere are shown. Areas of the lateral pain system that process the sensory-discriminative component of pain are coded in *blue*; areas of the medial pain system that process the affective-motivational component of pain are coded in *red*. The insula is anatomically and functionally positioned between the two systems. (From Seifert F, Maihofner C. Central mechanisms of experimental and chronic neuropathic pain: Findings from functional imaging studies. *Cell Mol Life Sci*. 2009;66:375–390.)

THE DESCENDING PAIN MODULATORY SYSTEM

The endogenous pain-modulating system is a complex network of brain cells that control nociceptive transmission in the spinal cord and brain stem by inhibitory and facilitating actions. This system is an anatomic network

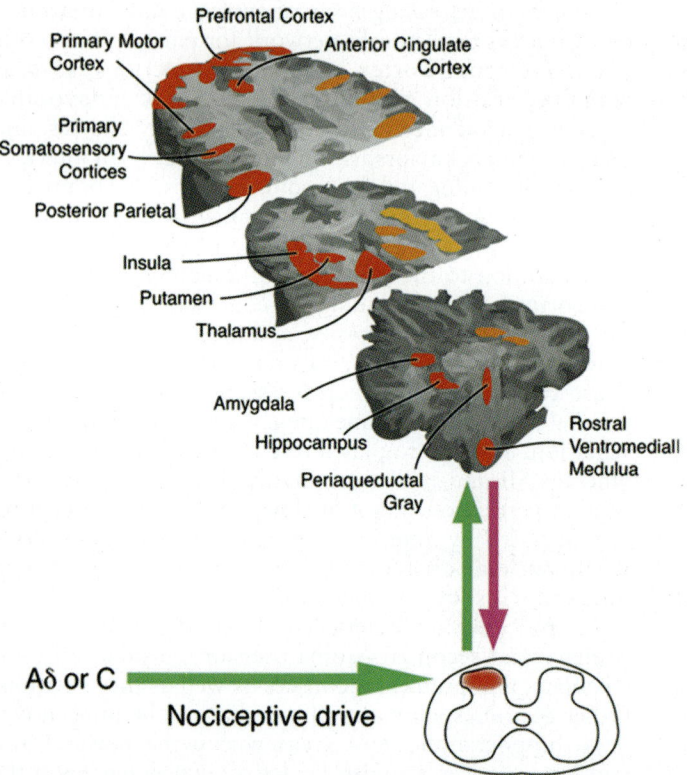

FIGURE 3.6 Neuroanatomy of pain processing. Main brain regions that activate during a painful experience, highlighted as bilaterally active but with increased activation on the contralateral hemisphere *(orange)*. (From Tracey I, Mantyh PW. The cerebral signature for pain perception and its modulation. *Neuron.* 2007;55(3):377–391. Copyright 2007, with permission from Elsevier.)

that enables a regulation of nociceptive processing (largely within the dorsal horn) in various circumstances to produce either facilitation or inhibition. There is evidence that several brain regions are involved in this descending modulation, including the frontal lobe, anterior cingulate cortex (ACC), insula, amygdala, hypothalamus, periaqueductal gray (PAG), nucleus cuneiformis (NCF), and rostral ventromedial medulla (RVM).[1] Figure 3.7 illustrates some of these key anatomic features.

Some neurons in the dorsal horn of the spinal cord are strongly inhibited when a nociceptive stimulus is applied to any part of the body outside their excitatory receptive fields.[25] One aspect of the inhibitory mechanism that modulates pain processing at the spinal cord level is termed *diffuse noxious inhibitory control* (DNIC), in which the activity of pain-signaling neurons in the spinal dorsal horn and in trigeminal nuclei is attenuated in response to noxious stimuli applied to a remote area of the body. Endogenous pain-modulating systems also include descending inhibitory projections that are coordinated in the rostroventral medulla and make up part of the spinal-bulbo-spinal DNIC pathway.[26] DNIC influences only convergent neurons: the other cell types that are found in the dorsal horn, including specific nociceptive neurons, are not affected by this type of control. In normal conditions, these inhibitions can be triggered only by conditioning stimuli, which are nociceptive. DNIC is sustained by a complex loop which involves supraspinal structures since, unlike segmental inhibitions, they cannot be observed in animals in which the cord has previously been transsected at the cervical level. The ascending and descending limbs of this loop travel through the ventrolateral and dorso-lateral funiculi, respectively. Expecta-

tions of pain relief can modulate DNIC responses.[27] Patients with chronic musculoskeletal pain may have impaired DNIC.[28] Nociceptive stimuli activate certain inhibitory controls that originate in the brainstem.[25] Since all convergent neurons are subject to DNIC, the transmission of nociceptive signals towards higher centers is probably under the influence of these controls.

DNIC has been identified as an advanced psychophysical measure, with high clinical relevancy, in the characterization of one's capability to modulate pain and consequently one's susceptibility to pain disorders. Preoperative DNIC testing may identify patients at risk for development of chronic postoperative pain.[29] A key mechanism of central pain modulation is the endogenous analgesia system, commonly evaluated by the DNIC test paradigm.[30] DNIC was calculated as the difference in pain rating between two identical noxious "test" stimuli applied first at baseline and then concomitantly with another "conditioning" remote noxious stimulus. A decrease in the test stimulus pain scores from baseline indicates efficient pain inhibition, expressed as a positive DNIC value. Granot et al.[30] described the test as the application of contact heat pain as the test stimulus to the nondominant forearm, with stimulation temperature at a psychophysical intensity score of 60 on a 0 to 100 numeric pain scale. The conditioning stimulus was a 60-second immersion of the dominant hand in cold (12°C, 15°C, 18°C), hot (44°C and 46.5°C), or skin temperature (33°C) water. The test stimulus was repeated on the nondominant hand during the last 30 seconds of the conditioning immersion. Endogenous analgesia extent was calculated as the difference between pain scores of the two test stimuli.

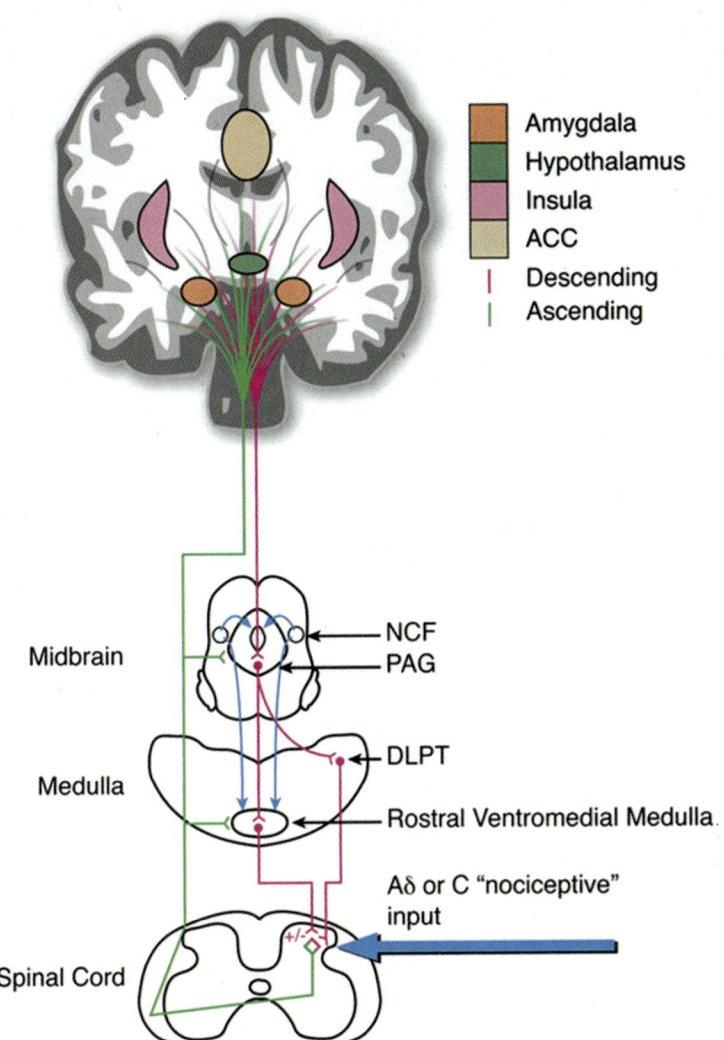

FIGURE 3.7 The descending pain modulatory system. NCF, Nucleus cuneiformis; PAG, periaqueductal gray; DLPT, dorsolateral pontine tegmentum; ACC, anterior cingulate cortex; +/−, pro- and antinociceptive influences, respectively. (With permission from Tracey I, Mantyh PW. The cerebral signature for pain perception and its modulation. *Neuron.* 2077;55:377–391. Copyright 2007, with permission from Elsevier.)

Augmented pain modulation, related to both sensitization of ascending pathways and deficiencies in pain descending inhibitory systems, has been suggested as the mechanism of several chronic pain disorders. Attenuated endogenous analgesia evaluated by DNIC test was found in temporomandibular disorder,[31] fibromyalgia,[32] tension-type headache,[33] and migraine.[34] This suggests that altered DNIC might be relevant in the pathogenesis of these disorders and other chronic pain states, including pain occurring in the patient with cancer.

References

1. Tracey I, Mantyh PW. The cerebral signature for pain perception and its modulation. *Neuron.* 2077;55:377–391.
2. Woolf CJ, Ma Q. Nociceptors—noxious stimulus detectors. *Neuron.* 2007;55:353–364.
3. Hucho T, Levine JD. Signaling pathways in sensitization: toward a nociceptor cell biology. *Neuron.* 2007;55:365–376.
4. Kim CH, Oh Y, Chung JM, Chung K. Changes in three subtypes of tetrodotoxin sensitive sodium channel expression in the axotomized dorsal root ganglion in the rat. *Neurosci Lett.* 2002;323:125–128.
5. Cummins TR, Sheets PL, Waxman SG. The roles of sodium channels in nociception: Implications for mechanisms of pain. *Pain.* 2007;131:243–257.
6. Gee NS, Brown JP, Dissanayake VU, et al. The novel anticonvulsant drug, gabapentin (Neurontin), binds to the alpha$_2$delta subunit of a calcium channel. *J Biol Chem.* 1996;271:5768–5776.
7. Lee Y, Lee CH, Oh U. Painful channels in sensory neurons. *Mol Cells.* 2005;20:315–324.
8. Voilley N, de Weille J, Mamet J, et al. Nonsteroid anti-inflammatory drugs inhibit both the activity and the inflammation-induced expression of acid-sensing ion channels in nociceptors. *J Neurosci.* 2001;21:8026–8033.
9. Hamilton SG, McMahon SB, Lewin GR. Selective activation of nociceptors by P2X receptor agonists in normal and inflamed rat skin. *J Physiol.* 2001;534:437–445.
10. Cockayne DA, Hamilton SG, Zhu QM, et al. Urinary bladder hyporeflexia and reduced pain-related behaviour in P2X3-deficient mice. *Nature.* 2000;407:1011–1015.
11. Meuser T, Pietruck C, Gabriel A, et al. 5-HT7 receptors are involved in mediating 5-HT-induced activation of rat primary afferent neurons. *Life Sci.* 2002;71:2279–2289.
12. Scholz J, Broom DC, Youn DH, et al. Blocking caspase activity prevents transsynaptic neuronal apoptosis and the loss of inhibition in lamina II of the dorsal horn after peripheral nerve injury. *J Neurosci.* 2005;25:7317–7323.
13. Pralong E, Pollo C, Bloch J, et al. Recording of ventral posterior lateral thalamus neuron response to contact heat evoked potential in patient with neurogenic pain. *Neurosci Lett.* 2004;367:332–3325.
14. Apkarian AV, Bushnell MC, Treede RD, et al.. Human brain mechanisms of pain perception and regulation in health and disease. *Eur J Pain.* 2005;9:463–84.
15. Casey KL. Forebrain mechanisms of nociception and pain: analysis through imaging. *Proc Natl Acad Sci U S A.* 1999;96:7668–7774.
16. Craig AD. Pain mechanisms: labeled lines versus convergence in central processing. *Annu Rev Neurosci.* 2003;26:1–30.

17. Ostrowsky K, Magnin M, Ryvlin P, et al. Representation of pain and somatic sensation in the human insula: a study of responses to direct electrical cortical stimulation. *Cereb Cortex.* 2002;12: 376–385.
18. Greenspan JD, Lee RR, Lenz FA. Pain sensitivity alterations as a function of lesion location in the parasylvian cortex. *Pain.* 1999;81:273–282.
19. Mayer EA, Naliboff BD, Craig AD. Neuroimaging of the brain-gut axis: from basic understanding to treatment of functional GI disorders. *Gastroenterology.* 2006;131:1925–1942.
20. Neugebauer V. Visceral pain and the black box called brain. *Pain.* 2008;138:5–6.
21. Shibasaki H. Central mechanisms of pain perception. *Suppl Clin Neurophysiol.* 2004;57:39–49.
22. Neugebauer V, Li W, Bird GC, et al. The amygdala and persistent pain. *Neurosci.* 2004;10:221–234.
23. Mohr C, Binkofski F, Erdmann C, et al. The anterior cingulate cortex contains distinct areas dissociating external from self-administered painful stimulation: a parametric fMRI study. *Pain.* 2005;114:347–357.
24. Neugebauer V. The amygdala: different pains, different mechanisms. *Pain.* 2007;127:1–2.
25. Villanueva L, Le Bars D. The activation of bulbo-spinal controls by peripheral nociceptive inputs: diffuse noxious inhibitory controls. *Biol Res.* 1995;28:113–125.
26. Millan MJ. Descending control of pain. *Prog Neurobiol.* 2002;66:355–474.
27. Goffaux P, Redmond WJ, Rainville P, Marchand S. Descending analgesia—when the spine echoes what the brain expects. *Pain.* 2007; 130:137–143.
28. Arendt-Nielsen L, Sluka KA, Nie HL. Experimental muscle pain impairs descending inhibition. *Pain.* 2008;140:465–471.
29. Yarnitsky D, Crispel Y, Eisenberg E, et al. Prediction of chronic postoperative pain: preoperative DNIC testing identifies patients at risk. *Pain.* 2008;138:22–28.
30. Granot M, Weissman-Fogel I, Crispel Y, et al. Determinants of endogenous analgesia magnitude in a diffuse noxious inhibitory control (DNIC) paradigm: do conditioning stimulus painfulness, gender and personality variables matter? *Pain.* 2008;136:142–149.
31. Maixner W, Fillingim R, Booker D, et al Sensitivity of patients with painful temporomandibular disorders to experimentally evoked pain. *Pain.* 1995;63:341–351.
32. Lautenbacher S, Rollman GB. Possible deficiencies of pain modulation in fibromyalgia. *Clin J Pain.* 1997;13:189–196.
33. Pielsticker A, Haag G, Zaudig M, et al. Impairment of pain inhibition in chronic tension-type headache. *Pain.* 2005;118: 215–223.
34. Sandrini G, Rossi P, Milanov I, et al. Abnormal modulatory influence of diffuse noxious inhibitory controls in migraine and chronic tension-type headache patients. *Cephalalgia.* 2006;26: 82–789.
35. Seifert F, Maihofner C. Central mechanisms of experimental and chronic neuropathic pain: Findings from functional imaging studies. *Cell Mol Life Sci.* 2009;66:375–390.

CHAPTER 4 ■ THE PROCESS OF PAIN IN THE CANCER PATIENT

"Pain is an unpleasant sensory and emotional experience associated with actual or potential tissue damage, or described in terms of such damage."[1] The sensory features and affective qualities of pain vary, depending on its origin, the previous experiences of the patient, and the environment that surrounds the patient. Its negative affective characteristics are related to the social and physical context in which pain occurs, as well as to cognitive processes such as the meaning of tissue trauma for the individual.

SENSORY COMPONENT OF CANCER PAIN

Tumor-associated pain is either nociceptive or neuropathic, or a combination of the two. Nociceptive pain is thought to be related to unhealed tissue injury of either somatic or visceral structures. Pain associated with injury to neural tissues is sustained by aberrant somatosensory processing in the peripheral or the central nervous system; it is labeled as neuropathic. An international survey of cancer pain characteristics and syndromes reported that pains thought to be nociceptive and caused by somatic injury occurred in 71.6% of patients, nociceptive visceral pain in 34.7%, and neuropathic pain in 39.7%.[2] Somatic nociceptive pain may be divided into superficial (cutaneous) and deep. Cutaneous pain usually is well localized, sharp, pricking, or burning. Deep tissue pain is usually reported as diffuse and dull or aching in quality. Visceral pain is usually poorly localized, often referred to the body surface, of long duration, and commonly described as "sickening."

Tumor involvement of the peripheral nervous system has many manifestations and can include lesions within the cerebrospinal fluid space, local invasion, compression of nerves, direct infiltration, perineural spread, and intraneural metastasis, although the last is quite rare.[3] Both myelinated and unmyelinated fibers and supporting tissues are destroyed by compression or invasion of nerves by tumor. Infiltration by a neoplasm is the prototypic tissue trauma stimulus. A remote neoplasm may produce indirect damage of unknown pathogenesis in peripheral nerves (eg, paraneoplastic syndrome). Tumor may also directly invade nerve.[4] Primary neural tumors also can lead to painful destruction of the parent nerve. Neural compression and the associated inflammatory changes can also lead to pain, especially when the nerve is confined by osseous structures, as, for example, where the dorsal root goes through the neural foramen.

Degenerative, regenerative, and other pathophysiologic processes are involved when a nerve is compressed or invaded.[5] The entire afferent neuron, dendrites, soma, and axon manifest biochemical changes that are both reactive and reparative. Eventually, the neuron loses its neuropeptides,[6] atrophies, and degenerates. Unmyelinated afferent neurons are particularly susceptible to this process. Neural degeneration after invasion or compression by cancerous tissue is probably similar to that seen after lesions of nerves induced by mechanical or other events. Changes occur not only in impulse transmission but also in the resting activity, as well as in responses to mechanical, thermal, and chemical stimulation.

SENSITIZATION OF NOCICEPTORS

Neoplasms contain, in addition to cancer cells, different cell types, such as inflammatory and neo-vascular cells, that are in proximity to primary afferent nociceptors (Fig. 4.1). Most of these cells belong to the immune system, including macrophages, neutrophils, and T-lymphocytes known to secrete various factors that sensitize or directly excite primary afferent neurons. These factors include prostaglandins, tumor necrosis factor (TNF), endothelins, interleukin-1 and -6, epidermal growth factor, transforming growth factor, and platelet-derived growth factor. Primary afferent neurons express receptors for many of these factors. Endothelins are a family of vasoactive peptides that are expressed at high levels by several types of tumor, including prostate cancer. Endothelins contribute directly to cancer pain by sensitizing or exciting nociceptors, because a subset of small, unmyelinated primary afferent neurons expresses endothelin-A receptors.[7] Angiogenesis and tumor growth are thought to be regulated by endothelins and prostaglandins that are produced by cancer cells.[8] These and many other factors, as well as others produced by cancer and inflammatory cells such as adenosine triphosphate (ATP), bradykinin, H^+, nerve growth factor (NGF), prostaglandins, and vascular endothelial growth factor (VEGF) sensitize or even excite adjacent nociceptors.[9] Endothelins released by cancer cells are detected by the nociceptor vanilloid receptor-1 (VR1), which is also sensitive to extracellular H^+. The tyrosine kinase receptor TrkA binds to NGF that has been released by macrophages.[10] Neurotransmitters, such as calcitonin gene-related peptide (CGRP), endothelin, histamine, glutamate, and substance P are liberated during nociceptor activation. Prostaglandins released from the peripheral terminals of sensory fibers during their activation can lead to vasodilatation, plasma extravasation, and the recruitment and activation of immune cells.

Tumor-related pain can be induced by tissue acidosis and other mechanisms. Decreases in tissue pH can be explained via several mechanisms. When inflammatory cells invade neoplastic tissues, they release protons that

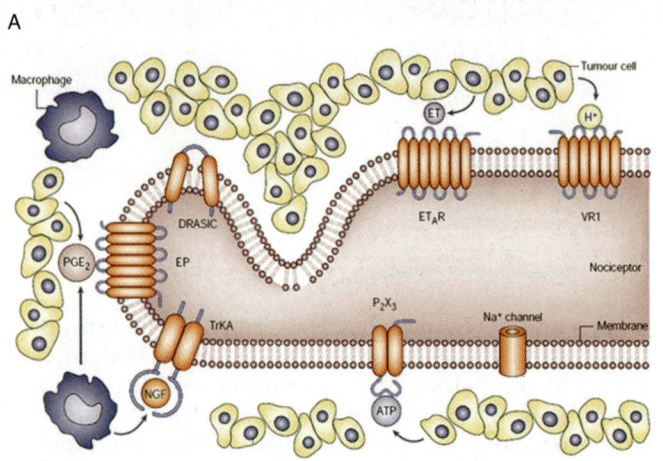
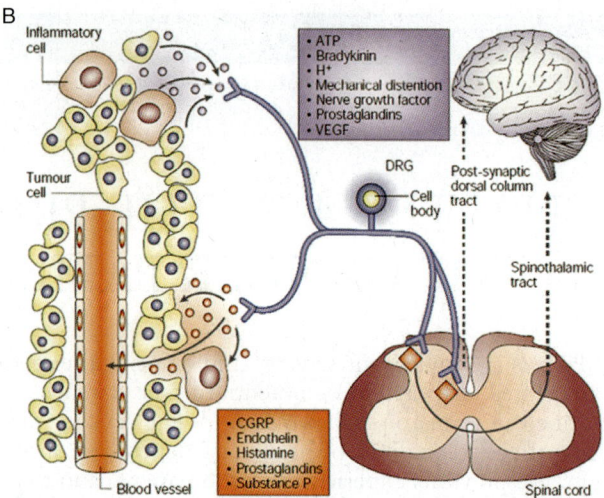

FIGURE 4.1 Detection by sensory neurons of noxious stimuli produced by tumors (**A**). Nociceptors *(pink)* use different receptors to detect and transmit signals about noxious stimuli produced by cancer cells *(yellow)* or other aspects of the tumor microenvironment. Vanilloid receptor-1 (VR1) detects H^+ produced by cancer cells, whereas endothelial-A receptors (ET_AR) detect endothelins (ET). Dorsal-root acid-sensing ion channel (DRASIC) detects mechanical stimuli as tumor growth distends sensory fibers. Other receptors expressed by sensory neurons include prostaglandin (PG) receptors, which detect PGE_2 (produced by cancer and inflammatory cells). Nerve growth factor (NGF) released by macrophages binds to tyrosine kinase receptor (TrkA). **B**: Tumor-nociceptor interface. In addition to cancer cells, tumors consist of inflammatory cells and blood vessels and are often adjacent to primary afferent nociceptors. Cancer cells and inflammatory cells release a variety of products, such as adenosine triphosphate (ATP), bradykinin, H^+, NGF, PG, and vascular endothelial growth factor (VEGF), that either excite or sensitize the nociceptor. Painful stimuli are detected by the nociceptors, the cell bodies of which lie in the dorsal root ganglion (DRG), and are transmitted to neurons in the spinal cord. The signal is then transmitted to higher centers of the brain. Cancer-associated pain signals seem to ascend to the brain by at least two main spinal-cord pathways, the spinothalamic tract and the dorsal column. Nociceptor activation results in the release of neurotransmitters, such as calcitonin gene–related peptide (CGRP), endothelin, histamine, glutamate, and substance P. Nociceptor activation also causes the release of PGs from the peripheral terminals of sensory fibers, which can induce plasma extravasation, recruitment and activation of immune cells, and vasodilatation.[9] VR1, Vanilloid receptor-1; ET_AR, endothelial-A receptor; ET, endothelin; DRASIC, dorsal-root acid-sensing ion channel; PG, prostaglandin; NGF, nerve growth factor; TrkA, tyrosine kinase receptor; ATP, adenosine triphosphate; VEGF, vascular endothelial growth factor; DRG, dorsal root ganglion; CGRP, calcitonin gene–related peptide. (Adapted from Mantyh PW et al. Molecular mechanisms of cancer pain. *Nat Rev Cancer* 2002;2(3):201–209. Copyright 2002, with permission from Macmillan Publishers, Ltd.)

generate local acidosis. Apoptosis commonly occurs in the tumor environment and contributes to acidosis, as apoptotic cells release intracellular ions, creating an acidic environment. The fall in pH can activate signaling by acid-sensing channels (including VR1) expressed on nociceptors. The generation of bone cancer pain may be dependent upon the tumor-induced release of protons and acidosis.[11] Tumor invasion of sensory fibers may also lead to pain, although tumors are not significantly innervated by sensory neurons.[12] However, rapid tumor growth may entrap and injure nerves, producing mechanical injury, compression, ischemia, or direct proteolysis. Tumor cells can also produce proteolytic enzymes that can cause injury to sensory and sympathetic fibers, leading to a neuropathic pain syndrome.

CAUSES OF PAIN IN THE CANCER PATIENT

Cancer pain is a mixture of acute pain, chronic pain, tumor-specific pain, and treatment-related pain, all compounded by ongoing psychological responses of distress and suffering. Almost all pain in cancer patients may be considered the result of one or more of three fundamental causes (Table 4.1): direct tumor involvement, cancer-directed therapy, and mechanisms unrelated to cancer or its treatment.

Complex patterns of pain that result from combinations of these categories are common in cancer patients; accurate diagnosis can be difficult. In addition, many elements that contribute to the challenge of controlling cancer-related and chronic noncancer pain (central sensitization, hyperalgesia, novel gene expression, synaptic remodeling, and behavioral adjustment) emerge promptly on persistent tissue injury.[13–14] Factors influencing the pain complaint include the primary tumor type, stage of disease, tumor site, and mood factors (anxiety and depression).[15–17] Vainio et al.[17] estimated the prevalence of pain in 1,840 patients with advanced cancer from seven hospices in Europe, the United States, and Australia. Twenty-four

TABLE 4.1

CAUSES OF PAIN IN ONCOLOGY PATIENTS

Cause	Example
Tumor	Invasion of nerves, bone, hollow organs
Indirect etiology	By infection
	By metabolic imbalance
	By vascular (venous or lymphatic) obstruction
Tumor therapy	Following surgical intervention
	Following chemotherapy
	Following radiation therapy
Unrelated to cancer	Diabetic peripheral neuropathic pain
	Migraine
	Fibromyalgia
	Pain problems associated with deactivation

TABLE 4.2

PREVALENCE OF PAIN (PERCENTAGE OF PATIENTS), BY PRIMARY SITE AMONG PALLIATIVE-CARE CANCER PATIENTS

Primary Site	None	Pain Level			N
		Mild	Moderate	Severe	
Prostate	17	22	20	41	41
Esophagus	29	21	13	38	24
Gynecologic	10	10	47	33	30
Colorectal	21	21	27	32	63
Lympho-hematologic	13	29	26	32	38
Head and neck	17	11	43	29	35
Lung	26	23	30	21	241
Breast	22	25	31	21	118
Stomach	26	30	26	17	53
Other or unknown	26	27	32	15	417
Total	24	24	30	21	1060

(From Vainio A, Auvinen A. Prevalence of symptoms among patients with advanced cancer: An international collaborative study. Symptom Prevalence Group. *J Pain Symptom Manage*. 1996;12:3–10. Copyright 1996, U.S. Cancer Pain Relief Committee.)

percent of the patients surveyed had no pain, 24% had mild pain, 30% had moderate pain, and 21% had severe pain. In addition, the prevalence of moderate or severe pain was highest in gynecological cancer and in head and neck cancer. Severe pain was most common in prostate cancer (Table 4.2). Van den Beuken-van Everdingen et al.,[18] in a meta-analysis of 52 studies, calculated the pooled prevalence of pain in oncology patients. The prevalence of pain in patients after curative treatment was 33%; in patients under anticancer treatment, 59%; in patients with advanced/metastatic/terminal disease, 64%; in patients at all disease stages, 53%. Of the patients with pain, more than one third graded their pain as moderate or severe. Pooled prevalence of pain was >50% in all cancer types, with the highest prevalence in head/neck cancer patients (70%).

Patients with advanced cancers often have multiple pain complaints at different sites; this is particularly true in patients with breast, lung, and prostate cancer when compared with gastrointestinal cancers.[16] Localization, etiology, and pathophysiologic mechanisms of pain syndromes associated with cancer were assessed by Grond et al. in a prospective study of 2,266 cancer patients.[19] Thirty percent of the patients presented with one, 39% with two, and 31% with three or more distinct pain syndromes. The overwhelming majority of patients had pain caused by cancer (85%); antineoplastic treatment was the primary cause in 17%; pain indirectly related to cancer disease was the cause in 9%, and 9% of cases were ascribed to noncancer etiologies. Pain was found to be originating from nociceptors in bone (35%), soft tissue (45%), visceral structures (33%), or neuropathy (34%). The pain was localized to the lower back (36%), abdominal region (27%), thoracic region (23%), lower limbs (21%), head (17%), and pelvic region (15%). The cancer site of origin did not markedly influence the pain's temporal characteristics, intensity, or etiology; not surprisingly, the site of origin of the cancer was a key factor in determining the body region and organ system involved in the pain.

In most patients with cancer, there is an association between number of metastases and the presence and magnitude of pain; breast and prostate cancers are the exceptions to this generalization. Neither the prevalence nor the severity of pain among breast cancer patients is related to the sites of overt metastases.[20–21] Pain was a common finding with or without metastatic disease, and it occurred in more than half of the patients. Patients with bone metastases usually reported bone pain; yet, significant percentages of patients (21% of breast and 22% of prostate patients) were asymptomatic even though they had imaging evidence for osseous metastasis.[22]

Pain syndromes may result from chemotherapy, radiation therapy, or surgery in the cancer patient. Postchemotherapy, painful peripheral neuropathy is well described with a variety of agents. Steroids are a common cause of chemotherapeutic toxicity; they are coadministered in many chemotherapeutic protocols. Osteonecrosis is a well-described complication of steroid use.[23] Morbidity is related to progressive joint damage that leads to decreased range of motion, pain with movement, and arthritis. Weight-bearing joints are most commonly involved, and joint replacement is often required to restore function and relieve pain. All of the joints of the upper extremity, as well as the vertebrae, can also be involved. Osteonecrosis usually develops within 3 years of steroid treatment, although cases of necrosis also have been reported after short-term use.[24] Osteonecrosis or avascular necrosis can occur after either intermittent or continuous steroid treatment. The most common site is the femoral head. Pain in the hip, thigh, or knee that is worse with movement is the predominant complaint. Localized tenderness may or may not be present. Humeral head disease presents with pain in the shoulder, upper arm, or elbow. Osteonecrosis may mimic bone tumor. Steroid therapy, as well as radiation and chemotherapy, can be the causes of this treatment complication. The imaged degree of bone involvement and the intensity of the associated pain are not highly correlated.

Combined medical and radiation therapies, both sequential and concurrent, are improving clinical outcomes with respect to tumor control, with enhanced patient survival and delay of recurrence. During the course of external radiation therapy, treatment generally influences normal function in tissues that have more rapid self-renewing proliferative index (eg, mucosal surfaces such as skin, head/neck, and esophagus) than other surface tissues that have less potential for self-renewal (eg, hair, nails, and surface glands). Injuries to these tissues are often self-limited and heal without specific intervention secondary to stem cell renewal. Acute effects from radiation therapy do not uniformly predict the late effects from treatment. Late effects generally affect tissues that have limited potential for self-renewal, and injury is often more permanent, requiring surgical debridement and possibly resulting in functional damage.

Radiation-induced neural damage and pain may become apparent some time after radiation therapy completion, confounding the diagnosis in some cases. Postsurgical pain syndromes come in many varieties, including postmastectomy, postamputation, postthoracotomy, and other chronic pain states. Treatments for head and neck cancer have the potential to increase pain and discomfort. Radical surgery, such as resection of portions of the tongue, palate, and mandible, and radical neck dissection cause major structural changes. Radiation therapy, which frequently is the primary therapy, may cause mucositis, xerostomia, loss of taste, and decreased quality of life. Subsequent late fibrosis of skin and soft tissues may lead to temperomandibular joint dysfunction and myofascial pain syndromes. Chua et al.[25] found that 65% of patients with head and neck cancers had continued pain despite the absence of tumor recurrence. In most cases, this was related to the effects of treatment. This incidence of oncologic treatment-related pain was also higher in this group than that reported for treated gastrointestinal tract and respiratory system cancers.

Both active cancer patients and cancer survivors may experience chronic nontumor-related pain. It is critical to distinguish between tumor-associated and nontumor-associated pain. Cancer survivors may manifest all the phenomena associated with chronic pain due to a benign disease and many of the same interdisciplinary treatment paradigms will be essential for their successful management. Pain associated with cancer and its treatment can be a real management challenge to the treating clinician. The prudent clinician realizes that pains may stem from multiple sites, have varying origins, make use of varied mechanisms, may have little or no relationship to the original tumor, and may change over time.

MYOGENIC PAIN

Muscle-related pain frequently occurs in an oncology patient population.[26] The debilitated cancer patient is particularly susceptible to muscle pain, because inactivity and deconditioning are known to be important etiological factors. Myofascial pain syndrome (MPS) is considered part of a distinct pain syndrome and diagnostic guidelines are partly based on the identification of *trigger points* (TrPs).[27] Signs and symptoms considered to be essential or associated with MPS include regional location of pain, trigger points, normal neurologic examination, reduced pain with local anesthetic or "spray and stretch," taut bands, tender points, palpable nodules, muscle ropiness, decreased range of motion, pain exacerbated by stress, and regional pain described as "dull," "achy," or "deep." Sensory or reflex abnormalities, scar tissue, and most test results were considered to be irrelevant to the diagnosis of MPS.[27] Trigger points may be defined as the presence of defined "exquisitely" painful triggers in a taut band of muscle, that produce characteristic patterns of referred pain on palpation and a local twitch response to mechanical stimulation or needling.

Muscle pain may also occur in patients treated with chemotherapeutic agents. The administration of paclitaxel (Taxol), a commonly used chemotherapeutic agent, results in a subacute myofascial pain syndrome in a large proportion of patients, impairing their physical function and quality of life.[28] This syndrome usually begins a few days after therapy and lasts for 3 to 7 days. In some patients, the pain can be severe and debilitating, resulting in a need for opioid therapy. The distribution of the pain complaint may be generalized in some patients and localized in others. Pain has been reported to be localized to the large axial muscles in the shoulders, paraspinal regions, pelvis, and thighs.[29] Based mainly on these clinical descriptions, this syndrome has been termed the paclitaxel-induced arthralgia/myalgia syndrome. Although the pathophysiology of this problem is unknown, animal studies suggest that paclitaxel may induce pathologic changes in small, presumably nociceptive, neurons within 24 to 48 hours of infusion, and that these pathologic changes may participate in the generation of the muscle pain reported by patients.[30-31] Other agents such as aromatase inhibitors, commonly used in the treatment of breast cancer, are frequently associated with arthralgias and myalgias that may be so severe as to necessitate a change in therapy.

Progressive disease may result in significant cachexia, weight loss, and muscle wasting. Severe muscle wasting can result in significant pain problems associated with deactivation as well as the risk of skeletal fractures. There are three pathways that contribute to muscle protein degradation: the lysosomal system, cytosolic proteases and the ubiquitin (Ub)-proteasome pathway.[32] The Ub-proteasome pathway seems to account for the majority of skeletal muscle degradation in cancer cachexia and is stimulated by several cytokines including tumor necrosis factor-α, interleukin-1β, interleukin-6, interferon-γ, and proteolysis-inducing factor. Cachexia is particularly severe in pancreatic cancer and contributes significantly to the poor quality of life and high mortality of these patients.

Direct tumor involvement of muscle may be associated with significant pain. Unlike cutaneous pain, for which there exists a plethora of experimental research and animal models, there is a relative lack of basic science and clinical data available for deep tissue pain. Convergent afferent input from skin, joints, and viscera to the spinothalamic tract and other ascending pain pathways may cause misinterpretation of information arising from Aδ- and C-fiber polymodal muscle nociceptors, as is the case with other types of referred pain. Pain in response to muscle injury is transmitted by the same basic pathways as those involved for other somatic structures. The neurophysiologic basis of local muscle pain is an increased impulse activity in muscle nociceptors.[33] Well-known sensitizers for muscle nociceptors are endogenous pain-producing substances such as bradykinin (BK), 5-HT, and K^+. Typically, muscle nociceptors respond to noxious local pressure or ischemia. Ischemia, lowered pH, and blood clotting cause kallidin, found in plasma cells, to split and liberate BK. 5HT is released after vascular injury, and muscle trauma or damage releases K^+. BK, 5-HT, and K^+ sensitize nociceptors. C nociceptors, when stimulated, release in the dorsal horn somatostatin, CGRP, and substance P. Substance P-mediated histamine release occurs from mast cells, causing vasodilation and increased vessel permeability, thereby releasing more BK, 5-HT, and prostaglandin E_2 (PGE_2). Proinflammatory cytokines such as TNF-α appear to play a role in the development of muscle-induced hyperalgesia.[34] Paraneoplastic necrotizing myopathy is characterized by a rapidly progressive, symmetric, predominantly proximal weakness that produces severe disability.[35] Muscle pathology demonstrates prominent necrosis with alkaline phosphatase staining of connective tissue and little inflammation. For certain tumors such as angioleiomyomas, pain fibers are located within the tumor parenchyma.[36]

Myogenic pain is usually characterized as aching and cramp-like. Localization of the pain may be difficult and the pain may be referred to other deep somatic structures. A simple examination of neck and shoulder range of motion can identify potential muscular causes of upper body pain. Examining the cervical spine for flexion, extension, lateral bend, and rotation and the shoulder girdles for forward elevation, and abduction of the upper extremity and functional (scapulohumeral and scapulothoracic motion) in external and internal rotation will help to point to muscles that may be contributing to the patient's pain. The examination of the trunk and lower extremities for potential myofascial problems may be achieved by determining range of motion and local tenderness and assists in diagnosis of pain in the cancer patient.

EMOTIONAL COMPONENT AND SUFFERING IN CANCER PATIENTS

The emotional mechanisms of cancer pain, as well as its sensory features, are the reasons that it generates suffering. Brain processing of pain in humans is based on multiple ascending pathways and brain regions that are involved in several pain components, such as sensory, immediate affective, and secondary affective dimensions.[37] The prefrontal cortex, anterior cingulate cortex, posterior parietal cortex, thalamus, and caudate are involved during evaluation of the spatial locations of noxious stimuli.[38] Brain mechanisms supporting discrimination of sensory features of pain extend far beyond the somatosensory cortices and involve frontal regions traditionally associated with affective processing and the medial pain system. These frontoparietal interactions are similar to those involved in the processing of innocuous information and may be critically involved in placing afferent sensory information into a personal historical context. Of course, most cancer patients suffer from a complex array of problems and not only pain. Nonetheless, sustained nociception in and of itself can produce suffering because of its ability to create negative emotional arousal and elicit stress responses.

Suffering has been described as a complex negative emotional and cognitive state characterized by perceived threat to the integrity of the self, perceived helplessness in the face of that threat, and apparent exhaustion of the psychosocial and personal resources for coping with that threat.[39] The perceived threat to the self may encompass the body, the psychosocial self or both. Suffering related to cancer is inherently emotional, unpleasant, complex, and enduring. The physician should recognize that, although suffering may be a consequence of pain, it is separate from pain and not a synonym for it. It differs from pain in that it entails additional cognitive and affective activities. Perceived helplessness (inability to cope, bankruptcy of physical, psychological or social resources) is an important aspect of suffering in most patients with incurable disease. Grief may progress when a cancer patient perceives the loss of a psychological or social resource, the loss of a body part or normal personal appearance, a valued job, or the ability to participate in a rewarding activity. In addition, suffering in the cancer patient sometimes involves a sense of separation from social support or alienation. These factors, combined with the emotional distress, fatigue, and stress associated with prolonged pain produce a complex state that is more than the pain itself. A study of 381 patients with advanced cancer revealed that 25% of patients were profoundly suffering.[40] We concur with the author of this study who stated that suffering is a multidimensional experience strongly related to physical symptoms, but with significant contributions from psychological distress, existential concerns, and interpersonal concerns.

PSYCHOLOGICAL FACTORS AND THE COMPLEXITIES OF CANCER PAIN

Patients who transform distress and global suffering into pain and other symptom expression are labeled *somatizers*, implying that mental processes and not tissue damage are responsible for the complaint of pain. Health care providers commonly view pain reported by cancer patients as somatogenic; chronic nonmalignant pain in patients who lack adequate objective physical pathology is often thought of as psychogenic.[41] It is not surprising, therefore, that providers tend to treat cancer pain with pharmacological, medical, or surgical modalities, whereas psychological factors are considered to be of secondary importance and do not receive adequate attention.[42]

Pain is always a complex experience entailing physiological, sensory, affective, cognitive and behavioral components (Fig. 4.2). The individual's perception of pain is dependent not only upon nociceptive input but also psychological modifiers such as fear, anxiety, anger, and depression. Pain requires consciousness and is always influenced by the environment as well as personal factors in the patient.

Turk et al.[41] studied the adaptation of cancer patients and noncancer chronic pain patients to persisting pain. The majority of the cancer patients, both with (81%) and

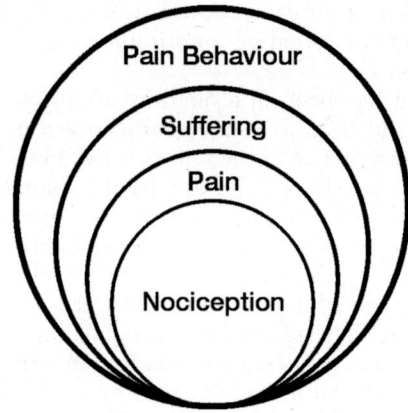

FIGURE 4.2 Components of pain.
(From Loeser JD. Perspectives on pain, clinical pharmacology and therapeutics. Turner P, ed. London: MacMillan, 1980:313–316.)

without (84%) metastatic disease, as well as the non–cancer chronic pain patients (85%), could be assigned to one of three psychosocial subgroups: dysfunctional (high levels of pain, perceived interference, affective distress, and low levels of perceived control and activity), interpersonally distressed (high levels of affective distress, negative responses from significant others, and low levels of perceived support) and adaptive copers (low levels of interference and affective distress, high levels of perceived control and activity). Such a classification scheme provides the clinician with insights into the management strategies that are most likely to be useful for each type of patient.

Psychological factors can play an important role in exacerbating pain. The belief that pain signifies disease is frequently identified in cancer patients,[43] and is associated with elevated pain intensity.[21,44] Speigel and Bloom[21] also reported that pain severity was predicted by the belief that pain is an indicator for disease progression, and, furthermore, that medication use can also predict pain severity. Patients who believe that their pain is a warning of underlying disease report greater pain than patients with non–tumor-associated interpretations, even though they have similar levels of disease progression.

The relationship between pain severity and the extent of disease is strongly influenced by psychological factors and is certainly not linear.[45] The relationships between physical pathology and pain in cancer have been the subject of studies with conflicting results/findings. Many patients with advanced cancer do not report pain at all. Twycross and Fairfield[46] reported that only 41 of 100 terminal-stage cancer patients reported pain from their disease. On the other extreme, Cleeland et al. reported that the majority of cancer patients with end-stage disease have pain that interferes with quality of life.[47] Front et al.[20] asserted that, for many cancer patients, pain reports did not correspond to the presence or location of bone metastases. Turk et al.[41] found that patients with cancer-related pain reported significantly higher levels of perceived disability and inactivity due to pain than did patients with pain of nonmalignant origin. Increased disability can be ascribed to the meanings patients attributed to their pain. Disease progression frequently means further deterioration of health and even impending death. Patients with cancer-related pain appeared to be more fearful of pain and reported significantly higher levels of cognitive and behavioral fear responses than did the patients with chronic pain that was not associated with cancer. Cancer patients seem to reflect and worry more about pain, avoid activities to prevent the initiation of pain, and generally feel more hopeless than the patients with chronic pain of nonmalignant origin.

References

1. Task Force on Taxonomy: *Classification of chronic pain. Descriptions of chronic pain syndromes and definitions of pain terms.* Seattle, Wash: IASP Press, 1986:S217.
2. Caraceni A, Portenoy RK. An international survey of cancer pain characteristics and syndromes. IASP Task Force on Cancer Pain. International Association for the Study of Pain. *Pain.* 1999;82:263–274.
3. Grisold W, Piza-Katzer H, Jahn R, et al. Intraneural nerve metastasis with multiple mononeuropathies. *J Peripher Nerv Syst.* 2000;5:163–167.
4. Gandhi D, Gujar S, Mukherji SK. Magnetic resonance imaging of perineural spread of head and neck malignancies. *Top Magn Reson Imaging.* 2004;15:79–85.
5. Vega F, Davila L, Delattre JY, et al. Experimental carcinomatous plexopathy. *J Neurol.* 1993;240:54–58.
6. Jessell T, Tsunoo A, Kanazawa I, et al. Substance P: depletion in the dorsal horn of rat spinal cord after section of the peripheral processes of primary sensory neurons. *Brain Res.* 1979;168:247–259.
7. Pomonis JD, Rogers SD, Peters CM, et al. Expression and localization of endothelin receptors: implications for the involvement of peripheral glia in nociception. *J Neurosci.* 2001;21:999–1006.
8. Asham EH, Loizidou M, Taylor I. Endothelin-1 and tumour development. *Eur J Surg Oncol.* 1998;24:57–60.
9. Mantyh PW, Clohisy DR, Koltzenburg M, et al. Molecular mechanisms of cancer pain. *Nat Rev Cancer.* 2002;2:201–209.
10. Julius D, Basbaum AI. Molecular mechanisms of nociception. *Nature.* 2001;413:203–210.
11. Clohisy DR, Mantyh PW. Bone cancer pain. *Clin Orthop Relat Res.* 2003:S279-88.
12. Mitchell BS, Schumacher U, Kaiserling E. Are tumours innervated? Immunohistological investigations using antibodies against the neuronal marker protein gene product 9.5 (PGP 9.5) in benign, malignant and experimental tumours. *Tumour Biol.* 1994;15:269–274.
13. Besson JM. The neurobiology of pain. *Lancet.* 1999;353:1610–1615.
14. Carr DB, Goudas LC. Acute pain. *Lancet.* 1999;353:2051–2058.
15. Glover J, Dibble SL, Dodd MJ, et al. Mood states of oncology outpatients: does pain make a difference? *J Pain Symptom Manage.* 1995;10:120–128.
16. Twycross R, Harcourt J, Bergl S. A survey of pain in patients with advanced cancer. *J Pain Symptom Manage.* 1996;12:273–282.
17. Vainio A, Auvinen A. Prevalence of symptoms among patients with advanced cancer: an international collaborative study. Symptom Prevalence Group. *J Pain Symptom Manage.* 1996;12:3–10.
18. Van den Beuken-van Everdingen MH, de Rijke JM, Kessels AG, et al. Prevalence of pain in patients with cancer: a systematic review of the past 40 years. *Ann Oncol.* 2007;18:1437–1449.
19. Grond S, Zech D, Diefenbach C, et al. Assessment of cancer pain: a prospective evaluation in 2266 cancer patients referred to a pain service. *Pain.* 1996;64:107–114.
20. Front D, Schneck SO, Frankel A, et al. Bone metastases and bone pain in breast cancer. Are they closely associated? *JAMA.* 1979;242:1747–1748.
21. Spiegel D, Bloom JR. Pain in metastatic breast cancer. *Cancer.* 1983;52:341–345.
22. Palmer E, Henrikson B, McKusick K, et al. Pain as an indicator of bone metastasis. *Acta Radiol.* 1988;29:445–449.
23. Talamo G, Angtuaco E, Walker RC, et al. Avascular necrosis of femoral and/or humeral heads in multiple myeloma: results of a prospective study of patients treated with dexamethasone-based regimens and high-dose chemotherapy. *J Clin Oncol.* 2005;23:5217–5223.
24. Taylor LJ. Multifocal avascular necrosis after short-term high-dose steroid therapy. A report of three cases. *J Bone Joint Surg Br.* 1984;66:431–433.
25. Chua KS, Reddy SK, Lee MC, et al. Pain and loss of function in head and neck cancer survivors. *J Pain Symptom Manage.* 1999;18:193–202.

26. Twycross R. Cancer pain classification. *Acta Anaesthesiol Scand.* 1997;41:141–145.
27. Harden RN, Bruehl SP, Gass S, et al. Signs and symptoms of the myofascial pain syndrome: a national survey of pain management providers. *Clin J Pain.* 2000;16:64–72.
28. Garrison JA, McCune JS, Livingston RB, et al. Myalgias and arthralgias associated with paclitaxel. *Oncology (Williston Park).* 2003;17:271–277;discussion 281–282, 286–288.
29. Rowinsky EK, Eisenhauer EA, Chaudhry V, et al. Clinical toxicities encountered with paclitaxel (Taxol). *Semin Oncol.* 1993;20:1–15.
30. Jimenez-Andrade JM, Peters CM, Mejia NA, et al. Sensory neurons and their supporting cells located in the trigeminal, thoracic and lumbar ganglia differentially express markers of injury following intravenous administration of paclitaxel in the rat. *Neurosci Lett.* 2006;405:62–67.
31. Peters CM, Jimenez-Andrade JM, Jonas BM, et al. Intravenous paclitaxel administration in the rat induces a peripheral sensory neuropathy characterized by macrophage infiltration and injury to sensory neurons and their supporting cells. *Exp Neurol.* 2007;203:42–54.
32. Melstrom LG, Melstrom KA, Jr., Ding XZ, et al. Mechanisms of skeletal muscle degradation and its therapy in cancer cachexia. *Histol Histopathol.* 2007;22:805–814.
33. Mense S. Nociception from skeletal muscle in relation to clinical muscle pain. *Pain.* 1993;54:241–289.
34. Schafers M, Sorkin LS, Sommer C. Intramuscular injection of tumor necrosis factor-alpha induces muscle hyperalgesia in rats. *Pain.* 2003;104:579–588.
35. Levin MI, Mozaffar T, Al-Lozi MT, et al. Paraneoplastic necrotizing myopathy: clinical and pathological features. *Neurology.* 1998;50:764–767.
36. Hasegawa T, Seki K, Yang P, et al. Mechanism of pain and cytoskeletal properties in angioleiomyomas: an immunohistochemical study. *Pathol Int.* 1994;44:66–72.
37. Price DD, Verne GN, Schwartz JM. Plasticity in brain processing and modulation of pain. *Prog Brain Res.* 2006;157:333–352.
38. Oshiro Y, Quevedo AS, McHaffie JG, et al. Brain mechanisms supporting spatial discrimination of pain. *J Neurosci.* 2007;27:3388–3394.
39. Chapman CR, Gavrin J. Suffering and its relationship to pain. *J Palliat Care.* 1993;9:5–13.
40. Wilson KG, Chochinov HM, McPherson CJ, et al. Suffering with advanced cancer. *J Clin Oncol.* 2007;25:1691–1697.
41. Turk DC, Sist TC, Okifuji A, et al. Adaptation to metastatic cancer pain, regional/local cancer pain and non-cancer pain: role of psychological and behavioral factors. *Pain.* 1998;74:247–256.
42. Turk DC, Fernandez E. On the putative uniqueness of cancer pain: do psychological principles apply? *Behav Res Ther.* 1990;28:1–13.
43. Potter VT, Wiseman CE, Dunn SM, et al. Patient barriers to optimal cancer pain control. *Psychooncology.* 2003;12:153–160.
44. Daut RL, Cleeland CS. The prevalence and severity of pain in cancer. *Cancer.* 1982;50:1913–1918.
45. Serlin RC, Mendoza TR, Nakamura Y, et al. When is cancer pain mild, moderate or severe? Grading pain severity by its interference with function. *Pain.* 1995;61:277–284.
46. Twycross RG, Fairfield S. Pain in far-advanced cancer. *Pain.* 1982;14:303–310.
47. Cleeland CS. The impact of pain on the patient with cancer. *Cancer.* 1984;54:2635–2641.
48. Loeser JD. Perspectives on pain. In: Clinical Pharmacology and Therapeutics. Turner P, ed. London: MacMillan, 1980:313–316.

CHAPTER 5 ■ ISSUES AFFECTING WELL-BEING IN CANCER PATIENTS

Cancer patients may experience a variety of symptoms as a result of their disease or its treatment. Common symptoms include fatigue, nausea, vomiting, pain, depression, and difficulty sleeping.[1] Although many cancer-related symptoms are the result of the disease, it has been increasingly recognized that neuropathy, fatigue, sleep disturbance, cognitive dysfunction, and affective symptoms can also be caused by cancer treatment.[2] Treatment-related symptoms may persist for extended periods and may even worsen, although the cancer itself is successfully treated.

Pain and symptom control are important components in comprehensive cancer care. Symptoms such as fatigue and sleep disturbances frequently occur together in patients who are receiving chemotherapy and radiation therapy.[3–4] In patients with advanced cancers, the primary cancer site strongly influences the development of symptom clusters. In a study of 1,366 cancer patients, Cheung et al.[3] noted that the most common primary cancer sites were gastrointestinal, lung, and breast and that the three most distressful symptoms were fatigue, poor general well-being, and decreased appetite.[3] Chow et al. found that anxiety and depression occurred together in patients with brain and bone metastases before and after palliative radiation therapy.[5–6]

Cancer patients frequently experience multiple symptoms that can independently predict changes in patient function, quality of life (QoL), treatment failures, and post-therapeutic outcomes.[7] Variance in QoL or functional outcomes is often determined by a set of symptoms.[8] Given et al.[9] demonstrated that pain and fatigue were independent and additive predictors of co-occurring symptoms. Patients with both pain and fatigue reported more symptoms overall than those who reported pain or fatigue alone or neither symptom. Symptom burden can be thought of as the sum of the severity and impact of symptoms reported by a significant proportion of patients with a given disease or treatment.[10] Studies investigating the multiplicity of symptoms experienced by cancer patients show that pain, fatigue, sleep disturbance, emotional distress, and poor appetite are almost universally found to be co-occurring.[11–13] These relatively nonspecific symptoms may not be monitored as closely as specific toxicities, and as a result, appropriate symptom management is often not addressed.[10]

Symptoms can vary independently. Symptom clusters may have different temporal patterns in response to treatment or disease progression.[14] Improvement in one symptom (eg, depression) may not correlate with improvement in another (eg, fatigue).[15] A National Institutes of Health statement on symptom management of pain, depression, and fatigue in cancer patients concluded that patients often were inadequately treated for these symptoms and that routine assessment should be mandatory.[16] Of course, we want all patients with cancer to experience optimal control of all symptoms from the time of diagnosis throughout the course of illness. Personal and cultural characteristics can sometimes make this goal problematic, but we believe that clinicians must make the effort to ameliorate all of the patient's symptoms as well as the underlying disease.

DEPRESSION IN CANCER PATIENTS

It is common for depressed patients to complain of a pervasive dysphoric mood, anhedonia, apathy and disinterest in normal activities, sleep problems, low energy, and, in severe cases, suicidal ideation. One fourth of all cancer patients meet criteria for major depressive syndrome at some point during their illness,[17] whereas the prevalence of depression in the patient population at large approximates 6% for outpatients and 11% for inpatients.[18–19] Craig and Abeloff[20] estimated an overall prevalence of depression at 53% for hospitalized cancer patients with varying primary sites and stages. Passik et al.[19] noted that depression is more associated with certain tumor types, such as pancreas and lung, than with others. The severity of depression has been correlated with pain, anxiety, disease type, and other health-related QoL issues.[21] Cancer pain, insomnia, fatigue, and depression and anxiety interact in complex ways; treatment plans must focus not only on the relief of specific symptoms to improve QoL but also on the impact of treatment on other symptoms. Depression seems to be more common with oropharyngeal (22% to 57%),[22] pancreatic (33% to 50%),[23] breast (1.5% to 46%),[24] and lung cancer patients (11% to 44%).[25–26] Significantly lower prevalence of depression has been reported in patients with colon (13% to 25%)[27] and gynecological (12% to 23%) cancers,[28–29] and lymphoma (8% to 19%).[30–31]

Depression has been described as an aggregation of mood disorders, as the evolving Diagnostic and Statistical Manual of Mental Disorders (DSM) classifications of the American Psychiatric Association indicate. To address the complexity of mood disorders, much of the classical thinking on depression attempted to force depressive syndromes (and patients) onto one or another continuum characterized by extremes at the poles.[32–33] Two common continua are reactive versus endogenous and neurotic versus psychotic depression. The various continua differ less than one might expect in basic characterizations of depression, and for our purposes, they are nearly equivalent. For simplicity, and because its language fits the cancer patient more readily, we describe the reactive–endogenous continuum that we use in our daily patient assessments.

Patients at the reactive pole usually link their depression to an event, a stressful situation, or a loss. In the cancer patient, the cancer diagnosis itself can serve as the precipitating event, as can the failure of an antineoplastic intervention, the loss of the ability to work, or mutilating and/or debilitating surgical procedures. Depressed cancer patients usually admit to anxiety, restlessness, irritability, problems falling asleep, and sometime to obsessional thinking or other obsessional problems. We have found that they will often not present depressive symptoms to their physician on the assumption that the physician is concerned only with the cancer itself. Those at the endogenous pole appear to develop depression without a precipitating cause. They tend to show marked slowing in motor responses, early-morning wakening with the most severe mood disturbance in the morning, weight loss, and feelings of hopelessness. One form of endogenous depression is bipolar mood disorder, in which patients shift between the extremes of depression and mania. A genetic predisposition for unipolar and bipolar depression clearly exists.[34] In such patients, the past history of depressive disorder is the best indicator of current endogenous depression. Most patients will fall between the polar extremes of reactive and endogenous depression.

DETECTING AND ASSESSING DEPRESSION IN THE CANCER PATIENT

Depression must be recognized and treated if the patient with pain from cancer is to be optimally managed (Table 5.1). If not identified and treated, depression has a significant negative impact on patient QoL, health care utilization,[22] and even disease outcome.[35]

Depression can be thought of as having two components: the psychological or "cognitive" component (eg, mood) and the physical or "somatic" component (eg, loss of appetite). All too often, depression goes unnoticed or unaddressed in the cancer patient.[36] Most physicians focus on somatic rather than psychological problems in patients with life-threatening illness, and some erroneously regard reactive depression in a patient who has received a diagnosis of cancer to be a normal response. Few oncologists or supporting consultants feel qualified to address depression, and for those who do, time limits on patient contact time make it difficult to engage in extensive questioning about psychological well-being. Patients and family members may add to the problem by assuming that care providers concern themselves solely with controlling the disease and wish to avoid the distractions that psychological management entails.

The symptom overlap between the psychiatric disorder, the toxicities of treatment, and the effects of the primary disease may render the diagnosis of depression difficult. Anxiety and depression may mimic physical symptoms of cancer or its treatments, and the emotional basis for distress can be overlooked. Chemotherapeutic agents (such as vincristine, vinblastine, L-asparaginase, procarbazine or cytoxin), biologic interventions such as interferon or interleukin, the antifungal agent amphotericin B, the toxic sequelae of whole-brain irradiation, and paraneoplastic syndromes can all lead to symptoms that resemble depression. Consequently, many of the physical symptoms of depression such as fatigue, diminished appetite, and weight loss also occur in emotionally healthy cancer patients.[37] In a study of the psychiatric morbidity among cancer patients, Alexander et al.[38] reported that psychiatric morbidity was less common in patients unaware of their cancer or in those who considered their treatment as curative. Aass et al.[39] noted that impaired social life, impaired professional work, and previous psychiatric problems were significantly correlated with depression, anxiety, physical function, fatigue, and pain in cancer patients. Depression, but not anxiety, increased in the presence of distant metastases, relapse, or progression and also increased when the diagnosis was made less than 1 month before assessment. They also found gender and age had no influence on the prevalence of depression. In a study of 148 postoperative breast cancer patients undergoing no active cancer treatment except hormones, Akechi et al.[40] found that biomedical factors (disease stage, performance status, and physical symptoms) were not significant determinants of psychiatric morbidity. In this study, family problems and coping responses were found to be more important.

It is widely known that depression exists in patients with cancer. The prevalence, however, varies widely by study and is often attributable to differences in assessment procedures.[41] Bukberg et al.[42] found that greater physical disability was associated with depression. The overall prevalence of depression was 42%, but a range of from 23% (in those with Karnofsky scores greater than 60) to 77% (in those with Karnofsky scores less than 40). Studies reporting the prevalence of depression in the terminally ill have ranged from 12.2% to 26%. Kadan-Lottick et al.[43] reported that 12% of patients with advanced cancer met criteria for a major psychiatric condition and 28% had accessed a mental health intervention for a psychiatric illness since the cancer diagnosis. Overall, these patients experienced major psychiatric disorders at a prevalence similar to the general population, but affected individuals have a

TABLE 5.1

DEPRESSION AND PAIN: IMPACTS ON CANCER PATIENTS

Component	Impact If Pain and Depression Present
Outcome and survival	Adversely affected
Recovery and compliance	Slower recovery and poorer compliance with health care and pain management
Medical evaluation and decision-making	Complicated
Pain	Pain can lead to reactive depression particularly in patients with life-threatening disease
Suffering	Augmented by serious disease, pain and depression
Suicide	Depression can lead to suicide

low rate of utilizing mental health services (services were not accessed by 55% of patients with major psychiatric disorders). In terminally ill cancer patients, the incidence of depression may be three times greater among patients who did not acknowledge their terminal prognosis.[44] Breitbart et al.[45] found a 17% prevalence of depression and a 17% prevalence for a desire for hastened death in a study of 92 terminally ill cancer patients. Chochinov et al.[46] noted that hopelessness significantly contributed to the prediction of suicidal ideation in terminally ill cancer patients even when the levels of depression were controlled.

Screening for depression should specifically address the cognitive/affective features, because these are not as readily confounded with treatment-associated toxicities. Several studies in palliative care patients have found that the single question "Are you depressed?" was the screening tool with the highest sensitivity and specificity and positive predictive value.[47-48] Cognitive/behavioral signs of depression include observable sadness, statements of pervasive despair, hopelessness or despondency, comments about being an unfair burden to others, expression of guilt or low self-esteem, and statements that life is and has been devoid of worth. Depressed patients also resist reassurances; for example, they tend to reject statements that a pain problem may not signal the progression of the disease. Depression has been studied in patients with cancer using a range of assessment methods. The methods (self-report, brief screening instruments, and structured clinical interviews) commonly used are the Hospital Anxiety and Depression Scale (HADS), Beck Depression Inventory (BDI), European Organization for Research and Treatment of Cancer Quality of Life Questionnaire, Patient Health Questionnaire (PHQ-9), and DSM-IV criteria. BDI is a 21-item test presented in multiple choice format designed to measure presence and degree of depression in adolescents and adults. Each of the 21 self-report items of the BDI attempts to assess a specific symptom or attitude that is specific for depressed patients. The BDI-II is a 1996 revision of the BDI.[49] Like the BDI, the BDI-II also contains 21 questions, and each answer is scored on a scale value of 0 to 3. The cutoffs used differ from the original: 0–13 represents minimal depression; 14–19 = mild depression; 20–28 = moderate depression; and 29–63 = severe depression. PHQ-9 contains a brief, nine-item patient self-report depression assessment specifically developed for use in primary care (Appendix J). The PHQ-9 has demonstrated usefulness as an assessment tool for the diagnosis of depression in primary care with acceptable reliability, validity, sensitivity, and specificity.[50] The nine items of the PHQ-9 come directly from the nine DSM-IV signs and symptoms of major depression. However, patients should not be diagnosed and treated solely on the basis of a PHQ-9 score, because differences in categorization of severity of depression exist between PHQ-9 and HADS.[51] Fann et al.[52] used a touch-screen version of the PHQ-9 as a screening tool to assess the prevalence and severity of depression in outpatients attending medical oncology, radiation oncology, and hematopoietic stem cell transplantation (HSCT) clinics. Among 342 patients enrolled, 33 (9.6%) at baseline (before oncologic care) and 69 (20.2%) at follow-up (during oncologic care, approximately 6 to 7 weeks later) triggered the full PHQ-9 by endorsing at least one cardinal symptom. Feasibility was high, with at least 97% completing the PHQ-2 and at least 96% completing the PHQ-9 when triggered with a mean completion time of about 2 minutes. Medical oncology patients had the highest percent of positive screens (12.9%) at baseline, whereas HSCT patients had the highest percent (30.5%) at follow-up. Using this method, 21 (6.1%) at baseline and 54 (15.8%) at follow-up of the total sample had moderate to severe depression.

In our practice, we routinely screen for depression by simply asking patients or their significant other the question "Are you depressed?" If the patient's response is affirmative, we routinely quantify the severity of depression and track treatment progress of depression using the Beck Depression Inventory. We believe that comprehensive cancer management must include diagnosis and treatment of depression.

CANCER-RELATED FATIGUE

Cancer-related fatigue (CRF) is a common, persistent, and subjective sense of tiredness related to cancer or to treatment for cancer that interferes with usual functioning.[53] Although fatigue is a common symptom during cancer treatment and in cancer survivors, it may also occur in patients before initiation of treatment.[54] It can also be a long-term (>5 years) problem in survivors.[55] Fatigue is a nonspecific symptom that may be found in association with most mental and physical disorders. By altering a person's ability to engage in meaningful personal, work, and social activities, CRF can have a major negative impact on QoL. Fatigue is frequently one of the initial symptoms experienced by patients, and tends to increase with the progression of cancer and cancer treatment. CRF differs from normal fatigue from overexertion or lack of sleep. In contrast to everyday or normal fatigue, CRF is characterized by feelings of tiredness and weakness despite adequate amounts of sleep and rest. In addition to the direct impact from cancer, various treatment modalities, particularly chemotherapy and radiation, are known to cause fatigue for many patients for an extended period of time.

It is estimated that fatigue is present at the time of diagnosis in approximately 50% of cancer patients.[56] It occurs in up to 75% of patients if bone metastases already are present. An estimated 60% to 96% of cancer patients in treatment experience fatigue, including 60% to 93% of patients on radiation therapy and 80% to 96% of patients on chemotherapy. Alexander et al.[57] reported on the prevalence of cancer-related fatigue syndrome in 300 disease-free breast cancer survivors. Diagnostic criteria were established in order to be considered a case of cancer-related fatigue. To fulfill these criteria, the subject must have experienced at least six of 11 fatigue-related symptoms on most days or every day for 2 weeks in the previous month. At least one of these symptoms must have been "significant fatigue, lack of energy, or an increased need to rest." The fatigue needs to be sufficiently severe to have had an impact on daily life. There must be evidence from the history, physical examination, or laboratory findings that the symptoms are a consequence of cancer or cancer therapy. Finally, the fatigue should not be "primarily a consequence of comorbid psychiatric disorders such as major depression, somatization disorder or delirium." The authors reported that fatigue occurred in 30% of women after breast cancer treatment and had significant effects on QoL and mood.

The pathogenesis of fatigue in patients with cancer is not well understood, but proposed mechanisms include the direct effects of cancer and the various modes of cancer treatment plus a wide variety of concomitant diseases (such as anemia, infections, dehydration, and electrolyte disorders), sleep disorders, chronic pain, immobility and lack of exercise, and a variety of psychosocial disorders.

Because of the high prevalence of anemia in oncology patients, the association of anemia with fatigue has been extensively studied. Sobrero et al.[58] reported that general scores for QoL, fatigue, and sensations of physical and functional well-being are significantly higher among patients with hemoglobin levels >12 g/dL.

Screening for fatigue is an important issue in the overall care of the oncology patient.[59] Criteria for screening for fatigue are listed in Table 5.2. Using these criteria, Cella et al.[60] assessed the prevalence of CRF in 379 patients who had been treated with chemotherapy, either alone or in combination with radiation therapy. Most of these patients had completed treatment more than 1 year previously. The prevalence in this study was 17%. At least 14 scales have been used to assess for fatigue.[61] Some of these include the Profile of Mood States (POMS) Fatigue subscale,[62] Functional Assessment Cancer Therapy Fatigue Subscale,[63] and Brief Fatigue Inventory.[64]

Once fatigue is identified, a detailed clinical evaluation should be performed. In addition to tiredness, patients may complain of lethargy, weariness, and physical and mental exhaustion (eg, loss of attention and concentration). It may also be described as a lack of energy, vigor, or vitality. Components of the evaluation should include details of the cancer including the type and duration of the treatment and its capacity to induce fatigue. Other components include documenting the characteristics of the fatigue such as when it started, what factors aggravate it, and so on. Emotional and psychological components should be identified, and the effect of the fatigue on the performance of normal, daily life activities should be determined. Then, various clinical organic conditions that can cause fatigue should be evaluated.

If a specific cause of CRF is identified (anemia, insomnia, depression, metabolic disorders, etc.), this should be treated first. Antidepressants and analgesics should be prescribed for patients with depression and pain. After common causes of anemia have been excluded, patients with low levels of hemoglobin should receive treatment with erythropoietic agents. Patients with sleep disorders should receive appropriate instructions for improving sleep quality or carefully prescribed drugs. Various nonpharmacologic interventions to ameliorate CRF have been suggested, including psychosocial interventions (eg, cognitive-behavioral therapy), complementary and alternative therapies (eg, massage), and physical exercise interventions (eg, aerobics). Exercise should be regarded as beneficial for individuals with CRF during and after cancer therapy.[65] Moderate exercise can be more effective than continuous rest.[66] Aerobic exercises can increase overall muscle tone, and it may be wiser to advise such exercise than rest.[67] Educating patients about fatigue is also extremely useful.[68] Kangas et al.[69] provide a comprehensive review of nonpharmacologic therapies for cancer-related fatigue.

There is no agreement on the best pharmacologic treatment for CRF. There is little evidence that methylphenidate is effective, although hematopoietic agents (erythropoietin, darbepoietin) appear to relieve fatigue associated with chemotherapy-induced anemia.[70] Antidepressant studies have shown mixed results.[71] Paroxetine seems to show benefit for fatigue primarily when it is a symptom of clinical depression. Bupropion, a norepinephrine/dopamine reuptake inhibitor, may have psychostimulant-like effects, and therefore may be more beneficial for treating fatigue. Modafinil has been used to treat fatigue associated with neurodegenerative disorders such as multiple sclerosis[72] and amyotrophic lateral sclerosis.[73] It is now being increasingly used for cancer-related symptoms targeted by psychostimulants. Preliminary evidence suggests that modafinil is efficacious in improving opioid-induced sedation, cancer-related fatigue, and depression.[74]

In our practice, we screen for fatigue issues in patient self-reporting in the Functional Assessment of Cancer Therapy-General (FACT-G) QoL survey. If fatigue is present, this will usually prompt a thorough investigation of the cause or causes of fatigue. In cancer survivors, if the symptom produces significant functional impairment and

TABLE 5.2

CRITERIA FOR CANCER-RELATED FATIGUE

Six (or more) of the following symptoms have been present every day or nearly every day during the same 2-week period in the past month, and at least one of the symptoms is *A1*, significant fatigue.
- A1. Significant fatigue, diminished energy, or increased need to rest, disproportionate to any recent change in activity level
- A2. Complaints of generalized weakness or limb heaviness
- A3. Diminished concentration or attention
- A4. Decreased motivation or interest to engage in usual activities
- A5. Insomnia or hypersomnia
- A6. Experience of sleep as unrefreshing or nonrestorative
- A7. Perceived need to struggle to overcome inactivity
- A8. Marked emotional reactivity (eg, sadness, frustration, or irritability) to feeling fatigued
- A9. Difficulty completing daily tasks attributed to feeling fatigued
- A10. Perceived problems with short-term memory
- A11. Postexertional malaise lasting several hours
- AND B. The symptoms cause clinically significant distress or impairment in social, occupational, or other important areas of functioning
- AND C. There is evidence from the history, physical examination, or laboratory findings that the symptoms are a consequence of cancer or cancer therapy
- AND D. The symptoms are not primarily a consequence of comorbid psychiatric disorders such as major depression, somatization disorder, somatoform disorder, or delirium

(Reprinted with permission from Cella D, Peterman A, Passik K, et al. Progress toward guidelines for the management of fatigue. *Oncology*. 1998;12(11A):369–377.)

the underlying cause(s) is or are correctable, we usually advocate a combination of supervised exercise therapy with low doses of modafinil.

CANCER CACHEXIA

Cancer cachexia occurs in the terminal phase of a malignancy and is associated with more than 20% of cancer deaths.[75] Cachexia is among the most debilitating and life-threatening aspects of cancer. Anorexia, involuntary weight loss, tissue wasting, poor performance, and ultimately death characterize cancer cachexia. In more than 20% of cancer patients, cachexia is the main cause of death.[76] The characteristic clinical picture of anorexia, tissue wasting, loss of body weight accompanied by a decrease in muscle mass and adipose tissue, and poor performance status that often precedes death has been named cancer-related anorexia/cachexia syndrome. In advanced cachexia, patients may demonstrate severe weight loss, anorexia, early satiety, weakness, anemia, and edema. Although anorexia frequently accompanies cachexia, the decrease in caloric intake alone cannot account for the body-composition changes seen in cachexia. Moreover, cachexia can occur even in the absence of anorexia.

Patients with hematological malignancies and breast cancer seldom have substantial weight loss, whereas most other solid tumors are associated with a higher frequency of cachexia. The highest prevalence of weight loss is seen amongst patients with solid tumors, eg, gastric, pancreatic, lung, colorectal, and head and neck.[77] Patients with upper gastrointestinal cancer are especially likely to suffer from substantial weight loss, and patients with pancreatic cancer have the highest frequency of developing a cachectic syndrome. In patients with pancreatic cancer, 80% of patients have at least 10% weight loss at diagnosis and the cachexia syndrome is present in 25%.[78] In a study of patients with advanced pancreatic cancer, Fearon et al.[78] identified weight loss (greater than 10%), evidence of systemic inflammation (defined by C-reactive protein greater than 10 mg/mL), and reduced food intake (less than 1500 kcal/day) as key features that impacted patients' function and survival.

Cachexia occurs as a result of a functional inability to ingest or use nutrients. It may be classified as primary and secondary. Primary cachexia occurs as a result of tumor-induced metabolic changes, whereas secondary cachexia is caused by factors that compromise dietary intake leading to malnutrition (eg, treatment-related toxicity such as nausea and vomiting, mechanical obstruction or malabsorption, and surgical interventions). Cachexia is a complex metabolic state with progressive weight loss and depletion of host reserves of adipose tissue and skeletal muscle. Cachexia should be suspected if involuntary weight loss of greater than 5% of premorbid weight occurs within a 6-month period.[79] Cachexia represents the clinical consequence of a chronic, systemic inflammatory response, with high hepatic synthesis of acute-phase proteins resulting in depletion of essential amino acids. This contrasts with starvation, when only fat metabolism is increased while the body tries to conserve lean body mass. Cachexia is a progressive wasting syndrome characterized by extensive loss of adipose tissue and skeletal muscle.

Loss of fat-free mass involves only skeletal muscle and not visceral protein reserves. In anorexia nervosa, depletion of adipose tissue exceeds that of lean body mass, whereas in cancer cachexia there is approximately equal loss from both compartments.[80] Furthermore, when a reduction in lean body mass eventually occurs during starvation, there is loss of visceral mass in proportion to loss of muscle mass, whereas in cachexia there is selective loss of skeletal muscle, with no change in the visceral protein compartment, even when the total weight loss reaches 30%.[81]

Cachexia has a detrimental effect on many aspects of a patient's QoL. Cachectic patients are likely to report decreased QoL scores, decreased levels of physical performance, increased risks of treatment failure, increased risks of treatment side effects, and an increased mortality rate.[77-78] Weight loss is a significant predictor of decreased survival in oncologic patients.[82] Weight loss and malnutrition are associated with poorer treatment tolerance and outcomes,[83] and poorer QoL.[84] Malnourished patients undergoing chemotherapy have a poor response to chemotherapy,[85-86] a reduced QoL,[83] and a higher rate of hospital readmission with a longer duration of hospital stay.[87]

Cancer cachexia is characterized by numerous metabolic abnormalities including inefficient substrate utilization, alterations in the balance of energy intake and expenditure, and the acute-phase protein response. These changes appear to be driven by proinflammatory cytokines, alterations of the neuroendocrine axis, and tumor-derived catabolic factors. These result in the loss of both fat and lean tissue. Tumor mechanisms in cachexia include the local secretion of proinflammatory cytokines that initiate the host systemic inflammatory response,[88] and the production of procachectic factors that have direct catabolic effects on host tissues (eg, proteolysis-inducing factor,[89] lipid mobilizing factor).[90] Mediators of cachexia also include hormones (eg, leptin), neuropeptides (eg, neuropeptide Y, melanocortin, melanin-concentrating hormone, orexin) and cytokines (eg, interleukin 1, interleukin 6, tumor necrosis factor a, interferon).[91] Host mechanisms involve an aberrant response to the tumor's presence, and include activation of both the systemic inflammatory response[88] and the neuroendocrine stress response.[92,93] The relative importance of different tumor and host mechanisms in the genesis of cachexia in individual patients and tumor types is unclear.

Treatment of primary cachexia has focused on nutritional supplements and the use of a variety of pharmacological agents (Fig 5.1). Pharmacologic agents include central-acting appetite stimulants, agents that interfere with the metabolic mediations that influence the cytokine response (thalidomide, corticosteroids), tumor-related factors (eicosapentaenoic acid [EPA]), fat metabolism (leptin, progestational drugs), and muscle tissue (steroid and nonsteroidal anabolics). Trials of conventional nutritional supplements in patients with cancer cachexia have failed to show any benefit in terms of weight gain or QoL.[94] Corticosteroids may improve the sensation of well-being and led to increased food intake, but this effect appears to be short-lived (only a few weeks).[95] Progestogens such as megestrol acetate and medroxyprogesterone acetate have also been used with limited effectiveness. The mechanism by which megestrol increases appetite is unknown. Berenstein and Ortiz[96] reviewed the efficacy and safety of

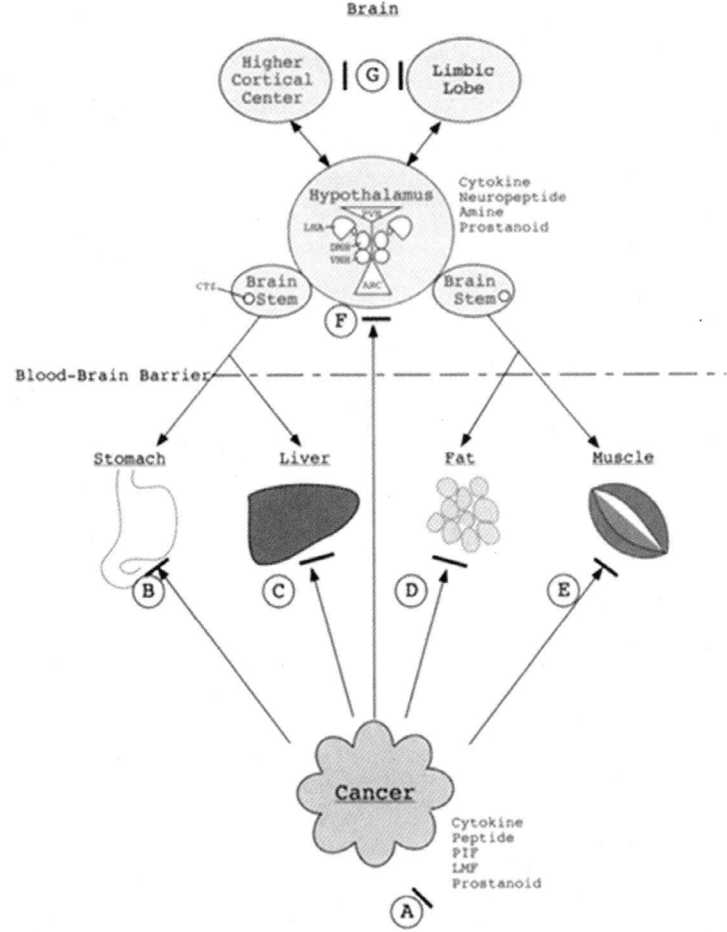

FIGURE 5.1 Pharmacological modalities for management of cancer anorexia-cachexia syndrome. Agents are classified as those established (first-line) or those unproven/investigational (second-line), depending on their site or mechanisms of action. (A) inhibitors of production/release of cytokines and other factors; (B) gastroprokinetic agents with or without antinausea effect; (C) blockers of Cori cycle; (D) (E) blockers of fat and muscle tissue wasting, respectively; (F) appetite stimulants with or without antinausea effect; (G) antianxiety/depressant drugs. First-line treatments: Glucocorticoids (F) (A); Progesterones (F) (A). Second-line treatments: Cannabinoids (F); Thalidomide (A); Cyproheptadine (F); β_2-adrenoceptor agonists (E); Branched-chain amino acids (E) (F); Nonsteroidal anti-inflammatory drugs (A) (F); Metoclopramide (B) (F); Others; Eicosapentaenoic acid (D) (E) (A); Anabolic steroids (E); 5'-deoxy-5-fluorouridine (A); Pentoxifylline (A); Melatonin (A); Hydrazine sulfate (C). These agents should be selected on an individual basis according to the cause of cachexia or the state of the patient. ARC, Arcuate nucleus of the hypothalamus; VMH, ventromedial nucleus of the hypothalamus; DMH, dorsomedial nucleus of the hypothalamus; LHA, lateral hypothalamic area; PVN, paraventricular nucleus of the hypothalamus; CTZ, chemoreceptor trigger zone; PIF, proteolysis-inducing factor; LMF, lipid mobilizing factor. (From Inui, A. Cancer Anorexia-cachexia syndrome: current issues in research and management. CA Cancer J Clin, 2002;52(2):72–91. Copyright 2002, American Cancer Society Reprinted with permission of John Wiley & Sons, Inc.)

megestrol in palliating anorexia-cachexia syndrome in patients with cancer, AIDS, and other underlying pathologies and concluded that megestrol improves appetite and weight gain in patients with cancer. Megestrol is typically prescribed in doses of 480 to 800 mg/day. Side effects include an increased risk of pulmonary embolism. EPA and docosahexaenoic acid (DHA) are added as liquid supplements to diets. However, Mazzotta et al.[97] noted no significant benefit of the effects of EPA and DHA on weight change, lean muscle mass change, survival, and QoL in cancer-associated anorexia-cachexia syndrome. Appetite stimulation and body weight gain may result from the use of marijuana and its derivatives.[98]

Evolving research is improving our understanding of the complex mechanisms associated with cancer cachexia. Treatment of this debilitating condition is limited and development of early and effective interventions aimed at preventing and reversing cachexia are required. Of concern to the clinician managing pain in the anorexic-cachectic cancer patient is the unpredictable pharmacology of opioids.[99] Advanced cachexia may impact the absorption of transdermal fentanyl, although studies are lacking.

References

1. Barsevick AM, Whitmer K, Nail LM, et al. Symptom cluster research: Conceptual, design, measurement, and analysis issues. *J Pain Symptom Manage.* 2006;31:85–95.
2. Cleeland CS, Bennett GJ, Dantzer R, et al. Are the symptoms of cancer and cancer treatment due to a shared biologic mechanism? A cytokine-immunologic model of cancer symptoms. *Cancer.* 2003;97:2919–2925.
3. Cheung WY, Le LW, Zimmermann C. Symptom clusters in patients with advanced cancers. *Support Care Cancer.* 2009.
4. Miaskowski C, Aouizerat BE, Dodd M, et al. Conceptual issues in symptom clusters research and their implications for quality-of-life assessment in patients with cancer. *J Natl Cancer Inst Monogr.* 2007:39–46.
5. Chow E, Fan G, Hadi S, et al. Symptom clusters in cancer patients with bone metastases. *Support Care Cancer.* 2007;15:1035–1043.
6. Chow E, Fan G, Hadi S, et al. Symptom clusters in cancer patients with brain metastases. *Clin Oncol (R Coll Radiol).* 2008;20:76–82.
7. Fan G, Filipczak L, Chow E. Symptom clusters in cancer patients: A review of the literature. *Curr Oncol.* 2007;14:173–179.
8. Gaston-Johansson F, Fall-Dickson JM, Bakos AB, et al. Fatigue, pain, and depression in pre-autotransplant breast cancer patients. *Cancer Pract.* 1999;7:240–247.
9. Given CW, Given B, Azzouz F, et al. Predictors of pain and fatigue in the year following diagnosis among elderly cancer patients. *J Pain Symptom Manage.* 2001;21:456–466.
10. Cleeland CS. Symptom burden: Multiple symptoms and their impact as patient-reported outcomes. *J Natl Cancer Inst Monogr.* 2007:16–21.
11. Cleeland CS, Mendoza TR, Wang XS, et al. Assessing symptom distress in cancer patients: The M.D. Anderson Symptom Inventory. *Cancer.* 2000;89:1634–1646.
12. Donnelly S, Walsh D, Rybicki L. The symptoms of advanced cancer: Identification of clinical and research priorities by assessment of prevalence and severity. *J Palliat Care.* 1995;11:27–32.
13. Grond S, Zech D, Diefenbach C, et al. Prevalence and pattern of symptoms in patients with cancer pain: A prospective evaluation of 1635 cancer patients referred to a pain clinic. *J Pain Symptom Manage.* 1994;9:372–382.
14. Wang XS, Fairclough DL, Liao Z, et al. Longitudinal study of the relationship between chemoradiation therapy for non-small-cell lung cancer and patient symptoms. *J Clin Oncol.* 2006;24:4485–4491.

15. Morrow GR, Hickok JT, Roscoe JA, et al. Differential effects of paroxetine on fatigue and depression: A randomized, double-blind trial from the University of Rochester Cancer Center Community Clinical Oncology Program. *J Clin Oncol.* 2003;21:4635–4641.
16. Program N. NIH State-of-the-Science Statement on symptom management in cancer: Pain, depression, and fatigue. *NIH Consens State Sci Statements.* 2002;19:1–29.
17. Breitbart W. Psychiatric management of cancer pain. *Cancer.* 1989;63:2336–2342.
18. Katon W, Sullivan MD. Depression and chronic medical illness. *J Clin Psychiatry.* 1990;51 Suppl:3-11.
19. Passik SD, Breitbart WS. Depression in patients with pancreatic carcinoma. Diagnostic and treatment issues. *Cancer.* 1996;78:615–626.
20. Craig TJ, Abeloff MD. Psychiatric symptomatology among hospitalized cancer patients. *Am J Psychiatry.* 1974;131:1323–1327.
21. Ell K, Sanchez K, Vourlekis B, et al. Depression, correlates of depression, and receipt of depression care among low-income women with breast or gynecologic cancer. *J Clin Oncol.* 2005;23:3052–3060.
22. Davies AD, Davies C, Delpo MC. Depression and anxiety in patients undergoing diagnostic investigations for head and neck cancers. *Br J Psychiatry.* 1986;149:491–493.
23. Joffe RT, Rubinow DR, Denicoff KD, et al. Depression and carcinoma of the pancreas. *Gen Hosp Psychiatry.* 1986;8:241–245.
24. Sachs G, Rasoul-Rockenschaub S, Aschauer H, et al. Lytic effector cell activity and major depressive disorder in patients with breast cancer: A prospective study. *J Neuroimmunol.* 1995;59:83–89.
25. Buccheri G. Depressive reactions to lung cancer are common and often followed by a poor outcome. *Eur Respir J.* 1998;11:173–178.
26. Montazeri A, Milroy R, Hole D, et al. Anxiety and depression in patients with lung cancer before and after diagnosis: Findings from a population in Glasgow, Scotland. *J Epidemiol Community Health.* 1998;52:203–204.
27. Fras I, Litin EM, Pearson JS. Comparison of psychiatric symptoms in carcinoma of the pancreas with those in some other intra-abdominal neoplasms. *Am J Psychiatry.* 1967;123:1553–1562.
28. Evans DL, McCartney CF, Nemeroff CB, et al. Depression in women treated for gynecological cancer: Clinical and neuroendocrine assessment. *Am J Psychiatry.* 1986;143:447–452.
29. Golden RN, McCartney CF, Haggerty JJ Jr, et al. The detection of depression by patient self-report in women with gynecologic cancer. *Int J Psychiatry Med.* 1991;21:17–27.
30. Devlen J, Maguire P, Phillips P, et al. Psychological problems associated with diagnosis and treatment of lymphomas. II: Prospective study. *Br Med J (Clin Res Ed).* 1987;295:955–957.
31. Devlen J, Maguire P, Phillips P, et al. Psychological problems associated with diagnosis and treatment of lymphomas. I: Retrospective study. *Br Med J (Clin Res Ed).* 1987;295:953–954.
32. Gray JA. *The neuropsychology of anxiety.* New York: Oxford University Press, 1982.
33. Gray JA. *The psychology of fear and stress,* 2nd ed. New York: Cambridge University Press, 1987.
34. Kandel ER. Disorders of mood: Depression, mania, and anxiety disorders. In: Kandel ER, Schwartz JH, Jessell TM, eds. *Principles of neural science,* 3rd ed. New York: Elsevier, 1991:869–886.
35. Spiegel D, Giese-Davis J. Depression and cancer: Mechanisms and disease progression. *Biol Psychiatry.* 2003;54:269–282.
36. Passik SD, Dugan W, McDonald MV, et al. Oncologists' recognition of depression in their patients with cancer. *J Clin Oncol.* 1998;16:1594–1600.
37. Endicott J. Measurement of depression in patients with cancer. *Cancer.* 1984;53:2243–2249.
38. Alexander PJ, Dinesh N, Vidyasagar MS. Psychiatric morbidity among cancer patients and its relationship with awareness of illness and expectations about treatment outcome. *Acta Oncol.* 1993;32:623–626.
39. Aass N, Fossa SD, Dahl AA, et al. Prevalence of anxiety and depression in cancer patients seen at the Norwegian Radium Hospital. *Eur J Cancer.* 1997;33:1597–1604.
40. Akechi T, Okuyama T, Imoto S, et al. Biomedical and psychosocial determinants of psychiatric morbidity among postoperative ambulatory breast cancer patients. *Breast Cancer Res Treat.* 2001;65:195–202.
41. Trask PC. Assessment of depression in cancer patients. *J Natl Cancer Inst Monogr.* 2004:80–92.
42. Bukberg J, Penman D, Holland JC. Depression in hospitalized cancer patients. *Psychosom Med.* 1984;46:199–212.
43. Kadan-Lottick NS, Vanderwerker LC, Block SD, et al. Psychiatric disorders and mental health service use in patients with advanced cancer: A report from the coping with cancer study. *Cancer.* 2005;104:2872–2881.
44. Chochinov HM, Tataryn DJ, Wilson KG, et al. Prognostic awareness and the terminally ill. *Psychosomatics.* 2000;41:500–504.
45. Breitbart W, Rosenfeld B, Pessin H, et al. Depression, hopelessness, and desire for hastened death in terminally ill patients with cancer. *JAMA.* 2000;284:2907–2911.
46. Chochinov HM, Wilson KG, Enns M, et al. Depression, Hopelessness, and suicidal ideation in the terminally ill. *Psychosomatics.* 1998;39:366–370.
47. Chochinov HM, Wilson KG, Enns M, et al. "Are you depressed?" Screening for depression in the terminally ill. *Am J Psychiatry.* 1997;154:674–676.
48. Lloyd-Williams M, Spiller J, Ward J. Which depression screening tools should be used in palliative care? *Palliat Med.* 2003;17:40–43.
49. Beck AT, Steer RA, Ball R, et al. Comparison of Beck Depression Inventories -IA and -II in psychiatric outpatients. *J Pers Assess.* 1996;67:588–597.
50. Kroenke K, Spitzer RL, Williams JB. The PHQ-9: Validity of a brief depression severity measure. *J Gen Intern Med.* 2001;16:606–613.
51. Cameron IM, Crawford JR, Lawton K, et al. Psychometric comparison of PHQ-9 and HADS for measuring depression severity in primary care. *Br J Gen Pract.* 2008;58:32–36.
52. Fann JR, Thomas-Rich AM, Katon WJ, et al. Major depression after breast cancer: A review of epidemiology and treatment. *Gen Hosp Psychiatry.* 2008;30:112–126.
53. Mock V, Atkinson A, Barsevick A, et al. NCCN Practice guidelines for cancer-related fatigue. *Oncology (Williston Park).* 2000;14:151–161.
54. Parsons CG, Danysz W, Quack G. Memantine is a clinically well tolerated N-methyl-D-aspartate (NMDA) receptor antagonist—a review of preclinical data. *Neuropharmacology.* 1999;38:735–767.
55. Bower JE, Ganz PA, Desmond KA, et al. Fatigue in long-term breast carcinoma survivors: A longitudinal investigation. *Cancer.* 2006;106:751–758.
56. Goedendorp MM, Gielissen MF, Verhagen CA, et al. Severe fatigue and related factors in cancer patients before the initiation of treatment. *Br J Cancer.* 2008;99:1408–1414.
57. Stasi R, Abriani L, Beccaglia P, et al. Cancer-related fatigue: Evolving concepts in evaluation and treatment. *Cancer.* 2003;98:1786–1801.
58. Alexander S, Minton O, Andrews P, et al. A comparison of the characteristics of disease-free breast cancer survivors with or without cancer-related fatigue syndrome. *Eur J Cancer.* 2009;45:384–392.
59. Sobrero A, Puglisi F, Guglielmi A, et al. Fatigue: A main component of anemia symptomatology. *Semin Oncol.* 2001;28:15–18.
60. Stone P, Richardson A, Ream E, et al. Cancer-related fatigue: Inevitable, unimportant and untreatable? Results of a multi-centre patient survey. Cancer Fatigue Forum. *Ann Oncol.* 2000;11:971–975.
61. Cella D, Davis K, Breitbart W, et al. Cancer-related fatigue: Prevalence of proposed diagnostic criteria in a United States sample of cancer survivors. *J Clin Oncol.* 2001;19:3385–3391.
62. Minton O, Stone P, Richardson A, et al. Drug therapy for the management of cancer related fatigue. *Cochrane Database Syst Rev.* 2008:CD006704.
63. Van Hooff ML, Geurts SA, Kompier MA, et al. "How fatigued do you currently feel?" Convergent and discriminant validity of a single-item fatigue measure. *J Occup Health.* 2007;49:224–234.
64. Yellen SB, Cella DF, Webster K, et al. Measuring fatigue and other anemia-related symptoms with the Functional Assessment of Cancer Therapy (FACT) measurement system. *J Pain Symptom Manage.* 1997;13:63–74.
65. Mendoza TR, Wang XS, Cleeland CS, et al. The rapid assessment of fatigue severity in cancer patients: Use of the Brief Fatigue Inventory. *Cancer.* 1999;85:1186–1196.
66. Cramp F, Daniel J. Exercise for the management of cancer-related fatigue in adults. *Cochrane Database Syst Rev.* 2008:CD006145.
67. Schmitz KH, Holtzman J, Courneya KS, et al. Controlled physical activity trials in cancer survivors: A systematic review and meta-analysis. *Cancer Epidemiol Biomarkers Prev.* 2005;14:1588–1595.
68. Knols R, Aaronson NK, Uebelhart D, et al. Physical exercise in cancer patients during and after medical treatment: A systematic review of randomized and controlled clinical trials. *J Clin Oncol.* 2005;23:3830–3842.

69. Wilkie DJ, Huang HY, Berry DL, et al. Cancer symptom control: Feasibility of a tailored, interactive computerized program for patients. *Fam Community Health*. 2001;24:48–62.
70. Kangas M, Bovbjerg DH, Montgomery GH. Cancer-related fatigue: A systematic and meta-analytic review of non-pharmacological therapies for cancer patients. *Psychol Bull*. 2008;134:700–741.
71. Breitbart W, Alici-Evcimen Y. Update on psychotropic medications for cancer-related fatigue. *J Natl Compr Canc Netw*. 2007;5:1081–1091.
72. Zifko UA, Rupp M, Schwarz S, et al. Modafinil in treatment of fatigue in multiple sclerosis. Results of an open-label study. *J Neurol*. 2002;249:983–987.
73. Lou JS. Fatigue in amyotrophic lateral sclerosis. *Phys Med Rehabil Clin N Am*. 2008;19:533–543, ix.
74. Prommer E. Modafinil: Is it ready for prime time? *J Opioid Manag*. 2006;2:130–136.
75. Tisdale MJ. Cachexia in cancer patients. *Nat Rev Cancer*. 2002;2:862–871.
76. Bruera E. ABC of palliative care. Anorexia, cachexia, and nutrition. *BMJ*. 1997;315:1219–1222.
77. Dewys WD, Begg C, Lavin PT, et al. Prognostic effect of weight loss prior to chemotherapy in cancer patients. Eastern Cooperative Oncology Group. *Am J Med*. 1980;69:491–497.
78. Fearon KC, Voss AC, Hustead DS. Definition of cancer cachexia: Effect of weight loss, reduced food intake, and systemic inflammation on functional status and prognosis. *Am J Clin Nutr*. 2006;83:1345–1350.
79. Inui A. Cancer anorexia-cachexia syndrome: Current issues in research and management. *CA Cancer J Clin*. 2002;52:72–91.
80. Tisdale MJ. Pathogenesis of cancer cachexia. *J Support Oncol*. 2003;1:159–168.
81. Fearon KC. The Sir David Cuthbertson Medal Lecture 1991. The mechanisms and treatment of weight loss in cancer. *Proc Nutr Soc*. 1992;51:251–265.
82. Bozzetti F. Screening the nutritional status in oncology: A preliminary report on 1,000 outpatients. *Support Care Cancer*. 2009;17:279–284.
83. Andreyev HJ, Norman AR, Oates J, et al. Why do patients with weight loss have a worse outcome when undergoing chemotherapy for gastrointestinal malignancies? *Eur J Cancer*. 1998;34:503–509.
84. O'Gorman P, McMillan DC, McArdle CS. Impact of weight loss, appetite, and the inflammatory response on quality of life in gastrointestinal cancer patients. *Nutr Cancer*. 1998;32:76–80.
85. Persson C, Glimelius B. The relevance of weight loss for survival and quality of life in patients with advanced gastrointestinal cancer treated with palliative chemotherapy. *Anticancer Res*. 2002;22:3661–3668.
86. Ross PJ, Ashley S, Norton A, et al. Do patients with weight loss have a worse outcome when undergoing chemotherapy for lung cancers? *Br J Cancer*. 2004;90:1905–1911.
87. Correia MI, Waitzberg DL. The impact of malnutrition on morbidity, mortality, length of hospital stay and costs evaluated through a multivariate model analysis. *Clin Nutr*. 2003;22:235–239.
88. Deans DA, Wigmore SJ, Gilmour H, et al. Elevated tumour interleukin-1beta is associated with systemic inflammation: A marker of reduced survival in gastro-oesophageal cancer. *Br J Cancer*. 2006;95:1568–1575.
89. Todorov P, Cariuk P, McDevitt T, et al. Characterization of a cancer cachectic factor. *Nature*. 1996;379:739–742.
90. Hirai K, Hussey HJ, Barber MD, et al. Biological evaluation of a lipid-mobilizing factor isolated from the urine of cancer patients. *Cancer Res*. 1998;58:2359–2365.
91. Ramos EJ, Suzuki S, Marks D, et al. Cancer anorexia-cachexia syndrome: Cytokines and neuropeptides. *Curr Opin Clin Nutr Metab Care*. 2004;7:427–434.
92. Barber MD, McMillan DC, Wallace AM, et al. The response of leptin, interleukin-6 and fat oxidation to feeding in weight-losing patients with pancreatic cancer. *Br J Cancer*. 2004;90:1129–1132.
93. Costelli P, Muscaritoli M, Bossola M, et al. IGF-1 is downregulated in experimental cancer cachexia. *Am J Physiol Regul Integr Comp Physiol*. 2006;291:R674-83.
94. Barber MD, Ross JA, Fearon KC. Cancer cachexia. *Surg Oncol*. 1999;8:133–141.
95. Tisdale MJ. Biology of cachexia. *J Natl Cancer Inst*. 1997;89:1763–1773.
96. Berenstein EG, Ortiz Z. Megestrol acetate for the treatment of anorexia-cachexia syndrome. *Cochrane Database Syst Rev*. 2005:CD004310.
97. Mazzotta P, Jeney CM. Anorexia-cachexia syndrome: A systematic review of the role of dietary polyunsaturated fatty acids in the management of symptoms, survival, and quality of life. *J Pain Symptom Manage*. 2008.
98. Martin BR, Wiley JL. Mechanism of action of cannabinoids: How it may lead to treatment of cachexia, emesis, and pain. *J Support Oncol*. 2004;2:305–314;discussion 314–316.
99. Balducci L, Extermann M. Management of the frail person with advanced cancer. *Crit Rev Oncol Hematol*. 2000;33:143–148.

CHAPTER 6 ■ CHARACTERISTICS OF CANCER PAIN

It is useful to develop a scheme for the classification of cancer-related pain. One example of such a scheme is presented in Table 6.1.

CHRONICITY

Acute pain is known to occur during and after certain diagnostic procedures and various anticancer therapies, particularly postoperative pain following surgical intervention,[1] pain during chemotherapy,[2] or radiation therapy[3] (Table 6.2). The course of acute pain is usually predictable and self-limiting, and the diagnosis of acute pain rarely is difficult. On the other hand, the assessment of patients with chronic pain tends to be much more difficult and complex. Onset of pain in these patients is often insidious, the precipitating factor less clear, and the course is prolonged and variable.

INTENSITY AND SEVERITY

It is common for health care workers to underestimate the severity of a patient's pain,[4,5] particularly when relying exclusively on their own observations. This is problematic, because pain is often undertreated when patients and physicians differ in their judgment of the pain's severity.[6] Although both severity and the degree of interference with function are crucial to the adequate assessment of pain, severity is the primary factor determining the impact of pain on the patient, and it drives the urgency and energy of the treatment process.[7] Thus, the consistent measurement of pain intensity helps assess patients' progress, provides outcome measures for research purposes, and should guide therapy.[8]

Patient self-report should always be the primary source of information for the measurement of pain-related issues. Observer ratings of symptom severity correlate poorly with patient ratings and are usually inadequate substitutes for patient reporting. Grossman et al.[4] found a low correlation between patients' visual analog scores for pain and those of health care providers. The discrepancies were most pronounced in those patients reporting severe pain. Although one can monitor some objective signs to clarify the manifestations and impact of certain symptoms, these signs only complement subjective assessment.

An assessment of pain intensity should include an evaluation of not only the present pain intensity but also pain at its least and worst. For research purposes, a variety of instruments are used to assess pain intensity. These instruments measure pain intensity alone, or in combination with different pain dimensions combined into a single composite score. Examples of these different dimensions include pain interference, pain affect, pain quality, and multidimension composite measures.[9] Pain interference refers to the extent to which pain interferes with important activities such as mood, sleep, and interaction with others. The most common measure of pain interference in cancer pain research is the interference scale of the Brief Pain Inventory. Examples of single rating scales include the visual analog scale, numeric rating scale, verbal rating scale, graphic rating scale, faces scale, and mechanical visual analog scale (Fig. 6-1). Typically, the scale involves placing a slash mark corresponding to intensity of pain on a 100 mm line ranging from "No pain," at one end, to the other end, "Pain as bad as it could possibly be." The VAS-I has consistently demonstrated sensitivity to changes in cancer pain associated with treatment or time and usually shows strong associations with other pain intensity ratings.[9] The VAS-I has also shown validity in its association with performance status, clinical setting (inpatient versus outpatient), measures of psychological distress, and measures of global quality of life.[9] Despite its validity in clinical trials, there is some evidence that patients with advanced disease have more difficulty in understanding and completing the VAS-I.[10] The Numerical Rating Scale of pain intensity (NRS-I) consists of a range of numbers (usually 0 to 10) and patients are asked to rate their pain intensity if 0 represents no pain and 10 the worst imaginable. NRS-I scales are used less often in research than VAS-I scales. For pain assessment in clinical settings, the VAS-I, VDS, and NRS-I approach equivalency,[11] so that clarity, ease of administration, and simplicity of scoring become justifiable criteria in response scale selection. In some clinical trials, NRS-I has proven more reliable than the VAS-I, especially with less educated patients.[12] Numerical scales work well as cancer clinical trial instruments, because they are easier to understand and easier to score.[13] NRS-I is also sensitive to changes in pain associated with radiation therapy[14] and physical therapy.[15] In our practice, we commonly use numerical rating scales for the assessment of pain intensity. Verbal rating scales of pain

TABLE 6.1

CRITERIA FOR PAIN CLASSIFICATION IN THE PATIENT WITH CANCER

Acute versus chronic
Severity of pain
Underlying mechanisms
Tumor type and stage of disease
Temporal patterns
Cancer pain syndromes

TABLE 6.2
ACUTE PAIN ASSOCIATED WITH CANCER MANAGEMENT

Procedure	Problem
Diagnostic procedures (venepuncture, lumbar puncture, angiography, endoscopy, biopsy)	Pain at site of procedure
Chemotherapy	Arthralgia
	Cardiomyopathy
	Extravasation of drug into tissues
	Gastrointestinal distress
	Mucositis
	Myalgia
	Pancreatitis
Radiation therapy	Esophagitis
	Itching
	Mucositis
	Painful fractures
	Pharyngitis
	Proctitis
	Skin burns
Surgical therapy	Postoperative pain
	Ileus, colic
	Urinary retention

intensity (VRS-I) consist of a list of descriptors (eg, none, some, moderate, severe) that represent varying degrees of pain intensity. Like VAS-I and NRS-I, VRS-I demonstrates sensitivity to changes in pain with treatment, tumor size and stage, analgesic use, disease stage, and anxiety about pain.[9]

There are excellent correlations between all three instruments. Research has shown that differences between categorical pain severity items are not linear.[16–17] For instance, when pain severity is rated at the midpoint or higher on numeric rating scales, patients report disproportionately more interference with daily function.[18] Many people, both with and without cancer, function quite effectively with a background level of mild pain that does not seriously impair or distract them. As pain severity increases to moderate intensity, a threshold is passed beyond which it is hard for the patient to ignore the pain. The pain now disrupts many aspects of the patient's life. When pain is severe, it becomes a primary focus of attention and prohibits most activities. Pain severity and the degree to which the patient's function is impaired are highly associated. As a way of delineating different levels of cancer pain severity, Serlin et al.[19] explored the relationship between numerical ratings of pain severity and ratings of pain's interference with such functions as activity, mood, and sleep. Based on the degree of interference with function, ratings of 1–4 correspond to mild pain, 5–6 to moderate pain, and 7–10 to severe pain. In a follow-up study in categorizing the severity of cancer pain, Paul et al.[20] confirmed a nonlinear relationship between cancer pain severity and interference with function and that the boundary between a mild and a moderate level of cancer pain was at 4. However, they failed to confirm the boundary between moderate and severe cancer pain, and reported that a rating of 7 was in the moderate category and ratings >7 in the severe category.

In assessment of pain intensity, our practice is simply to use a numeric rating scale. In the interpretation of severity, we correlate the patient's average and worst ratings with a functional assessment.

PATHOPHYSIOLOGY/MECHANISMS

The distinction between nociceptive (both somatic and visceral) and neuropathic pain is fundamental in assessment because it influences therapy. In principle, pain results from stimulation of nociceptors or by lesions of

A Visual Analog Scale

NO PAIN ──────────────────────── WORST PAIN EVER

B Numeric Rating Scale

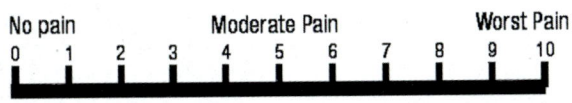

C Verbal Descriptor Scale

None   Mild   Moderate   Severe

FIGURE 6.1 Common scales for measuring pain intensity. The visual analog scale (**A**) requires the patient to place a mark on the scale to indicate level of pain. This mark is then measured from the zero reference point (no pain) and the distance recorded as the score. The numeric rating scale (**B**) may be administered verbally or visually. The verbal descriptor scale (**C**) requires the patient to report pain intensity using simple intensity descriptors (eg, "no pain," "mild pain," "moderate pain," "severe pain").

afferent peripheral or central nerve fibers. Pain is nociceptive if the sustaining mechanisms are related to ongoing tissue pathology. Pain is neuropathic when there is evidence that the pain stems from injury to neural tissues and aberrant somatosensory processing in the periphery or in the central nervous system. Physical influences such as pressure, traction, compression, and tumor infiltration, as well as metabolic or chemical disturbances, can produce pain. Obviously, classification by physiologic mechanism would be ideal, but sufficient information to do this is not currently available.

Tumor Involvement of Encapsulated Organs

Tumors of the liver, both primary and secondary, are the most frequent examples of tumors of encapsulated organs. These can enlarge the organ to several times the normal size. Since the organ capsule of connective tissue grows less rapidly than the tumor, the intracapsular pressure rises as capsular distention develops. In addition, tumor infiltrates the capsule locally, producing dull, and, on rare occasion, stabbing pains. The massive growth of the organ not only stimulates intracapsular nociceptors, but it also irritates larger nerves by pressure or traction on the tissue suspending the organ. Similar organ-enlarging processes in the spleen and kidneys do not lead to pain to the same extent as in the liver, perhaps because of the more stable suspension or embedding of these organs, which are farther away from the midline with its abundant nerve pathways. Kidney tumors produce pain only when the kidney has been almost completely destroyed and the tumor has invaded the pararenal tissue, or when it destroys the renal pelvis. Extrarenal tumor compression on the kidney or ureter can result in severe flank pain (Fig. 6-2).

The brain is also an encapsulated organ. Its unique feature is that the bony skull prevents any generalized enlargement after puberty. Pain arises not by destruction of parenchyma but by the increase of intracranial pressure with stimulation of the meningeal and blood vessel nociceptors. Such an increase of intracranial pressure occurs with space-occupying tumor growth or in focal or generalized brain edema. Focally, edema can develop around neoplasms or damaged brain from trauma or vascular compromise. Generalized edema develops in diffuse metastatic invasion of the meninges due to disturbance of the circulation of cerebrospinal fluid (CSF). Such a tumor invasion of the leptomeninges is frequent in malignant lymphomas. However, metastatic invasion of the leptomeninges can also occur in patients with solid tumors, eg, bronchial and breast carcinoma, and malignant melanoma, with the predominant symptom being headache (Fig. 6-3). In such cases, tumor infiltration of cranial nerves may also occur and lead to focal pain.

Tumor Infiltration of Peripheral Nerves

Infiltration by tumor tissue is the quintessential tissue trauma stimulus. Indirect damage of unknown pathogenesis might also occur to peripheral nerves in the context of tumor-related conditions (eg, paraneoplastic syndromes). Tumor tissue often infiltrates the perineural cleft, but this does not regularly cause pain. Painful entrapment of the brachial plexus or individual nerves can occur, especially in extensive breast carcinomas and their recurrences or in chest wall metastases of bronchial carcinomas. The perineural cleft widens with tumor infiltration, and infiltration of the tumor into the nerve itself is common. Degenerative changes of the axis cylinders are sometimes

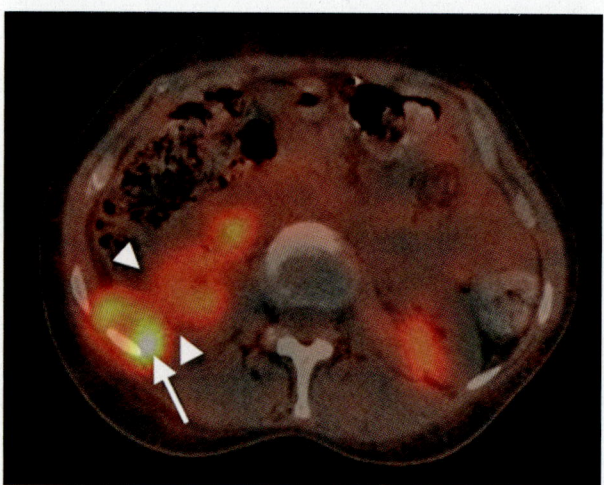

FIGURE 6.2 PET CT scan of 56-year-old woman with metastatic breast cancer. The patient presented complaining of severe right flank pain requiring large doses of oral opioids for pain control. PET CT scan of abdomen shows lateral border *(arrow heads)* of normal right kidney with large hyperintense mass *(arrow)* compression. PET, Positron-emission tomography; CT, computed tomography.

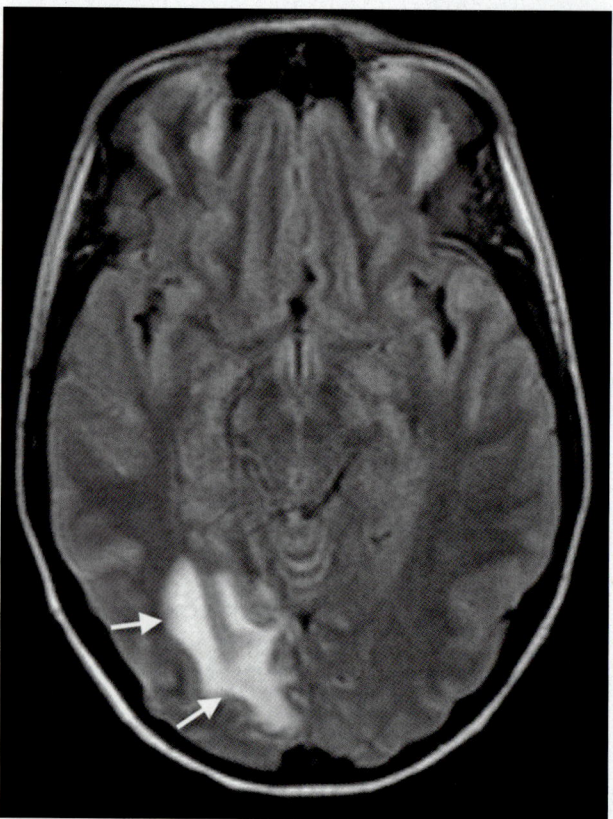

FIGURE 6.3 MRI of brain of a 35-year-old woman with ER-negative, PR-negative, HER-2/neu-negative right breast infiltrating ductal carcinoma who presented complaining of severe headaches, photophobia, and worsening nausea and vomiting. MRI shows tumor with reactive edema *(arrows)*.

visible with conventional screening methods. Tumor compression regularly elicits pain when the affected nerve cannot give way (eg, a spinal nerve).

Tumor Infiltration of Soft Tissues

Tumor infiltration of soft tissues can cause pain utilizing the mechanisms described above, as with massive infiltration of the retroperitoneum. In addition, infiltration and destruction of mobile structures (eg, the skeletal musculature and tendons and ligaments) can lead to pain via disturbance of function. Here, the tumor spreads in the interstitium and destroys blood vessels, lymphatics, and nerves.

Tumor Infiltration of Bone

Infiltration of bone is the most frequent cause of pain in cancer patients. This applies to primary and secondary neoplasias originating from the bone marrow as well as to neoplasms of the bone itself. Such tumors cause pain when they lead to an elevation of the intraosseous pressure, to loss of stability, or to a lesion of the periosteum resulting in periosteal elevation, or with the release of chemical mediators that sensitize nociceptors. The transducers that generate nociception in finely myelinated and unmyelinated axons reside in the bone marrow, in the bone, and in the periosteum.

Metastases frequently lead to extensive bone destruction. Vertebral spread of tumor may involve intervertebral foramina, where nerve root compression can be an additional source of pain (Fig. 6-4). Further spread posteriorly leads to encroachment of the spinal cord and the spinal nerves. In bone, the metastases primarily localized in the bone marrow result in osteolysis or osteosclerosis. Necroses and hemorrhages occur frequently in bone metastases and doubtless play a role in the etiology of pain. The hemorrhages probably result from microfractures. Metastatic bone disease is discussed in additional detail in the section "Bone Metastases."

Tumor Infiltration of Abdominal Hollow Organs

Tumors and their sequelae in the bronchial tree tend to be indolent, whereas those in abdominal hollow organs frequently lead to pain. This applies to all primary and secondary intestinal tumors. There is significant variability in the generation of pain from intestinal tumors. Pain can be caused by ulcerations, motility disorders, dilatations, and disorders of blood flow. In accordance with the extent of the lymphatic tissue, large tumors with extensive ulceration and hemorrhage occur in malignant lymphomas of the gastrointestinal tract. Perineural tumor infiltration, arteritis, or perineural inflammatory reactions are common in tumors of the abdominal and urogenital hollow organs.

Tumor Infiltration and Inflammation of Serous Mucosa

Pleural carcinomatosis does not usually lead to pain, probably because of the development of pleural effusion, which prevents the pleurae from rubbing together. Peritoneal carcinosis is more frequently associated with pain, and this may be the first symptom of cancer. It stems from either direct contact of the metastases with peripheral nerves or an inflammatory reaction elicited by carcinomatosis with disorders of visceral motility. Acute inflammatory reactions of the peritoneum with the clinical picture of an "acute abdomen," and possibly with empyema, appear after tumor-induced perforation or penetration of hollow viscera.

Tumor-Induced Necroses in Solid Organs

Specific necroses can produce typical pain symptoms in the pancreas. Such necroses, with the typical clinical picture of autodigestive pancreatitis, can occur with pancreatic metastases of a bronchial carcinoma. The autodigestion probably results from tumorous destruction of the parenchyma in conjunction with tumor infiltration and stenoses of the excretory ducts.

Tumor-Induced Occlusions of Blood Vessels

Invasion of the lymphatics and blood vessels is part of the biology of malignant neoplasias and is the precondition for metastasis. Generally, small and peripheral vessels are involved, obstruction of which does not result in any appreciable disorder of the circulation. Larger veins occasionally become infiltrated and occluded. This can lead to edema and pain in the affected area of venous drainage. Infiltration of larger arteries is rare.

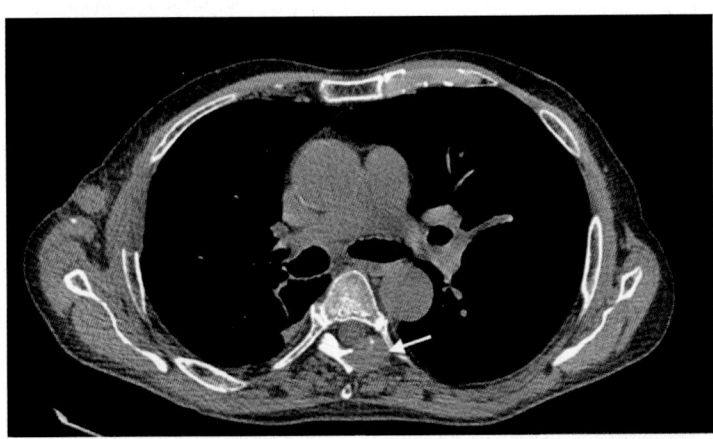

FIGURE 6.4 A 61-year-old man with metastatic squamous cell carcinoma of the larynx. One year after diagnosis, the patient presented complaining of mid-thoracic back and left-sided chest pain. CT of the chest revealed extensive destruction of the left lamina with encroachment of the T6 foramen. *Arrow* shows tumor encroachment.

PATTERNS OF CANCER PAIN

Cancer patients may have constant or intermittent pain as discussed above. The term "breakthrough pain" (BTP) was introduced by Portenoy and Hagen in 1990[21] and refers to sudden increases in the base level of pain or different but recurring pains. Breakthrough pain is defined as transitory exacerbation of pain that occurs in addition to otherwise stable persistent pain or one that interrupts a tolerable background level of pain. The estimated prevalence of breakthrough pain in cancer patients may be as high as 65%.[22] The cause and anatomic site of BTP is often, but not always, the same as that of the baseline persistent pain.[23] The majority of breakthrough pains are usually associated with tumor, but Portenoy et al.[21] reported that tumor therapy was the cause in 14% of cases and 4% were unrelated to either the cancer or its treatment. Typical features of breakthrough pain include rapid onset (the time from onset of BTP to peak severity is usually within 3 to 5 minutes), short duration (approximately 30 minutes), and significant intensity (described usually as severe or excruciating). Breakthrough pain can be assigned to one of three categories:

1. Incident pain: pain directly related to an event or activity, such as turning in bed, weight-bearing, a bowel movement, coughing, swallowing meals, and so on. Often, incident pain is well defined and predictable, so that physicians can anticipate and treat the problem prophylactically.
2. End-of-dose failure: pain that emerges because of too much time between doses of medication. One can predict this pattern for the individual patient and readily prevent it by using time-contingent dosing at an appropriate interval. The key is monitoring symptoms in relation to the dosing schedule.
3. Spontaneous pain: pain that occurs spontaneously without relationship to particular events or procedures. These pains are more difficult because of their unpredictable nature and their often fleeting character. In some cases, adjunctive analgesics effectively provide relief. Longer-lasting pains require rapid-onset analgesics. Increasing the dose of the time-contingent opioids will often increase the overall side effects of these medications.

Cancer-related breakthrough pain has a profound impact on both quality of life and health economics.[24,25] Uncontrolled or poorly controlled pain of any etiology is strongly associated with impairment of sleep, walking, daily activities, enjoyment of life, and relationships with others. It also is correlated with worsening of anxiety and depression, dissatisfaction with opioid therapy, and poor medical outcomes.[26] In addition, patients with cancer-related BTP or uncontrolled pain are likely to use more health care resources, have more pain-related hospitalizations and emergency department visits, and have greater direct and indirect treatment costs than those without breakthrough pain.[25]

CANCER PAIN SYNDROMES

Tables 6-3 to 6-6 list the common pain syndromes in the patient with cancer. Table 6-7 lists the prevalence of painful manifestations of cancer and their common etiologies. Bone, viscera, and nerve are the most common sites of metastases associated with chronic cancer pain.

TABLE 6.3

PAIN SYNDROMES DUE TO TUMOR INVOLVEMENT

Primary Etiology	Pathophysiology	Characteristics of Pain	Other Symptoms and Signs
A. Tumor Invasion of Bone Vertebral body metastases			
Subluxation of atlas	Metastasis of odontoid process of axis → fracture of atlas → compression of spinal cord or brainstem	Severe neck pain radiating to back and top of skull, aggravated by flexion and other movements	Progressive sensory, somatomotor, and autonomic dysfunction beginning in upper extremity
C7-T1 metastases	Cancer of breast and lung → hematogenous spread or more frequently tumor originating in brachial plexus or paravertebral space → spread to adjacent vertebra and epidural space	Constant, dull, aching pain in paraspinal area radiating to both shoulders; unilateral radicular pain with radiation to shoulder and medial (ulnar) aspect of limb	Tenderness on percussion of spinous process; paresthesia and numbness in ulnar distribution of limb; progressive weakness of triceps and hand; Horner's syndrome indicating sympathetic involvement
Thoracic metastases	Frequent site of metastasis from breast, prostate, and other tumors	Dull, aching pain; unilateral or bilateral chest wall component	Possible long tract signs from impending epidural and spinal cord compression
L1 metastases	Frequent site of metastasis from breast, prostate, or other tumors	Dull, aching pain in mid-back with reference to regions of one or both sacroiliac joints and superior iliac crest; radicular pain with girdle-like distribution anteriorly or to both paraspinal areas in the sacroiliac region	Possible numbness and weakness in the back; pain exacerbated by lying or sitting and relieved by standing

(continued)

TABLE 6.3			
CONTINUED			
Primary Etiology	Pathophysiology	Characteristics of Pain	Other Symptoms and Signs
Sacral metastases	Another frequent site of metastasis from breast, prostate, or other tumors	Dull, aching pain in the low back and/or coccygeal region exacerbated by lying or sitting and relieved by walking. Possible radicular component if S1 roots involved.	Perianal sensory loss and bowel and bladder dysfunction and impotence
Base of the skull metastases			
Jugular foramen	Metastasis to jugular foramen with involvement of cranial nerves IX–XII	Occipital pain with reference to the vertex and one or both shoulders and arms, exacerbated by head movement	Tenderness of occipital condyle and often ptosis, hoarseness, dysarthria, dysphagia and neck and shoulder weakness
Clivus syndrome	Metastasis to clivus of sphenoid bone and basilar portion of occipital bone	Progressively severe vertex headache exacerbated by neck flexion	Dysfunction of lower (VII–XII) cranial nerves, which begins unilaterally but extends bilaterally
Sphenoid sinus	Metastasis to the sphenoid sinus on one or both sides	Severe bifrontal headache radiating to both temples with intermittent retro-orbital pain	Nasal stuffiness or sense of fullness in the head associated with diplopia
Cavernous sinus	Metastasis to cavernous sinus syndrome from breast, prostate, and lung	Unilateral frontal headache and dull aching pain in supraorbital and facial region	Dysfunction of CN III–VI, diplopia, ophthalmoplegia, papilledema
Occipital condyle	Metastasis from breast, lung, prostate	Severe localized continuous unilateral occipital pain aggravated by neck flexion	CN XII paralysis → paralysis of tongue; weakness of sternocleidomastoid, stiff neck
Other bone involvement			
Pelvis	Metastasis from breast, prostate, and other tumors	Dull, aching pain in sacrum, hips, or pubis	Extension to sacral plexus with consequent motor, sensory, and/or autonomic changes
Long bones	Metastasis from breast, prostate, or other tumors	Dull, aching, severe pain localized to site of tumor that may be referred (eg, reference to knee from hip metastasis); pathologic fracture produces severe pain on movement	
B. Tumor Involvement of Nerves, Plexus, or Spinal Cord			
Peripheral, cranial, or spinal neuropathy	Infiltration, compression, or damage to nerve	Dull, aching, burning pain associated with bouts of lancinating pain in distribution of affected nerve or nerves; hyperpathia	Hypoesthesia, dysesthesia, motor, and/or autonomic dysfunction and reflex changes
Brachial plexus	Compression, infiltration, or damage of brachial plexus by metastatic tumor or lower cervical and upper thoracic vertebra or Pancoast's tumor	Progressively more severe, dull, aching pain which is first located in the shoulder and arm and vertebral border of scapula and later extends to medial part of arm, elbow, forearm, and hand	Paresthesia, dysesthesia, hypoesthesia; subjective numbness and progressive muscle weakness in C7, C8, and T1 distribution, often Horner's syndrome and anhidrosis of the ipsilateral face
Lumbosacral plexus	Compression, infiltration, or damage of lumbar and sacral plexus by cancer of the prostate, bladder, uterus, cervix, or colon from extension of tumor into adjacent lymph nodes and bone	Radicular pain either in groin and anterior thigh (L1, L2, and L3 nerve involvement) or down the posterior aspect of leg to the heel (L5, S1, and S2 distribution) or dull, aching midline pain in the perianal area (S2, S3, S4 distribution)	Paresthesia followed by numbness and dysesthesia and progressive motor and sensory loss in the areas supplied by the involved nerves

(continued)

TABLE 6.3 CONTINUED

Primary Etiology	Pathophysiology	Characteristics of Pain	Other Symptoms and Signs
Complex Regional Pain Syndrome Type II	Compression, infiltration, or damage of major nerve or plexuses	Severe burning pain not limited to a segmental or peripheral nerve distribution; aggravated by touch and emotional stress	Hyperalgesia, vasomotor, and sudomotor disturbances and other symptomatology of causalgia
Leptomeningeal carcinomatosis	Tumor infiltration of the cerebrospinal leptomeninges with or without invasion of the meninges of the brain	Pain in 40% of patients of two types: headache, with or without neck stiffness; and pain in the low back and buttock regions	Malignant cells in cerebrospinal fluid, elevated protein and low glucose levels
Epidural spinal cord compression	Tumor compression of cervical, thoracic, or lumbosacral parts of spinal cord and involvement of vertebra or roots of spinal nerves	Local dull, aching pain, and tenderness in the region of involved vertebral body or radicular pain, which is unilateral with cervical or lumbosacral compression and bilateral with thoracic cord compression	Depend on site of epidural compression, include motor weakness progressing to paraplegia, sensory loss, and loss of bowel and bladder function
C. Tumor Involvement of Viscera			
Obstruction of hollow viscus or of ductal system of solid viscus	Contraction of smooth muscle under isometric conditions → intense distension of smooth muscles	Diffuse, poorly localized, dull, aching, or colicky pain referred to abdominal wall or chest wall	Dyspnea and cough with thoracic viscera; abdominal distension, nausea, vomiting with abdominal visceral pathology
Rapid tumor growth in solid viscus	Rapid growth of hepatic, splenic, or kidney tumors → rapid distension and stretching of investing fascia → stimulation of mechanical nociceptors	Dull, aching, poorly localized pain referred to midline (liver) or in one side in lower thoracic and upper lumbar segments	Symptomatology of visceral dysfunction
D. Other Types of Tumor Involvement			
Tumor involvement of blood vessels			
Infiltration	Perivascular lymphangitis and vasospasm	Burning pain in the areas supplied by the affected vessels	Signs of vasoconstriction or ischemia
Obstruction of large vein	Venous engorgement → progressive edema → distension of fascial compartments and soft tissue	Severe headache with obstruction of veins to head; pain in limbs with obstruction in axilla or pelvis	Edema and cyanosis of affected part
Obstruction of large artery	Ischemia in tissues with liberation of algesic substances	Progressively severe, burning pain	Paresthesia, pallor of affected part
Necrosis or ulceration of mucous membrane	Necrosis, infection, and inflammation of mucous membrane → algesic substances → lowering of nociceptors' threshold	Excruciating local or referred pain depending on site of lesion	Signs of infection or inflammation

From Fitzgibbon D, Chapman C. Cancer Pain, Assessment and Diagnosis. In Loeser JD, ed. *Bonica's Management of Pain*, 3rd edition. Philadelphia: Lippincott Williams & Wilkins, 2000:635–637.

TABLE 6.4

PAIN SYNDROMES ASSOCIATED WITH CANCER THERAPY

Primary Etiology	Pathophysiology	Characteristics of Pain	Other Symptoms and Signs
A. Postsurgical Syndromes			
Post-thoracotomy Post–radical neck resection Postmastectomy	Partial injury or complete severance of nerves during operation → damage to nerve membrane or neuroma formation, which becomes hypersensitive to pressure and norepinephrine → abnormal sensory input to CNS (peripheral-central mechanisms)	Continuous, burning or dull, aching pain with occasional bout of lancinating pains in the areas supplied by affected nerves, aggravated by touch, movement, or emotional stress with catecholamine release	Dysesthesia, hyperesthesia in the scar area with hypoesthesia in the surrounding zone. Frequently associated with restricted activities in affected area 2° to myofascial component.
Postamputation pain	Persistent nociception in stump and loss of sensory input to neuraxis → deafferentation (peripheral-central mechanism)	Constant aching or burning pain in stump or in phantom limb or cramping "proprioceptive" pain characterized by abnormal position of missing part of limb; also lancinating pain	Sudomotor and vasomotor changes in stump. Persistent phantom limb pain.
B. Postchemotherapy Pain			
Peripheral neuropathy	Symmetrical polyneuropathy caused by Vinca alkaloids (peripheral mechanism)	Constant burning pain in the hand and/or feet	Dysesthesia and paresthesia. May be associated with large fiber signs (ataxia, motor weakness)
Aromatase inhibitors	Possible central mechanism secondary to estrogen deprivation. Preclinical data suggests estrogen role in articular chondrocyte production.	Diffuse muscle aching and joint pains and stiffness	May increase risk of osteoporosis problems including fractures
Steroid	Diffuse myalgias and pseudorheumatism arthralgias caused by withdrawal of steroid medication (peripheral mechanism)	Diffuse pain and tenderness in affected muscles and joints	Fatigue and general malaise; these and the pain disappear with reinstitution of steroid medication
Aseptic necrosis of bone	Aseptic necrosis of humoral head or femoral head as complication of chronic steroid therapy (peripheral mechanism)	Dull, aching pain in the shoulder or knee	Limitation of joint movement with inability to use arm or hip joint → frozen shoulder or impaired hip
Mucositis	Drug produces biochemical changes in mucous membranes and other structures (peripheral mechanisms)	Severe, excruciating pain in mouth, throat, nasal passages, and gastrointestinal tract	Difficulty or inability to eat, drink, or even talk
C. Postradiation therapy pain			
Radiation fibrosis of brachial or lumbosacral plexus	Radiation-induced fibrosis of connective tissue surrounding plexus and consequent injury to nerve structures develops 6 months to 20 years following therapy → deafferentation (peripheral-central mechanisms)	Progressively increasing, severe, diffuse, burning pain in a part or the entire limb, which occurs after other symptomatology	Numbness, paresthesia, dysesthesia, and motor weakness in distribution of C5 and C6 in the upper limb or in lower limb
Radiation myelopathy	Damage to spinal cord → Brown-Sequard syndrome progresses to complete transverse myelopathy (central pain)	Pain that is localized or referred to peripheral structures	Dysesthesia and other symptomatology of myelopathy
Painful peripheral nerve tumors	Radiation induces nerve sheath tumors 4 to 20 years after therapy	Progressively severe, burning, aching pain in distribution of involved nerves	Progressive neurologic deficit
Postherpetic neuralgia	Induced by radiation or after herpes zoster in the area of tumor pathology	Continuous burning pain associated with intermittent lancinating pain	Dysesthesia, hypoesthesia, and hyperpathia

From Fitzgibbon D, Chapman C. Cancer Pain, Assessment and Diagnosis. In Loeser, JD, ed. *Bonica's Management of Pain*, 3rd edition. Philadelphia: Lippincott Williams & Wilkins, 2000:637.

TABLE 6.5

PAIN SYNDROMES CAUSED BY CANCER-INDUCED PATHOPHYSIOLOGIC CHANGES

Primary Etiology	Pathophysiology	Characteristics of Pain	Other Symptoms and Signs
A. Paraneoplastic syndromes	Autoimmune and inflammatory disorder with loss of neurons in affected areas	Visceral: $2°$ to chronic gastrointestinal pseudo-obstruction, Sensory: $2°$ to neuronopathy. Often asymmetrical or multifocal. Upper extremities often affected first.	Related to sensory neuronopathy, paraneoplastic limbic encephalitis, and paraneoplastic cerebellar degeneration. Sensory loss in face, abdomen, chest. Ataxia. Proximal weakness lower extremities. Dermatomyositis.
B. Debility, constipation, bed sores, rectal or bladder spasm, gastric distension	Related to specific lesions depending on involved site	Local or referred pain	Related to specific pathophysiology

From Fitzgibbon D, Chapman C. Cancer Pain, Assessment and Diagnosis. In Loeser JD, ed. *Bonica's Management of Pain*, 3rd edition. Philadelphia: Lippincott Williams & Wilkins, 2000:637–638.

TABLE 6.6

PAIN SYNDROMES UNRELATED TO CANCER

Primary Etiology	Pathophysiology	Characteristics of Pain	Other Symptoms and Signs
A. Examples: arthritis, osteoporosis	Pathology of affected part	Local or referred pain	Related to specific pathophysiology
B. Myalgia Fibromyalgia	Fibromyalgia—central sensitization	Fibromyalgia—widespread muscle aching and soreness	Fibromyalgia—sleep disturbance, fatigue, depression; tender points; viscerosomatic pain syndromes
Myofascial pain syndrome	Myofascial—predominantly peripheral	Myofascial—discrete aching and soreness; reproducible usual or spontaneous pain	Myofascial—often referred (segmental) to different, usually distal, site; trigger points

TABLE 6.7

PREVALENCE OF PAINFUL MANIFESTATIONS OF CANCER AND COMMON ETIOLOGIES

Primary Site of Cancer	Approximate Incidence of Pain (%)	Common Pain Syndromes
Oropharynx	55–80	Postradical neck dissection syndrome Infection
Colon-rectum	45–95	Bone metastasis Perineal pain syndrome Lumbosacral plexopathy Epidural spinal cord compression
Pancreas	70–100	Abdominal visceral pain
Liver/biliary tract	65–100	Abdominal visceral pain
Lung	55–90	Bone metastasis Epidural spinal cord compression Brachial plexopathy Post-thoracotomy syndrome
Breast	55–100	Brachial plexopathy Postmastectomy syndrome Bone metastasis Epidural spinal cord compression Leptomeningeal carcinomatous

(continued)

TABLE 6.7

CONTINUED

Primary Site of Cancer	Approximate Incidence of Pain (%)	Common Pain Syndromes
Uterus-cervix and ovary	40–100	Lumbosacral plexopathy
Prostate	55–100	Bone metastasis
		Base of skull syndromes
		Vertebral body syndromes
		Epidural spinal cord compression
Urinary tract	60–100	Lumbosacral plexopathy
		Epidural spinal cord compression
Lymphoma and leukemia	5–75	Leptomeningeal carcinomatosis
		Bone pain
		Mucositis
Sarcoma and primary bone tumors	75–90	Postamputation pain (stump, phantom limb)
		Epidural spinal cord compression

From Fitzgibbon D, Chapman C. Cancer Pain, Assessment and Diagnosis. In Loeser JD, ed. *Bonica's Management of Pain*, 3rd edition. Philadelphia: Lippincott Williams & Wilkins, 2000:638.

References

1. De Leon-Casasola OA, Myers DP, Donaparthi S, et al. A comparison of postoperative epidural analgesia between patients with chronic cancer taking high doses of oral opioids versus opioid-naive patients. *Anesth Analg.* 1993;76:302–307.
2. Chapman CR, Donaldson GW, Jacobson RC, et al. Differences among patients in opioid self-administration during bone marrow transplantation. *Pain.* 1997;71:213–223.
3. Allison RR, Vongtama V, Vaughan J, et al. Symptomatic acute mucositis can be minimized or prophylaxed by the combination of sucralfate and fluconazole. *Cancer Invest.* 1995;13:16–22.
4. Grossman SA, Sheidler VR, Swedeen K, et al. Correlation of patient and caregiver ratings of cancer pain. *J Pain Symptom Manage.* 1991;6:53–57.
5. Peteet J, Tay V, Cohen G, et al. Pain characteristics and treatment in an outpatient cancer population. *Cancer.* 1986;57:1259–1265.
6. Cleeland CS, Gonin R, Hatfield AK, et al. Pain and its treatment in outpatients with metastatic cancer. *N Engl J Med.* 1994;330:592–596.
7. Cleeland CS, Syrjala KL. How to assess cancer pain. In: Turk D, Melzack R, eds. *Pain assessment.* New York: Guilford Press, 1992:360–387.
8. Jacox A, Carr DB, Payne R. New clinical-practice guidelines for the management of pain in patients with cancer. *N Engl J Med.* 1994;330:651–655.
9. Jensen MP. The validity and reliability of pain measures in adults with cancer. *J Pain.* 2003;4:2–21.
10. Bruera E, Kuehn N, Miller MJ, et al. The Edmonton Symptom Assessment System (ESAS): A simple method for the assessment of palliative care patients. *J Palliat Care.* 1991;7:6–9.
11. Jensen MP, Karoly P, Braver S. The measurement of clinical pain intensity: A comparison of six methods. *Pain.* 1986;27:117–126.
12. Ferraz MB, Quaresma MR, Aquino LR, et al. Reliability of pain scales in the assessment of literate and illiterate patients with rheumatoid arthritis. *J Rheumatol.* 1990;17:1022–1024.
13. Moinpour CM, Feigl P, Metch B, et al. Quality of life end points in cancer clinical trials: review and recommendations. *J Natl Cancer Inst.* 1989;81:485–495.
14. Trotti A, Johnson DJ, Gwede C, et al. Development of a head and neck companion module for the quality of life–radiation therapy instrument (QOL-RTI). *Int J Radiat Oncol Biol Phys.* 1998;42:257–261.
15. Smith WB, Gracely RH, Safer MA. The meaning of pain: cancer patients' rating and recall of pain intensity and affect. *Pain.* 1998;78:123–129.
16. Wallenstein SL. Measurement of pain and analgesia in cancer patients. *Cancer.* 1984;53:2260–2266.
17. Wallenstein SL, Heidrich G, Kaiko R, et al. Clinical evaluation of mild analgesics: the measurement of clinical pain. *Br J Clin Pharmacol.* 1980;10 Suppl 2:319S-327S
18. Cleeland CS. Effects of attitudes on cancer pain control. In: Straton Hill JC, Fields WS, eds. *Drug treatment of cancer pain in a drug oriented society.* New York: Raven Press, 1989:81–89.
19. Serlin RC, Mendoza TR, Nakamura Y, et al. When is cancer pain mild, moderate or severe? Grading pain severity by its interference with function. *Pain.* 1995;61:277–284.
20. Paul SM, Zelman DC, Smith M, et al. Categorizing the severity of cancer pain: further exploration of the establishment of cutpoints. *Pain.* 2005;113:37–44.
21. Portenoy RK, Hagen NA. Breakthrough pain: definition, prevalence and characteristics. *Pain.* 1990;41:P 273-81.
22. Caraceni A, Portenoy RK. An international survey of cancer pain characteristics and syndromes. IASP Task Force on Cancer Pain. International Association for the Study of Pain. *Pain.* 1999;82:263–274.
23. Svendsen KB, Andersen S, Arnason S, et al. Breakthrough pain in malignant and non-malignant diseases: a review of prevalence, characteristics and mechanisms. *Eur J Pain.* 2005;9:195–206.
24. Fortner BV, Demarco G, Irving G, et al. Description and predictors of direct and indirect costs of pain reported by cancer patients. *J Pain Symptom Manage.* 2003;25:9–18.
25. Fortner BV, Okon TA, Portenoy RK. A survey of pain-related hospitalizations, emergency department visits, and physician office visits reported by cancer patients with and without history of breakthrough pain. *J Pain.* 2002;3:38–44.
26. Gureje O, Von Korff M, Simon GE, Gater R. Persistent pain and well-being: A World Health Organization study in primary care. *JAMA.* 1998;280:147–151.

CHAPTER 7 ■ TUMOR PROCESSES AND PAIN

Nociceptive processes and the perception of pain are influenced by biologic factors such as primary tumor type, stage of disease, and tumor site, as well as psychological factors such as anxiety and depression.[1-3] With the onset of metastatic disease, approximately one in three patients report significant pain. Although pain tends to reflect the presence of metastases, this is not uniformly the case.[4-5]

Tumor-induced pain may occur early in a disease or at an advanced stage. It is rarely one of the early indicators of the onset of disease, and, as such, is not a significant problem for the majority of patients at that stage. Only 5% to 10% of patients with solid tumors at diagnosis report pain at a level that interferes with mood and activity. However, new onset pain may be the concern that prompts the patient to seek medical consultation. Vuorinen et al.[6] found that 28% of newly diagnosed unselected cancer patients reported pain. Pain is much more common as disease progresses. Cleeland et al.[7] reported that the majority of patients with end-stage disease have pain of a severity that interferes with several aspects of the patient's quality of life (QoL). Daut and Cleeland[8] found that pain was an early symptom of cancer in 40% to 50% of patients with cancer of the breast, ovary, prostate, colon, or rectum, and in about 20% of patients with cancer of the uterus or cervix.

Knowledge of the natural history of a malignant disease facilitates understanding of the pain processes and is important in determining the nature and timing of all aspects of treatment. In addition, treatments can be painful and clinicians should differentiate treatment-associated pain from tumor pain. This chapter describes the more common neoplastic processes that cause pain and how they affect different systems within the body. We describe the basic pathophysiology of different tumor types, as well as the common treatments that may influence pain management and QoL issues.

BREAST CANCER

Breast cancer is a major health problem. It is by far the most frequent cancer of women (23% of all cancers), with 1.15 million new cases in 2002, ranking second overall when both sexes are considered together.[9] More than half of the cases are in industrialized countries—about 361,000 in Europe (27.3% of cancers in women) and 230,000 in North America (31.3%). Incidence rates are high in most of the developed areas (except for Japan, where it is third after colorectal and stomach cancers), with the highest age-standardized incidence in North America (99.4 per 100,000).[10] The prognosis from breast cancer is generally good, the average estimated survival rate in developed countries is 73% and in developing countries 57%.[9] As a result, breast cancer ranks as the fifth cause of death from cancer overall, although still the leading cause of cancer mortality in women (14% of female cancer deaths). Because of its high incidence and relatively good prognosis, breast cancer is the most prevalent cancer in the world today; there are an estimated 4.4 million women alive who have had breast cancer diagnosed within the last 5 years.[9] It is estimated that 1.5% of the US female population are survivors of breast cancer.[11]

The major influences on breast cancer risk appear to be certain reproductive factors, body size or obesity, alcohol, physical activity, exogenous hormones (oral contraceptives, hormone replacement therapy), and, possibly, diet. However, the etiology of this disease is not well known, and the most important risk factor, exposure to endogenous and exogenous estrogen throughout life, cannot explain the heterogeneity of prognoses nor the clinical features of patients. Women with germline mutations in the genes *BRCA1* and BRCA2 have a lifetime risk of developing breast cancer of up to 80% and may account for up to 10% of breast cancer cases in developed countries.[12] Women who received thoracic radiation therapy for Hodgkin disease after menarche and before 30 years of age also have a substantial increased risk of breast cancer.[13]

The origin of breast cancers is thought to be the epithelial cells that line the terminal duct lobular unit. Cancer cells that do not penetrate the basement membrane of the elements of the terminal duct lobular unit and the draining ducts are classified as in situ or and are thought to be noninvasive. Invasive breast cancers manifest dissemination of cancer cells outside the basement membrane of the ducts and lobules into the surrounding normal tissues. The histologic types of breast cancer include: carcinoma, ductal, lobular, nipple, and other (undifferentiated). The adverse prognostic factors for patients who have early-stage breast cancer include increasing tumor size and nodal involvement. The breast lymphatics drain via three major routes: axillary, transpectoral, and internal mammary. Intramammary lymph nodes are considered with, and coded as, axillary lymph nodes for staging purposes. Metastases to any other lymph node are considered distant. The diagnosis of breast cancer by triple assessment (clinical, radiologic, and pathologic, increasingly with core biopsy) is established in the context of multidisciplinary management. Positron-emission tomography (PET) scanning is useful in the evaluation of primary lesions, as well as regionally metastatic and systemic metastases of breast cancer. Fluorodeoxyglucose (FDG)-PET in conjunction with magnetic resonance imaging (MRI) offers useful treatment-planning data for patients clinically suspected of having recurrent axillary or supraclavicular breast cancer. FDG-PET can confirm the diagnosis of metastases in patients with indeterminate MRI findings. It also has been reported to reveal unsuspected metastases outside the axilla.[14] FDG-PET is better than bone scintigraphy for the detection of osteolytic breast cancer metastases.[15] Contrast-enhanced MRI is useful for the detection of the cancer that is occult on mammography or sonography, multifocal or multicentric disease in patients with a known primary, residual disease in patients with positive margins after breast-conserving surgery, response to neoadjuvant chemotherapy, unknown primary in patients with axillary lymph node metastases, early disease in high-risk *BRCA1/2* patients, and recurrence in patients after completion of radiation therapy.[16] Despite its improved accuracy, contrast-enhanced MRI is not recommended for general screening because of its expense and limited availability. MRI screening may be used for women with a 20% or greater lifetime risk of developing breast cancer.[17]

Therapeutic strategies for patients with breast cancer depend upon various prognostic variables that include size of the primary neoplasm, the presence and extent of axillary lymph node metastases, pathological stage of disease after primary therapy, and the presence or absence of receptor (estrogen, progesterone) activity. Breast-conserving surgery by wide local excision is currently the preferred option, with mastectomy predominantly reserved for tumors not suitable for wide local excision and for patients who request it. Removal of axillary nodes provides prognostic information, guides adjuvant therapy, and may achieve local control. Biopsy of the sentinel lymph node is accepted as the standard of care in early breast cancer, with removal of the first lymph node or nodes that drain the tumor. Radiation therapy is the mainstay of local and regional treatment for breast cancer in women treated both by breast-conserving surgery and by mastectomy. After primary treatment with breast-conserving surgery and radiation, 10% to 20% of patients will have local recurrence in the breast within 1 to 9 years. Between 10% and 25% of these will have locally extensive or metastatic disease. After radical surgery and postoperative radiation, loco-regional recurrences occur in <10%.[18]

Endocrine manipulation with tamoxifen, ovarian ablation, or both are the preferred options with endocrine-responsive tumors. Hormone receptor status is a well-established prognostic and predictive factor. A meta-analysis of seven cooperative group adjuvant therapy trials confirmed the role of estrogen receptor (ER) status as a prognostic factor.[19] Women who had ER-negative tumors showed a peak annual hazard of recurrence 1 to 2 years after surgery of 18.5%. The hazard declined rapidly thereafter to a rate of 1.4% in years 8 through 12. Approximately two thirds of women with breast cancer have ER-positive disease. The selective estrogen modulator, tamoxifen, is the standard first-line therapy for women with ER positive breast cancer. For postmenopausal women, third-generation nonsteroidal aromatase inhibitors are useful alternatives. Aromatase inhibitors and tamoxifen have different spectra of side effects. Tamoxifen causes more vasomotor symptoms, thromboembolism, and strokes, whereas aromatase inhibitors are associated with more arthralgias, bone thinning, and fracture. For some patients the arthralgia associated with an aromatase inhibitor, which is probably caused by estrogen suppression, may lead to discontinuation of therapy. Patients taking aromatase inhibitors should have bone mineral density measured at baseline.

Overexpression of transmembrane peptide growth factor receptors, such as epidermal growth factor receptor (EGFR) or the human epidural receptor 2 (HER2) has been associated with poor prognosis and resistance to hormonal therapy.[20] HER2 is amplified and overexpressed in 15% to 30% of newly diagnosed breast cancers and is associated with more aggressive behavior.[21] HER2-positive breast cancers manifest resistance to tamoxifen therapy, presumably as a result of cross-talk between intracellular signaling pathways.[22] The antibody trastuzumab (Herceptin), which targets HER2 and is generally given for 12 months, reduces the risk of relapse by a further 35% to 52%.[23] Biopsies of tumors from breast cancer patients who have relapsed on an antiestrogen show a functional estrogen receptor,[24] although women who have become refractory to tamoxifen can respond to further endocrine manipulation with an aromatase inhibitor or fulvestrant (Faslodex).[25] Because the ER remains functional and can interact with growth factor signaling pathways, there is a strong rationale for combining novel signal transduction inhibitors with endocrine therapy rather than using them independently. Combining hormonal therapy with angiogenesis inhibitors may be an alternative strategy. Angiogenesis is critical to tumor growth and is principally mediated via tumor secretion of vascular endothelial growth factor (VEGF). The successful use of a monoclonal antibody against VEGF (bevacizumab, Avastin) in combination with chemotherapy has been demonstrated in the treatment of breast cancer.[26] A large number of endocrine/targeted combinations are currently in clinical trials and may offer improvement in outcomes for women with ER-positive breast cancer.

Deaths from breast cancer have decreased in the recent years, in part because of improved screening techniques, surgical interventions, understanding of the pathogenesis of the disease, and utilization of traditional chemotherapies in a more efficacious manner. Combination chemotherapy is superior to single agents, and anthracycline-containing regimens are superior to the combination of cyclophosphamide, methotrexate, and fluorouracil (5-FU).[27] Compared with single-chemotherapy agents for metastatic breast cancer, combination regimens show a statistically significant advantage for tumor response and time to progression in women with metastatic breast cancer, a modest improvement in overall survival, and significantly worse toxicities.[28] Anthracycline (doxorubicin or epirubicin)-based chemotherapy reduces mortality by 38% for women younger than 50 years and 20% for women aged 50 to 69 years.[29] Taxanes are now fundamental in the treatment of early and advanced breast cancer. The addition of a taxane (docetaxel or paclitaxel) to anthracycline-based chemotherapy reduces the relative risk of death further, by about 15%.[30] However, tumors vary in their sensitivity to these agents; resistance can be acquired or de novo resistance can occur. Epothilones and associated analogs are novel microtubule-stabilizing agents that induce apoptosis and promote cell death. Research now supports the efficacy of epothilones in breast cancer patients who have progressed on taxanes and anthracyclines.[31] Combined endocrine therapy–chemotherapy is the standard adjuvant treatment in high-risk patients with endocrine-responsive tumors.

Widespread metastasis is characteristic of breast cancer and can involve any organ in the body, most commonly bone, lung, liver, and brain. Metastases characteristically appear within a few years of the onset of the primary lesion, but late recurrence (sometimes many years later in bone) is well described. Although metastatic disease may be asymptomatic, the most common site of metastases—bone—typically hurts. Between 40% and 60% of patients with breast cancer will have metastasis to bone, and, in many of these patients, the involved bones (vertebrae, femoral and humoral shafts, the acetabular area) are those that are involved with motion. Moreover, patients with metastatic breast cancer to bone as their only site of metastatic disease have median survival expectations of 27 to 29 months, during which time pain may be the chief manifestation of disease. Even patients with pulmonary metastases have median survivals of the order of 18 to 23 months,[32] and patients with only unilateral pleural involvement on the order of 44 months.[33] Metastatic breast cancer may be currently incurable, but it certainly is treatable. Survival of patients with metastatic disease has been improving over the decades as treatments have improved. For many women, treatment now resembles that for a chronic disease, with sequential use of different chemotherapy and hormonal therapies to control disease and maintain quality of life. Metastatic breast cancer in many women has become a chronic relapsing and remitting disease that may transiently respond to an array of cytotoxic and endocrine therapies.

Long interactions are likely between clinicians and patients with metastatic breast cancer. This disease in patients with metastatic breast cancer usually follows one of two patterns: an indolent course or disease not immediately life-threatening, and that which is rapidly progressing or with extensive vital organ disease. Treatment planning, both of the disease itself and of the associated pain, mandates understanding of the natural history and its variances in breast cancer.

Table 7.1 lists some of the common causes of pain in patients with breast cancer.

LUNG CANCER

Worldwide, the most common cancer is lung cancer, and it is the leading cause of cancer-related mortality in Western countries. Lung cancer has been the most common cancer in the world since 1985, and, by 2002, there were 1.35 million new cases, representing 12.4% of all new cancers.[9]

TABLE 7.1

CAUSES OF PAIN IN PATIENTS WITH BREAST CANCER

Etiology	Class	Example
Tumor-related	Bone metastases	Axial skeleton fracture
	Neural metastases	Brachial plexopathy
		Epidural metastases with spinal cord compression
		Meningeal carcinomatosis
		Peripheral tumor-induced nerve entrapment
	Visceral metastases	Bowel obstruction
		Liver capsule distention
		Peritoneal irritation
		Pleural effusion and encasement
Treatment-induced	Surgical issues:	
	Wound healing	
	Infection	
	Postmastectomy syndrome lymphedema	
	Radiation issues:	
	Wound healing	
	Lymphedema	
	Chronic scarring (chest, axilla)	
	Chemotherapy-induced:	
	Peripheral neuropathy	
	Mucositis	
	Arthralgia/myalgia	
Pre-existing conditions	Chronic nonmalignant pain	Fibromyalgia, migraine, nonspecific low back pain

It was also the most common cause of death from cancer, with 1.18 million deaths, or 17.6% of the world total. Almost half (49.9%) of the cases occur in the developing countries of the world. Lung cancer remains a highly lethal disease. Survival at 5 years measured by the Surveillance, Epidemiology, and End Results Program (SEER) program in the United States is 15%, the best recorded at the population level. The average survival in Europe is 10%, not much better than the 8.9% observed in developing countries.

A practical classification used by clinicians separates lung cancer into two distinct subgroups: small-cell lung cancer (SCLC) and nonsmall cell lung cancer (NSCLC) (Fig. 7.1). NSCLC is responsible for 80% to 85% of all lung cancers, and SCLC the remaining 15% to 20%. SCLC is associated very strongly with smoking. It tends to arise centrally, presenting in the main-stem or lobular bronchi. SCLC probably arises from the basal neuroendocrine Kulchitsky cells. The tumor tends to metastasize early to hilar, mediastinal, and distant sites. The disease is often associated with paraneoplastic syndromes, including the syndrome of inappropriate secretion of antidiuretic hormone (SIADH), ectopic adrenocorticotropic hormone (ACTH) production with Cushing syndrome, and Eaton-Lambert syndrome, a rare neuromuscular disorder characterized by progressive muscular weakness, autonomic dysfunction, and absent deep tendon reflexes. There are three subcategories of SCLC: oat-cell, small-cell, and combined oat-cell carcinoma. NSCLC is a heterogeneous aggregate of histologies. The most common histologies are epidermoid or squamous carcinoma, adenocarcinoma, and large-cell carcinoma. These histologies are often classified together because approaches to diagnosis, staging, prognosis, and treatment are similar. Adenocarcinoma is the predominant histologic subtype in many countries.

Lung cancers that occur in the apex of the chest and invade apical chest wall structures are called *superior sulcus* tumors or *Pancoast* tumors (Fig. 7.2). The classic description of such cases involves a syndrome of pain radiating down the upper extremity as a manifestation of brachial plexus involvement. With improvements in imaging, earlier diagnosis, and a more detailed understanding of the anatomy, a tumor can be classified as a Pancoast tumor when it invades any of the structures at the apex of the chest, including the most superior ribs or periosteum, the lower nerve roots of the brachial plexus, the sympathetic chain near the apex of the chest, or the subclavian vessels. These tumors are now divided into anterior, middle, and posterior compartment tumors, depending on the location of the chest wall involvement in relation to the insertions of the anterior and middle scalene muscles on the first rib. A syndrome of pain radiating down the arm is no longer a prerequisite for an apical tumor to be designated a Pancoast tumor.[34] The presence of Horner syndrome is associated with poor survival.[35]

Staging procedures include history, physical examination, routine laboratory evaluations, chest x-ray, and chest computed tomography (CT) (contrast enhanced). The CT scan should extend inferiorly to include the liver and adrenal glands. MRI scans of the thorax and upper abdomen do not appear to yield advantages over CT scans.[36] The combination of CT scanning and PET scanning has greater sensitivity and specificity than CT scanning

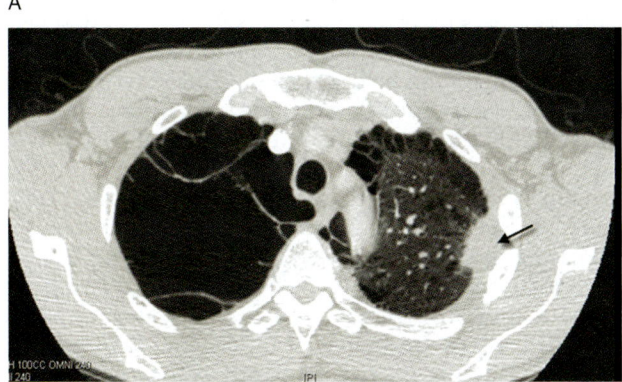

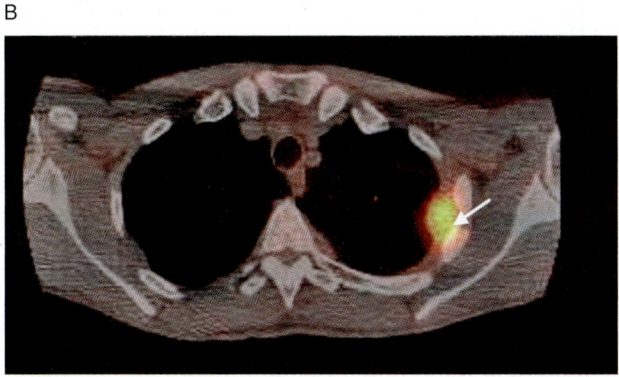

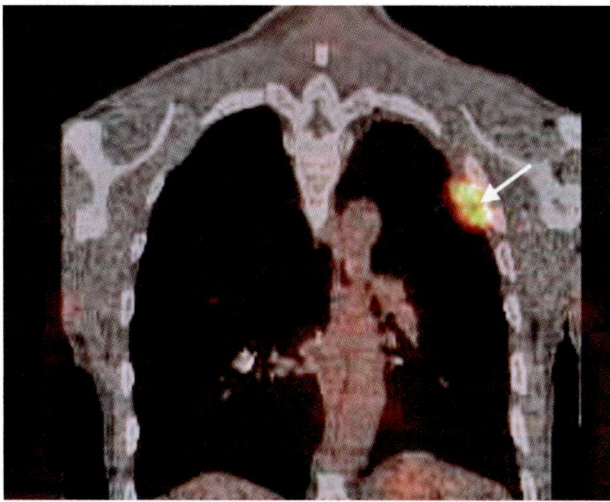

FIGURE 7.1 **A:** A 53-year-old man with stage IV nonsmall cell lung cancer. Axial CT chest shows a mass in the left upper lobe *(arrow)*. Extensive right upper lobe emphysematous changes are also present. Hypermetabolic uptake within the area of the mass are seen on axial PET CT (**B**) and on coronal PET CT (**C**). PET, Positron-emission tomography; CT, computed tomography.

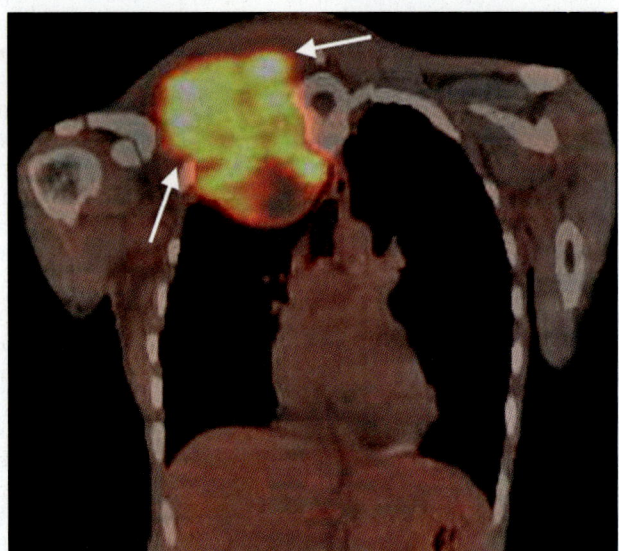
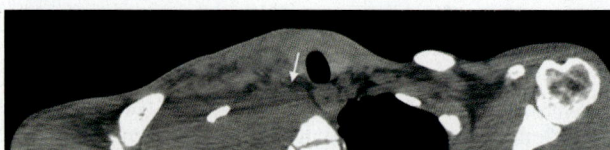

FIGURE 7.2 A 38-year-old woman with severe pain in right upper chest, back, and upper extremity. Patient was diagnosed with Pancoast tumor from a lung adenocarcinoma. Coronal PET CT (**A**) shows marked FDG uptake *(arrows)* in right upper chest and supraclavicular region. CT (**B**) shows the large supraclavicular mass *(arrows)* with destruction of the first rib *(arrow heads)*. PET, Positron-emission tomography; CT, computed tomography; FDG, fluorodeoxyglucose.

alone.[37] Patients at risk for brain metastases may be staged with CT or MRI scans.

Complete evaluation of a patient with newly diagnosed SCLC is similar. Although the prevalence of brain metastases at diagnosis varies, the brain is a common site of treatment failure; therefore, evaluation of the brain before treatment is usually required. Untreated SCLC is aggressive, with a median survival of 2 to 4 months after diagnosis.[38] SCLCs are relatively sensitive to cytotoxic chemotherapy and radiation therapy. Chemotherapy is used for most patients, either as adjuvant therapy for the few patients eligible for surgery, or as primary therapy for patients with inoperable tumors. Surgery is usually limited to patients with smaller tumors without evidence of nodal involvement or spread outside the hemithorax of origin. The benefit of surgery in conjunction with chemotherapy in terms of survival for patients with limited stage disease is uncertain. The role of radiation therapy in extensive disease is less established than in patients with limited-stage disease.[39] Patients with limited-stage SCLC should be treated with combined concurrent chemoradiotherapy. Patients eligible to receive early concurrent chemoradiotherapy should be treated with accelerated hyperfractionated radiation therapy concurrently with platinum-based chemotherapy.[40] Because brain metastases are so common with this disease, patients with either limited-stage or extensive-stage SCLC with a clinical response should be offered prophylactic cranial radiation.[40] Many patients respond to primary therapy but relapse after remissions of varying duration. The prognosis of patients who relapse is poor. Chemotherapy regimens usually involve platinum-etoposide combinations in patients with limited stage disease and platinum-based regimens in patients with extensive-stage disease.

For early-stage and locally advanced NSCLC (stages I through III), a multimodality treatment approach is appropriate, because it improves survival. Treatment options include surgery (lobectomy, pneumonectomy, or segmental, wedge, or sleeve resection as appropriate), radiation therapy with curative intent (for potentially operable tumors in patients with medical contraindications to surgery), and adjuvant chemotherapy with or without other modalities after curative. In general, patients with an early-stage NSCLC without mediastinal nodal involvement (stage I and II) are treated primarily with surgery, whereas those with a locally advanced lung cancer with mediastinal nodal involvement (stages IIIA and IIIB) are treated with chemotherapy and radiation. Approximately 40% of patients with newly diagnosed NSCLC have stage IV disease.[41] Chemotherapy improves survival and palliates disease-related symptoms in patients with good performance status. Palliative chemotherapy typically involves a cisplatin-based or carboplatin-based regimen. Bevacizumab (Avastin) improves survival combined with carboplatin and paclitaxel (Taxol) in a clinically selected subset of patients with stage IV NSCLC and good performance status (nonsquamous histology, lack of brain metastases, and no hemoptysis).[41] Clinical trials show efficacy for agents such as docetaxel (Taxotere) and pemetrexed (Alimta) in the second line setting for refractory disease.[42] Preliminary data also shows some efficacy for erlotinib (Tarceva) in patients with advanced NSCLC.[43] Recurrent NSCLC may be treated with chemotherapy or radiation therapy.

Radiation therapy may be effective in palliating symptomatic local involvement with NSCLC, such as tracheal, esophageal, or bronchial compression; bone or brain metastases; pain; vocal cord paralysis; hemoptysis; or superior vena cava syndrome. In some cases, endobronchial laser therapy and/or brachytherapy has been used to alleviate proximal obstructing lesions.[44] Thoracic radiation therapy is an effective treatment modality to relieve symptoms from intrathoracic disease, either after disease progression during chemotherapy or in patients who are not candidates for or decline chemotherapy.

Paraneoplastic syndromes frequently are associated with lung cancers, in particular SCLS. Paraneoplastic syndrome implies the ability of certain tumors to produce signs and symptoms at a distance from the site of the primary tumor or its metastases. These syndromes are typically caused by ectopic hormone production or immune-mediated tissue destruction caused by neural antigen expression from cancer cells. Cancer cachexia and SIADH occur in approximately 40% of cases. Cushing syndrome can result from increased serum and tissue levels of immunoreactive ACTH. Often seen in patients with NSCLC, hypercalcemia is uncommon in patients with SCLC. About 10% of all lung cancer patients have hypercalcemia, and this is not associated with bone metastases in 10% to 15%. Humoral hypercalcemia of malignancy is more common in NSCLC, and especially squamous cell carcinoma. Malignancy-associated hyponatremia is commonly associated with production of arginine vasopressin (AVP) by tumor cells. A significant proportion of the new cases of syndrome of SIADH in elderly smokers are due to SCLC. The neurological syndromes associated with lung cancer can be rare disorders such as subacute cerebellar degeneration, optic neuritis and retinopathy, subacute necrotizing myelopathy, and peripheral neuropathy. Paraneoplastic neurologic syndromes also include Lambert-Eaton myasthenic syndrome.

Pain is a major symptom in the patient with lung cancer.[45-46] The duration of pain before diagnosis can vary. Huhti et al.[47] reported that 20% of patients had pain for more than 6 months before the diagnosis. Portenoy et al.[48] found that the median duration of pain experienced by lung cancer outpatients was 4 weeks, but there was a wide range, from 1 week to 177 weeks. Ischia et al.[49] found that 30% of patients with locally advanced disease had pain for more than 6 months before the diagnosis was established. Lung cancer can cause pain either locally by invasion of the parietal pleura, ribs and chest soft tissue, thoracic spinal column and cord, or brachial plexus, or remotely by its propensity to metastasize. Nociceptive or somatic pain is the major pathophysiologic subtype in lung cancer pain (weighted mean prevalence 73%; range: 75% to 86%), but in approximately one third of cases, the pain is a visceral or neuropathic subtype (weighted mean prevalence 32% and 30%, respectively).[45,50-52] Watson and Evans[51] reported that the three main causes of pain in 221 lung cancer patients were skeletal metastatic disease (34%), Pancoast tumor (31%), and chest wall disease (21%) and together comprised 78% of tumor-related problems in these patients. The chest area is the most common site of pain in patients with small-cell lung cancer. Patients often complain of pain that is poorly localized, dull in character, which may radiate to the neck or back, and is exacerbated by coughing. Mercadante et al.[45] reported that patients with advanced lung cancer commonly reported chest wall (including ribs and shoulder blade) pain, followed by lower extremities and lumbar regions, then abdomen and upper extremities, and the head area.

PROSTATE CANCER

Prostate cancer is an age-associated disease. Over 70% of all cases of prostate cancer are diagnosed in men over 65 years of age, and the median age of men with prostate cancer is 79 years.[53-54] The risk of developing prostate cancer increases from 1 in 45 for those aged 40 to 59 years to 1 in 7 for those aged 60 years or older.[55] This is the fifth most common cancer in the world and the second most common in men (11.7% of new cancer cases overall, 19% in developed countries, and 5.3% in developing countries).[9]

The prognosis is relatively good; it is a less prominent cause of mortality, with 221,000 deaths per year (5.8% of cancer deaths in men and 3.3% of all cancer deaths).

Prostate cancers (95%) are almost all adenocarcinomas. The remaining 5% are squamous cell carcinoma, signet-ring carcinoma, transitional carcinoma, neuroendocrine carcinoma, or sarcoma. Prostate adenocarcinoma typically invades regional structures, including the seminal vesicles, urinary bladder, or surrounding tissues. Distant metastases can arise from lymphatic spread or hematogenous dissemination, which is usually to bone. Tumor aggressiveness can be determined by an examination of the microscopic pattern of the cancer cells. The most commonly used tumor grading system is the Gleason grading, which assigns a grade for each prostate cancer from 1 (least aggressive) to 5 (most aggressive) based on the degree of architectural differentiation of the tumor. Tumors often show multiple different grade "patterns" within the prostate or even a single core biopsy. To account for this, the Gleason score is obtained by assigning a primary grade to the most predominant grade present and a secondary grade to the second most predominant grade. An exception to this is in the case where the highest (most aggressive) pattern present in a biopsy is not either the most predominant or second most predominant pattern; in this situation, the Gleason score is obtained by combining the most predominant pattern grade with the highest grade. The Gleason score is then displayed as, for example, 3 + 4, where 3 would be the most common pattern of tumor and 4 the second most common pattern (or highest pattern) of tumor seen in the core. Given that the individual Gleason value can range from 1 to 5, the added values (Gleason scores or "sums") can range from 1 + 1 to 5 + 5 or from 2 to 10. Generally, Gleason scores of 2 to 4 are uncommon; the majority of biopsied tumors range from 5 to 10. The regional lymph nodes for the prostate are the pelvic nodes below the bifurcation of the common iliac arteries. Distant lymph nodes are outside the confines of the true pelvis. They are the aortic (para-aortic, periaortic, lumbar), common iliac, inguinal, superficial inguinal (femoral), supraclavicular, cervical, scalene, and retroperitoneal nodes.

Serum prostate-specific antigen (PSA), digital rectal examination (DRE), and transrectal ultrasonography (TRUS) are the three major diagnostic tools for prostate cancer. PSA is an organ-specific glycoprotein which originates in the cytoplasm of ductal cells of the prostate. Its function is the liquefaction of seminal fluid. PSA is prostate tissue-specific, but not tumor-specific. This limits its utility, because elevated PSA levels may also be the sign of benign disorders such as benign prostatic hyperplasia (BPH), or prostatitis. Moreover, there is no consensus as to what PSA level constitutes disease recurrence following prostatectomy. Nonetheless, rising PSA levels are a cause of concern in a patient who has had prostate cancer. Men presenting initially with PSA <1.0 ng/mL may not have to be rescreened for a period of 8 years. With a PSA in the range of 1.0 to 2.9 ng/mL, prostate biopsies may detect many cancers, with a proportion of 20% to 30% showing aggressive patterns by Gleason score.[56]

Prostate gland neoplasms can lead to local rectal, urethral, suprapubic, and penile pain due to expansion and inflammation of the prostate. Pain referred to the back, lower extremities, and abdominal area can result from tu-

TABLE 7.2

CAUSES OF PAIN IN PROSTATE CANCER

Causes of Pain	Examples/Clinical Syndromes
Bone metastasis	Single metastasis to pelvis or long bone
	Vertebral body metastasis, spinal cord compression
	Base-of-skull metastasis, cranial nerve palsies
	Perineal pain syndromes
Soft tissue metastasis	Lumbosacral plexopathy
	Pelvic tension "myalgia"
Pelvic visceral pain	"Prostatitis" pain

(From Payne R. Pain management in the patient with prostate cancer. *Cancer*. 1993;71 (3 Suppl):1131–1137. Copyright 1993 American Cancer Society. This material is reproduced with permission of Wiley-Liss, Inc., a subsidiary of John Wiley & Sons, Inc.)

mor growth within the pelvis. Distant bone pain with associated neurological dysfunction can be found with long bone, vertebral, and skull metastases (Table 7.2).

Prostate cancer has a predilection for bone: the majority of patients with metastatic disease will have bone pain (Fig. 7.3). Vital organs are rarely the sites of metastasis, and disease progression is usually slow. Rapid evolution can be seen with spinal cord compression due to vertebral metastasis and collapse, or epidural metastasis, or with ureteral obstruction secondary to retroperitoneal lymph node metastases.

The majority of symptomatic patients with prostate cancer present either bone pain, other bone-related symptoms, or symptoms related to urethral obstruction. Clinical syndromes can be identified by the site of bony involvement, the development of mechanical instability secondary to fractures, and by the neurologic dysfunction caused by tumor infiltration of contiguous neurologic structures. Metastases to bones of the hip and pelvis often produce local pain that is exacerbated by movement, especially during weight bearing. The syndrome of perineal pain consists of perineal and perirectal pain that is accentuated by pressure on the perineal region, such as that caused by sitting or lying prone. Such a patient may not be able to sit or lie flat because of the pain. Invasion of the parasympathetic sacral innervation to bladder and bowel may lead to early incontinence. Local spread of tumor from the prostate into other pelvic and abdominal structures often produces visceral and neuropathic pain, particularly if the lumbosacral plexus is involved. Stage IV prostate cancer includes patients with locally advanced tumors (T4, indicating invasion of the bladder, rectum, pelvic wall), involvement of lymph nodes (N1) or presence of distant metastasis (M1), which includes nonregional lymph-nodes or metastasis to other organs, usually bones. Imaging studies of some patients may not reveal metastatic disease, although patients may present with a high PSA. A PSA level above 20 ng/mL is highly suggestive of advanced disease, and a level >50 ng/mL is virtually diagnostic of metastatic disease.

Patients with clinically localized prostate cancer may be considered candidates for interstitial prostate brachytherapy, but practitioners differ with respect to which risk groups are offered this approach. Some practitioners will use this treatment option for low-risk disease only, whereas others will treat both low- and intermediate-risk patients. Before initiating therapy, a transrectal ultrasound-based volume study is performed to assess prostate volume and to determine the number of needles and corresponding radioactive seeds, the isotope, and the isotope strength necessary for the procedure. Radioactive needles are implanted via a transperineal approach under guidance of transrectal ultrasound or magnetic resonance imaging. Common regimens employ 120 Gy (palladium)

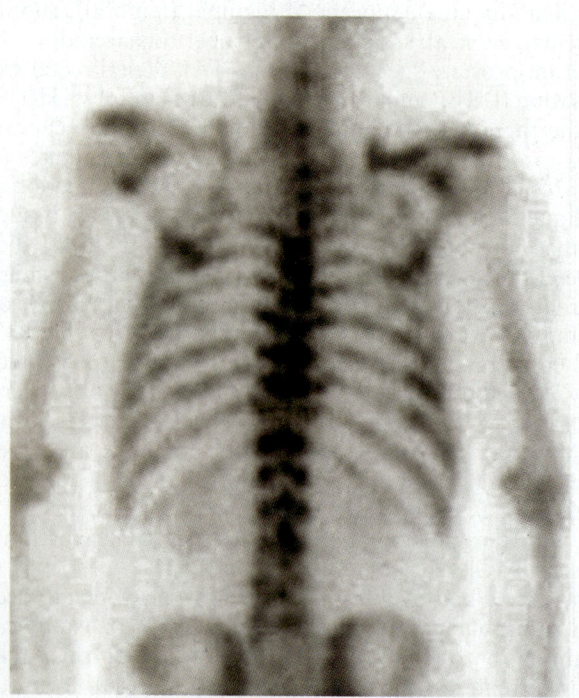

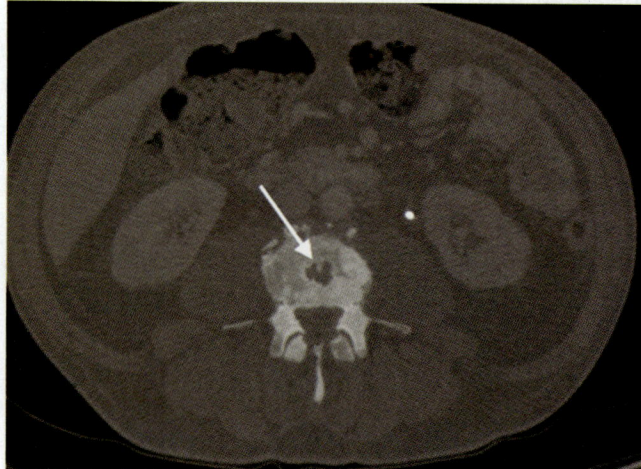

FIGURE 7.3 A 61-year-old man with castration-resistant prostate adenocarcinoma with extensive skeletal metastases. Patient complained of diffuse achy back pain. Bone scan (**A**) shows diffuse tracer uptake throughout the spine. Axial CT of lumbar spine (**B**) shows an osteoblastic lesion in the vertebral body *(arrow)*. CT, Computed tomography.

or 140 Gy (^{125}I), with postoperative dosimetry performed for each patient. Radical prostatectomy involves removal of the entire prostate and the attached seminal vesicles with the ampulla of the vas deferens. The procedure may be performed using a retropubic or perineal incision or by using a laparoscopic or robotic-assisted technique. Depending on tumor characteristics and the patient's sexual function, either nerve-sparing or nonnerve-sparing surgery is performed. Pelvic lymphadenectomy may be performed concurrently particularly for patients at higher risk for nodal involvement.

Five-year relative survival rates are a function of the stage at diagnosis: from 80% or more when malignancy is confined to the prostate to about 25% where bone metastases have already occurred. Adenocarcinoma of the prostate is dependent on hormonal stimulation (by testosterone) until a very late stage of the disease, at which point new clones of hormone-independent cells arise.[57] Treatment starts with hormone manipulation while the disease is hormone sensitive. Androgen deprivation therapy is the mainstay of initial therapy for systemic disease, whether it is biochemical recurrence (ie, PSA-rise only) after definitive localized therapy or overt metastatic disease. Though hormone manipulation can control the disease for several years, eventually addition of cytotoxic medication is required due to development of hormone-independent tumor cells. For patients with localized or local advanced prostate cancer, neoadjuvant and adjuvant hormone therapy combined with prostatectomy or radiation therapy is associated with significant clinical benefits.[58] First-line hormone therapy consists of blocking testosterone synthesis, either by orchiectomy or by using a gonadotrophin-releasing hormone analog (aLHRH) such as leuprolide (Lupron). The most common side effects of leuprolide are hot flushes, decreased libido, sexual impotence, and osteopenia. Because therapy is associated with low testosterone levels, additional problems may occur. Low testosterone levels have been shown to affect mood and self-esteem. Androgen deprivation therapy may be associated with an increased risk of depression. In a pilot cross-sectional study of 45 men, 13% of men receiving androgen deprivation therapy had major depressive disorder, eight times the normal rate of depression {Pirl, 2002 #2318}. Men with a previous history of depression were more likely to develop a major depressive disorder. Furthermore, cognitive issues, particularly in older men, may occur with therapy.[59]

Patients who want to try to maintain sexual function (seldom possible with use of an aLHRH) could try to use nonsteroidal androgen receptor blockers such as Cyproterone first, although the effectiveness of treatment may not be as good.[60] Hormone manipulation is effective, but not curative in 80% to 85% of cases. Chemotherapy has a well-recognized role in the management of hormone-refractory prostate cancer but results are not impressive. Chemotherapeutic agents in use include estramustine, 5-FU, cyclophosphamide, doxorubicin, mitoxantrone, and docetaxel. In a review of chemotherapy for hormone-refractory prostate cancer, Mike et al.[61] noted that only studies using docetaxel reported a significant improvement in overall survival compared to best standard of care, although the increase was small (<2.5 months). The mean percentage of patients achieving at least a 50% reduction in PSA compared to baseline was as follows: estramustine 48%, 5-FU 20%, doxorubicin 50% (one study only), mitoxantrone 33%, and docetaxel 52%. Pain relief was reported in 35% to 76% of patients receiving either single agents or combination regimens. A regime of docetaxel given every three weeks significantly improved pain relief compared to mitoxantrone plus prednisone. All chemotherapeutic agents, either as single agents or in combination, were associated with toxicities, the major ones being myelosuppression, gastrointestinal toxicity, cardiac toxicity, neuropathy, and alopecia. QoL was significantly improved with docetaxel compared to mitoxantrone plus prednisone.

External beam radiation therapy for the treatment of locoregional prostate cancer yields similar survival rates to radical prostatectomy (10-year survival: 90% to 95%, 60% to 70%, and 50% to 60% in T1, T2, and T3-stages, respectively).[62] Postoperative radiation therapy in high-risk prostate cancer may improve the local and distant disease-free survival of patients. The relative role of radiation therapy in metastatic disease is to deal with isolated symptoms, which may persist despite systemic treatment. Palliative radiation provides pain relief in up to 80% of prostate cancer patients with single or at most a few sites of localized bone pain.[63] A single large hemibody radiation field (typically 8 Gy) is as effective in the alleviation of pain for patients with widespread bone metastasis[64-65] compared to the more standard treatment of fractionated therapy of 30 Gy delivered in 10 treatment fractions over 2 weeks,[66] although patients receiving a single treatment fraction have a higher rate of retreatment and less acute toxicity. Bisphosphonates should be considered for patients with metastatic prostate cancer for the treatment of refractory bone pain and prevention of skeletal events.[67] In addition, androgen deprivation can be considered a risk factor for the development of osteopenia, osteoporosis, and bone fracture, which can be mitigated by appropriate bisphosphonate therapy.[68]

COLORECTAL CANCER

Colorectal cancer is a common malignancy in the Western world and is responsible for about 10% of all cancer deaths in both Europe and the United States.[69] Approximately 30% of all patients with colorectal cancer have metastatic disease at diagnosis, and 50% of early-stage patients will eventually develop metastatic or advanced disease[70] (Fig. 7.4). In terms of incidence, colorectal cancers rank fourth in frequency in men and third in women. Survival estimates (in men) at 5 years are 65% in North America, 54% in Western Europe, 34% in Eastern Europe, and 30% in India. The overall relatively good prognosis means that mortality is about one half that of incidence, whereas prevalence is second only to that of breast cancer worldwide, with an estimated 2.8 million persons alive with colorectal cancer within 5 years of diagnosis.[9]

There are strong correlations between risk of colon cancers and consumption patterns of meat,[71] fat (specifically animal fat),[72] and fiber.[73] In addition, physical inactivity, excess body weight, and a central deposition of adiposity have a major influence on risk of colon cancer.[74] Adenocarcinoma (>90%) is the most common histologic

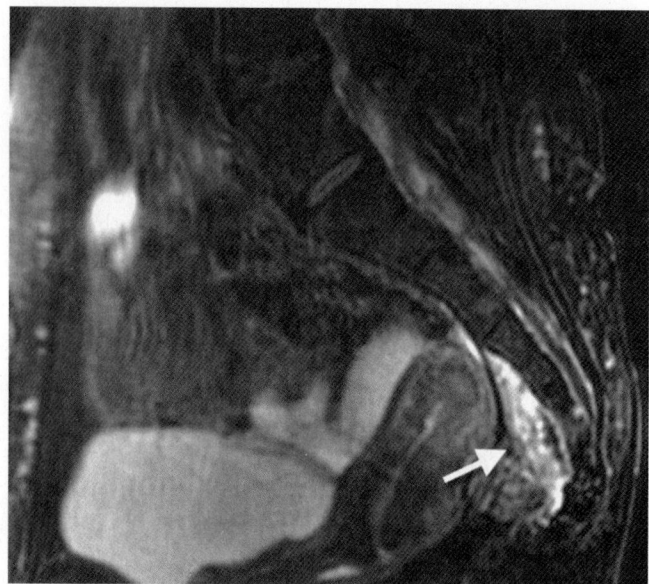

FIGURE 7.4 A 52-year-old woman with pelvic recurrence of rectal cancer (T3 N0 M0). Patient was initially treated with abdominoperineal resection and adjuvant chemoradiation. Three years later, patient presented with increasing pelvic pain and dyspareunia with an elevated CEA level. Axial MRI shows a 2-cm soft-tissue mass behind the uterus, extending from the coccyx to the level of mid-S3 (arrow). This mass was surgically resected with a posterior exenteration, sacrectomy, and rectus myocutaneous flap. CEA, carcinoembryonic antigen; MRI, magnetic resonance imaging.

type, followed by carcinoid tumors, leiomyosarcomas, and lymphoma. Spread to regional lymph nodes is usually correlated with depth of invasion by the primary tumor and its grade of differentiation. Tumors apparently confined to the bowel wall may have nodal spread in 10% to 20%. Hematogenous spread via portal venous transmission is usually to the liver. Age is one of the strongest risk factors for colon cancer, particularly age over 50 years.[75] Higher-risk groups include patients with a family history of colorectal cancer or adenomatous polyps, a past history of successful resection of colorectal cancer or adenomatous polyp, and a long-standing history of ulcerative colitis or Crohn disease. More than 95% of colorectal cancers arise in benign adenomatous polyps (adenomas) that develop in the large bowel over several years.[76] Tumors are staged with the TNM universal system or a modification of the Dukes system for colorectal cancer. The Astler and Coller–modified Dukes staging system uses the following designations: A, a tumor limited to the mucosa; B1, tumors extending into the muscularis propria that do not breach the serosa; B2, tumors that penetrate the bowel wall without lymph node or distant metastases; and C, tumors with regional lymph node involvement without distant metastases. Many allocate cancer with distant metastases or local spread into other organs as stage D. The stage-related 5-year survival of cancers reported in different series is as follows: A, 85% to 95%; B, 60% to 80%; C, 30% to 60%; and D, less than 5%.

Metastatic spread to the liver is most common (65%); extra-abdominal metastases in the lungs (25%) and brain and bone (10%) are less frequent. Approximately one in five patients has metastatic colorectal cancer at diagnosis, which, at best, is associated with a 5-year survival rate of just 10%.[77] Recurrences usually appear within 2 years (about 70%) and almost all (90%) within 5 years.

Complete resection of all malignant tissue offers the only reasonable chance of cure or long-term survival and is the treatment of choice for most patients with colorectal cancer. The goal of surgery is a wide resection of the involved segment of bowel together with the removal of its lymphatic drainage. The surgical approach to rectal cancers is determined by the location and size of the tumor. Radical surgery for rectal cancer is associated with potential mortality as well as significant morbidity associated with poor bowel or sexual function, and possibly a stoma. An abdominoperineal resection is reserved for patients without such a margin or for some with large bulky tumors deep in the pelvis, extensive local spread of rectal cancer, or a poorly differentiated cancer. In patients who underwent a low anterior resection for rectal cancer, bowel continuity was classically restored with a straight colorectal anastomosis. In 1986, J-pouch coloanal anastomosis was developed in order to increase colonic reservoir function and improve QoL.

There is no well-defined role for radiation therapy in colon cancer. The response rates to chemotherapy (usually 5-FU) in recurrent and metastatic cancer remain poor and of limited duration. In addition to staging systems, independent prognostic factors include histologic type, histologic grade, serum carcinoembryonic antigen (CEA) level, and extramural venous invasion. Elevated CEA levels are found in a variety of cancers other than colonic, such as breast, lung, pancreas, stomach, and ovary. Postoperative serum CEA testing should be performed every 3 months in patients with stage II or III disease for at least 3 years after diagnosis.[78] Because 5-FU therapy may falsely elevate CEA values,[79] adjuvant treatment should probably be completed before initiation of surveillance. Patients who are at higher risk of recurrence and who are surgical candidates should undergo annual CT scanning of the chest and abdomen for 3 years after primary treatment. FDG-PET has utility in the initial staging of colorectal cancer and for evaluation of recurrent disease. Contrast-enhanced CT and FDG-PET imaging appear to increase the sensitivity, specificity, and accuracy for staging. Contrast-enhanced CT increases the spatial localization, and FDG-PET adds functional information.[80]

Ten years ago, 5-FU was the only treatment for metastatic colorectal cancer. With the development of new drug combinations, both the response rate and median overall survival have doubled, approaching 50% and 20 months, respectively.[81] Neoadjuvant chemotherapy may be used with the goal of inducing tumor shrinkage so that the disease becomes resectable and thereby potentially curable. Chemotherapy plus newer biologic agents such as bevacizumab or cetuximab might additionally improve survival.[82] Both oxaliplatin combined with bolus and continuous infusion 5-FU plus leucovorin (FOLFOX) and irinotecan combined with bolus and continuous infusion 5-FU plus leucovorin (FOLFIRI) are recognized as standard first-line therapies for metastatic colorectal cancer, with FOLFOX emerging as the preferred upfront treatment option in the United States.[77] Colorectal cancer can lead to severe pain from bowel obstruction, rupture of a viscus or from metastatic disease, most often in the liver.

Preoperative or postoperative radiotherapy with concurrent chemotherapy is the standard of care for patients with Stage II and III rectal cancer. Patients with locoregional recurrence have a poor prognosis. The median overall survival in some series was just over 2 years from the time of recurrence, with an estimated 3-year survival rate of 41%.[83] Yu et al.[83] reported on the patterns of locoregional recurrence after surgery and radiation therapy or chemoradiation in 554 patients with rectal cancer. The estimated 5-year locoregional control rate was 91%. Thirty-six patients had locoregional recurrences at 43 sites. There were 28 (65%) in-field, 7 (16%) marginal, and 8 (19%) out-of-field recurrences. Of the in-field recurrences, nearly 80% occurred in the low pelvic and presacral regions. Fifteen (56%) occurred in the low pelvis, 6 (22%) in the presacral region. Presacral tumors may cause significant low back pain (Fig. 7.4). With disease progression and sacral infiltration, patients may experience severe lower extremity pain from nerve root involvement and bladder/bowel dysfunction. In patients with a history of colorectal cancer complaints of back pain in combination with neurological symptoms, pain persisting and gradually worsening over time and coccygeal pain that fails to resolve should prompt further investigations such as pelvic MRIs and/or PET CT scans.

HEAD AND NECK CANCER

Head and neck cancer (oral cavity, pharynx, and larynx) is the eighth most common cause of cancer-related deaths worldwide.[84] In the United States, 47,560 new head and neck carcinomas were diagnosed in 2008, and this disease accounts for 5% of all newly diagnosed cases of cancer.[85] These cancers comprise 5% of all cancer cases worldwide and result in 6% of cancer deaths in men and 3% in women.[9] The majority of cases present with potentially curable but locally advanced disease. Despite advances in the treatment of these patients, long-term disease-free survival and overall survival remain poor. Approximately 40% to 60% of patients develop local recurrences, and 20% to 30% will be diagnosed with distant metastatic disease.[86] Patients with head and neck cancers are at increased risk of developing a second primary cancer of the oral cavity and pharynx, esophagus, larynx and lung; these cancers are largely due to shared risk factors such as tobacco and alcohol.[87] The 5-year survival for head and neck cancer patients is approximately 50% and only 20% if these patients develop a second primary cancer.[87]

Squamous cell carcinomas arise from tissues lined by squamous epithelium. Squamous cell carcinomas of the head and neck, regardless of site, share similar etiologies, pathogenesis, and response to therapy. In addition, the lymphoid tissues, neuroendocrine cells, melanocytes, and minor salivary glands may give rise to neoplasms. Such tumors are biologically distinct from squamous cell carcinomas and have different natural histories. Approximately 90% to 95% of oropharyngeal neoplasms are squamous cell carcinomas of the head and neck. Most oropharyngeal cancers originate from the base of the tongue and tonsils, and more than 90% of these are squamous cell carcinomas (Fig. 7.5). The majority (60%) of patients present with stage III/IV poor-prognosis disease.

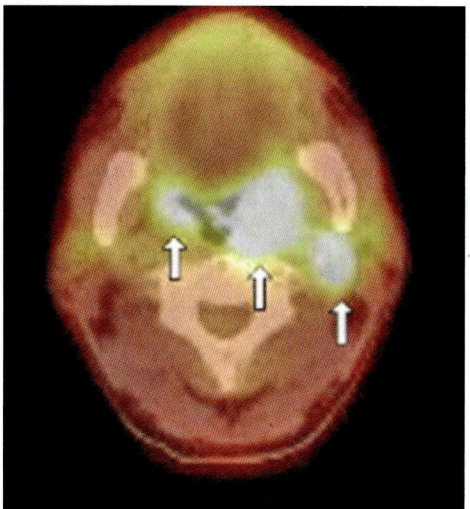

FIGURE 7.5 A 58-year-old man with bilateral squamous cell carcinoma of the tonsils treated with concurrent radiation therapy and cetuximab. Patient had a long history of alcohol and tobacco abuse. Presented initially with a debilitating and progressive sore throat. **A:** CT head shows a 2.0- × 2.9-cm left tonsillar mass *(arrows)*. **B:** PET CT shows bilateral tonsillar masses *(arrows)*. CT, Computed tomography; PET, positron-emission tomography.

Nasopharyngeal carcinoma is a unique form of head and neck cancer. It occurs at high frequencies in China and Southeast Asia. Nasopharyngeal cancer is a rare malignant disease in the Western world, with an incidence well under 1 per 100,000 persons per year in whites from North America and other Western countries. By contrast, the highest incidence is found among Southern Chinese (approximately 25 to 30 per 100,000 persons per year), especially those of Cantonese origin.[88] The average age at diagnosis for this cancer is in the sixth decade of life, but a significant proportion of patients are diagnosed earlier, in their 20s and 30s. Nasopharyngeal carcinoma tends to metastasize early; distant metastases are found in 5% to 10% of patients at the time of initial diagnosis.[89]

Presenting signs and symptoms for head and neck cancers vary with the location of the primary tumor. Nasopharyngeal cancer frequently presents late with nodal neck metastasis. Nasal cavity and paranasal sinuses tumors often present with epistaxis or nasal obstruction. Diagnosis may be delayed as local symptoms may be attributable to other causes such Eustachian tube obstruction or cranial nerve dysfunction. Oral cavity cancers can present as nonhealing, painful ulcers. Laryngeal tumors may present as persistent hoarseness. Later symptoms include dysphagia, chronic cough, hemoptysis, stridor, and respiratory distress. Tumors of the oropharynx and supraglottic larynx usually present late with cervical lymph node enlargement, pain, otalgia, dysphagia, or dysphonia. Endoscopy with biopsy, such as laryngopharyngoscopy, is often used to facilitate the evaluation of the primary tumor. Approximately 15% to 30% of patients present with early-stage disease, and 60% to 80% present with locoregionally advanced disease. Distant metastasis at the time of presentation is not common, but preferential sites include the lung, mediastinal lymph nodes, bones, and liver. PET has a higher sensitivity than CT scan to detect occult metastasis.[90-91]

Treatment of patients with locoregionally advanced or unresectable squamous cell carcinoma of the head and neck is complex and associated with significant toxicities. Local recurrences without evidence of distant metastases may be salvaged surgically if the primary therapy was radiation therapy or with radiation therapy if the primary therapy was surgery. Locally advanced, unresectable disease is best treated with concurrent chemotherapy and radiation therapy,[92] particularly if patients have adequate functional status.

Surgery and radiation therapy are the primary treatment modalities for squamous cell carcinoma of the head and neck. Treatment options for cancers of the larynx present a somewhat unique situation because of patients' desire to preserve vocal ability. In 1991, induction chemotherapy followed by radiotherapy became a standard treatment option for patients with advanced cancer of the larynx who wanted to preserve their voices.[93] Normally these patients would have been treated with a total laryngectomy and postoperative radiation. A functioning larynx was preserved in 62% of surviving patients treated with chemotherapy, and survival in the chemotherapy group was not significantly different from that in the surgery group. Induction therapy with cisplatin and fluorouracil followed by radiation therapy with concurrent cisplatin is an alternative standard of care to preserve the larynx when total laryngectomy would otherwise have been required.[94]

The focus of surgery for head and neck cancer is on conservation of organ function and reconstruction. The debilitating effect of neck dissection on shoulder and neck function is diminished with less radical procedures such as modified comprehensive neck dissection and selective dissection. Selective neck dissection, in which only the anatomical regions that are most likely to contain involved nodes are removed, is used with increasing frequency. Tissue reconstruction to correct surgical defects has improved with the use of tissue whose characteristics are similar to those of the native organ. Radial forearm skin provides tissue in the oral cavity and pharynx to allow articulatory and gustatory functions. Reconstruction of mandibular defects is performed with bone grafts taken from the iliac crest or fibula, with excellent functional results. Oral intake may be resumed after partial or total glossectomy in patients in whom the tongue bulk was replaced with the use of microvascular flaps from the rectus abdominus muscle.[92]

Advantages of radiation therapy include preservation of facial appearance. Radiation of lymph nodes can be included with little added morbidity compared with the added morbidity of extensive neck dissection, and medically unfit patients may tolerate radiation therapy better than radical surgery. Radiation therapy to the head and neck is commonly associated with both acute and late toxicities. Commonly observed acute toxicities are mucositis, stomatitis, and dermatitis. In general, the acute toxicities of radiotherapy are increased with the addition of concurrent chemotherapy. Acute hospital admissions may be required for treatment of dehydration and associated confusion, and for pain management because of severe oropharyngeal mucositis. Late toxic effects (dependent on the location treated) may include chronic xerostomia, loss of taste, dysphagia, skin depigmentation and muscle scarring, trismus, feeding-tube dependence, weight loss and lack of appetite, aspiration risk, and thyroid dysfunction (hypothyroidism). The consequences of radiation-induced mucositis include pain, dysphagia including feeding tube dependency, dehydration, micronutrient deficiencies, weight loss, and potentially life-threatening aspiration.[95]

Chemotherapy alone is not curative treatment but may be used as palliation for patients with metastatic disease. In general, chemotherapy may be administered as neoadjuvant therapy, concurrently with radiation (resulting in radiosensitization and better tumor control), or as an adjuvant after surgery. The cytotoxic drugs most commonly used to treat head and neck cancer are methotrexate, cisplatin, carboplatin, 5-FU, paclitaxel, and docetaxel. Most chemotherapy regimens have included combinations of platinum-based agents such as cisplatin with 5-FU. Induction chemotherapy with carboplatin and paclitaxel before concurrent chemoradiation reduced distant progression while maintaining high locoregional control of disease in patients with locoregionally advanced head and neck cancer.[96] Therapy for patients with distant metastases is only palliative.

In head and neck cancer treatment, QoL issues and assessment of QoL outcomes are especially important for patients and their caregivers because of the potential impact on important functions such as speech, swallowing, and breathing, as well as cosmesis and communication.[97] QoL assessment in these patients may predict survival.[98] In a study of 570 patients with head and neck cancer, Terrell et al.[97] noted that the presence of a feeding tube was a strong negative predictor of quality of life, as were multiple medical comorbid conditions, including the presence of a tracheotomy tube, previous chemotherapy, laryngectomy status, previous neck dissection, and radiation therapy (in descending order of severity).

Patients treated for head and neck cancer suffer from a number of symptom domains: physical symptoms linked to diet and feeding, communication disorders, pain and their general state of health; psychological symptoms including depression, irritability, loss of self-esteem, and social symptoms including relationship difficulties with partner (sexual disorders) or with other family members, loss of work, and sense of uselessness, resulting in a negative impact on their daily lives.[99] The likelihood of experiencing treatment-related chronic pain approaches 40% in the first year after treatment and at least 15% at 5 years.[100-102] Logan et al.[103] studied pain levels among 5-year survivors of head and neck cancer patients and noted a 43% prevalence of pain. All patients in this study had received radiation therapy. Depression was also a significant independent predictor of function-related pain. In addition, the authors noted that the presence of metallic taste significantly contributed to the level of both function-related pain and spontaneous pain. Metallic taste and the presence of taste phantoms (taste sensations in the absence of stimulation) are likely proxies for oral structural damage from radiation therapy to this region.[104-105] Furthermore, burning mouth is associated with the presence of metallic taste phantoms, suggesting a link between oral pain and taste phantoms.[106] Curative doses of radiation therapy for head and neck cancer can result in trismus (and associated pain problems) in a high percentage of patients, independent of other treatment modalities.[107]

Head and neck cancers pose a unique set of management issues that complicate treatment of the disease itself. Pain is a likely concomitant that has a major impact upon quality of life. These patients are particularly in need of a multidisciplinary management team.

CERVICAL CANCER

Cancer of the cervix is the second most common cancer among women worldwide and the seventh most common cancer among women in developed countries[9] (Fig. 7.6). It is much more common in developing countries, where 83% of cases occur and where cervical cancer accounts for 15% of female cancers, with a risk before age 65 of 1.5%. In developed countries, cervical cancer accounts for only 3.6% of new cancers, with a cumulative risk (0 to 64 yrs) of 0.8%. Despite decreased incidence and mortality rates of cervical cancer in the United States,[108] racial/ethnic and geographic disparities persist. Black and Hispanic women have higher rates of cervical cancer incidence and mortality than other groups; in the United States, it is the sixth most common cancer among black and Hispanic women and the 13th most common among white women.[109-110]

Mortality rates are substantially lower than incidence. Worldwide, the ratio of mortality to incidence is 55%.

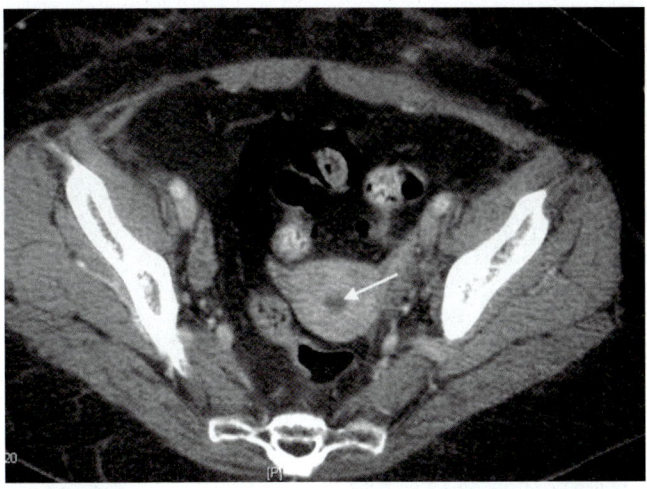

FIGURE 7.6 A 36-year-old woman with Stage IIIB cervical squamous cell carcinoma. Axial CT shows a cervical mass with central necrosis (arrow). CT, Computed tomography.

Survival rates vary between regions, with quite good prognosis in low-risk regions (74% in the United States Surveillance, Epidemiology, and End Results [SEER] program and 63% in European registries).[9] Even in developing countries, where many cases present at relatively advanced stage, survival rates are fair.

The decline in mortality and incidence of cervical cancer is attributable in large part to the widespread use of cervical cytology screening, and the decline is most notable in squamous cell carcinomas, which are detected more readily with the Papanicolaou (Pap) test than adenocarcinomas.[111] Oncogenic human papillomavirus (HPV) infections are responsible for abnormal cervical cytology, cervical dysplasia, and cervical cancer. Clinical trials with the vaccine have shown efficacy approaching 100%.[112-113] We expect, therefore, that the incidence of this disease is going to further decrease wherever the vaccine is utilized. However, various cofactors that vary by race/ethnicity, such as tobacco use and high parity, have been implicated that may facilitate the progression from HPV infection to cervical cancer.[114] In addition, low socioeconomic status varies by race/ethnicity and is associated with increased rates of cervical cancer, most likely because of reduced access to care.[115]

Approximately 80% of cervical cancers are squamous cell, and 15% are adenocarcinomas. This malignancy spreads primarily by direct extension to adjacent tissues and by lymphatic dissemination. Less frequently, hematogenous spread to lungs, liver, and bone occurs (Fig. 7.7). Lymphatics are the main pathway of dissemination for gynecologic malignancies and, in particular, those with preferential regional spread. The cervix drains by preureteral, postureteral, and uterosacral routes into the regional lymph nodes: parametrial, paracervical, hypogastric (obturator), common iliac, external iliac, internal iliac, sacral, and presacral. The common sites of distant spread include the aortic (para-aortic, periaortic), lateral aortic and mediastinal nodes, lungs, and skeleton. In patients with locally advanced disease (stages IIB to IVA), 24% have para-aortic disease.[116] The presence of lymph node metastasis is an important issue in patients with cervical cancer as it influences 5-year survival and affects treatment planning.[117]

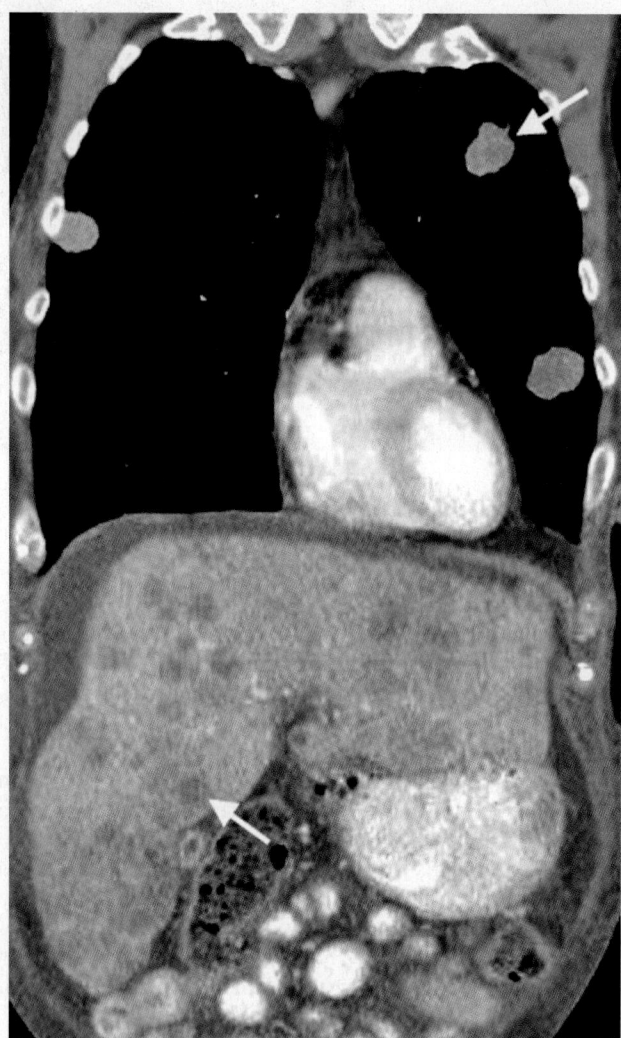
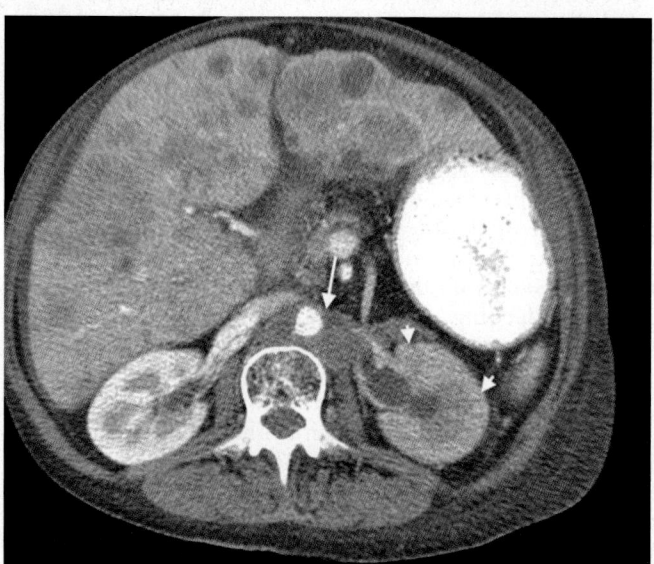

FIGURE 7.7 A 59-year-old woman with metastatic cervical cancer. Coronal CT (**A**) shows extensive liver and lung metastases *(arrows)*. Axial CT abdomen (**B**) shows extensive retroperitoneal mass encasing the abdominal aorta *(arrow)* with narrowing of the left renal artery and vein and left-sided hydronephrosis *(arrow heads)*. CT, Computed tomography.

In particular, identification of para-aortic nodal status allows modification of therapy (usually extended-field radiation therapy) with improved survival.[118-119] Detection of para-aortic lymph node metastases may be difficult using standard imaging techniques such as abdomino-pelvic CT scanning, which has a sensitivity of only 34%.[116] We have observed a patient with metastatic cervical cancer who complained of persistent severe back pain; CT imaging of the abdomen and pelvis did not reveal evidence of any retroperitoneal lymphadenopathy. However, at subsequent exploratory surgery, the patient had extensive adenopathy encasing the abdominal aorta. Because of the suboptimal sensitivity of both CT and MRI imaging in detecting nodal metastases, aortic lymphadenectomy has been considered a staging procedure.[116] However, Rose et al.[120] demonstrated that PET scanning accurately predicted both the presence and absence of pelvic and para-aortic nodal metastatic disease. Although MRI is superior to CT in defining the extent of disease in the cervix and parametria,[121] it remains relatively inaccurate in assessing lymphadenopathy. Compared to conventional MRI, higher powered MRI (3 tesla) using diffusion-weighted imaging resulted in better sensitivity (83% vs. 25%) and similar sensitivity (99% vs. 98%) in detecting lymph node metastases in patients with cervical cancer.[122]

Although CT and MRI of the pelvis have been extensively used. FDG-PET appears to be better for imaging of cervical carcinoma.[123] Most primary tumors, except for very small lesions, are readily seen on PET images and exhibit intense FDG uptake. FDG-PET has relatively poor spatial resolution and is unable to reliably visualize parametrial invasion or involvement of adjacent organs. FDG-PET may be superior to conventional imaging methods for detecting metastatic disease, particularly lymph node metastasis, but it is not useful for staging of the primary tumor.[124]

Treatment of invasive cervical cancer is influenced by the stage of the disease. Five-year survival rates vary between 92% for stage I disease and 17% for stage IV disease.[53] The International Federation of Gynaecology and Obstetrics system of staging (FIGO staging) is based on the anatomical extent of disease and on clinical evaluation. Surgery remains the preferred management for women with early disease who are good surgical candidates, especially younger patients who wish to preserve ovarian or reproductive function. Some of the advances in surgical management of this disease are surgical staging (which includes sentinel node biopsy and nodal debulking); minimal access and robotic radical hysterectomy; fertility-preserving surgery; nerve-sparing radical hysterectomy; total mesometrial resection based on developmentally defined surgical anatomy; and supraradical hysterectomy.[125] The superiority of these new developments over the standard treatment has not yet been demonstrated by controlled prospective trials. In a disease-based treatment option model, patients are laparoscopically staged, a sentinel lymph node is histopathologically explored, and different treatment options ranging from uterus preserving surgery to primary exenteration are presented. The concept of sentinel lymph node biopsy in cervical cancer is not yet fully established.[126] Removal of para-aortic, superficial intercavoaortic, and paracaval nodes is adequate to evaluate the extent of periaortic disease. The median number of nodes typically removed from this area for an accurate staging is 13 (range: 8 to 23).[127] Aortic lymphadenectomy is a part of surgical staging of patients with locally advanced disease and in planning the extension of radiation therapy.

Microinvasive cervical cancer has limited metastatic potential and likely curable by nonradical treatment. Treatment is directed at preserving fertility and preventing the potential complications of radical treatment. Surgical treatment involves conization or simple hysterectomy (dependent on fertility requirements). Lymphadenectomy is not necessary. With depth of invasion, the incidence of lymph and vascular space invasion and the risk of pelvic node metastases increases. Patients can be treated by primary radical hysterectomy, modified radical hysterectomy with pelvic lymphadenectomy, or primary radiation therapy. Radical vaginal trachelectomy and laparoscopic pelvic lymphadenectomy may be an option where preservation of fertility is desired.[128]

Early invasive carcinoma of the cervix can be treated with intracavitary radioactive sources alone, which should be considered in patients who are at increased risk of operative mortality because of age or medical status. With more advanced stages of cervical cancer, treatment protocols vary. Combinations of surgery and radiation therapy are often used. Neoadjuvant chemotherapy is also an option particularly in the treatment of bulky Stage Ib-IIa cervical cancer.[129] The rationales for the use of neoadjuvant chemotherapy are several. Tumor size reduction may reduce pelvic distortion by tumor mass and facilitate subsequent radiation therapy. Size reduction is also associated with a simplification of surgical procedures and the possible transformation of inoperable tumor to radically resectable ones. Effective cytotoxic treatment options for advanced cervical cancer are exceedingly limited. Cisplatin-based combination chemotherapy, the most commonly used cytotoxic therapy, has produced response rates ranging from 20% to 30% and overall survival of less than 10 months.[130]

Radiation therapy has long played a major role in the treatment of locally advanced cervical cancer. Standard treatment for advanced cervical cancer is radical external-beam radiation therapy plus brachytherapy. It is important that appropriate dosing is administered to the central tumor and the pelvic side wall nodes. Intracavitary brachytherapy (ICBT) is an integral component of standard radiation therapy for cervical cancer and enables delivery of high dose radiation to the central tumor volume with relative sparing of surrounding normal organs, such as the bladder and rectum. Extended-field radiation therapy with concomitant cisplatin and ICBT produces significant acute toxicity but relatively low long-term toxicity.[131]

Concurrent cisplatin-based chemo-radiation is now considered the treatment of choice in locally advanced, metastatic, and recurrent cervical cancer.[132] The recurrence rate of cervical cancer is between 10% and 20% for FIGO stages Ib-IIa and 50% to 70% in locally advanced cases (stages IIb-IVa).[133] Unfortunately, the 5-year survival for patients with recurrent or persistent cervical cancer is less than 5%.[134] Treatment of recurrent disease depends on previous treatment, site or extent of recurrence, disease-free interval and patient's performance status. Chemotherapy is appropriate for patients with recurrent, metastatic, or persistent carcinoma of the cervix for whom treatment with potentially curative intent is no longer amenable. The combination of cisplatin and topotecan may prolong survival in this patient group; although the response time is typically short.[134] Several single-agent regimens have been tested, but none has been found to be superior to cisplatin. Both topotecan and paclitaxel in combination with cisplatin have yielded superior response rates and progression-free survival without diminishing patient quality of life.[135] However, only the combination of cisplatin and topotecan has improved overall survival.[136]

Pelvic exenteration may be considered in selected cases of central pelvic recurrence after radiation therapy, when there is no evidence of distant metastases. In cases of tumor involvement of pelvic wall, exenteration is no longer feasible. Pelvic exenteration involves removal of the bladder, urethra, genital organs (including vulva/vagina), parts of the perineum and anus/rectum. This may be modified according to the caudal extension of tumor and with regard to leaving a pelvic organ in situ (anterior or posterior exenteration). This extensive procedure can result in significant changes to the patient's self-perception of body image and result in significant lifestyle changes.

Most cervical cancer patients are diagnosed at a relatively young age, and most live for many years with the sequelae of the disease and its treatment. Early detection and improved treatment programs significantly affect survival.[137] In survivors treated with surgery alone or a combination of therapies, the most frequent symptoms are crampy pain in the abdomen or belly (17%), urinary leakage (15%), menopausal symptoms (18%), and problems with sexual activity.[138] Patients treated with radiation may be more associated with reduced QoL than patients treated with surgery or chemotherapy.[139] These problems may persist even after 2 to 10 years.[140] In patients treated with radiation, problems with bowel or bladder function are not unusual. Patients may report frequent urination and urge incontinence, fecal leakage, severe diarrhea, and dyspareunia.[141] Others complications of treatment include vesicovaginal and rectal-vaginal fistulas which may be associated with intractable pelvic pain. Postradiation vesicovaginal fistulas are difficult to surgically repair because of poor vascularity and tissue healing.[142]

Cervical cancer is a potentially preventable disease. Invasive cervical cancer is often asymptomatic, although patients may report vaginal discharge and postcoital vaginal bleeding. In some cases, patients present with advanced disease that extends beyond the cervix and involves pelvic lymph nodes, resulting in lower extremity edema, deep venous thrombosis, or ureteral obstruction. Cervical cancer often recurs in a local or regional distribution, in the form of pelvic or para-aortic adenopathy, but it may also metastasize to distant sites, such as the lungs and bone. Because local recurrence is often a component of relapse, patients may have pelvic pain and lower-extremity edema due to lymphatic obstruction; they may eventually die from ureteral obstruction. Some patients have a local pelvic relapse without evidence of distant disease. Most patients with recurrent cervical cancer have disease at both local and distant sites.

Cervical cancer can cause somatic, visceral, or neuropathic pain. Local invasion of somatic structures within the pelvis such as the pelvic side wall or the obturator muscles may cause pelvic pain or pain with hip movement. In addition, infiltration of the sacrum or presacral region may result in severe back pain. Visceral pain may ensue from bladder or bowel infiltration. Pain from the cervix is typically felt over the lower back and sacral area and can also be referred to the hypogastrium. Malignant infiltration of the adjacent lumbosacral plexus may result in severe neuropathic pain. Tumor invasion of the bladder may manifest with a variety of urinary symptoms (including dysuria, frequency, and hematuria) and deep pelvic pain. Retroperitoneal lymphadenopathy in the pelvis or abdomen may manifest as complaints of back or pelvic pain. Advanced cervical cancer may present with unilateral edema, sciatic nerve pain, and ureteral obstruction suggesting unresectable pelvic side wall extension.

OVARIAN CANCER

Ovarian carcinomas are a heterogeneous group of neoplasms and are traditionally subclassified based on type and degree of differentiation. Ovarian cancer is the sixth most common cancer and the seventh cause of death from cancer in women (4.0% of cases and 4.2% deaths). Incidence rates are highest in developed countries, with rates in these areas exceeding 9 per 100,000, except for Japan (6.4 per 100,000).[9]

More than 90% of ovarian cancers arise from cells that make up the epithelial layer that covers the surface of the ovaries. Germ cell tumors (5% of total) and stromal tumors (5% of total) constitute the remainder. Stromal tumors arise in the hormonally active cells within the connective tissue stroma of the ovary. The most lethal gynecologic malignancy in the United States, with approximately 22,000 new cases and 16,000 deaths occurring annually, is the epithelial ovarian cancer. The incidence of ovarian cancer increases with age and peaks in the eighth decade. Epithelial ovarian cancer is infrequent before the age of 40 years. The median age of diagnosis is 63 years and 48% of patients are 65 years old or older.[143] The germline mutation in the gene *BRCA1* increases the lifetime risk of ovarian cancer to 40%, whereas in women with germline mutations in *BRCA2*, the lifetime risk increases to 10%–20%.

Most women are diagnosed with ovarian cancer after the disease has already disseminated throughout the abdominal cavity. Three fourths of ovarian carcinomas are not discovered until they have reached an advanced stage.[144] Frequent presenting symptoms include abdominal discomfort, poorly localized pain, abdominal fullness, changes in bowel habits, early satiety, dyspepsia, and bloating. Occasionally, patients may present with bowel obstruction due to intra-abdominal masses or shortness of breath due to pleural effusion. Early-stage ovarian cancer is usually asymptomatic, and the diagnosis is often incidental, although such patients may occasionally present with dyspareunia or pelvic pain due to ovarian torsion. The primary assessment of a pelvic mass includes serum CA-125 level as a marker for a possible epithelial ovarian cancer (Fig. 7.8). False-positive results can be associated with peritoneal inflammation, such as endometriosis, adenomyosis, pelvic inflammatory disease, menstruation, uterine fibroids, or benign cysts. Increased CA-125 levels can be seen with other malignancies as well; but the most marked elevations (>1500 U/mL) are found exclusively with ovarian cancer.

Cytoreductive surgery is the primary treatment of patients with advanced ovarian cancer. The goal of surgery is not only to document the extent of disease but also to perform surgical cytoreduction or tumor debulking. Cytoreductive surgery for ovarian cancer is most often performed at the time of diagnosis (primary cytoreduction). It is also performed during primary chemotherapy (interval cytoreduction) and after disease recurrence (secondary cytoreduction). Early stage surgery usually involves total abdominal hysterectomy, bilateral salgingo-oophorectomy, omentectomy, random peritoneal biopsies including the paracolic gutters, and plevic para-aortic lymph node sampling.[145] In younger patients wanting to conserve fertility with localized, unilateral tumors (stage I) and favorable histology, unilateral salpingo-oophorectomy may not be associated with a significantly higher risk of recurrence. Wedge biopsy of the contralateral ovary should be performed, if the contralateral ovary is not normal on inspection. Advanced stage disease surgery includes total abdominal hysterectomy and bilateral salpingo-oophorectomy with omentectomy, as well as staging biopsies. Progression of disease within the abdomen may compromise the intestinal lumen resulting in intestinal obstruction and necessitate surgical relief of the obstruction. The most common site of obstruction is the small intestine.

Most patients in remission are followed with a combination of pelvic examinations, abdominal CT scans, and serum CA-125 levels. CA-125 can accurately predict tumor relapse and should be performed at each follow-up visit. CT scans should be performed if there is clinical or CA-125 evidence for progressive disease.

The use of radiation therapy in the management of ovarian cancer is controversial. Systemic therapy for ovarian cancer consists of a combination of a platinum agent (cisplatin or carboplatin) and a taxane (paclitaxel or docetaxel)l. Although the majority of patients achieve clinical complete remission after six cycles of chemotherapy, the relapse rate stands at over 50%.[146] Median survival time for patients after recurrence is approximately 2 years. New treatment approaches for patients with advanced ovarian cancer include consolidation and maintenance therapy, intraperitoneal administration of cytotoxic agents, new combination chemotherapy regimens, the development of new cytotoxic agents, and molecular-targeted therapies. Women with optimally debulked stage II ovarian cancer may benefit from a combination of

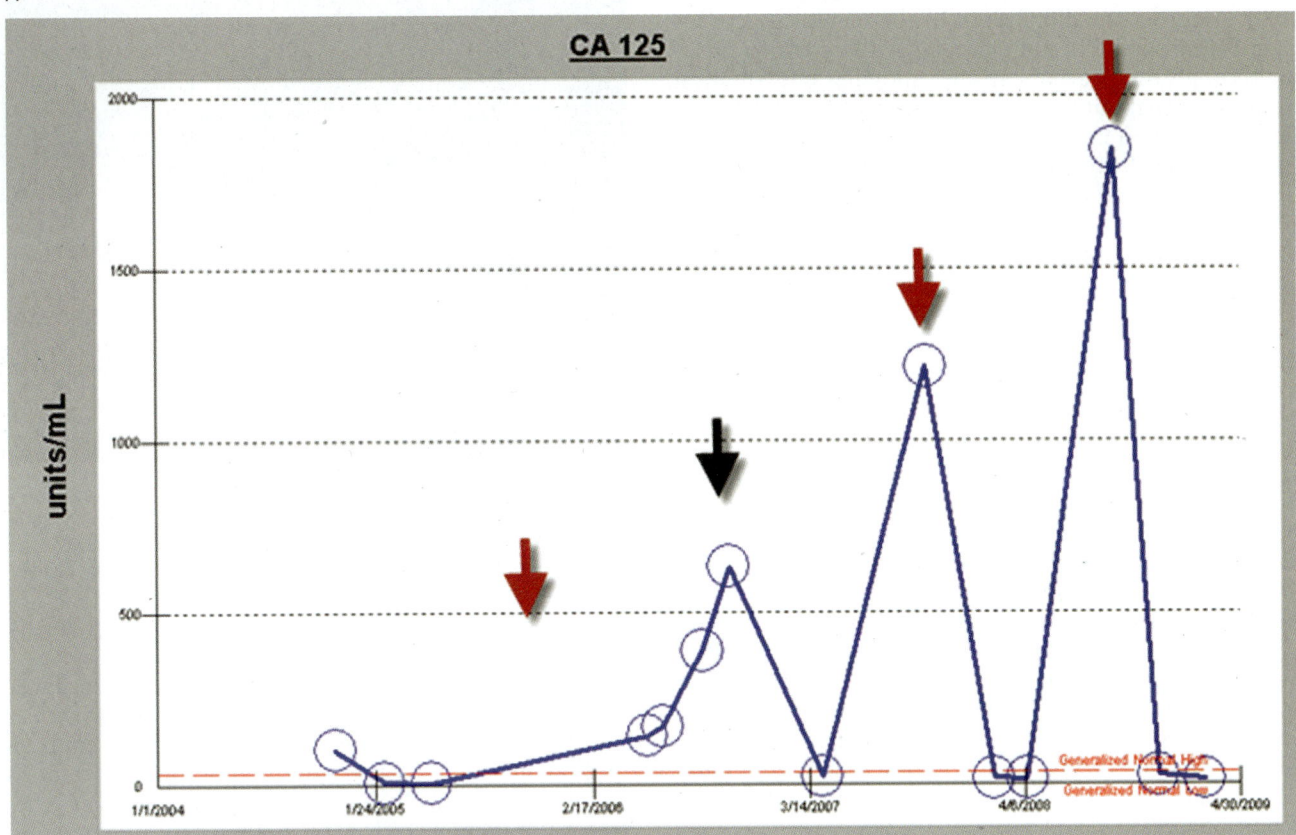

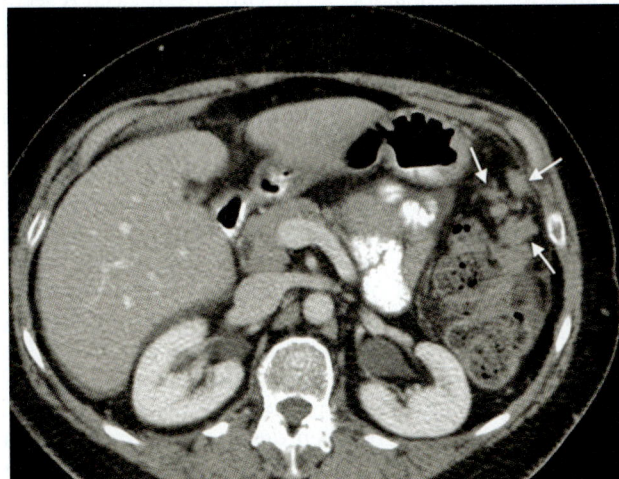

FIGURE 7.8 A 59-year-old woman with recurrent ovarian carcinoma. She was originally diagnosed with ovarian cancer in 2002. She was initially treated with TAH-BSO, omentectomy and a sigmoid resection with end-to-end reanastomosis. Her disease was very responsive to chemotherapy and responses were assessed by serial measurements of CA-125 (**A**). She received six cycles of taxotere and carboplatin in April of 2005 for recurrence *(red arrow)*. She received pelvic radiation therapy for pelvic recurrence in April of 2006 *(black arrow)*. Additional six cycles of taxotere and carboplatin in October of 2007. Patient completed six cycles of carboplatin and taxotere with amifostine after a CT scan showed disease recurrence in August 2008. Axial CT (**B**) shows several foci of soft tissue density in the left anterior omentum, adjacent to the left colon suggestive of metastatic disease. CT, Computed tomography.

intravenous and intraperitoneal chemotherapy. The combination of IV and IP chemotherapy is associated with a clinically significant benefit in survival, although it may increase toxicity compared to IV chemotherapy alone.[147]

The majority of patients with ovarian cancer achieve a clinical complete remission with first-line chemotherapy, but the disease will recur in most. Systemic therapy for recurrent ovarian cancer is not curative. No evidence either supports or refutes the use of more than one line of chemotherapy in patients with platinum-refractory or platinum-resistant recurrence.[148] The 5-year survival rate for patients with advanced ovarian cancer is approximately 30%. Most patients with ovarian cancer will respond to platinum-taxane combination chemotherapy. The issue of how many treatment regimens to use in patients with advanced ovarian cancer is controversial. Since subsequent chemotherapies have low response rates, patients need to decide whether to continue chemotherapy or receive supportive care only.

The prevalence of pain associated with ovarian cancer resembles the prevalence rates in populations with other solid tumors.[149] Ovarian cancer spreads by intraperitoneal, lymphatic, and locally invasive pathways. Lymphatic pathways for tumor spread include the abdominal retroperitoneum to the groin via the inguinal/femoral canals or across the diaphragm to the pleural space. Intraperitoneal spread of tumor begins with extension of tumor through the ovarian capsule, allowing implantation of tumor throughout the abdomen. Intraperitoneal metastases are common in the omentum and diaphragm, but no organ is spared, and concomitant ascites is frequent. Portenoy et al.[149] noted that pain, fatigue, and psychological distress were the most prevalent symptoms in patients with advanced (stage III or IV) ovarian cancer. Women usually describe frequent or almost constant, moderate to severe intensity pain as occurring in the abdomino-pelvic or lower back region. Pain in the lower extremities due to invasion of the lumbosacral plexus by tumor or from lymphedema secondary to iliac vessel occlusion is common as the disease advances.

PANCREATIC CANCER

The incidence of pancreatic carcinoma in Europe and North America has remained unchanged in the past 30 years. It is estimated that 9 to 10 cases per 100,000 will occur per annum, with slightly increased male:female and black:white ratios. In Western countries, pancreatic cancer is now the fifth most common cause of cancer-related deaths.[150] Risk factors for cancer of the pancreas include age (50 years and older), male sex, race (black), smoking, a diet high in meats and fat, presence of diabetes or chronic pancreatitis, and a family history.

Histologically, the pancreatic parenchyma is divided in two components: the exocrine portion, which is composed of ducts and acini, and the endocrine component, which is composed of hormone-secreting cells arranged in islets (islets of Langerhans). Pancreatic cancer usually arises in the exocrine component of the gland, and almost all of these tumors exhibit ductal differentiation. Tumors arising in the epithelium lining the pancreatic duct represent 85% of all pancreatic tumors, with the acinar cell tumors comprising less than 1% of them. Tumors arising from the islets of Langerhans are called islet cell tumors and comprise 1% to 2% of all pancreatic cancers. Only 23% of patients with cancer of the exocrine pancreas will survive for 1 year, and about 4% will survive for 5 years.

The majority of patients with pancreatic adenocarcinoma have an advanced stage of disease when the diagnosis is first established. The prognosis for these patients is poor, with a 1-year survival rate of 20% and a 5-year survival rate of less than 5%. Local tumor extension commences in the peripancreatic fat tissue by direct invasion of lymphatic channels and the perineural spaces. Tumors located in the pancreatic head commonly infiltrate the duodenum, stomach, gall bladder, and peritoneum (Fig. 7.9). Body and tail tumors often invade the liver, spleen, and left adrenal gland. Lymphatic spread to adjacent and distant lymph nodes occurs before hematogenous spread. The organs most likely to be invaded are liver, peritoneum, lungs, adrenals, kidneys, bones, and brain, in descending order. Early, relatively limited disease is painful in one third to two thirds of patients; this increases to over 80% with advanced pancreatic cancer.[151–152]

Many factors contribute to the generation and perpetuation of pancreatic cancer pain (Table 7.3). Extensive

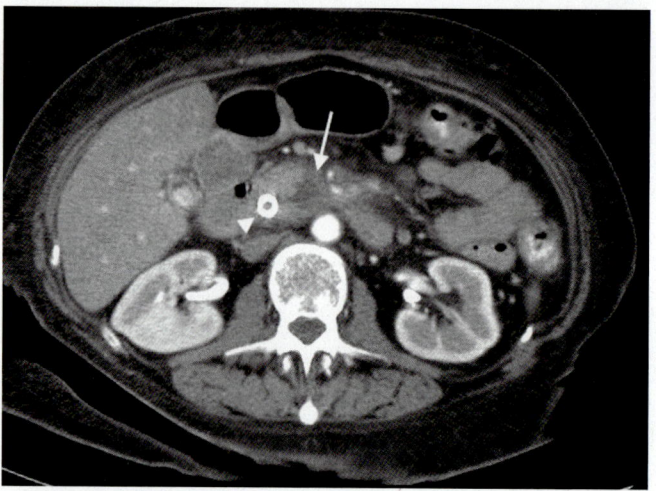

FIGURE 7.9 A 59-year-old woman with intractable epigastric pain secondary to pancreatic adenocarcinoma. CT shows a 2.3- × 2.4-cm mass in the head of the pancreas encompassing the superior mesenteric artery *(arrow)*. There is also a stent in the common bile duct *(arrow head)*. CT, Computed tomography.

macrophage infiltration accompanies pancreatic cancer.[153] This is associated with upregulation of nerve growth factor (NGF) which is correlated with both the extent of perineural invasion of the tumor and the reported pain intensity.[154] It is likely that macrophages and other inflammatory or immune cells play an important role in pain associated with pancreatic cancer; they are commonly seen in large numbers in association with this disease. A second mechanism that may be involved in pancreatic cancer pain is the apparent sprouting (in precancerous and early stage pancreatic cancer) and then destruction (in late stage disease) of sensory and sympathetic fibers that innervate the pancreas. Disease progression is associated with an increase in the density of CGRP sensory fibers.[155] This increase in density of CGRP fibers may represent NGF-induced sprouting; macrophages are known to elaborate NGF. As pancreatic cancer evolves, the central area of head, body and tail of the pancreas, containing CGRP fibers, gradually becomes necrotic, resulting in destruction of the distal ends of the sensory and sympathetic fibers that had innervated these regions of the pancreas.[155] Peripheral nerve damage can produce neuropathic pain. The extensive sprouting and then destruction of sensory and sympathetic fibers may contribute to the sensitization and activation of the nerve fibers innervating the pancreas.

The most common presenting symptom of patients with pancreatic adenocarcinoma of the pancreatic head is jaundice. Pain due to pancreatic cancer is usually upper abdominal, but it can also involve the lower abdomen or even be diffuse[156] (Table 7.3). Back pain is present with the abdominal pain in one half of cases, but only 5% to 10% of patients report back pain as their only complaint.[157] In one series, 67% of patients could not describe their pain location better than as over their "diffuse abdomen."[157] Pain can also be generated by direct infiltration of pancreatic afferent nerves, pancreatic duct obstruction with retention pancreatitis, biliary obstruction, or duodenal infiltration resulting in bowel obstruction. The pain often is aggravated by eating. Tumors of the head of the pan-

TABLE 7.3

PANCREATIC CANCER PAIN SYNDROMES

Pain Due to Tumor Involvement	Pain Due to Cancer Therapies
Visceral pain: • Pancreatic gland infiltration • Gastric infiltration • Duodenal infiltration • Liver metastases: capsule distention, diaphragmatic irritation • Biliary tree distention • Bowel obstruction (duodenal, peritoneal carcinomatosis) • schemic abdominal pain due to mesenteric vessel involvement	Postoperative pain syndromes: • Delayed gastric emptying • Wound dehiscence or nonhealing
Somatic pain: • Retroperitoneal involvement (direct, nodal) • Parietal peritoneum and abdominal wall involvement • Abdominal distention due to ascites • Bone metastases and vertebral compression	Procedure-related pain: • Biliary prosthesis complications • Externalized drains
Neuropathic pain: • Radiculopathy from retroperitoneal spread or bone metastatic involvement • Lumbosacral plexopathy • Epidural spinal cord compression	Postchemotherapy pain syndromes: • Liver chemoembolization • Mucositis Postradiation pain syndromes: • Radiation enteritis

(From Caraceni A, Portenoy RK. Pain management in patients with pancreatic carcinoma. *Cancer*. 1996;78 (3Suppl):639–653. Copyright 1996 American Center Society. This material is reproduced with permission of Wiley Liss, Inc., a subsidiary of John Wiley & Sons, Inc.)

creas have been said to cause epigastric pain with right-flank radiation, whereas pain from tumors in the tail have left-sided radiation.[158] Back pain in the lumbosacral junction is very common and may be the first symptom in 10% to 30% of cases. Back pain may be relieved by sitting and aggravated by lying flat. This pain is probably caused by retroperitoneal tumor involvement, and celiac plexus block may not relieve it.

Pancreatic pain often has a devastating impact. It is frequently accompanied by depression, loss of appetite, and digestive disorders. The pain certainly contributes to the rapid decline in function that characterizes this disease.[157–159] As disease progresses, malignant ascites can develop resulting in significant abdominal pain due to distension. Malignant ascites is one of the poor prognostic factors for pancreatic cancer, and causes serious symptoms and treatment-related toxicity.[160]

The only potentially curative treatment available at this time is complete surgical resection. A resectable pancreatic tumor cannot manifest extrapancreatic disease or tumor extension to the celiac axis and superior mesenteric artery. Pancreaticoduodenectomy is the standard procedure in pancreatic surgery, because most pancreatic ductal carcinomas arise in the head of the pancreas. For many years, the classical Whipple procedure was the surgical procedure of choice for tumors located in the head of the pancreas.[161] It consists of the resection of the pancreatic head and duodenum along with a distal gastrectomy, cholecystectomy, removal of the common bile duct and proximal jejunum, and en bloc resection of regional lymph nodes.[162] Other surgical procedures include a pylorus-sparing pancreaticoduodenectomy, distal pancreatectomy for tumors located in the pancreatic body or tail, and total pancreatectomy and segmental resection for rare indications.

Advanced or metastatic pancreatic cancer is an incurable disease. The main treatment is chemotherapy with cytotoxic agents. Responses remain low; 5% to 25% of patients have a partial response, life prolongation is significantly achieved versus best supportive care, and clinical benefit is observed in 40% to 60% of patients. Rarely do patients survive for more than 2 years, and no patient is cured. The standard cytotoxic treatment is with gemcitabine. The addition of other agents, such as erlotinib, cisplatin, irinotecan, oxaliplatin and taxanes, in combination with gemcitabine, has shown higher response rates, but overall survival has not significantly increased.[163] Symptomatic treatment is critical in the management of pancreatic cancer and metastatic disease. Stenting of the bile or pancreatic ducts and/or bypass surgery for obstructive jaundice or gastric outlet/duodenal obstruction can ameliorate symptoms and signs and improve quality of life.

RENAL CELL CANCERS

Renal cell carcinoma (RCC) encompasses a histologically diverse group of solid tumors, contributing to about 3% of all adult neoplasms.[69] Mortality from RCC appears not to have decreased significantly and may even be rising.[164] The most common histologic subtypes are clear-cell and papillary RCC. Other histologic subtypes include chromophobe RCC, collecting duct carcinoma, and unclassified RCC. Most RCCs now are discovered as incidental radiographic findings discovered during workup of unrelated conditions.[165] RCC originates in the renal cortex. RCCs comprise 85% to 90% of renal masses that are radiologically demonstrated to be solid. Von Hippel-Lindau disease is a familial multiple-cancer syndrome in which there is a predisposition to a variety of cancers including RCC. There are no effective serum tumor markers for diagnosis of RCC at this time. Almost one third of patients have overt metastases at the time of initial diagnosis. Although clear-cell RCCs account for only 80% of primary malignant renal tumors, 90% of the tumors that metastasize are derived from the conventional clear type. The classical clinical presentation of flank pain, hematuria, and a palpable flank mass is relatively uncommon (approximately 5% to 10% of cases).

The tumor can extend directly into the perinephric fat, ipsilateral adrenal gland, or adjacent musculature, and, less frequently, the liver, spleen, pancreas, and colon. Rarely, the tumor may invade the renal collecting system. RCC has a propensity for extending, as tumor thrombus, into the tributaries of the renal veins and subsequently to the main renal vein, the inferior vena cava, the hepatic veins, and potentially the right atrium. Hematogenous metastases are more common and occur earlier than lymphatic dissemination, the former most commonly to the lungs and bone, but essentially to any organ, including the subcutaneous tissues and skeletal muscle. Common sites for metastases include the lung (50% to 60% of patients with metastases), bone (30% to 40%), liver (30% to 40%), and brain (5%). Unusual sites of metastases are typical of renal cancer, however, and may involve virtually any organ site, including the thyroid, pancreas, skeletal muscle, and skin or underlying soft tissue (Fig. 7.10). The regional lymph nodes of the kidney are renal hilar, paracaval, aortic (para-aortic, periaortic, lateral aortic), and retroperitoneal. Papillary RCC are less likely to metastasize than clear-cell RCC, but metastatic lesions may have a worse prognosis than clear-cell metastases.

Surgical resection is the principal treatment for renal-cell carcinomas. Radical nephrectomy includes resection of kidney, perirenal fat, and ipsilateral adrenal gland. The procedure is considered "radical" when it includes excision of the perirenal fat, including the ipsilateral adrenal gland, and a lymph node dissection. The dissection involves the region from the diaphragmatic crus to the aortic bifurcation of the ipsilateral, and possibly the contralateral aspects of the IVC or the aorta. The ideal extent and potential benefit of lymphadenectomy remain controversial. In 10% to 20% of patients, nodal involvement is found at surgery although clinically evident distant metastases cannot be found.[166–167] However, almost all such patients subsequently relapse with distant metastases despite their lymphadenectomy.[167] Although an occasional patient may be cured by resection of a lymph node metastasis, in most patients the benefit of lymphadenectomy is limited to the prognostic information it provides. RCC is extremely radioresistant, but palliative radiation therapy is considered appropriate for brain and bone metastases. Local recurrence in the nephrectomy bed occurs in approximately 20% to 40% of patients, typically in the first 5 years after nephrectomy;[168] the risks appear highest when resection margins are not tumor-free.

Survival is primarily determined by the anatomical extent of the tumor, ie, the pathologic stage. Patients with low-stage, low grade, and often incidentally detected renal

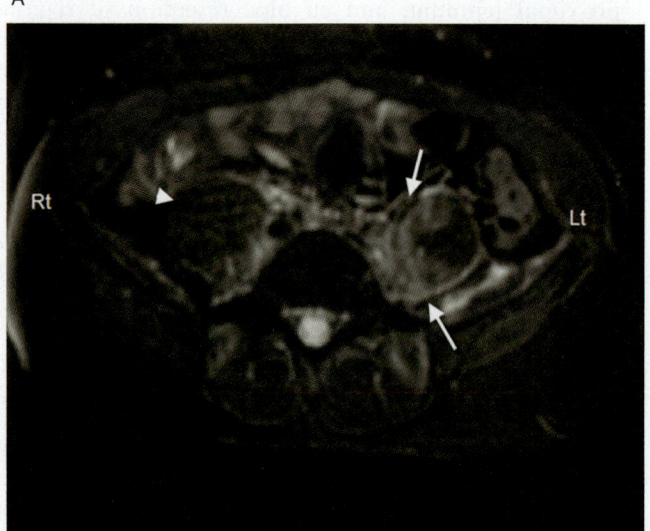
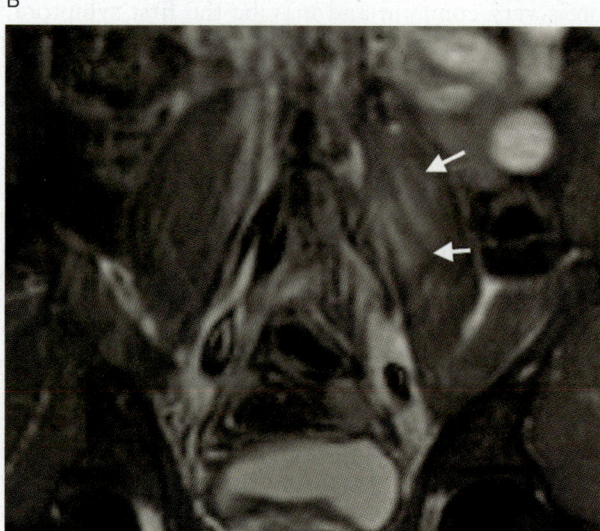

FIGURE 7.10 A 43-year-old man with metastatic renal cell carcinoma. Patient previously underwent a left radical nephrectomy. Two years later, patient presented complaining of severe left hip and thigh pain. On examination, the patient had severe pain with left hip flexion and internal rotation. Axial T1 MRI (**A**) shows patchy irregular signal within left psoas muscle *(arrows)* suggestive of recurrent disease. Normal psoas muscle is outlined on right *(arrow heads)*. Coronal STIR (**B**) shows abnormal signal within left psoas *(arrows)*. Patient's pain was attributed to locally recurrent disease within the psoas muscle with upper lumbar plexus involvement. MRI, magnetic resonance imaging.

tumors have a favorable long-term prognosis. Patients with organ-confined disease that is resected completely usually have better outcomes than those with nodal involvement or distant metastases. For patients with clinically localized disease, the 5-year relative survival rates range from 90% for patients with organ-confined disease to 62% for patients with regional spread, and for patients with distant metastases 9%.[169] Twenty to 30 percent of patients with localized tumors relapse after radical nephrectomy. Local recurrences occur in 5%, whereas lung metastases are the most common sites of distant relapse, occurring in 50% to 60% of patients.[170-171] After nephrectomy, the median time before a relapse is 15 to 18 months, and 85% of relapses occur within 3 years.[170-171] In metastatic RCC, surgery does not usually alter disease progression.[172]

Metastatic RCC is generally resistant to standard chemotherapy, radiation therapy, and hormonal therapy. Response rates of <10% have been reported with frequently used chemotherapeutic agents (gemcitabine, fluorouracil, capecitabine, vinblastine).[173] High dose cytokine therapy (interferon[INF]-α, interleukin[IL]-2) is used for advanced cases of RCC but is associated with significant toxicity and relatively poor responses.[174] A better understanding of the molecular biology of RCC has identified the vascular endothelial growth factor (VEGF) and platelet-derived growth factor signaling pathways as rational targets for anticancer therapy. The multitargeted receptor tyrosine kinase inhibitors sunitinib (Sutent) and sorafenib (Nexavar) have both demonstrated improved efficacy as second-line therapy in patients with RCC.[175] Sunitinib is also considered first-line treatment for advanced and/or metastatic RCC. Bevacizumab (Avastin) may also be beneficial for patients with advanced disease.[176] Bone metastasis from RCC is relatively resistant to standard forms of treatment such as radiation and chemotherapy.[177] Metastatic RCC to bone may result in significant morbidity including severe, persistent pain, pathologic fractures, and spinal compression from vertebral disease. Bone metastases from RCC are classically lytic with a higher risk of fracture than with metastases from other cancers.

In a study of symptom burden among patients with RCC, Harding et al.[178] reported that patients who were diagnosed with either localized or metastatic disease and underwent surgery, had a high symptom prevalence. The symptoms most apparent among the localized RCC patients included irritability, pain, fatigue, worry, and sleep disturbance, whereas the metastatic-stage patients also had symptoms related to treatment and disease progression, including weakness and shortness of breath. Patients treated with IL-2 or in combination with INFα-2b may manifest depressive symptoms early in treatment.[179] Patients treated with IL-2 or INFα-2b may report sleep disturbance, loss of appetite, depressed activity levels, loss of interest in usual activities, and mood and cognitive disorders.[180-181]

RCC is a challenging disease in many different aspects. The disease is difficult to diagnose early. Cure of disease depends on successful surgical resection which is the only known effective treatment for localized disease. Advanced disease has limited treatment options and is associated with significant morbidity. The most successful existing medical therapies for metastatic disease are based on nonspecific stimulation of the immune system, but these therapies induce durable remissions in only a minority of patients.[182] Pain management can be challenging throughout the course of treatment.

MULTIPLE MYELOMA

Myeloma is a general term for a group of plasma cell dyscrasias. Incidence rates increase with age, particularly after age 40 years, and are higher in men, particularly African American men.[183] Myeloma constitutes 0.8% of all cancers worldwide. Incidence rates vary from 0.4 to 5 per 100,000. It is very rare in persons under 40 years of age.[9] The 5-year survival rate for patients with myeloma is 15% to 20%. Multiple myeloma is the ninth most common cause of cancer death among U.S. women and the fourteenth most common cause of cancer death among U.S. men, accounting for approximately 2% of cancer deaths for each gender.[183]

The spectra of disease ranges from solitary plasmacytoma, asymptomatic, or smoldering myeloma, to the generalized and classic types of multiple myeloma. MGUS (monoclonal gammopathy of undetermined significance) is a precursor condition and is considered a premalignant disorder in which a clone of plasma cells produces a monoclonal paraprotein. Patients with MGUS most often progress to the typical form of symptomatic multiple myeloma, but they may also develop amyloidosis or macroglobulinemia instead.

Multiple myeloma is a malignant disorder characterized by the proliferation of a single clone of plasma cells derived from B cells in the bone marrow. Normally, plasma cells produce immunoglobulins to resist infection. Immunoglobulin consists of two linked heavy chains with one light chain attached to each. Monoclonal myeloma plasma cells overproduce M protein (abnormal IgG, IgM, IgA, IgE, or IgD). The M protein is named in reference to its monoclonal characteristics. It may be found in serum or urine and is detected by electrophoresis or immunofixation. Multiple myeloma cells also produce abnormal light chain proteins (κ or λ), known as Bence Jones protein. The immunoglobulin disorder is IgG in 52%, IgA in 21%, free κ in 9%, free λ in 7%, negative M protein in 7%, biclonal in 2%, IgD in 2%, and IgM in 0.5%. Excessive M protein level causes hyperviscosity; excessive light chain proteins can cause end-organ damage (especially renal); and invasive bone lesions may cause bone pain, osteoporosis, and hypercalcemia. Up to 20% of patients with multiple myeloma lack heavy-chain expression in the M protein and are considered to have light-chain multiple myeloma. The M protein in these patients is always detected in urine but can be absent in serum, even by multiple myeloma immunofixation, making it imperative that protein electrophoresis and multiple myeloma immunofixation are always performed on both serum and urine in all patients in whom multiple myeloma is suspected. Myeloma is characterized by a large increase in M protein, which appears as a "spike" on electrophoresis. Diagnosis depends on the identification of abnormal monoclonal plasma cells in the bone marrow, M protein in the serum or urine, evidence of end-organ damage, and a clinical picture consistent with multiple myeloma. The clinical and laboratory abnormalities in myeloma are shown in Table 7.4.

TABLE 7.4
CLINICAL AND LABORATORY ABNORMALITIES IN MYELOMA

Clinical/Laboratory Features	Proportion of Patients with Abnormality (%)
Anemia <12 g/dL	72
Bone lesions (lytic lesion, pathologic fractures, or severe osteopenia)	80
Renal failure (serum creatinine =2 mg/dL	19
Hypercalcemia (≥11 mg/dL)	13
Monoclonal protein in serum protein electrophoresis	82
Monoclonal protein on serum protein immunofixation	93
Monoclonal protein on serum plus urine protein immunofixation (or serum immunofixation plus serum free light-chain assay)	97
Type of M protein:	
IgM	52
IgA	21
Light-chain only	16
Increased ≥10% clonal bone marrow plasma cells	96

(From Kyle RA, Rajkumar SV. Criteria for diagnosis, staging, risk stratification, and response assessment of multiple myeloma. *Leukemia*. 2009;23:3–9. Copyright 2009. Reprinted by permission from Macmillan Publishers Ltd.)

Multiple myeloma produces a constellation of disease manifestations, including osteolytic lesions due to uncoupled bone metabolism, anemia and immunosuppression due to loss of normal hematopoietic stem cell function, and end-organ damage due to monoclonal multiple myeloma immunoglobulin secretion. The most common presenting symptoms of multiple myeloma are fatigue, bone pain, and recurrent infections. Anemia is present in 70% of patients at diagnosis. Hypercalcemia is found in one fourth of patients, whereas the serum creatinine level is elevated in almost one half. Conventional radiography shows skeletal abnormalities in approximately 80% of patients. The M protein can be detected by serum protein electrophoresis in 82% of patients and by multiple myeloma immunofixation in 93%. However, the spectrum of presentation of multiple myeloma is broad. At one end of this spectrum are the entities of plasmacytoma, smoldering (asymptomatic) or indolent multiple myeloma, and all multiple myeloma arising from MGUS manifested with focal bone marrow involvement. These patients have a serum M protein at less than "myeloma levels" and unrelated clinical symptoms and signs. Smoldering multiple myeloma patients are typically asymptomatic but have a high risk of progression to multiple myeloma. On the other end of the spectrum is full blown, aggressive multiple myeloma which is characterized by disseminated disease, with multiorgan plasmacytic infiltration, paraproteinemia, and multiple myeloma immune dysfunction and related organ or tissue impairment. Frequently, there is invasion of the adjacent bone, which destroys skeletal structures and results in severe bone pain and fractures.

POEMS (polyneuropathy, organomegaly [most commonly liver, lymph nodes, and spleen], endocrinopathy [commonly elevated estrogens, diabetes mellitus, hypothyroidism, hyperprolactinemia, hypoparathyroidism], monoclonal gammopathy, and skin changes [commonly diffuse hyperpigmentation]) is a rare multisystemic disease that occurs in a setting of a plasma cell dyscrasia. All cases of POEMS syndrome are associated with a plasma cell disorder. Although the pathogenesis is not well understood, overproduction of VEGF probably secreted by plasma cells may be responsible.[184] The syndrome is seen in association with osteosclerotic myeloma, MGUS, and Waldenstrom macroglobulinemia, but not with classic multiple myeloma. Polyneuropathy associated with POEMS syndrome is bilateral and symmetrical involving both motor and sensory nerves. The neuropathy typically begins distally and spreads proximally. Demyelination and axonal degeneration occurs more frequently in the small rather than large, myelinated nerves.[185] Treatment of POEMS syndrome is difficult although the combination of bevacizumab (anti-VEGF monoclonal antibody) and thalidomide, followed by autologous stem cell transplant may be helpful.[186]

Multiple myeloma is a fatal hematologic malignancy associated with clonal expansion of malignant plasma cells within the bone marrow and the development of a destructive osteolytic bone disease. The principal cellular mechanisms involved in the development of myeloma bone disease are an increase in osteoclastic bone resorption and a reduction in bone formation[187] (Fig. 7.11). Skeletal lesions may also be detected by MRI, PET or CT. CT and MRI scans are more sensitive than conventional radiography in detecting bone and bone marrow involvement.[188] Among asymptomatic multiple myeloma patients with normal x-rays, up to 50% may have tumor-related abnormalities on MRI of the lower spine. One or more of these studies are indicated when symptomatic areas show no abnormality on routine radiographs. The goal of imaging is to provide an accurate assessment of the extent of

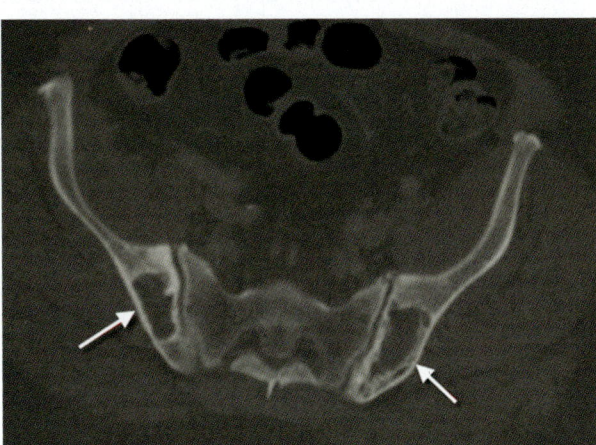
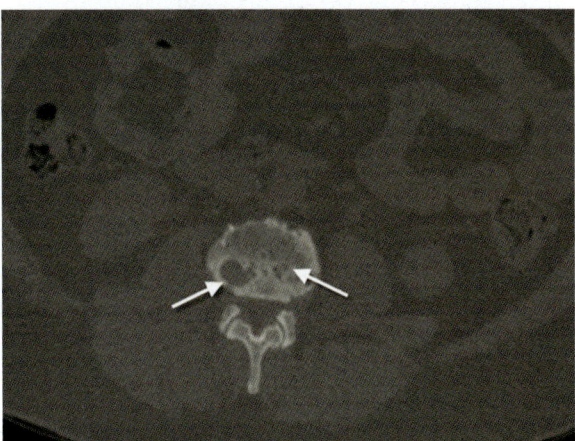

FIGURE 7.11 A 63-year-old man with multiple myeloma complaining of bilateral hip, buttock, and low back pain. CT scans show extensive lytic involvement *(arrows)* of both ilia (**A**) and vertebral body (**B**). CT, Computed tomography.

disease throughout the skeleton. Traditionally, this is done with a whole body radiographic bone survey. Patients with presumed solitary plasmacytoma of bone or soft tissue (extramedullary) plasmacytoma should have a survey and MR imaging to ensure there is only one lesion present.

Despite many significant advances in the understanding of the biology of multiple myeloma, it remains an incurable disease, and destructive osteolytic bone lesions are a major cause of morbidity. Typically, median survival is approximately 3 years[189]; some patients with multiple myeloma can live longer than 10 years. Corticosteroids, thalidomide and its analogue lenalidomide (Revlimid), and bortezomib (Velcade) are used in patients with multiple myeloma. The use of thalidomide is limited by adverse effects of sedation, constipation, neuropathy, and thromboembolism.[190] Thalidomide-associated neuropathy is not always reversible and may require discontinuation of the drug.[191] Lenalidomide does not produce significant sedation, constipation, or neuropathy, but does lead to significant myelosuppression, unlike thalidomide.[190] Single-agent bortezomib has been shown to provide significantly greater efficacy than high-dose dexamethasone, and bortezomib has also been investigated in combination with other agents commonly used to treat myeloma, including thalidomide and lenalidomide, with high overall and complete response rates.[192] As an alternative to standard-dose chemotherapy, a variety of more intense treatment strategies have been developed that involve the administration of high doses of chemotherapy and/or total body irradiation (TBI) followed by autologous or allogeneic hematopoietic stem cell transplantation. For patients who are candidates, high-dose therapy followed by autologous stem cell transplantation results in higher complete response rates and improved long-term survival compared to treatment with standard doses of chemotherapy alone. Rotta et al.[193] showed the median time to progression after transplantation was 3 years and a 5-year overall survival of 64%. Surgical fixation of fractures or impending fractures of long bones may be needed. Local radiation should be limited to patients with disabling pain who have a well-defined focal process that has not responded to analgesics and/or chemotherapy.

SARCOMAS OF SOFT TISSUE AND BONE

Sarcomas are cancers derived from primitive mesenchymal cells. Soft-tissue sarcomas are a rare and diverse group of malignant neoplasms of mesodermal tissue origin. They comprise less than 1% of all cancers, with an overall incidence of 30 to 40 per million per year.[194] Although sarcomas are a rare tumor, we discuss this tumor type because local recurrence of these tumors and surgical treatments of these tumors are frequently painful (Fig. 7.12).

The World Health Organization has defined approximately 50 tumor subtypes relevant to soft-tissue sarcomas[195]; the more common subtypes are malignant fibrous histiocytoma, liposarcoma, leiomyosarcoma, synovial sarcoma, malignant peripheral nerve sheath tumor, and rhabdomyosarcoma. Bone sarcomas are also rare, with osteosarcoma being the most common primary bone sarcoma. The most common bone sarcomas are osteosarcoma, chondrosarcoma, Ewing sarcoma, chordoma, and malignant fibrous histiocytoma/fibrosarcoma.[196] Osteosarcoma and Ewing sarcoma occur in childhood and chondrosarcoma occurs more frequently in older adults. Ewing

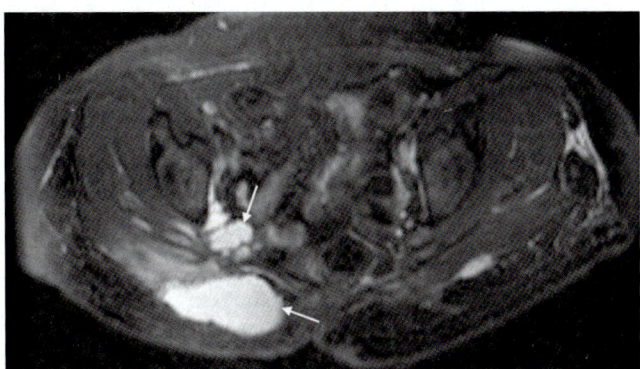

FIGURE 7.12 A 37-year-old woman with recurrent sacral chordoma complaining of pain in the right buttock and lower extremity. Axial fat-suppressed T2 MRI of pelvis. Multiple lobulated masses predominantly in the right gluteal area *(arrows)*. MRI, magnetic resonance imaging.

sarcoma is the second most common bone malignancy in children. Ewing sarcoma represents a family of tumors consisting of typical and atypical Ewing sarcoma and peripheral neuroectodermal tumor (PNET). Soft-tissue sarcomas arise predominantly in the extremities, although they may arise anywhere in the body. Approximately 40% arise in the lower extremities and girdle (predominantly thigh), 20% in the upper extremities and girdle, 10% in the trunk, 20% in the retroperitoneal and intraperitoneal sites, and 10% in the head and neck.[197] One third of malignant tumors that arise in the retroperitoneum are sarcomas, and approximately 15% of soft-tissue sarcomas arise in the retroperitoneum. Retroperitoneal sarcomas are malignant tumors arising from mesenchymal cells, which are usually located in muscle, fat, and connective tissues. Retroperitoneal sarcomas have varying clinical courses depending on their histologic subtype and grade. Bone sarcomas can arise in any bone and within any region of bone. Approximately 45% of osteosarcomas arise in the femur. Chondrosarcomas are also commonly seen in the femur and pelvis. Ewing sarcoma has a predilection for long tubular bones and the pelvis. Malignant fibrous histiocytoma of bone occurs most often in the knee region. Chordomas are the most common primary neoplasm of the adult spine, excluding lymphoproliferative tumors. Most are found in the clivus or saccrococcygeal regions but they can also occur in the cervical and lumbosacral vertebrae. Chondrosarcomas are most commonly seen in the thoracic spine but can be seen at all levels and occur usually in middle age.

The natural history of soft-tissue sarcoma varies with the histologic subtype, but is one of local recurrence, usually at the primary site, or of pulmonary metastases. The dominant pattern of metastasis is hematogenous; lymph node metastasis is rare (less than 5%). Bone metastases are unusual. Other potential sites of metastasis include the brain and the liver. Visceral and retroperitoneal sarcomas show a propensity to metastasize to the liver and peritoneum. Osteosarcoma and Ewing sarcoma share a tendency for early distant spread with metastases of osteosarcoma involving lungs in over 80%. In both osteosarcoma and Ewing sarcoma, outcomes after local or metastatic recurrence are poor, with overall survival rates of only approximately 10% to 20%.

MRI is the preferred modality for evaluating soft-tissue lesions particularly of the extremities. It provides superior soft-tissue contrast. In general, sarcomas tend to be FDG-avid, and consequently PET scanning is very helpful in initial diagnosis or recurrence. However, the role of PET scanning in sarcoma management, particularly after treatment, is not clear.[198] Contrast-enhanced CT is preferred for evaluation of retroperitoneal sarcomas. Osteosarcoma may present with both lytic and sclerotic changes; Ewing tumors are usually lytic. MRI is the essential tool to define intramedullary tumor extent, soft-tissue component and relationship of the tumor to vessels and nerves and is superior to CT for these purposes. Chest CT scans are preferred for routine follow-up of patients at risk for metastases.

Untreated, sarcomas run a relentless course, with local and often systemic disease progression. Distant metastases occur most often to the lung. Some patients with pulmonary metastases may survive for long periods after surgical resection. Patients with unresectable pulmonary metastases or extrapulmonary metastatic sarcoma have a uniformly poor prognosis and are best treated with systemic chemotherapy. The cornerstone of therapy for patients who have primary soft-tissue sarcoma is margin-negative resection. Adjuvant radiation therapy has been shown to reduce the risk of recurrence for high-grade extremity and trunk soft-tissue sarcomas,[199] although its role for retroperitoneal sarcomas is not clear. A randomized trial of preoperative versus postoperative radiation therapy demonstrated that there was an increased risk of wound complications with preoperative treatment but that the long-term morbidity was less because the treatment volumes were smaller.[200] Preoperative treatment has been adopted routinely by some centers.

The goal of bone sarcoma surgery is complete tumor removal. With primary extremity osteosarcomas, the rate of local control with chemotherapy and surgical resection is more than 90%.[201] By contrast, in osteosarcoma lesions of the head and neck, spine, and pelvis, local control with surgery and chemotherapy is less favorable. Advances in imaging techniques and in biomedical engineering as well as positive effects of preoperative chemotherapy have led to a major shift away from amputation towards limb-salvage surgery. Endoprostheses and implantation of allografts are commonly used. If unavoidable, a planned marginal excision is not associated with an increased risk of relapse, especially if this includes a resectable fascial plane or barrier such as periosteum or perineurium, compared with a true wide excision, provided it is combined with adjuvant radiation therapy. In osteosarcoma and Ewing tumors, local therapy alone is not sufficient, as 80% to 90% even of patients with seemingly localized disease will develop metastases and die if chemotherapy is not included as part of multidisciplinary treatment.[202] Treatment regimens encompassing primary (neoadjuvant) induction chemotherapy, followed by local therapy (surgery and/or radiation therapy) and then adjuvant chemotherapy lead to cure in approximately two thirds of patients with seemingly localized disease.[203-204] Neoadjuvant chemotherapy allows preparation for local therapy and assessment of histologic tumor response, an important prognostic factor in both osteosarcoma and Ewing tumors. The total duration of therapy is usually 8 to 12 months. Combinations of doxorubicin, cisplatin, high-dose methotrexate, and ifosfamide are considered the most active agents against osteosarcoma.[204] Standard chemotherapy against Ewing sarcoma is usually based on a combination of vincristine, doxorubicin (adriamycin), cyclophosphamide, and actinomycin.[205] One of the most important developments in sarcoma therapy has been the introduction of imatinib (Gleevec) for the treatment of gastrointestinal stromal tumor (GIST).[206] GIST is a rare mesenchymal tumor of the gastrointestinal tract. GIST is largely driven by activating mutations in the proto-oncogene *KIT*, a receptor tyrosine kinase. Imatinib is a protein tyrosine kinase inhibitor and is the treatment of choice for advanced inoperable or metastatic GIST. Activating mutations in the platelet-derived growth factor receptor *a* (PDGFRA) gene may also drive GIST. Since PDGFRA is also an imatinib substrate, some tumors without *KIT* mutations respond to imatinib, owing to the inhibition of PDGFRA. However, resistance to imatinib typically develops within 2 years, with the need for further therapy and the possible use of sunitinib (Sutent) in combination with imatinib for imatinib-refractory GIST.[207]

Local recurrence rates vary depending on the anatomic site. In extremity lesions one third of patients will have locally recurrent disease with a median disease-free interval of 18 months.[208] Treatment results for extremity local recurrence may approach those for primary disease. Isolated pulmonary metastases may be resected with 20% to 30% 3-year survival rates. Chemotherapy has a limited role in the primary management of most types of soft-tissue sarcoma. The efficacy of chemotherapy appears to be marginal in localized resectable soft-tissue sarcoma with respect to local recurrence, distant recurrence, overall recurrence, and overall survival.[209] However, there are diseases where chemotherapy substantially improves outcome, namely rhabdomyosarcoma and the Ewing family tumors including soft tissue Ewing sarcoma and primitive neuroectodermal tumor (PNET).

The primary symptom of a patient with a malignant bone tumor is pain, which often occurs at rest or at night. The pathophysiology of bone cancer pain has been described in detail by Sabino and Mantyh.[210] In animal models, tumor cells grow within the bone; they come into contact with, injure, and then destroy the distal processes of sensory fibers that innervate the bone marrow and mineralized bone. Sensory fibers were observed at and within the leading edge of the tumor. However, in the deep stromal regions of the tumor, sensory nerve fibers displayed a discontinuous and fragmented appearance and ultimately were undetectable by microscopy. These data correlate well with observations in humans, where sensory innervation of solid tumors is sparse and, when present, is usually associated with the blood vessels near the leading edge of the growing tumor.[211-213] Most soft-tissue sarcomas present as a painless lesion but location of the tumor influences pain. Approximately one third of patients with soft-tissue sarcoma of the chest present with pain associated with a mass.[214] Although soft-tissue sarcomas grow in a centrifugal fashion and compress normal structures, impingement on bone or neurovascular structures rarely causes pain. Similarly, retroperitoneal sarcomas are almost always observed as a large asymptomatic mass and infrequently present with obstructive gastrointestinal symptoms or neurologic symptoms related to lumbosacral plexus compression.

PRIMARY CNS NEOPLASMS

Central nervous system (CNS) tumors are a mixed group of neoplasms that vary widely by site of origin, morphologic features, genetic alterations, growth potential, extent of invasiveness, tendency for progression and recurrence, and treatment response. Primary malignant tumors of the CNS represent about 2% of all cancers in adults but account for significant morbidity and mortality.[215] Malignant tumors of the brain and spinal cord together account for approximately 2.2% of all cancer-related deaths.[216] Approximately 11 to 12 persons per 100,000 in the United States are diagnosed with a primary brain tumor each year, and 6 to 7 per 100,000 are diagnosed with a primary malignant brain tumor.[217] In the United States, the median age at diagnosis among all adults diagnosed with a primary brain tumor between 1998 and 2002 was 57 years.

Primary CNS tumors may be classified as gliomas or ngliomas. The most common gliomas are astrocytomas, oligodendrogliomas, and ependymomas. Nongliomas consist of benign tumors, such as meningiomas and pituitary adenomas, as well as malignant tumors such as medulloblastomas, and primary CNS lymphomas. Gliomas account for 40% of all tumors and 78% of malignant tumors. High-grade (malignant) glial neoplasms can arise either alone (primary glioblastoma) or from a preexisting low-grade tumor (secondary glioblastoma). Gliomas may be heterogenous, so that low-grade tumor elements may be immediately adjacent to highly malignant cells. The malignant astrocytomas—anaplastic astrocytoma and glioblastoma multiforme—are the most common glial tumors. At least 80% of malignant gliomas are glioblastomas[218] (Fig. 7.13). Gliomas can occur anywhere in the brain but usually affect the cerebral hemispheres. The peak age at onset for anaplastic astrocytomas is in the fourth or fifth decade, whereas glioblastomas usually present in the sixth or seventh decade. Most patients die of the disease, with median survival of about 3 years for anaplastic astrocytoma and 1 year for glioblastoma. It is rare for primary brain tumors to metastasize outside of the central nervous system. The major problem with gliomas is their propensity to spread by infiltration; as such, they are not localized and cannot be successfully treated by surgical excision alone. Primitive neuroectodermal tumors, such as medulloblastoma, as well as CNS germ cell tumors, and primary CNS lymphoma, frequently spread via the subarachnoid space to the leptomeninges. Ionizing radiation is the only unequivocal risk factor that has been identified for glial and meningeal neoplasms.[218] Irradiation of the cranium can increase the incidence of meningiomas by a factor of 10 and the incidence of glial tumors by a factor of 3 to 7.

Brain tumors can lead to pain whether they are intrinsic to the brain, involve the skull base, involve the vault bones of the skull, or occur in the pituitary gland. The other presenting symptoms of an intrinsic brain tumor are related to mass effect, parenchymal infiltration, and tissue destruction. Headache, the most common presenting symptom, can be related to increased intracranial pressure or to irritation of the dura or blood vessels at the base of the brain. It occurs in approximately one third of patients with intrinsic tumors. New onset of headaches in a patient who has not previously had headaches is characteristic, especially if the headaches are more severe in the morning and are associated with nausea, vomiting, or localizing or lateralizing neurologic deficits. In patients with preexisting headaches, a change in the characteristics of the headaches or an increase in their frequency and/or intensity can also herald the presence of an intracranial mass. Typically, the headache is diffuse, but it can accurately indicate the hemisphere in which the tumor is located.[219] Seizures occur in approximately one third of patients with gliomas, especially in patients with low-grade tumors. Altered mental status may develop in 15% to 20% of patients with gliomas.

Mass lesions of the pituitary gland, most commonly adenomas of the gland itself, but occasionally metastasis or other pathology, can lead to a characteristic midline vertex headache or can result in diffuse headaches. Large

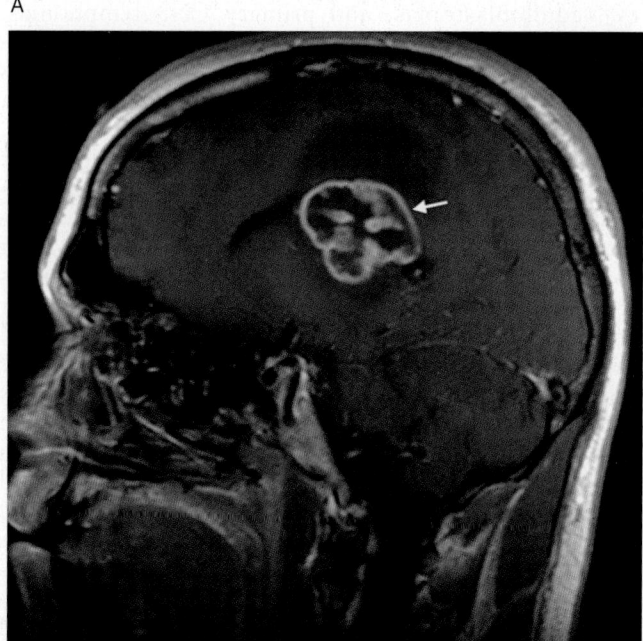
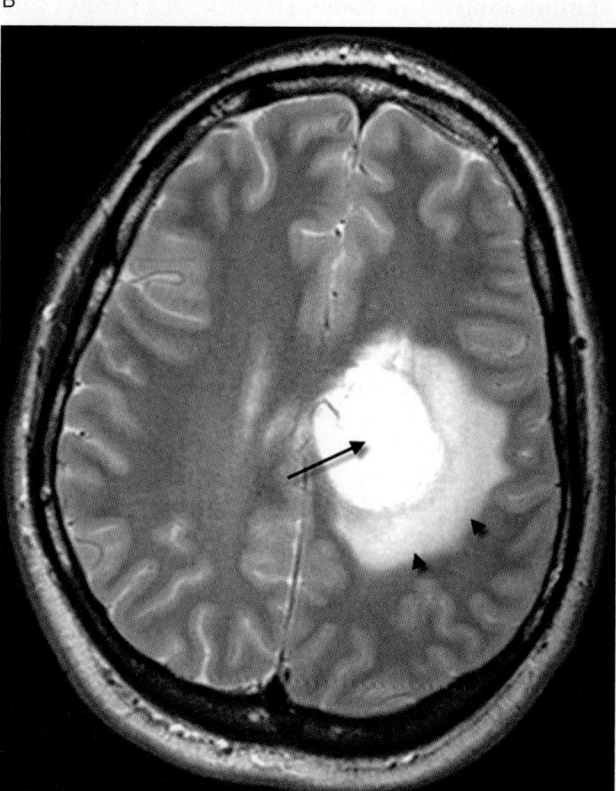

FIGURE 7.13 MRI of 24-year-old man complaining of mild headaches and right-sided hemiplegia. Surgical biopsy revealed a glioblastoma multiforme. **A:** Sagittal T1 MRI with gadolinium enhancement shows a large cyst with peripheral enhancement centered in the left corona radiata *(arrow)*. **B:** Axial T2 MRI shows the cyst *(arrow)* with associated edema *(arrow heads)*, partial effacement of the left lateral ventricle, and significant midline shift. MRI, magnetic resonance imaging.

tumors in the pituitary may compress the optic nerves or chiasm and lead to visual field defects, of which the patient may be unaware. Some of the adenomas are hormonally active; others are not but may interfere with pituitary hormone production. Apoplexy is a sudden neurologic impairment usually due to a vascular process. Classical pituitary apoplexy is a clinical syndrome characterized by sudden headache, vomiting, visual impairment, and meningismus caused by the rapid enlargement of a pituitary adenoma, usually caused by hemorrhagic infarction of the tumor.[220] Altered mental status and hormonal dysfunction also occur. Visual symptoms may include both visual acuity impairment and visual field impairment from involvement of the optic nerve or chiasm and ocular motility dysfunction from involvement of the cranial nerves traversing the cavernous sinus. Male patients and patients with functional adenoma had a higher probability of developing apoplexy.[221]

Brain tumors, intrinsic or extrinsic to the brain parenchyma, can lead to increased intracranial pressure due to the presence of a mass inside the closed box of the skull or to hydrocephalus from obstruction of cerebrospinal fluid (CSF) flow. In either case, the patient may complain of constant, diffuse headache which is characteristically worse in the morning or on lying down. Appropriate surgical intervention, rather than analgesics is the best method of dealing with the complaint of headache pain. Tumors involving the base of the skull may lead to both diffuse and focal headache as they involve osseous, dural, muscular, or neural tissues. Commonly associated lesions in this area include meningiomas, chordomas, and neurofibromas as well as malignant tumors such as carcinomas or sarcomas.

Spinal cord neoplasms are an uncommon cause of back pain. However, the most common presenting complaint of patients with primary tumors of the spinal cord is pain. Pain at rest or at night can serve as clues suggesting that further investigation is justified. In Weinstein's study, approximately 85% of patients with primary spinal tumors complained of pain; 60% complained of axial pain and 25% complained of radicular symptoms.[222] Spinal cord tumors may be intradural or extradural. Extradural tumors account for approximately 60% of spinal cord neoplasms. The most common primary extramedullary spinal cord tumors are derived from sheath cells covering the spinal nerve roots (schwannomas and neurofibromas) or meningial cells located along the spinal-cord surface (meningiomas). Local or radicular pain is the most common presenting symptom in patients with these tumors, and has highest incidence with tumors located in the lumbar spine. Paresthesia and numbness are common symptoms, and hypoesthesia or anesthesia at and below a level of the spinal cord is often evident on clinical examination. Glial tumors, such as astrocytomas and ependymomas, represent up to 80% of intramedullary spinal tumors. The majority of intramedullary spinal cord gliomas are low-grade, and they have a 5-year survival exceeding 70%.[223] Patients with intramedullary neoplasms most often present with myelopathic symptoms of insidious onset. Localized pain and upper-extremity paresthesia are the initial symptoms in 50% to 90% of the adult population with cervical intramedullary tumors.[224] Thoracic intramedullary tumors can present with lower extremity sensory loss that extends proximally with upper motor neuron signs in the lower extremities. Radicular pain becomes more prominent with intramedullary tumors of the lumbosacral spine affecting the nerve roots in the cauda equina. At the time of diagnosis, astrocytomas may be observed as elongated cysts extending several levels from the tumor location. Intramedullary spinal cord metastasis is a very uncommon complication of systemic cancer. Intramedullary metastases most often affect the conus and cervical levels of the spinal cord. Such metastases are predominantly associated with lung cancer.[225]

For years, contrast-enhanced CT has been the gold standard for the diagnosis of brain tumors because of its ability to detect a brain lesion, accurately define its dimension and relation with surrounding brain structures, assess surrounding edema, and define the presence of other lesions. CT has now been largely replaced by MRI studies, which are characterized by higher contrast resolution associated with multiplanar views. MRI is also the procedure of choice in the evaluation of intramedullary and extramedullary spinal cord lesions. However, this evaluation can be challenging, because the small size of the spinal cord makes tumor measurements difficult. Definitive diagnosis usually requires a surgical biopsy or resection with histologic examination. The characteristic appearance of an astrocytoma on MRI is that of a diffuse, nonenhancing mass that is hypointense on T1-weighted images and best seen on T2-weighted images as a bright outline. MRI may be supplemented by PET, particularly in patients who are presumed to have high-grade gliomas, which are characterized by increased FDG uptake.[226] FDG-PET, magnetic resonance (MR) spectography, and MR perfusion studies may also be helpful in distinguishing recurrent tumor from radiation necrosis.[227]

Mortality from CNS cancer has remained remarkably consistent over the past 20 years. Prognosis for most persons in whom a CNS malignancy is diagnosed remains poor. The age-adjusted 5-year relative survival was 30.8% from 1989 to 1996 in the United States, only a modest improvement from the 22.5% for those with tumors diagnosed between 1974 and 1976.[228] Survival differs only minimally by sex and race, but substantial age differences are apparent. For those aged 44 or younger at diagnosis, the average 5-year relative survival rate is 58.7%. Corresponding survival rates for ages 45 to 54 years, 55 to 64 years, 65 to 74 years, and 75 or older are 23.0%, 10.2%, 6.5%, and 3.6%, respectively.[228] Children, who tend not to develop high-grade glioblastomas, generally fare better than adults. Among those aged 19 years or younger, 5-year relative survival is 65%.

The goals of brain tumor surgery are to obtain tissue for histologic diagnosis and analysis of molecular markers, to reduce mass effect while preserving neurologic function, to reduce tumor size, and to treat hydrocephalus, if present. Surgery remains the initial therapy for nearly all patients with brain tumors and can be curative for most benign tumors, including meningiomas. Stereotactic techniques allow for biopsy specimens to be obtained from nearly any part of the brain, including the brainstem. Surgery for patients with intramedullary spinal tumors involves maximum safe resection and often, in situations of low-grade tumors, observation if a complete or near-complete resection is performed.[229] External beam radiotherapy is an essential component of treatment for many patients with brain tumors. It can be curative for some patients and prolongs survival for most. Radiation is often the primary treatment modality for patients with metastatic brain tumors, epidural spinal cord compression, and leptomeningeal metastases. Stereotactic radiosurgery techniques are beneficial for well-circumscribed lesions such as meningioma or limited brain metastases. Increasingly, stereotactic reradiation is administered for spinal cord tumors through radiosurgery technology in patients. The patients who appear to benefit most from this treatment are those with a primary spinal tumor with severe tumor-associated pain[230] or as a primary treatment for lesions not amenable to open surgical techniques, in lesions located in previously irradiated sites, or as an adjunct to surgery.[231]

Primary tumors of the adult CNS are among the most chemotherapy-resistant of neoplasms. Survival time after brain tumor diagnosis is a function of histologic type, age of the patient, and Karnofsky performance status. Relative survival is lowest for patients with glioblastoma. Less than one third of these patients survive longer than a year.[217] The most commonly used chemotherapeutic agent is temozolomide, which penetrates the intact blood-brain barrier and produces benefit in many patients with gliomas. Nitrosoureas, such as carmustine and lomustine, also have modest antitumor activity, especially in patients with oligodendroglioma, but they have been replaced by Temodar because of its lower incidence of side effects and its oral route of administration. Platinum-based drugs have antitumor efficacy for medulloblastomas and germ cell tumors, and high-dose methotrexate regimens result in clear clinical benefit for patients with primary CNS lymphomas. The success of high-dose chemotherapy and local administration of chemotherapy into a brain tumor has generally been modest: Gliadel leads to an increased survival of 12 weeks, which is the same as Temodar.[232] In a cohort of 22 patients with recurrent low-grade spinal gliomas, Chamberlain[229] demonstrated modest efficacy with acceptable toxicity with a 2-year progression free survival of 27%. New classes of drugs, including antiangiogenesis agents such as Avastin, topoisomerase inhibitors such as CPT11, and signal transduction inhibitors such as Iressa, are currently being evaluated in large, multicenter clinical trials.[233-234]

CNS tumors are a heterogeneous group of neoplasms, each with its own biology, treatment, and prognosis. In spite of advances in diagnosis, monitoring, and treatment of these tumors, morbidity from both the disease and its treatments is significant. Survival remains poor and presents a significant therapeutic challenge. Long before death, CNS tumors are likely to effect a major decrease in QoL. From the perspective of pain management, headache, both at the time of diagnosis and as a complication of craniotomy remain the major issues for most patients. Such headaches can be difficult to control with medications as well as surgical therapy.

BRAIN METASTASES

Brain metastases occur in 20% to 40% of patients with cancer, most commonly in the setting of widely disseminated disease (Fig. 7.14). They are a major cause of morbidity and mortality and are more common than primary brain tumors. Brain metastases occur most commonly in the setting of widely disseminated cancer. Brain metastases occur in 20% to 40% of patients with cancer, being symptomatic during life in 60% to 75% of these or discovered incidentally on CT/MRI and at autopsy.[235] The majority of these tumors metastasize from lung carcinoma, breast carcinoma, melanoma, renal cell carcinoma, gastrointestinal carcinoma, uterine/vulvar carcinoma, or unknown primary carcinoma.[236] In contrast, the propensity of cancers of the prostate, ovary, thyroid, and sarcomas to spread to the brain is low. The overwhelming majority of brain metastases are propagated hematogenously.

Metastatic lesions may occur anywhere within the brain parenchyma: the cerebral hemispheres, brain stem, or cerebellum. The occurrence of metastases in the different locations is roughly proportional to their relative mass and blood flow: 80% of patients have lesions located in the cerebral hemispheres, 15% in the cerebellum, 5% in the brainstem, and, rarely in basal ganglia, pineal gland, and hypophysis.[237] The highest incidence of parenchymal metastasis occurs near the junction of the temporal, parietal, and occipital lobes along the gray-white matter interface, probably because of embolic spread from terminal middle cerebral artery branches.[238]

In a series of 729 patients with brain metastases, the median duration from diagnosis of cancer to presentation with a brain metastasis was 12 months, ranging from 3 months for patients with NSCLC to 53 months for patients with breast carcinoma.[236] The median duration from presentation with brain metastases to death was 4 months, ranging from 3 months for patients with SCLC to 13 months for patients with prostate carcinoma. Median survival from presentation with brain metastases to death was 5 months for patients with single lesions and 3 months for patients with multifocal intracranial disease. The majority of patients who develop brain metastases (which is always indicative of Stage IV disease) have a relatively short survival, despite the fact that initial treatment of the intracranial mass lesion is often effective. The short survival is usually the result of progressive systemic disease.

The clinical presentation is similar to the presentation of any intracranial mass lesion. Symptoms and signs depend on the affected neuroanatomic structures. Some lesions present slowly with progressive headache or cognitive dysfunction. Others present acutely with seizures. Often, the patient may present with combinations of headaches, nausea, and/or vomiting and seizures. Many patients may manifest some form of neurologic and/or neurocognitive impairment which can cause emotional difficulties and affect QoL. Altered mental status or impaired cognition are common. Some patients may have no symptoms or signs, metastases being discovered on routine staging work-up of their neoplasm. The prognosis for these patients also is poor; without therapeutic intervention the natural course is one of progressive neurological deterioration with a median survival time of 1 month.[239]

Contrast-enhanced MRI is the gold standard for diagnosis of intracranial metastases. There are no pathognomonic features on CT or MRI that distinguish brain metastases from primary malignant brain tumors or non-neoplastic conditions: therefore, a tissue diagnosis by biopsy should be always obtained in patients without a known primary tumor before undergoing radiation therapy and/or chemotherapy for brain metastasis.[240] With a known primary lesion, newly discovered brain lesions are metastatic in more than 90% of cases.

Treatment options for brain metastases include whole brain radiation therapy (WBRT), neurosurgery, stereotactic radiosurgery, or a combination of all three. Steroids may be used to control tumor-associated edema and alleviate neurologic symptoms, including headache. Most patients are successfully managed with starting doses of 4 to 8 mg of dexamethasone per day, with higher doses (16 mg/day) reserved for patients who present with severe headaches, significant focal deficits, or somnolence.[241] Conventional chemotherapy (topotecan, cisplatin, paclitaxel) has a limited role, because these drugs do not penetrate the blood-brain barrier. In contrast, temozolomide (Temodar) readily crosses the blood-brain barrier. WBRT is the standard of care in patients with multiple brain metastases; surgery and stereotactic radiosurgery play a role when there are isolated or limited metastases. Radiosurgery, alone or in conjunction with WBRT, yields results which are comparable to those reported after surgery

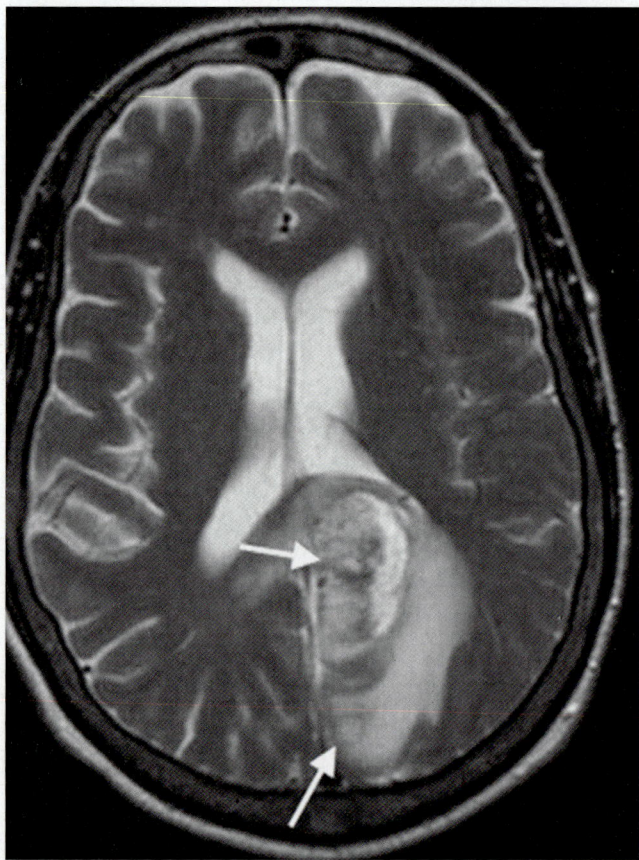

FIGURE 7.14 A 63-year-old woman with metastatic breast cancer presented with mental status changes. T2 axial MRI shows 2.7- × 3.4- × 4.1-cm left deep parietal rim enhancing lesion with surrounding vasogenic edema. There is a smaller 1.1- × 1.0- × 1.4-cm occipital lesion posterior to this lesion. MRI, magnetic resonance imaging

followed by WBRT, provided that the lesion's diameter does not exceed 3 to 3.5 cm.[240]

Whole brain radiation can cause brain injury and neurologic complications. Long-term survivors of brain metastases treated with radiation are at risk for dementia and progressive memory loss.[242] Radiation predominantly causes vascular endothelial damage and demyelination of white matter which can lead to white matter necrosis. Li et al.[243] found that, 6 months after whole brain radiation, neurocognitive function preceded and predicted decline in QoL, as measured by activities of daily living, with delayed recall (memory) being the most predictive test. The presence of metastasis to the brain alters the management of most malignancies and reduces the life expectancy of the patient regardless of the treatments that can be utilized. These factors are likely to influence the management strategies for pains associated with the primary disease or metastases elsewhere in the body.

TUMOR MARKERS

A biomarker is a characteristic objectively measured and evaluated to indicate normal or pathogenic biological processes or pharmacologic response. Genomics, proteomics, and metabolomics have been employed to develop molecular signatures for disease diagnosis, prognosis, and therapeutic efficacy.

Tumor-associated antigens discovered by these strategies have been employed to develop passive (humoral) as well as active immunotherapy strategies to stimulate the immune system. Biomarker development and validation, in parallel with therapeutics, can speed development times through accurate screening of patient populations. The substitution of surrogate markers that correlate well with clinical outcomes facilitates treatment development. The term *tumor marker* is applied to all substances of biochemical character produced by either tumor cells or a host organism, and whose presence may be detected in the serum or other biological fluids. A tumor marker can be defined as a molecule that indicates the likely presence of cancer or that provides information about the likely future behavior of a cancer. Ideally, its serum concentrations should be high even in presence of small tumors, making it useful for both early diagnosis of disease and early detection of relapse. Markers can be used to screen for early malignancy. They can also be a diagnostic or prognostic aid, predicting therapeutic efficacy, maintaining surveillance following surgical removal of the primary tumor, and monitoring therapy in advanced malignancy. Some examples of prognostic tumor markers are shown in Table 7.5.

Tumor markers also can be helpful in the postoperative follow-up of patients diagnosed with malignancy. Examples of markers used for surveillance in this fashion are listed in Table 7.6.

Treatment decisions can be guided by markers. For example, molecular biomarkers in breast cancer may help in the selection of optimal therapy. ER positive patients may receive hormonal therapy such as tamoxifen or Arimidex, HER2-positive patients may receive immunotherapy such as Herceptin, and *BRCA1* patients such chemotherapy as anthracyclines or taxanes.[244] Markers can also frequently be used to monitor treatment in patients with advanced disease. Steadily increasing marker levels indicate treatment failure and imply the need to switch to alternative treatments. (The role of CA-125 has been discussed in "Ovarian Cancer" and PSA is discussed in "Prostate Cancer.")

CA19-9 is a monoclonal antibody generated against a colon carcinoma cell line to detect a monosialoganglioside found in patients with gastrointestinal adenocarcinoma. It is found to be elevated in 21% to 42% of cases of gastric cancer, 20% to 40% of colon cancer, and 71% to 93% of pancreatic cancer, and has been proposed to differentiate benign from malignant pancreatic disease; however, the specificity and sensitivity of CA19-9 is inadequate for reliable diagnosis in pancreatic cancer if used alone.[245] Patients with cervical adenocarcinoma sometimes show elevated CA19-9 levels.[246] CA19-9 levels seem to predict long-term outcome for patients with pancreatic cancer.[247] Preoperative CA19-9 levels correlate with disease stage, whereas a postoperative decrease in CA19-9 and a postoperative CA19-9 value of less than 200 U/mL are strong independent predictors of survival.

Alpha-fetoprotein (AFP), a homolog of albumin, is thought to act as a carrier protein in the fetus. AFP is a normal fetal serum protein synthesized by the liver, yolk sac, and gastro-intestinal tract that shares sequence

TABLE 7.5

PROGNOSTIC TUMOR MARKERS IN MALIGNANCY

Cancer	Marker Abbreviation	Marker
Breast	ER	Estrogen receptor
	HER-2/neu	Human epidermal growth factor receptor 2
	CA 15-3	Cancer antigen 15-3
Colorectal	CEA	Carcinoembryonic antigen
Nonseminomatous germ cell	AFP	α-fetoprotein
	hCG	human chorionic gonadotropin
Ovarian	CA-125	Cancer antigen 125
Prostate	PSA	Prostate-specific antigen
Trophoblastic disease	hCG	Human chorionic gonadotropin

TABLE 7.6
TUMOR MARKERS USED FOR POSTOPERATIVE AND THERAPY SURVEILLANCE

Cancer	Marker Abbreviation	Marker
Breast	CA 15-3	Cancer antigen 15-3
	BRCA-1	Breast cancer gene 1
	BRCA-2	Breast cancer gene 2
	CEA	Carcinoembryonic antigen
Colorectal	CEA	Carcinoembryonic antigen
Ovarian	CA 125	Cancer antigen 125
Prostate	PSA	Prostate-specific antigen
Thyroid (differentiated)	Thyroglobulin	
Trophoblastic	hCG	Human chorionic gonadotropin

homology with albumin. AFP is a marker for hepatocellular and germ cell (nonseminoma) carcinoma. Human chorionic gonadotropin (HCG), a glycoprotein, is secreted at low levels by the pituitary, producing measurable plasma levels. The serum concentration may increase with patient age, particularly in postmenopausal women. HCG is expressed at very high concentrations by the placenta and trophoblastic tumors, including choriocarcinoma of the testis. All gestational trophoblastic tumors produce HCG, and it is a valuable marker in these tumors, screening reliably in all cases and indicating poor responses to treatment. The level correlates with tumor mass and thus has prognostic value. HCG is extremely sensitive, being elevated in women with minute amounts of tumor. Lactate dehydrogenase (LDH) is expressed in many tissues and increased levels may be caused by a wide variety of diseases. Despite its lack of specificity, LDH is a useful marker, especially for staging of seminoma.

CEA is an oncofetal antigen, and increased serum levels of CEA are frequently found in a variety of benign diseases and cancers, including ovarian carcinoma. CEA was one of the first antigens to be described and exploited clinically. It is a complex glycoprotein that is associated with the plasma membrane of tumor cells, from which it may be released into the blood. The American Society for Clinical Oncology recommends that CEA is the only marker of choice for monitoring the response of metastatic colorectal disease to systemic therapy at present.[248] Although CEA was first identified in colon cancer, an abnormal CEA blood level is specific neither for colon cancer nor for malignancy in general. Elevated CEA levels are found in a variety of cancers other than colonic, including pancreatic, gastric, lung, and breast. It is also detected in benign conditions, including cirrhosis, inflammatory bowel disease, chronic lung disease, and pancreatitis. The frequency of increased concentration in ovarian carcinoma varies with the histological type and disease stage, generally being higher in patients with mucinous ovarian cancers and with metastatic disease. The sensitivity of CEA as a marker to detect ovarian cancer is approximately 25%, and the positive predictive value of an increased CEA concentration is only 14%.[249] Although CEA is not a marker for early diagnosis owing to its low sensitivity, CEA can be useful in determining treatment response in ovarian cancer patients.

References

1. Glover J, Dibble SL, Dodd MJ, et al. Mood states of oncology outpatients: does pain make a difference? *J Pain Symptom Manage.* 1995;10:120–128.
2. Twycross R, Harcourt J, Bergl S. A survey of pain in patients with advanced cancer. *J Pain Symptom Manage.* 1996;12:273–282.
3. Vainio A, Auvinen A. Prevalence of symptoms among patients with advanced cancer: an international collaborative study. Symptom Prevalence Group. *J Pain Symptom Manage.* 1996;12:3–10.
4. Serlin RC, Mendoza TR, Nakamura Y, et al. When is cancer pain mild, moderate or severe? Grading pain severity by its interference with function. *Pain.* 1995;61:277–284.
5. Spiegel D, Bloom JR. Pain in metastatic breast cancer. *Cancer.* 1983;52:341–345.
6. Vuorinen E. Pain as an early symptom in cancer. *Clin J Pain.* 1993;9:272–278.
7. Cleeland CS. The impact of pain on the patient with cancer. *Cancer.* 1984;54:2635–2641.
8. Daut RL, Cleeland CS. The prevalence and severity of pain in cancer. *Cancer.* 1982;50:1913–1918.
9. Parkin DM, Bray F, Ferlay J, et al. Global cancer statistics, 2002. *CA Cancer J Clin.* 2005;55:74–108.
10. Jemal A, Clegg LX, Ward E, et al. Annual report to the nation on the status of cancer, 1975–2001, with a special feature regarding survival. *Cancer.* 2004;101:3–27.
11. Hewitt M, Breen N, Devesa S. Cancer prevalence and survivorship issues: Analyses of the 1992 National Health Interview Survey. *J Natl Cancer Inst.* 1999;91:1480–1486.
12. McPherson K, Steel CM, Dixon JM. ABC of breast diseases. Breast cancer–epidemiology, risk factors, and genetics. *BMJ.* 2000;321:624–628.
13. Travis LB, Hill D, Dores GM, et al. Cumulative absolute breast cancer risk for young women treated for Hodgkin lymphoma. *J Natl Cancer Inst.* 2005;97:1428–1437.
14. Hathaway PB, Mankoff DA, Maravilla KR, et al. Value of combined FDG PET and MR imaging in the evaluation of suspected recurrent local-regional breast cancer: Preliminary experience. *Radiology.* 1999;210:807–814.
15. Cook GJ, Houston S, Rubens R, et al. Detection of bone metastases in breast cancer by 18FDG PET: Differing metabolic activity in osteoblastic and osteolytic lesions. *J Clin Oncol.* 1998;16:3375–3379.
16. Singletary SE. Multidisciplinary frontiers in breast cancer management: A surgeon's perspective. *Cancer.* 2007;109:1019–1029.
17. Murphy CD, Lee JM, Drohan B, et al. The American Cancer Society guidelines for breast screening with magnetic resonance imaging: An argument for genetic testing. *Cancer.* 2008;113:3116–3120
18. Kalaja VV. Recurrent or metastatic breast cancer: ESMO clinical recommendations for diagnosis, treatment and follow-up. *Ann Oncol.* 2007;18 Suppl 2:ii, 9–11.
19. Saphner T, Tormey DC, Gray R. Annual hazard rates of recurrence for breast cancer after primary therapy. *J Clin Oncol.* 1996;14:2738–2746.

20. Kurokawa H, Lenferink AE, Simpson JF, et al. Inhibition of HER2/neu (erbB-2) and mitogen-activated protein kinases enhances tamoxifen action against HER2-overexpressing, tamoxifen-resistant breast cancer cells. *Cancer Res.* 2000;60:5887–5894.
21. Slamon DJ, Clark GM, Wong SG, et al. Human breast cancer: Correlation of relapse and survival with amplification of the HER-2/neu oncogene. *Science.* 1987;235:177–182.
22. Schiff R, Massarweh S, Shou J, et al. Breast cancer endocrine resistance: How growth factor signaling and estrogen receptor coregulators modulate response. *Clin Cancer Res.* 2003;9:447S–54S.
23. Smith I, Procter M, Gelber RD, et al. Two-year follow-up of trastuzumab after adjuvant chemotherapy in HER2-positive breast cancer: A randomised controlled trial. *Lancet.* 2007;369:29–36.
24. Johnston SR, Lu B, Dowsett M, et al. Comparison of estrogen receptor DNA binding in untreated and acquired antiestrogen-resistant human breast tumors. *Cancer Res.* 1997;57:3723–3727.
25. Dowsett M, Nicholson RI, Pietras RJ. Biological characteristics of the pure antiestrogen fulvestrant: Overcoming endocrine resistance. *Breast Cancer Res Treat.* 2005;93 Suppl 1:S11–8.
26. Miller KD, Chap LI, Holmes FA, et al. Randomized phase III trial of capecitabine compared with bevacizumab plus capecitabine in patients with previously treated metastatic breast cancer. *J Clin Oncol.* 2005;23:792–799.
27. Guarneri V, Conte PF. The curability of breast cancer and the treatment of advanced disease. *Eur J Nucl Med Mol Imaging.* 2004;31 Suppl 1:S149–61.
28. Carrick S, Parker S, Wilcken N, et al. Single agent versus combination chemotherapy for metastatic breast cancer. *Cochrane Database Syst Rev.* 2005:CD003372.
29. Early Breast Cancer Trialist's Collaborative Group (EBCTCG). Effects of chemotherapy and hormonal therapy for early breast cancer on recurrence and 15-year survival: An overview of the randomised trials. *Lancet.* 2005;365:1687–717.
30. De Laurentiis M, Cancello G, D'Agostino D, et al. Taxane-based combinations as adjuvant chemotherapy of early breast cancer: A meta-analysis of randomized trials. *J Clin Oncol.* 2008;26:44–53.
31. Atzori F, Fornier M. Epothilones in breast cancer: Current status and future directions. *Expert Rev Anticancer Ther.* 2008;8:1299–311.
32. Swenerton KD, Legha SS, Smith T, et al. Prognostic factors in metastatic breast cancer treated with combination chemotherapy. *Cancer Res.* 1979;39:1552–1562.
33. Smalley RV, Lefante J, Bartolucci A, et al. A comparison of cyclophosphamide, adriamycin, and 5-fluorouracil (CAF) and cyclophosphamide, methotrexate, 5-fluorouracil, vincristine, and prednisone (CMFVP) in patients with advanced breast cancer. *Breast Cancer Res Treat.* 1983;3:209–220.
34. Shen KR, Meyers BF, Larner JM, et al. Special treatment issues in lung cancer: ACCP evidence-based clinical practice guidelines (2nd ed). *Chest.* 2007;132:290S–305S.
35. Detterbeck FC, Jones DR, Rosenman JG. Pancoast tumors. In: Detterbeck FC, Rivera MP, Socinski MA, Rosenman JG, eds. *Diagnosis and treatment of lung cancer: an evidence-based guide for the practicing clinician.* Philadelphia, Pa:WB Saunders, 2001:233–243.
36. Webb WR, Gatsonis C, Zerhouni EA, et al. CT and MR imaging in staging non–small cell bronchogenic carcinoma: Report of the Radiologic Diagnostic Oncology Group. *Radiology.* 1991;178:705–713.
37. Vansteenkiste JF, Stroobants SG, De Leyn PR, et al. Lymph node staging in non–small-cell lung cancer with FDG-PET scan: A prospective study on 690 lymph node stations from 68 patients. *J Clin Oncol.* 1998;16:2142–2149.
38. Samson DJ, Seidenfeld J, Simon GR, et al. Evidence for management of small cell lung cancer: ACCP evidence-based clinical practice guidelines (2nd ed). *Chest.* 2007;132:314S–323S.
39. Murren JR, Turrisi AT, Pass HI. Small cell lung cancer. In: DeVita VTJ, Hellman S, Rosenberg SA, eds. *Cancer: principles and practice of oncology,* 7th ed. Philadelphia, Pa: Lippincott, Williams & Wilkins, 2005:810–843.
40. Simon GR, Turrisi A. Management of small cell lung cancer: ACCP evidence-based clinical practice guidelines (2nd ed). *Chest.* 2007;132:324S–339S.
41. Socinski MA, Crowell R, Hensing TE, et al. Treatment of non–small cell lung cancer, stage IV: ACCP evidence-based clinical practice guidelines (2nd ed). *Chest.* 2007;132:277S–289S.
42. Fathi AT, Brahmer JR. Chemotherapy for advanced stage non–small cell lung cancer. *Semin Thorac Cardiovasc Surg.* 2008;20:210–216.
43. Carlson JJ, Reyes C, Oestreicher N, et al. Comparative clinical and economic outcomes of treatments for refractory non–small cell lung cancer (NSCLC). *Lung Cancer.* 2008;61:405–415.
44. Miller JI Jr, Phillips TW. Neodymium:YAG laser and brachytherapy in the management of inoperable bronchogenic carcinoma. *Ann Thorac Surg.* 1990;50:190–5;discussion 195–6.
45. Mercadante S, Armata M, Salvaggio L. Pain characteristics of advanced lung cancer patients referred to a palliative care service. *Pain.* 1994;59:141–145.
46. Sebastian P, Varghese C, Sankaranarayanan R, et al. Evaluation of symptomatology in planning palliative care. *Pall. Med.* 1993;7:27–34.
47. Huhti E, Sutinen S, Reinila A, et al. Lung cancer in a defined geographical area: history and histological types. *Thorax.* 1980;35:660–667.
48. Portenoy RK, Miransky J, Thaler HT, et al. Pain in ambulatory patients with lung or colon cancer. Prevalence, characteristics, and effect. *Cancer.* 1992;70:1616–1624.
49. Ischia S, Ischia A, Luzzani A, et al. Results up to death in the treatment of persistent cervico-thoracic (Pancoast) and thoracic malignant pain by unilateral percutaneous cervical cordotomy. *Pain.* 1985;21:339–355.
50. Grond S, Zech D, Diefenbach C, et al. Assessment of cancer pain: a prospective evaluation in 2266 cancer patients referred to a pain service. *Pain.* 1996;64:107–114.
51. Watson PN, Evans RJ. Intractable pain with lung cancer. *Pain.* 1987;29:163–173.
52. Wilkie DJ, Huang HY, Reilly N, et al. Nociceptive and neuropathic pain in patients with lung cancer: a comparison of pain quality descriptors. *J Pain Symptom Manage.* 2001;22:899–910.
53. Jemal A, Siegel R, Ward E, et al. Cancer statistics, 2007. *CA Cancer J Clin.* 2007;57:43–66.
54. Yancik R. Population aging and cancer: a cross-national concern. *Cancer.* 2005;11:437–441.
55. Crawford ED. Epidemiology of prostate cancer. *Urology.* 2003;62:3–12.
56. Schroder FH, Carter HB, Wolters T, et al. Early detection of prostate cancer in 2007. Part 1:PSA and PSA kinetics. *Eur Urol.* 2008;53:468–477.
57. Feldman BJ, Feldman D. The development of androgen-independent prostate cancer. *Nat Rev Cancer.* 2001;1:34–45.
58. Kumar S, Shelley M, Harrison C, et al. Neo-adjuvant and adjuvant hormone therapy for localised and locally advanced prostate cancer. *Cochrane Database Syst Rev.* 2006:CD006019.
59. Mohile SG, Mustian K, Bylow K, et al. Management of complications of androgen deprivation therapy in the older man. *Crit Rev Oncol Hematol.* 2009;70:235–255.
60. Schroder FH. Cyproterone acetate—mechanism of action and clinical effectiveness in prostate cancer treatment. *Cancer.* 1993;72:3810–3815.
61. Mike S, Harrison C, Coles B, et al. Chemotherapy for hormone-refractory prostate cancer. *Cochrane Database Syst Rev.* 2006:CD005247.
62. Koukourakis MI, Touloupidis S. External beam radiotherapy for prostate cancer: current position and trends. *Anticancer Res.* 2006;26:485–494.
63. Olson KB, Pienta KJ. Pain management in patients with advanced prostate cancer. *Oncology (Williston Park).* 1999;13:1537–49;discussion 1549–50 passim.
64. Kaasa S, Brenne E, Lund JA, et al. Prospective randomised multicenter trial on single fraction radiotherapy (8 Gy × 1) versus multiple fractions (3 Gy × 10) in the treatment of painful bone metastases. *Radiother Oncol.* 2006;79:278–284.
65. Manas A, Casas F, Ciria JP, et al. Randomised study of single dose (8 Gy vs. 6 Gy) of analgesic radiotherapy plus zoledronic acid in patients with bone metastases. *Clin Transl Oncol.* 2008;10:281–287.
66. Hartsell WF, Scott CB, Bruner DW, et al. Randomized trial of short-versus long-course radiotherapy for palliation of painful bone metastases. *J Natl Cancer Inst.* 2005;97:798–804.
67. Yuen KK, Shelley M, Sze WM, et al. Bisphosphonates for advanced prostate cancer. *Cochrane Database Syst Rev.* 2006:CD006250.
68. Saad F, Adachi JD, Brown JP, et al. Cancer treatment-induced bone loss in breast and prostate cancer. *J Clin Oncol.* 2008;26:5465–5476.
69. Jemal A, Siegel R, Ward E, et al. Cancer statistics, 2006. *CA Cancer J Clin.* 2006;56:106–130.
70. Midgley R, Kerr D. Colorectal cancer. *Lancet.* 1999;353:391–399.
71. Armstrong B, Doll R. Environmental factors and cancer incidence and mortality in different countries, with special reference to dietary practices. *Int J Cancer.* 1975;15:617–631.

72. Prentice RL, Sheppard L. Dietary fat and cancer: consistency of the epidemiologic data, and disease prevention that may follow from a practical reduction in fat consumption. *Cancer Causes Control.* 1990;1:81–97;discussion 99–109.
73. McKeown-Eyssen G. Epidemiology of colorectal cancer revisited: are serum triglycerides and/or plasma glucose associated with risk? *Cancer Epidemiol Biomarkers Prev.* 1994;3:687–695.
74. Giovannucci E. Modifiable risk factors for colon cancer. *Gastroenterol Clin North Am.* 2002;31:925–943.
75. Merlin F, Prochilo T, Tondulli L, et al. Colorectal cancer treatment in elderly patients: An update on recent clinical studies. *Clin Colorectal Cancer.* 2008;7:357–363.
76. Itzkowitz SH. Gastrointestinal adenomatous polyps. *Semin Gastrointest Dis.* 1996;7:105–116.
77. Desch CE, Benson AB 3rd, Somerfield MR, et al. Colorectal cancer surveillance: 2005 update of an American Society of Clinical Oncology practice guideline. *J Clin Oncol.* 2005;23:8512–8519.
78. Moertel CG, Fleming TR, Macdonald JS, et al. An evaluation of the carcinoembryonic antigen (CEA) test for monitoring patients with resected colon cancer. *JAMA.* 1993;270:943–947.
79. Wald C, Scheirey CD, Tran TM, et al. An update on imaging of colorectal cancer. *Surg Clin North Am.* 2006;86:819–847.
80. Saletti P, Cavalli F. Metastatic colorectal cancer. *Cancer Treat Rev.* 2006;32:557–571.
81. Macarulla T, Ramos FJ, Elez E, et al. Update on novel strategies to optimize cetuximab therapy in patients with metastatic colorectal cancer. *Clin Colorectal Cancer.* 2008;7:300–308.
82. O'Neil BH, Goldberg RM. Innovations in chemotherapy for metastatic colorectal cancer: An update of recent clinical trials. *Oncologist.* 2008;13:1074–1083.
83. Yu TK, Bhosale PR, Crane CH, et al. Patterns of locoregional recurrence after surgery and radiotherapy or chemoradiation for rectal cancer. *Int J Radiat Oncol Biol Phys.* 2008;71:1175–1180.
84. Choong N, Vokes E. Expanding role of the medical oncologist in the management of head and neck cancer. *CA Cancer J Clin.* 2008;58:32–53.
85. Jemal A, Siegel R, Ward E, et al. Cancer statistics, 2008. *CA Cancer J Clin.* 2008;58:71–96.
86. Seiwert TY, Cohen EE. State-of-the-art management of locally advanced head and neck cancer. *Br J Cancer.* 2005;92:1341–1348.
87. Chuang SC, Scelo G, Tonita JM, et al. Risk of second primary cancer among patients with head and neck cancers: A pooled analysis of 13 cancer registries. *Int J Cancer.* 2008;123:2390–2396.
88. Lo KW, To KF, Huang DP. Focus on nasopharyngeal carcinoma. *Cancer Cell.* 2004;5:423–428.
89. Lee AW, Poon YF, Foo W, et al. Retrospective analysis of 5037 patients with nasopharyngeal carcinoma treated during 1976–1985: Overall survival and patterns of failure. *Int J Radiat Oncol Biol Phys.* 1992;23:261–270.
90. Ng SH, Yen TC, Liao CT, et al. 18F-FDG PET and CT/MRI in oral cavity squamous cell carcinoma: A prospective study of 124 patients with histologic correlation. *J Nucl Med.* 2005;46:1136–1143.
91. Teknos TN, Rosenthal EL, Lee D, et al. Positron emission tomography in the evaluation of stage III and IV head and neck cancer. *Head Neck.* 2001;23:1056–1060.
92. Forastiere A, Koch W, Trotti A, et al. Head and neck cancer. *N Engl J Med.* 2001;345:1890–900.
93. The Department of Veterans Affairs Laryngeal Cancer Study Group. Induction chemotherapy plus radiation compared with surgery plus radiation in patients with advanced laryngeal cancer. *N Engl J Med.* 1991;324:1685–1690.
94. Pfister DG, Laurie SA, Weinstein GS, et al. American Society of Clinical Oncology clinical practice guideline for the use of larynx-preservation strategies in the treatment of laryngeal cancer. *J Clin Oncol.* 2006;24:3693–704.
95. Rosenthal DI, Trotti A. Strategies for managing radiation-induced mucositis in head and neck cancer. *Semin Radiat Oncol.* 2009;19:29–34.
96. Salama JK, Stenson KM, Kistner EO, et al. Induction chemotherapy and concurrent chemoradiotherapy for locoregionally advanced head and neck cancer: a multi-institutional phase II trial investigating three radiotherapy dose levels. *Ann Oncol.* 2008;19:1787–1794.
97. Terrell JE, Ronis DL, Fowler KE, et al. Clinical predictors of quality of life in patients with head and neck cancer. *Arch Otolaryngol Head Neck Surg.* 2004;130:401–408.
98. Karvonen-Gutierrez CA, Ronis DL, Fowler KE, et al. Quality of life scores predict survival among patients with head and neck cancer. *J Clin Oncol.* 2008;26:2754–2760.
99. Babin E, Sigston E, Hitier M, et al. Quality of life in head and neck cancers patients: Predictive factors, functional and psychosocial outcome. *Eur Arch Otorhinolaryngol.* 2008;265:265–270.
100. Connelly ST, Schmidt BL. Evaluation of pain in patients with oral squamous cell carcinoma. *Pain.* 2004;5:505–510.
101. Kolokythas A, Connelly ST, Schmidt BL. Validation of the University of California San Francisco Oral Cancer Pain Questionnaire. *Pain.* 2007;8:950–953.
102. Rogers SN, Miller RD, Ali K, et al. Patients' perceived health status following primary surgery for oral and oropharyngeal cancer. *Int J Oral Maxillofac Surg.* 2006;35:913–919.
103. Logan HL, Bartoshuk LM, Fillingim RB, et al. Metallic taste phantom predicts oral pain among 5-year survivors of head and neck cancer. *Pain.* 2008;140:323–331.
104. Halyard MY, Jatoi A, Sloan JA, et al. Does zinc sulfate prevent therapy-induced taste alterations in head and neck cancer patients? Results of phase III double-blind, placebo-controlled trial from the North Central Cancer Treatment Group (N01C4). *Int J Radiat Oncol Biol Phys.* 2007;67:1318–1322.
105. Lees J. Incidence of weight loss in head and neck cancer patients on commencing radiotherapy treatment at a regional oncology centre. *Eur J Cancer Care (Engl).* 1999;8:133–136.
106. Grushka M, Epstein JB, Gorsky M. Burning mouth syndrome. *Am Fam Physician.* 2002;65:615–620.
107. Louise Kent M, Brennan MT, Noll JL, et al. Radiation-induced trismus in head and neck cancer patients. *Support Care Cancer.* 2008;16:305–309.
108. Sherman ME, Wang SS, Carreon J, et al. Mortality trends for cervical squamous and adenocarcinoma in the United States: Relation to incidence and survival. *Cancer.* 2005;103:1258–1264.
109. Espey DK, Wu XC, Swan J, et al. Annual report to the nation on the status of cancer, 1975–2004, featuring cancer in American Indians and Alaska Natives. *Cancer.* 2007;110:2119–2152.
110. McDougall JA, Madeleine MM, Daling JR, et al. Racial and ethnic disparities in cervical cancer incidence rates in the United States, 1992–2003. *Cancer Causes Control.* 2007;18:1175–1186.
111. Smith HO, Tiffany MF, Qualls CR, et al. The rising incidence of adenocarcinoma relative to squamous cell carcinoma of the uterine cervix in the United States—a 24-year population-based study. *Gynecol Oncol.* 2000;78:97–105.
112. Ault KA. Human papillomavirus vaccines: An update for gynecologists. *Clin Obstet Gynecol.* 2008;51:527–532.
113. Markowitz LE, Dunne EF, Saraiya M, et al. Quadrivalent human papillomavirus vaccine: Recommendations of the Advisory Committee on Immunization Practices (ACIP). *MMWR Recomm Rep.* 2007;56:1–24.
114. Castellsague X, Munoz N. Cofactors in human papillomavirus carcinogenesis—role of parity, oral contraceptives, and tobacco smoking. *J Natl Cancer Inst Monogr.* 2003;20–28.
115. Benard VB, Johnson CJ, Thompson TD, et al. Examining the association between socioeconomic status and potential human papillomavirus-associated cancers. *Cancer.* 2008;113:2910–2918.
116. Heller PB, Maletano JH, Bundy BN, et al. Clinical-pathologic study of stage IIB, III, and IVA carcinoma of the cervix: Extended diagnostic evaluation for paraaortic node metastasis—A Gynecologic Oncology Group study. *Gynecol Oncol.* 1990;38:425–430.
117. Kodama J, Seki N, Nakamura K, et al. Prognostic factors in pathologic parametrium–positive patients with stage IB-IIB cervical cancer treated by radical surgery and adjuvant therapy. *Gynecol Oncol.* 2007;105:757–761.
118. Rubin SC, Brookland R, Mikuta JJ, et al. Para-aortic nodal metastases in early cervical carcinoma: Long-term survival following extended-field radiotherapy. *Gynecol Oncol.* 1984;18:213–217.
119. Vigliotti AP, Wen BC, Hussey DH, et al. Extended field irradiation for carcinoma of the uterine cervix with positive periaortic nodes. *Int J Radiat Oncol Biol Phys.* 1992;23:501–509.
120. Rose PG, Adler LP, Rodriguez M, et al. Positron emission Tomography for evaluating para-aortic nodal metastasis in locally advanced cervical cancer before surgical staging: A surgicopathologic study. *J Clin Oncol.* 1999;17:41–45.
121. Subak LL, Hricak H, Powell CB, et al. Cervical carcinoma: Computed tomography and magnetic resonance imaging for preoperative staging. *Obstet Gynecol.* 1995;86:43–50.
122. Lin G, Ho KC, Wang JJ, et al. Detection of lymph node metastasis in cervical and uterine cancers by diffusion-weighted magnetic resonance imaging at 3T. *J Magn Reson Imaging.* 2008;28:128–135.

123. Sahdev A, Sohaib SA, Wenaden AE, et al. The performance of magnetic resonance imaging in early cervical carcinoma: A long-term experience. *Int J Gynecol Cancer.* 2007;17:629–636.
124. Reinhardt MJ, Ehritt-Braun C, Vogelgesang D, et al. Metastatic lymph nodes in patients with cervical cancer: Detection with MR imaging and FDG PET. *Radiology.* 2001;218:776–782.
125. Dornhofer N, Hockel M. New developments in the surgical therapy of cervical carcinoma. *Ann N Y Acad Sci.* 2008;1138:233–252.
126. Levenback CF. Status of sentinel lymph nodes in cervical cancer. *Gynecol Oncol.* 2007;107:S18–9.
127. Benedetti-Panici P, Maneschi F, Scambia G, et al. Lymphatic spread of cervical cancer: An anatomical and pathological study based on 225 radical hysterectomies with systematic pelvic and aortic lymphadenectomy. *Gynecol Oncol.* 1996;62:19–24.
128. Milliken DA, Shepherd JH. Fertility preserving surgery for carcinoma of the cervix. *Curr Opin Oncol.* 2008;20:575–580.
129. Benedetti-Panici P, Greggi S, Colombo A, et al. Neoadjuvant chemotherapy and radical surgery versus exclusive radiotherapy in locally advanced squamous cell cervical cancer: Results from the Italian multicenter randomized study. *J Clin Oncol.* 2002;20:179–188.
130. Del Campo JM, Prat A, Gil-Moreno A, et al. Update on novel therapeutic agents for cervical cancer. *Gynecol Oncol.* 2008;110:S72–6.
131. Sood BM, Gorla GR, Garg M, et al. Extended-field radiotherapy and high-dose-rate brachytherapy in carcinoma of the uterine cervix: Clinical experience with and without concomitant chemotherapy. *Cancer.* 2003;97:1781–1788.
132. Tambaro R, Scambia G, Di Maio M, et al. The role of chemotherapy in locally advanced, metastatic and recurrent cervical cancer. *Crit Rev Oncol Hematol.* 2004;52:33–44.
133. Benedet JL, Odicino F, Maisonneuve P, et al. Carcinoma of the cervix uteri. *Int J Gynaecol Obstet.* 2003;83 Suppl 1:41–78.
134. Hirte HW, Strychowsky JE, Oliver T, et al. Chemotherapy for recurrent, metastatic, or persistent cervical cancer: a systematic review. *Int J Gynecol Cancer.* 2007;17:1194–204.
135. Pectasides D, Kamposioras K, Papaxoinis G, et al. Chemotherapy for recurrent cervical cancer. *Cancer Treat Rev.* 2008;34:603–613.
136. Robati M, Holtz D, Dunton CJ. A review of topotecan in combination chemotherapy for advanced cervical cancer. *Ther Clin Risk Manag.* 2008;4:213–218.
137. Gatta G, Capocaccia R, Coleman MP, et al. Toward a comparison of survival in American and European cancer patients. *Cancer.* 2000;89:893–900.
138. Korfage IJ, Essink-Bot ML, Mols F, et al. Health-related quality of life in cervical cancer survivors: A population-based survey. *Int J Radiat Oncol Biol Phys.* 2008.
139. Vistad I, Fossa SD, Dahl AA. A critical review of patient-rated quality of life studies of long-term survivors of cervical cancer. *Gynecol Oncol.* 2006;102:563–572.
140. Moore KN, Gold MA, McMeekin DS, et al. Vesicovaginal fistula formation in patients with Stage IVA cervical carcinoma. *Gynecol Oncol.* 2007;106:498–501.
141. Yancik R, Ries LG, Yates JW. Ovarian cancer in the elderly: An analysis of Surveillance, Epidemiology, and End Results Program data. *Am J Obstet Gynecol.* 1986;154:639–647.
142. Argento M, Hoffman P, Gauchez AS. Ovarian cancer detection and treatment: current situation and future prospects. *Anticancer Res.* 2008;28:3135–3138.
143. Baekelandt MM, Castiglione M. Endometrial carcinoma: ESMO clinical recommendations for diagnosis, treatment and follow-up. *Ann Oncol.* 2008;19 Suppl 2:ii19–20.
144. Ozols RF. Systemic therapy for ovarian cancer: Current status and new treatments. *Semin Oncol.* 2006;33:S3–11.
145. Trimble EL, Christian MC. National Cancer Institute-United States strategy regarding intraperitoneal chemotherapy for ovarian cancer. *Int J Gynecol Cancer.* 2008;18 Suppl 1:26–28.
146. Fung-Kee-Fung M, Oliver T, Elit L, et al. Optimal chemotherapy treatment for women with recurrent ovarian cancer. *Curr Oncol.* 2007;14:195–208.
147. Portenoy RK, Kornblith AB, Wong G, et al. Pain in ovarian cancer patients. Prevalence, characteristics, and associated symptoms. *Cancer.* 1994;74:907–915.
148. Rosewicz S, Wiedenmann B. Pancreatic carcinoma. *Lancet.* 1997;349:485–489.
149. Korfage IJ, Essink-Bot ML, Mols F, et al. Health-related quality of life in cervical cancer survivors: A population-based survey. *Int J Radiat Oncol Biol Phys.* 2009;73:1501–1509.
150. Vistad I, Fossa SD, Kristensen GB, Dahl AA. Chronic fatigue and its correlates in long-term survivors of cervical cancer treated with radiotherapy. *BJOG.* 2007;114:1150–1158.
151. Greenwald HP, Bonica JJ, Bergner M. The prevalence of pain in four cancers. *Cancer.* 1987;60:2563–2569.
152. Krech RL, Walsh D. Symptoms of pancreatic cancer. *J Pain Symptom Manage.* 1991;6:360–367.
153. Emmrich J, Weber I, Nausch M, et al. Immunohistochemical characterization of the pancreatic cellular infiltrate in normal pancreas, chronic pancreatitis and pancreatic carcinoma. *Digestion.* 1998;59:192–198.
154. Schneider MB, Standop J, Ulrich A, et al. Expression of nerve growth factors in pancreatic neural tissue and pancreatic cancer. *J Histochem Cytochem.* 2001;49:1205–1210.
155. Lindsay TH, Jonas BM, Sevcik MA, et al. Pancreatic cancer pain and its correlation with changes in tumor vasculature, macrophage infiltration, neuronal innervation, body weight and disease progression. *Pain.* 2005;119:233–246.
156. Singh SM, Longmire WP Jr, Reber HA. Surgical palliation for pancreatic cancer. The UCLA experience. *Ann Surg.* 1990;212:132–139.
157. Kelsen DP, Portenoy RK, Thaler HT, et al. Pain and depression in patients with newly diagnosed pancreas cancer. *J Clin Oncol.* 1995;13:748–755.
158. Saltzburg D, Foley KM. Management of pain in pancreatic cancer. *Surg Clin North Am.* 1989;69:629–649.
159. Passik SD, Breitbart WS. Depression in patients with pancreatic carcinoma. Diagnostic and treatment issues. *Cancer.* 1996;78:615–626.
160. Yonemori K, Okusaka T, Ueno H, et al. FP therapy for controlling malignant ascites in advanced pancreatic cancer patients. *Hepatogastroenterology.* 2007;54:2383–2386.
161. Bramhall SR, Allum WH, Jones AG, et al. Treatment and survival in 13,560 patients with pancreatic cancer, and incidence of the disease, in the West Midlands: An epidemiological study. *Br J Surg.* 1995;82:111–115.
162. Whipple AO, Parsons WB, Mullins CR. Treatment of carcinoma of the ampulla of Vater. *Ann Surg.* 1935;102:763–779.
163. Stathopoulos GP, Androulakis N, Souglakos J, et al. Present treatment and future expectations in advanced pancreatic cancer. *Anticancer Res.* 2008;28:1303–1308.
164. Murai M, Oya M. Renal cell carcinoma: Etiology, incidence and epidemiology. *Curr Opin Urol.* 2004;14:229–233.
165. Cohen HT, McGovern FJ. Renal-cell carcinoma. *N Engl J Med.* 2005;353:2477–2490
166. Herrlinger A, Schrott KM, Schott G, et al. What are the benefits of extended dissection of the regional renal lymph nodes in the therapy of renal cell carcinoma? *J Urol.* 1991;146:1224–1227.
167. Phillips E, Messing EM. Role of lymphadenectomy in the treatment of renal cell carcinoma. *Urology.* 1993;41:9–15.
168. Chin AI, Lam JS, Figlin RA, et al. Surveillance strategies for renal cell carcinoma patients following nephrectomy. *Rev Urol.* 2006;8:1–7.
169. Hollingsworth JM, Miller DC, Daignault S, et al. Rising incidence of small renal masses: A need to reassess treatment effect. *J Natl Cancer Inst.* 2006;98:1331–1334.
170. Rabinovitch RA, Zelefsky MJ, Gaynor JJ, et al. Patterns of failure following surgical resection of renal cell carcinoma: Ifor adjuvant local and systemic therapy. *J Clin Oncol.* 1994;12:206–212.
171. Sandock DS, Seftel AD, Resnick MI. A new protocol for the followup of renal cell carcinoma based on pathological stage. *J Urol.* 1995;154:28–31.
172. Chan DY, Marshall FF. Surgery in advanced and metastatic renal cell carcinoma. *Curr Opin Urol.* 1998;8:369–373.
173. Motzer RJ, Russo P. Systemic therapy for renal cell carcinoma. *J Urol.* 2000;163:408–417.
174. Motzer RJ, Mazumdar M, Bacik J, et al. Effect of cytokine therapy on survival for patients with advanced renal cell carcinoma. *J Clin Oncol.* 2000;18:1928–1935.
175. Oudard S, George D, Medioni J, et al. Treatment options in renal cell carcinoma: past, present and future. *Ann Oncol.* 2007;18 Suppl 10:x25–31.
176. Melichar B, Koralewski P, Ravaud A, et al. First-line bevacizumab combined with reduced dose interferon-alpha2a is active in patients with metastatic renal cell carcinoma. *Ann Oncol.* 2008;19:1470–1476.
177. Weber K, Doucet M, Kominsky S. Renal cell carcinoma bone metastasis—elucidating the molecular targets. *Cancer Metastasis Rev.* 2007;26:691–704.

178. Harding G, Cella D, Robinson D Jr, et al. Symptom burden among patients with renal cell carcinoma (RCC): Content for a symptom index. *Health Qual Life Outcomes.* 2007;5:34.
179. Capuron L, Ravaud A, Dantzer R. Early depressive symptoms in cancer patients receiving interleukin 2 and/or interferon alfa-2b therapy. *J Clin Oncol.* 2000;18:2143–2151.
180. Denicoff KD, Rubinow DR, Papa MZ, et al. The neuropsychiatric effects of treatment with interleukin-2 and lymphokine-activated killer cells. *Ann Intern Med.* 1987;107:293–300.
181. Valentine AD, Meyers CA, Kling MA, et al. Mood and cognitive side effects of interferon-alpha therapy. *Semin Oncol.* 1998;25:39–47.
182. Curti BD. Renal cell carcinoma. *JAMA.* 2004;292:97–100.
183. Alexander DD, Mink PJ, Adami HO, et al. Multiple myeloma: a review of the epidemiologic literature. *Int J Cancer.* 2007;120 Suppl 12:40–61.
184. Dispenzieri A. POEMS syndrome. *Blood Rev.* 2007;21:285–299.
185. Koike H, Iijima M, Mori K, et al. Neuropathic pain correlates with myelinated fibre loss and cytokine profile in POEMS syndrome. *J Neurol Neurosurg.* Psychiatry 2008;79:1171–1179.
186. Ohwada C, Nakaseko C, Sakai S, et al. Successful combination treatment with bevacizumab, thalidomide and autologous PBSC for severe POEMS syndrome. *Bone Marrow Transplant.* 2008;43:739–740
187. Edwards CM, Zhuang J, Mundy GR. The pathogenesis of the bone disease of multiple myeloma. *Bone.* 2008;42:1007–1013.
188. Dinter DJ, Neff WK, Klaus J, et al. Comparison of whole-body MR imaging and conventional X-ray examination in patients with multiple myeloma and implications for therapy. *Ann Hematol.* 2008;88:457–464
189. Rajkumar SV, Kyle RA. Multiple myeloma: Diagnosis and treatment. *Mayo Clin Proc.* 2005;80:1371–1382.
190. Shah SR, Tran TM. Lenalidomide in myelodysplastic syndrome and multiple myeloma. *Drugs.* 2007;67:1869–1881.
191. Barlogie B, Tricot G, Anaissie E, et al. Thalidomide and hematopoietic-cell transplantation for multiple myeloma. *N Engl J Med.* 2006;354:1021–1030.
192. Richardson PG, Hideshima T, Mitsiades C, et al. The emerging role of novel therapies for the treatment of relapsed myeloma. *J Natl Compr Canc Netw.* 2007;5:149–162.
193. Rotta M, Storer BE, Sahebi F, et al. Long-term outcome of patients with multiple myeloma after autologous hematopoietic cell transplantation and nonmyeloablative allografting. *Blood.* 2008;113:3383–3391.
194. Jemal A, Tiwari RC, Murray T, et al. Cancer statistics, 2004. *CA Cancer J Clin.* 2004;54:8–29.
195. World Health Organization Classification of Tumours. Pathology and genetics of tumours of soft tissue and bone. Lyon, France, IARC Press, 2002.
196. Sundaresan N, Rosen G, Boriani S. Primary malignant tumors of the spine. *Orthop Clin North Am.* 2009;40:21–36.
197. Clark MA, Fisher C, Judson I, et al. Soft-tissue sarcomas in adults. *N Engl J Med.* 2005;353:701–711.
198. Iagaru A, Masamed R, Chawla SP, et al. F-18 FDG PET and PET/CT evaluation of response to chemotherapy in bone and soft-tissue sarcomas. *Clin Nucl Med.* 2008;33:8–13.
199. Khanfir K, Alzieu L, Terrier P, et al. Does adjuvant radiation therapy increase loco-regional control after optimal resection of soft-tissue sarcoma of the extremities? *Eur J Cancer.* 2003;39:1872–1880.
200. O'Sullivan B, Davis AM, Turcotte R, et al. Preoperative versus postoperative radiotherapy in soft-tissue sarcoma of the limbs: A randomised trial. *Lancet.* 2002;359:2235–2241.
201. Bielack SS, Kempf–Bielack B, Heise U, et al. Combined modality treatment for osteosarcoma occurring as a second malignant disease. Cooperative German-Austrian-Swiss Osteosarcoma Study Group. *J Clin Oncol.* 1999;17:1164.
202. Bielack SS, Machatschek JN, Flege S, et al. Delaying surgery with chemotherapy for osteosarcoma of the extremities. *Expert Opin Pharmacother.* 2004;5:1243–1256.
203. Grier HE, Krailo MD, Tarbell NJ, et al. Addition of ifosfamide and etoposide to standard chemotherapy for Ewing's sarcoma and primitive neuroectodermal tumor of bone. *N Engl J Med.* 2003;348:694–701.
204. Heinrich MC, Owzar K, Corless CL, et al. Correlation of kinase genotype and clinical outcome in the North American Intergroup Phase III Trial of imatinib mesylate for treatment of advanced gastrointestinal stromal tumor: CALGB 150105 Study by Cancer and Leukemia Group B and Southwest Oncology Group. *J Clin Oncol.* 2008;26:5360–5367.
205. Hopkins TG, Marples M, Stark D. Sunitinib in the management of gastrointestinal stromal tumours (GISTs). *Eur J Surg Oncol.* 2008;34:844–850.
206. Lewis JJ, Brennan MF. Soft-tissue sarcomas. *Curr Probl Surg.* 1996;33:817–872.
207. Pervaiz N, Colterjohn N, Farrokhyar F, et al. A systematic meta-analysis of randomized controlled trials of adjuvant chemotherapy for localized resectable soft-tissue sarcoma. *Cancer.* 2008;113:573–581.
208. Sabino MA, Mantyh PW. Pathophysiology of bone cancer pain. *J Support Oncol.* 2005;3:15–24.
209. Barron SA, Heffner RR Jr. Weakness in malignancy: Evidence for a remote effect of tumor on distal axons. *Ann Neurol.* 1978;4:268–274.
210. Chamary VL, Robson T, Loizidou M, et al. Progressive loss of perivascular nerves adjacent to colorectal cancer. *Eur J Surg Oncol.* 2000;26:588–593.
211. Seifert P, Spitznas M. Tumours may be innervated. *Virchows Arch.* 2001;438:228–231.
212. Arndt CA, Crist WM. Common musculoskeletal tumors of childhood and adolescence. *N Engl J Med.* 1999;341:342–352.
213. Bielack SS, Kempf-Bielack B, Delling G, et al. Prognostic factors in high-grade osteosarcoma of the extremities or trunk: An analysis of 1,702 patients treated on neoadjuvant cooperative osteosarcoma study group protocols. *J Clin Oncol.* 2002;20:776–790.
214. Gross JL, Younes RN, Haddad FJ, et al. Soft-tissue sarcomas of the chest wall: Prognostic factors. *Chest.* 2005;127:902–908.
215. Buckner JC, Brown PD, O'Neill BP, et al. Central nervous system tumors. *Mayo Clin Proc.* 2007;82:1271–1286.
216. Schor NF. Pharmacotherapy for adults with tumors of the central nervous system. *Pharmacol Ther.* 2008;121:253–264
217. Fisher JL, Schwartzbaum JA, Wrensch M, et al. Epidemiology of brain tumors. *Neurol Clin.* 2007;25:867–890, vii.
218. DeAngelis LM. Brain tumors. *N Engl J Med.* 2001;344:114–123.
219. Forsyth PA, Posner JB. Headaches in patients with brain tumors: A study of 111 patients. *Neurology* .1993;43:1678–1683.
220. Randeva HS, Schoebel J, Byrne J, et al. Classical pituitary apoplexy: Clinical features, management and outcome. *Clin Endocrinol (Oxf).* 1999;51:181–188.
221. Mou C, Han T, Zhao H, et al. Clinical features and immunohistochemical changes of pituitary apoplexy. *J Clin Neurosci.* 2009;16:64–68.
222. Weinstein JN. Surgical approach to spine tumors. *Orthopedics.* 1989;12:897–905.
223. Raco A, Esposito V, Lenzi J, et al. Long-term follow-up of intramedullary spinal cord tumors: a series of 202 cases. *Neurosurgery.* 2005;56:972–81;discussion 972–81.
224. Schwartz TH, McCormick PC. Intramedullary ependymomas: Clinical presentation, surgical treatment strategies and prognosis. *J Neurooncol.* 2000;47:211–218.
225. Nguyen NC, Sayed MM, Taalab K, et al. Spinal cord metastases from lung cancer: Detection with F-18 FDG PET/CT. *Clin Nucl Med.* 2008;33:356–358.
226. Sasaki M, Kuwabara Y, Yoshida T, et al. A comparative study of thallium-201 SPET, carbon-11 methionine PET and fluorine-18 fluorodeoxyglucose PET for the differentiation of astrocytic tumours. *Eur J Nucl Med.* 1998;25:1261–1269.
227. Palumbo B. Brain tumour recurrence: Brain single-photon emission computerized tomography, PET and proton magnetic resonance spectroscopy. *Nucl Med Commun.* 2008;29:730–735.
228. Gurney JG, Kadan-Lottick N. Brain and other central nervous system tumors: Rates, trends, and epidemiology. *Curr Opin Oncol.* 2001;13:160–166.
229. Chamberlain MC. Temozolomide for recurrent low-grade spinal cord gliomas in adults. *Cancer.* 2008;113:1019–1024.
230. Wowra B, Zausinger S, Drexler C, et al. CyberKnife radiosurgery for malignant spinal tumors: Characterization of well-suited patients. *Spine.* 2008;33:2929–2934.
231. Gerszten PC, Burton SA, Ozhasoglu C. CyberKnife radiosurgery for spinal neoplasms. *Prog Neurol Surg.* 2007;20:340–358.
232. Hart MG, Grant R, Garside R, et al. Chemotherapeutic wafers for high grade glioma. *Cochrane Database Syst Rev.* 2008:CD007294.
233. Pedeboscq S, L'Azou B, Passagne I, et al. Cytotoxic and apoptotic effects of bortezomib and gefitinib compared to alkylating agents on human glioblastoma cells. *J Exp Ther Oncol.* 2008;7:99–111.

234. Poulsen HS, Grunnet K, Sorensen M, et al. Bevacizumab plus irinotecan in the treatment patients with progressive recurrent malignant brain tumours. *Acta Oncol.* 2009;48:52–58.
235. Arnold SM, Patchell RA. Diagnosis and management of brain metastases. *Hematol Oncol Clin North Am.* 2001;15:1085–107, vii.
236. Nussbaum ES, Djalilian HR, Cho KH, et al. Brain metastases. Histology, multiplicity, surgery, and survival. *Cancer.* 1996;78:1781–1788.
237. Delattre JY, Krol G, Thaler HT, et al. Distribution of brain metastases. *Arch Neurol.* 1988;45:741–744.
238. Kindt GW. The pattern of location of cerebral metastatic tumors. *J Neurosurg.* 1964;21:54–57.
239. Zimm S, Wampler GL, Stablein D, et al. Intracerebral metastases in solid-tumor patients: Natural history and results of treatment. *Cancer.* 1981;48:384–394.
240. Soffietti R, Ruda R, Mutani R. Management of brain metastases. *J Neurol.* 2002;249:1357–1369.
241. Vecht CJ, Hovestadt A, Verbiest HB, et al. Dose-effect relationship of dexamethasone on Karnofsky performance in metastatic brain tumors: A randomized study of doses of 4, 8, and 16 mg per day. *Neurology.* 1994;44:675–680.
242. DeAngelis LM, Delattre JY, Posner JB. Radiation-induced dementia in patients cured of brain metastases. *Neurology.* 1989;39:789–796.
243. Li J, Bentzen SM, Li J, et al. Relationship between neurocognitive function and quality of life after whole-brain radiotherapy in patients with brain metastasis. *Int J Radiat Oncol Biol Phys.* 2008;71:64–70.
244. James CR, Quinn JE, Mullan PB, et al. BRCA1, a potential predictive biomarker in the treatment of breast cancer. *Oncologist.* 2007;12:142–150.
245. Locker GY, Hamilton S, Harris J, et al. ASCO 2006 update of recommendations for the use of tumor markers in gastrointestinal cancer. *J Clin Oncol.* 2006;24:5313–5327.
246. Borras G, Molina R, Xercavins J, et al. Tumor antigens CA 19.9, CA 125, and CEA in carcinoma of the uterine cervix. *Gynecol Oncol.* 1995;57:205–211.
247. Ferrone CR, Finkelstein DM, Thayer SP, et al. Perioperative CA19-9 levels can predict stage and survival in patients with resectable pancreatic adenocarcinoma. *J Clin Oncol.* 2006;24:2897–902.
248. Yamashita K, Watanabe M. Clinical significance of tumor markers and an emerging perspective on colorectal cancer. *Cancer Sci.* 2009;100:195–199.
249. Tuxen MK, Soletormos G, Dombernowsky P. Tumor markers in the management of patients with ovarian cancer. *Cancer Treat Rev.* 1995;21:215–245.

CHAPTER 8 ■ BONE METASTASES

Compared to other organs, bone has a dynamic and complex structure that provides a suitable environment for cancer cells. Skeletal involvement, a frequent and troublesome complication affecting many patients with neoplastic disease, is the third most common metastatic site after the lung and liver.[1] Metastatic cancer may invade bone in 30% to 70% of patients.[2] Up to 85% of patients dying from breast, prostate, or lung cancer demonstrate bone involvement at autopsy.[3] Bone pain is the most common cause of pain due to cancer.[4–6] Pain from bone metastases affects 28% of hospice inpatients, 34% of patients in a cancer pain clinic,[7] and 45% of home-based advanced-cancer patients. Bone disease frequently gives rise to complications that have a significant impact on a patient's quality of life, because osteolytic bone disease is a major source of pain and causes difficulty in ambulation, neurological deficits, and pathological fractures. Fractures are common in patients with myeloma and breast cancer, and long bones are more frequently involved.[8]

Bone metastases most commonly affect the axial skeleton. The axial skeleton contains the red marrow in adults, which suggests that properties of the circulation, cells, and extracellular matrix within this region could assist in the formation of bone metastases. The drainage of blood to the skeleton via the vertebral-venous plexus may, at least in part, explain the tendency of breast and prostate cancers, as well as those arising in kidney, thyroid, and lung, to produce metastases in the axial skeleton and limb girdles. The vertebral-venous plexus is certainly not the entire explanation of why these cancers metastasize to the skeleton. Molecular and cellular biologic characteristics of the tumor cells and tissues to which they metastasize are of major importance and influence the pattern of metastatic spread.

Bone metastases from carcinomas of the breast, lung, prostate, kidney, and thyroid are the most frequent (Table 8.1), whereas tumors of the gastrointestinal tract rarely (<10%) produce bone metastases. The prevalence of skeletal disease is greatest in breast and prostate carcinoma, reflecting both the high incidence and the relatively long clinical course of these tumors. These two cancers alone probably account for more than 80% of cases of metastatic bone disease. Survival from the time of diagnosis varies among different tumor types. The median survival time from diagnosis of bone metastases from prostate cancer or breast cancer is measurable in years. By contrast, the median survival time from the diagnosis of advanced lung cancer is typically measured in months. Coexisting nonosseous metastatic disease is important in determining prognostic differences between patients with bone metastases from the same type of tumor. Additionally, for patients with advanced breast cancer and metastatic disease confined to the skeleton at first relapse, the probability of survival is influenced by the subsequent development of metastases at extraosseous sites. Multiple myeloma is a malignant proliferation of plasma cells involving more than 10% of the bone marrow. The bone complications associated with multiple myeloma include bone pain, pathologic fractures, hypercalcemia of malignancy, and spinal cord compression. The principal pathophysiology of bone disease in multiple myeloma is a shift in the balance of bone remodeling toward bone resorption.

The radiological appearance of bone metastases are typically labeled *lytic*, *sclerotic*, or "mixed." When bone resorption predominates with little new bone formation, focal bone destruction occurs and the metastases have a lytic appearance. Lytic lesions are most common in multiple myeloma, melanoma, breast, lung, thyroid, renal, and gastrointestinal malignancies. Conversely, in bone metastases characterized by increased osteoblastic activity, the lesions appear sclerotic. Progressive waves of bone resorption result in the destruction of skeletal elements and focal osteolysis. Osteosclerotic metastases formed by uncoupled bone formation represent the deposition of new bone either on quiescent bone surfaces or arising from stromal condensations within the marrow cavity.[9] Metastases from prostate carcinoma especially, but also those of breast, lung, carcinoid, and medullablastoma tumors, produce sclerotic lesions (Fig 8.1). Some tumors characteristically demonstrate a purely lytic radiographic appearance, such as multiple myeloma, lung cancer, and renal carcinoma,

TABLE 8.1

FREQUENCY OF BONE METASTASES IN CANCER

Primary Site	Bone Metastases (%)
Breast	50–85
Prostate	50–75
Lung	30–50
Kidney	30–50
Thyroid	39
Pancreas	5–10
Colon/Rectum	5–10
Stomach	5–10
Liver	8
Ovary	2–6

(Adapted from Nystrom JS, Weiner JM, Heffelfinger-Juttner J, et al. Metastatic and histologic presentations in unknown primary cancer. *Semin Oncol*. 1977;4:53–58.)

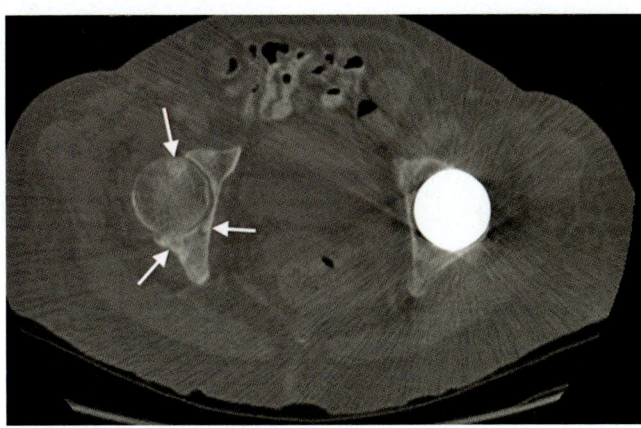

FIGURE 8.1 A 79-year-old woman with metastatic breast cancer. She presented complaining of new-onset right-groin pain. CT scan of pelvis revealed extensive osteosclerotic bone metastases in the right acetabulum and head of femur *(arrows)*. Patient had a previous left hemiarthroplasty. CT, Computed tomography.

and these are more prone to pathologic fracture. Other tumors have a blastic radiographic appearance. Prostate cancer cells produce osteoblast stimulatory factors, probably specific growth factors or acid phosphatase.[10] In this case, new bone forms directly on trabecular bone surface before osteoclastic resorption.[11] The resulting sclerotic metastases are less prone to fracture because of locally increased bony mass. Breast metastases exhibit a mixed picture of both lytic and sclerotic areas.[12] These different mechanisms correspond to typical radiological features showing mixed lytic and sclerotic metastases, osteolytic metastases, or sclerotic metastases, respectively.

Skeletal metastases may arise from direct invasion from the primary tumor or by extension from a secondary site, such as a lymph node. True lymphatic spread to the skeleton is rare. Direct invasion is usually accompanied by a detectable soft-tissue mass, an unusual feature of metastases that occur by hematogenous spread. The left sides of the vertebral bodies are more frequently affected by direct invasion from local lymph nodes, because the left-sided lymph nodes are closer to bone than the right-sided ones.[13] Hematogenous spread is far more frequent than lymphatic spread or direct invasion. The venous route, especially via the Batson paravertebral plexus, appears to be more important for hematogenous spread than the arterial route. The distribution of the Batson venous plexus, as well as the overall skeletal vascularity, results in a predilection for hematogenous spread to the axial skeleton and the proximal long bones.

MOLECULAR BASIS OF SKELETAL METASTASES

The biology of cancer is complex, with multiple different actions, reactions, and molecular pathways interacting to facilitate the passage of tumor cells from their primary source to distant sites. The biologic consequence of skeletal metastases is complex and has been reviewed by Choong.[14]

Bone tissue is under continuous renewal owing to two opposite activities of bone cells, the bone-resorbing osteoclasts and the bone forming osteoblasts. These processes are normally tightly coupled; as old bone is resorbed by osteoclasts, the same amount of new bone is formed by osteoblasts. Alteration of this tightly regulated balance leads to uncoupling and a net event of accelerated bone loss or increased bone formation. Uncoupling in metastatic bone disease occurs only at sites of tumor implantation. Bone lesions can be either osteolytic or osteogenic depending on which cells are stimulated predominantly by tumor cells. Activation of osteoclasts by tumor cells is required to facilitate expansion of the metastasis in the mineralized matrix. Previously, it was assumed that tumor cells themselves degraded bone to cause osteolysis, but there is now ample evidence that tumors drive bone degradation by stimulating osteoclastic activity.[15] Bone resorption around metastatic foci is predominantly mediated by osteoclasts. Osteoclast differentiation and activation are regulated at the local level by the relative expression of receptor activator of nuclear factor-κB ligand (RANKL) and osteoproteregin (OPG). RANKL and OPG are mainly produced by the osteoblast lineage. RANKL acts directly on osteoclast precursors and mature osteoclasts through its receptor RANK to increase osteoclast differentiation and activation. The relative expression of RANKL and OPG is modulated by proinflammatory cytokines (TNFα, TNFβ, IL-1, IL-6) and eicosanoids released by tumor cells.[16] Tumor cells also can produce parathyroid hormone-related protein (PTHrP), which has been shown to increase RANKL and decrease OPG expression in stromal cells and appears to be particularly important in the development of osteolytic lesions in metastatic bone disease. PTHrP also has anabolic properties and could be in part responsible for osteoblastic-type reactions in prostate cancer. PTHrP can facilitate tumor bone metastasis either by enhancing metastatic potentials of malignant cells directly via autocrine, paracrine, and intracrine mechanisms, or by converting bone to a much more fertile environment for tumor growth via tumor and bone interactions[17] (Fig 8.2). Prostate cancer is by far the most common neoplasm that produces focal osteogenesis in bone tissue. A number of growth factors have been identified including insulin-like growth factors (IGFs), fibroblast growth factors (FGF), transforming growth factor β (TGFβ), vascular endothelial growth factor (VEGF), and others. Osteoblastic metastases can be caused by tumor-secreted endothelin-1 (ET-1).

CHARACTERISTICS OF METASTATIC BONE PAIN

The painful symptoms of bony metastases can vary from muscle spasms to paroxysms of stabbing pain. Hematologic malignancies (especially acute leukemias) may produce a syndrome of generalized and migrating bone pain as a result of marrow infiltration.[18] Limb pain is the most common presentation, and local bone tenderness (especially on long bone diaphyses) is a frequent finding. The vertebrae are the most common sites of bone metastases. The thoracic spine is affected in more than 66% of cases,

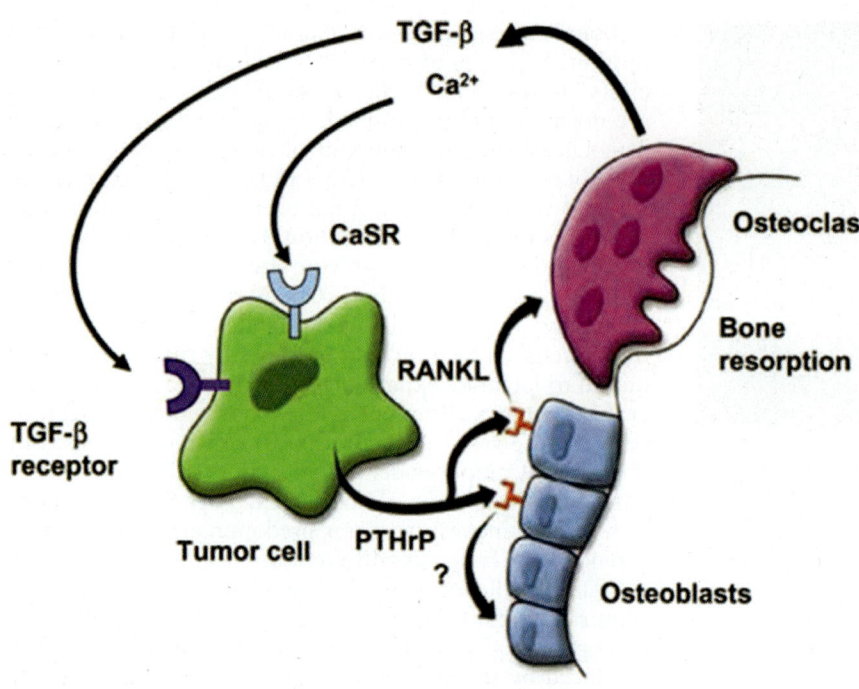

FIGURE 8.2 PTHrP and the cycle of bone metastasis. Tumor cells secrete PTHrP which stimulates bone resorption via receptor activator nuclear factor-κB ligand (RANKL) expression in osteoblastic cells. Bone resorption results in release of growth factors such as TGFβ and calcium from the extracellular matrix. Calcium and TGFβ both feed back to tumor cells to increase PTHrP production. PTHrP, Parathyroid hormone related protein; TGFβ, transforming growth factor fl. (From Liao J, McCauley LK. Skeletal metastasis: Established and emerging roles of parathyroid hormone related protein (PTHrP). *Cancer Metastasis Rev.* 2006; 25(4):559–571. With permission from Springer Science+Business Media.)

the lumbosacral spine in 20% and the cervical spine in 10%. Multiple vertebral lesions are common. Pain from metastases involving T12 and L1 often is referred to the iliac crest or sacroiliac joint unilaterally or bilaterally. Patients with tumor invasion of the upper cervical vertebrae may present with pain in the neck that is referred to the occipital region and skull vertex. Neck flexion typically exacerbates the pain.

Osteolytic bone metastases commonly lead to bone pain, pathologic fractures, hypercalcemia, or more rarely, swelling or neurological symptoms and signs. The vertebrae, pelvis, ribs, femur and skull are the sites most frequently involved.[1] Pain gradually develops during a period of weeks or months, becoming progressively more severe. The pain is usually well localized in a particular area and is often strongest at night or on weight bearing. Patients describe the pain as dull in character, constant in presentation and gradually progressive in intensity. Pain increases with pressure on the involved area. Continuous pain may be moderate on resting and then increase with different movements or positions, such as standing, walking or sitting. Breakthrough pain can result from weight-bearing or instability due to incipient or actual pathological fractures. Although the locus of bone pain usually corresponds to the site of the underlying lesion, characteristic patterns of referral to noncontiguous cutaneous areas occurs; for example, hip pain due to a hip lesion may be referred to the knee.

CLINICAL CONSEQUENCES OF SKELETAL METASTASES

Skeletal metastases are the cause of significant morbidity: pain, impaired mobility, hypercalcemia, pathologic fracture, spinal cord or nerve root compression, and bone marrow infiltration. On average, a patient with metastatic disease will experience a skeletal-related event every 3 to 6 months.[19] However, the occurrence of these morbid events is not regular, with events clustering around periods of progression and becoming more frequent as the disease becomes more extensive and the treatment options reduce. Spinal instability is the cause of back pain in 10% of cancer patients.[20] Metastatic destruction of bone reduces its load-bearing capabilities, initially producing trabecular disruption and microfractures and subsequently total loss of bony integrity. Rib fractures and vertebral collapse are most common, resulting in loss of height, kyphoscoliosis, and a degree of restrictive lung disease. However, the fracture of a long bone or epidural extension of tumor into the spine causes the most disability. The probability of developing a pathologic fracture increases with the duration of metastatic involvement. It is therefore, paradoxically, more common in patients with disease confined to bone who have a relatively good prognosis. Because a fracture is so devastating to a cancer patient, it is important to predict which metastatic sites are at risk of fracture for a particular patient, to use surgery prophylactically, and to administer long-term bisphosphonates.[21]

Bone metastases are the most common cause of cancer-related pain.[22] The pathophysiologic mechanisms of pain in patients with bone metastases are still not fully understood, but advances in basic research suggest that the mechanisms involved probably include tumor-induced osteolysis, tumor production of growth factors and cytokines, direct infiltration of nerves, stimulation of ion channels, and local tissue production of endothelins and nerve growth factors.[23] The presence or intensity of pain does not correlate with the type of tumor, location, number and size of metastases, gender, or age of patients.[24] Although about 80% of patients with breast cancer will develop osteolytic or osteoblastic metastases, about two thirds of demonstrated sites of bone metastases are painless.[25] Different sites of bone metastases are associated with distinct clinical pain syndromes. Common sites of metastatic involvement associated with pain are the base of skull (in association with cranial nerve palsies, neuralgias, and headache), vertebral metastases (producing neck and back pain with or without neurologic complications secondary to epidural extension), and pelvic and femoral lesions (producing pain in the back and lower limbs, often associated with mechanical instability and incident pain).

Hypercalcemia is probably the most common complication of malignancy, and closely related to tumor morbidity. It affects 10% to 40% of the oncology population during the course of their illness.[26] The extent of metastatic bone disease does not correlate with hypercalcemia.[27] Though some non-PTHrP factors could also be involved, PTHrP appears to play a central role in cancer-associated hypercalcemia. The majority of hypercalcemia patients have high levels of PTHrP.[17] Multiple tumors produce PTHrP and high production of PTHrP is often detected in the serum or urine of cancer patients. Measuring serum or urinary PTHrP could be a simple and useful way for early tumor detection, imaging, and prognostic evaluation.

Fractures are common through lytic lesions in weight-bearing bones. Damage to both cortical and trabecular bone is structurally important. Radiological features that may predict imminent fracture include large, predominantly lytic lesions that erode the cortex. The main complications of vertebral metastases are vertebral collapse, radiculopathy, and metastatic epidural spinal cord compression (MESCC). Collapse of vertebral bodies is particularly frequent in the thoracic spine metastases. Back pain is a frequent symptom in patients with advanced cancer and in 10% of cases is a result of spinal instability. The pain, which can be severe, is mechanical in origin, and frequently the patient is only comfortable when lying still. Radiculopathies can occur at any level; patients feel the pain in the spine, deep in the muscles innervated by the affected nerve root, and in the corresponding dermatome. MESCC is a serious complication of vertebral metastases (see "Vertebral Metastases").

CLINICAL IMAGING

Detection of metastatic disease is a function of the type of primary tumor and the imaging methodology. For some types of tumor, such as breast carcinoma, skeletal metastases are readily identifiable by imaging studies. For other conditions, such as chordoma, disseminated skeletal metastases are often evident at autopsy but rarely apparent during the patient's life. Metastases are classified based on x-ray and computed tomography (CT) morphology, differentiating between osteolytic metastases (approximately 50% of skeletal metastases), osteoblastic metastases (approximately 35% of skeletal metastases) primarily from prostate cancer, mixed metastases (approximately 15% from breast, cervical, colon, and thyroid cancer) and periosteal metastases, which rarely occur as a result of lung cancer. The development of skeletal metastases tends to occur most often in hematopoietic active bone marrow which in adults is predominantly found in the axial skeleton including the skull and the proximal portion of the humerus and femur. As a result, localization of metastases preferentially occurs in the axial skeleton (80%), on the femur (40%), and the skull and pelvis (20%). Other less common sites include the ribs and the sternum (25% to 30%).

Various modalities are used for whole-body imaging of the musculoskeletal system, including radiography, bone scintigraphy (Fig 8.3), CT, magnetic resonance imaging (MRI), and positron-emission tomography-computed tomography (PET-CT). Only pronounced destruction of bone with loss of bone mineral content exceeding 50% is readily visible in radiographic examinations.[28] Skeletal scintigraphy utilizing technetium (^{99m}Tc)-marked phosphate complexes has been the largely unrivaled method of choice since the 1980s for the basic bone-related diagnosis, and this modality, with its 95% sensitivity rate, has also been shown to be a reasonable screening examination method for malignant solid tumors.[29] Skeletal scintigraphy is still the diagnostically most valuable and most cost-effective method that enables whole body examinations of almost all patients with high sensitivity. One limitation of skeletal scintigraphy is its lack of specificity. Phosphate accumulates not only in malignant processes but also in patients with infection, fractures, arthrosis, arthritis and osteomyelitis, as well as benign bone tumors. The three-dimensional representation of the skeletal system using single photon-emission computed tomography (SPECT) increases the specificity of skeletal scintigraphy, because this method demonstrates a clearly improved anatomic localization of the accumulation evidenced by skeletal scintigraphy. CT is definitely more sensitive than radiography, and it is the image modality of choice to evaluate the extent of destruction of trabecular and cortical bone and to assess stability and fracture risk. Multislice CT (MS-CT) is frequently used in oncologic imaging, and, in the detection of bone destruction, CT is far more sensitive than radiography. Multislice CT is of particular importance in the evaluation of the stability of skeletal metastases.

MRI allows bone marrow components, such as hematopoietic and fat cells, to be visualized. Moreover, tumor infiltration into the spinal canal and paravertebral soft tissues is clearly depicted. Compared with other imaging modalities like radiography, CT, or bone scintigraphy, it is the most sensitive technique for the detection of pathologies restricted to the bone marrow, even if trabecular bone is not destroyed. For MRI bone metastases screening, the combination of unenhanced T1-weighted spin echo and turbo-STIR (Short T1 Inversion Recovery) sequences is highly sensitive in discriminating benign from malignant marrow disorders.[30] On T1-weighted sequences, tumor spread is identified by replacement of normal fat-containing marrow, resulting in a hypointense signal. Fat-suppressed sequences, such as STIR, depict neoplastic lesions by virtue of the hyperintense signal owing to increased content of water within the tumor cells. However, osteoblastic metastases may be depicted in STIR sequences with variable signal intensities from hypointense in dense sclerotic lesions to hyperintense when more cellular components are present. The unique soft-tissue contrast of MRI allows precise assessment of tumor infiltration within the bone marrow and even diffuse infiltration of the bone marrow with neoplastic cells,

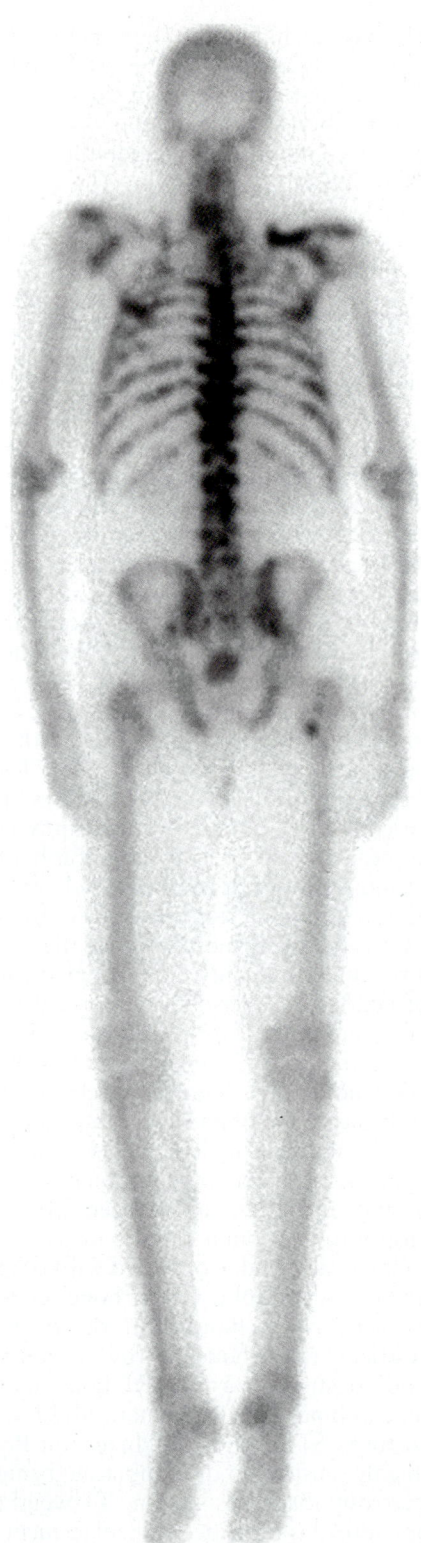

FIGURE 8.3 A 65-year-old man with metastatic prostate cancer. Patient complained of diffuse pain throughout his spine. Postero-anterior (PA) view of bone scan shows diffuse uptake of tracer throughout the vertebral column, right clavicle, bilateral scapular tips, bilateral sacroiliac regions, and right lesser trochanter.

even when not associated with focal bone destructions or formation of new bone. Diagnostic sensitivity of radiography in the detection of myeloma manifestations is low and allows diagnosis only at advanced stages of the disease,

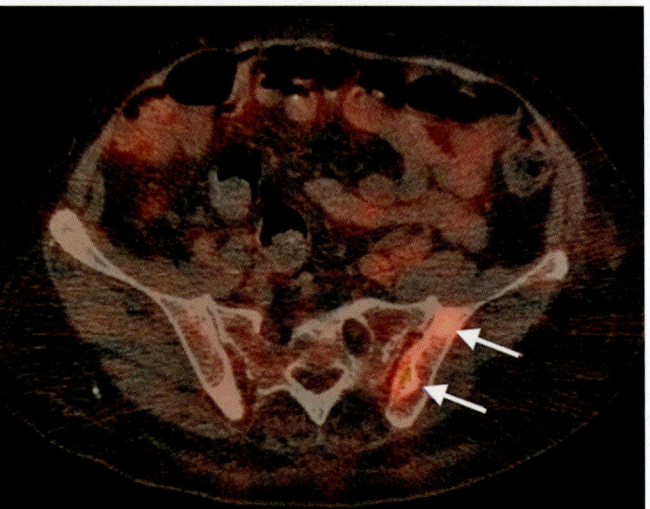

FIGURE 8.4 Axial PET-CT in a 77-year-old woman with ER-positive bone dominant metastatic breast cancer showing hypermetabolic bone lesions in left ilium (arrows). PET-CT, Positron-emission tomography-computed tomography; ER, estrogen receptor.

when at least 50% of the bone mineral content has been lost. Whole-body MRI may be the diagnostic test of choice in this patient group.[31]

A significant advance has been the implementation of PET. PET has been successfully utilized in combination with CT as a functional, morphological examination method in the routine clinical evaluation of oncologic patients. PET has been established as a modern nuclear medicine clinical method. For the purpose of oncologic diagnosis, ^{18}F-FDG is most often used because this PET tracer is a marker of enhanced glucose uptake characteristic of malignant cells. The ^{18}F-FDG tracer is not tumor-specific and also accumulates in infected tissue. FDG-PET imaging can be useful for detecting many types of neoplastic, infectious, and inflammatory processes. Any process that results in greater glucose utilization than background activity demonstrates greater activity. Many malignant and benign neoplasms can be detected with PET imaging because they demonstrate higher rates of glycolysis than background tissues. The degree of enhanced glycolysis depends on the tumor type; therefore, the utility of PET imaging depends on whether the specific cell type uses glucose in sufficient quantities to allow differentiation from the surrounding tissues. The standard uptake value (SUV) is a semiquantitative index used to enumerate glucose metabolism in a given region of tissue. The integration of multislice CT into combined PET-CT imaging allows for the acquisition of high-resolution diagnostic CT data in addition to the anatomic PET data (Fig 8.4). In addition to ^{18}F-FDG-PET, the substance ^{18}F-fluoride is utilized more frequently as an osteotropic radiotracer that, in comparison with bisphosphonates marked with ^{99m}Tc, exhibits a higher osteal uptake and, in addition, leads to a better contrast between osteal and nonosteal structures, owing to increased renal clearance.

PROGNOSIS

The impact of bone metastases is difficult to assess because incidence is influenced by the sensitivity of diagnos-

TABLE 8.2

INCIDENCE AND PROGNOSIS OF BONE METASTASES

Tumor	Incidence of Bone Metastases in Patients with Advanced Disease (%)	Median Survival from Diagnosis of Bone Metastases (Months)
Breast	65–75	19–25
Prostate	65–75	12–53
Lung	30–40	6–7
Bladder	40	6–9
Renal cell	20–25	12
Thyroid	60	48
Melanoma	14–45	6

(From Selvaggi G, Scagliotti GV. Management of bone metastases in cancer: a review. *Crit Rev Oncol Hematol.* 2005;56(3):365–378. With permission from Elsevier.)

TABLE 8.3

KARNOFSKY PERFORMANCE STATUS

Grade	Performance Level
100	Normal, no complaints, no evidence of disease
90	Able to carry on normal activity; minor signs or symptoms of disease
80	Normal activity with effort; some signs or symptoms of disease
70	Cares for self; unable to carry on normal activity or to do active work
60	Requires occasional assistance, but is able to care for most of his or her needs
50	Requires considerable assistance and frequent medical care
40	Disabled, requires special care and assistance
30	Severely disabled, hospitalization indicated; death not imminent
20	Very sick, hospitalization necessary, active supportive treatment necessary
10	Moribund, fatal processes, progressing rapidly
0	Dead

(From Karnofsky DA, et al. Use of nitrogen mustard in the palliative treatment of cancer. *Cancer.* 1948;1:635-656. Copyright 1948 American Cancer Society. Reproduced with permission of Wiley-Liss, Inc., a subsidiary of John Wiley & Sons, Inc.)

tic tools and by the length of patient survival. In general, the prognosis for patients presenting with bone metastases is poor (Table 8.2).

Patients with fewer metastases or solitary lesions appear to have a better outlook than those with multiple metastatic deposits. Once tumor cells spread to the skeleton, the disease is usually incurable, and it may be best to shift the focus of treatment to palliation. Patients suffering from metastatic breast disease survive 34 months on average after detection of the first metastasis, with a range of 1 to 90 months.[32] Survival with metastatic prostate cancer averages 24 months, and lung cancer patients have a prognosis of less than 1 year.[3]

Prognosis in patients with metastatic disease is related to the interval between primary diagnosis and the development of metastases, as well as the current Karnofsky performance status (Table 8.3). The Karnofsky score after palliative irradiation reliably predicts survival.[33] Other factors that predict survival include the site of the primary disease and whether single or multiple bone metastases are present.[34–39] No one has, as yet, developed a classification system, such as a staging system, that can predict the overall prognosis and subsequent patterns of metastatic spread from multiple factors. Staging systems currently in use predict probability of disease control and patterns of failure.

The presence of distant metastases in patients with prostate carcinoma increases with the advancing stage of disease, occurring in 21% of patients with Stage A_2 (T_{1b}) and B (IT_2) disease, 40% of patients with Stage C (T_3) disease, and 62% of patients with Stage D_1 (T_4) disease presentations.[36] The risk for the subsequent development of distant metastases diminishes significantly when the primary tumor is controlled. Survival rates after an isolated recurrence of disease in the prostate depend upon the initial stage of the disease and the disease-free interval from initial treatment. With or without associated local recurrence of the prostate carcinoma, the survival rate is significantly worse when distant metastases are present. The survival rates at 5 and 10 years after pelvic recurrence alone equal 50% and 22%, respectively; with distant metastases, the survival rate at 5 years is 20% and at 10 years <5%.[36,–39] Age significantly influences the 5-year survival rate for patients with prostate carcinoma, independent of race and extent of disease. In prostate carcinoma patients older than 75 years, 5-year survival rates are only 74% with localized disease, 55% with regional disease, and 29% with distant metastases. By contrast, the 5-year survival rates are 86% *(P < .01)*, 73% *(P < .01)*, and 31% *(P < .05)*, respectively, in patients 65 to 74 years of age.[37,40]

The distribution of metastases on bone scans also has prognostic significance. Patients with metastatic carcinoma survive significantly longer if their metastases respond to salvage hormone therapy and do not spread beyond the pelvis or lumbar spine. Diffuse bone metastases tend to occur in patterns of anaplastic histologic features, visceral metastases, and lymph node metastases.[39]

After the diagnosis of metastasis to bone, the median survivals are 12 months for patients with breast carcinoma, 6 months for patients with prostate carcinoma, and 3 months for patients with lung carcinoma. The median survival rate is 48 months when metastases are confined to the skeletal system in patients with breast carcinoma, but it decreases to only 9 months if visceral metastases also are present.[38,41]

SACRAL INSUFFICIENCY FRACTURE

Insufficiency fractures represent a special category of stress fractures that occur in bones with reduced mineral content and elastic resistance. They are often observed in postmenopausal women, in patients who have had high doses of steroids, or in patients who have had exposure to radiation.[42] Radiation has a direct effect on bone and an indirect effect associated with vascular changes.[43] The

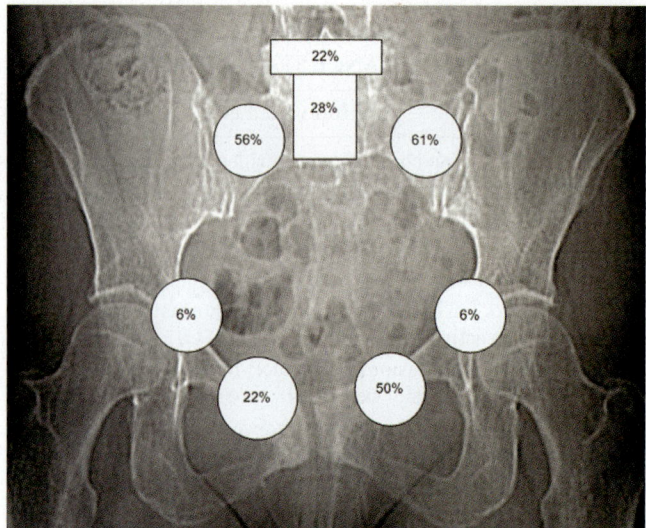

FIGURE 8.5 Distribution of insufficiency fractures. (Modified from Ikushima H, Osaki K, Furutani S, et al. Pelvic bone complications following radiation therapy of gynecologic malignancies: Clinical evaluation of radiation-induced pelvic insufficiency fractures. *Gynecol Oncol.* 2006; 103(3):1100–1104. Copyright 2006, with permission from Elsevier.)

incidence of fracture varies from 8.2% to 17.9% in gynecologic patients who receive radiation therapy.[44–46] One of the main factors responsible for the late effects on irradiated bone is injury of the microvasculature of mature bone. Microcirculation occlusion ultimately results in an increase of susceptibility of stress fracture. Common areas for insufficiency fractures include weight-bearing areas such as the sacral ala, sacral body, and pubic limb (Fig 8.5). The sacral ala is particularly susceptible because of its weight-bearing role. Findings on conventional radiographs are usually subtle and may be misleading. Bone window CT scan is the definitive diagnostic examination for showing fracture lines in many cases of insufficiency fracture. MRI also has a high sensitivity in revealing the edema associated with fracture. The fractures always show increased uptake on radionuclide bone scans (Fig 8.6). The "H" or "Honda" sign on an isotope bone scan is considered diagnostic in the right clinical setting, but this sign is often not present.[47] The diagnostic criteria of sacral insufficiency fracture included regionally increased activity of sacroiliac joint or sacrum or other pelvic bone on bone scintigraphy and/or findings of T1-hypointense and T2-hyperintense lesion without soft-tissue mass on

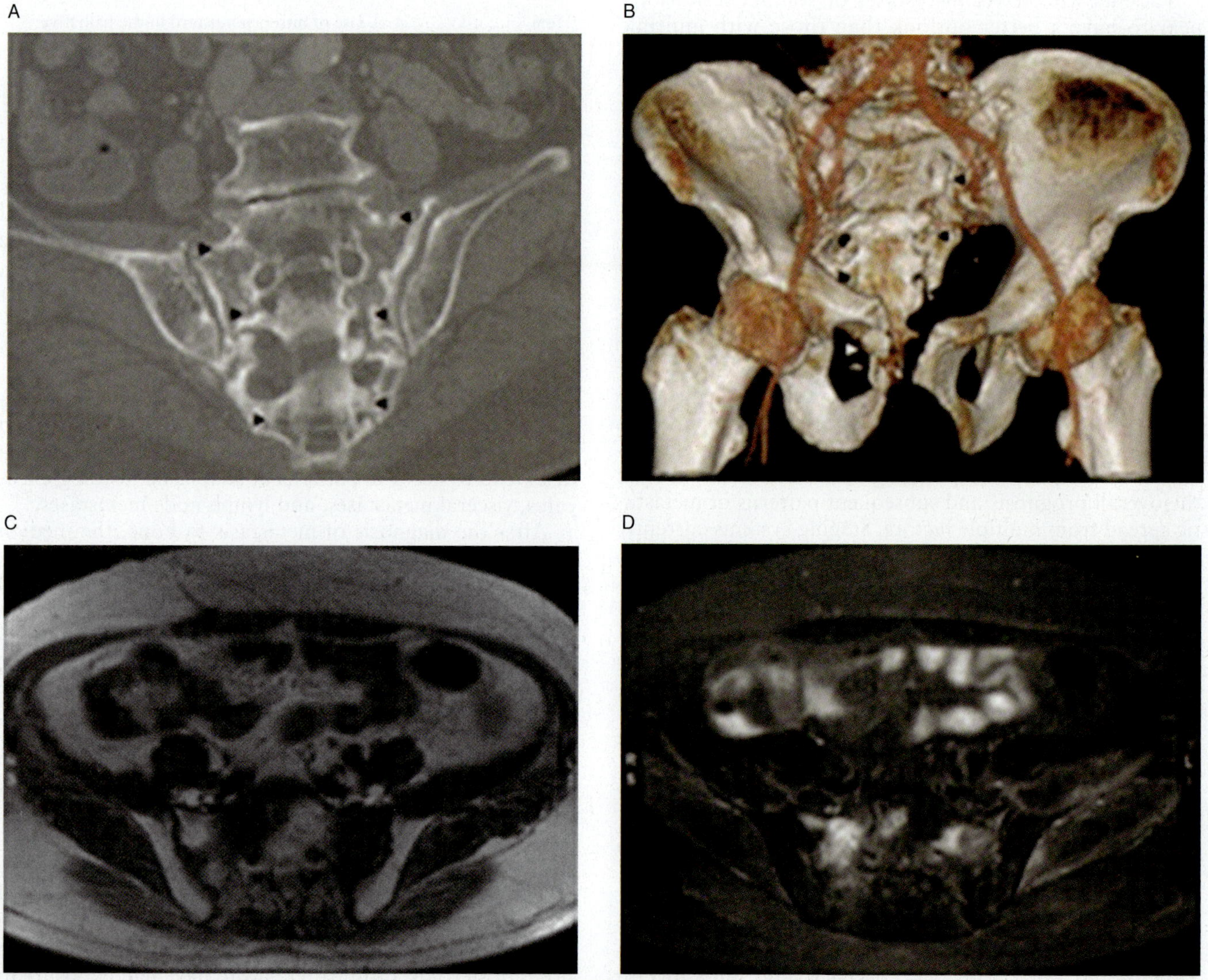

FIGURE 8.6 Imaging of insufficiency fractures. **A:** Coronal plane of CT. **B:** three-dimensional reconstructed image of CT. **C:** T1-weighted image of MRI, **D:** T2-weighted image of MRI, *(Continued on next page)*

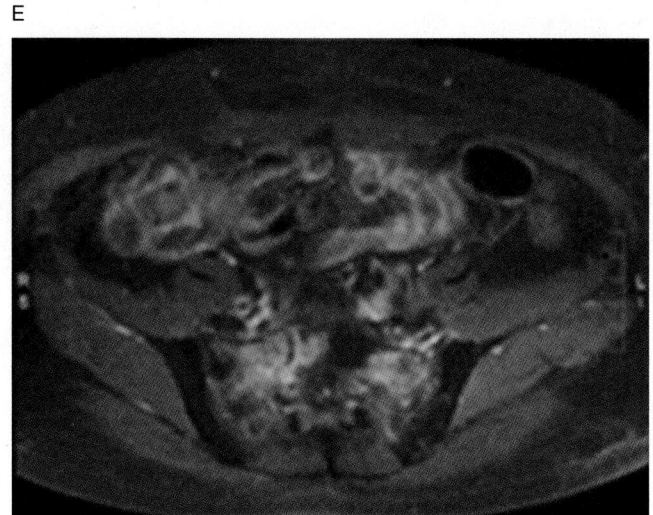 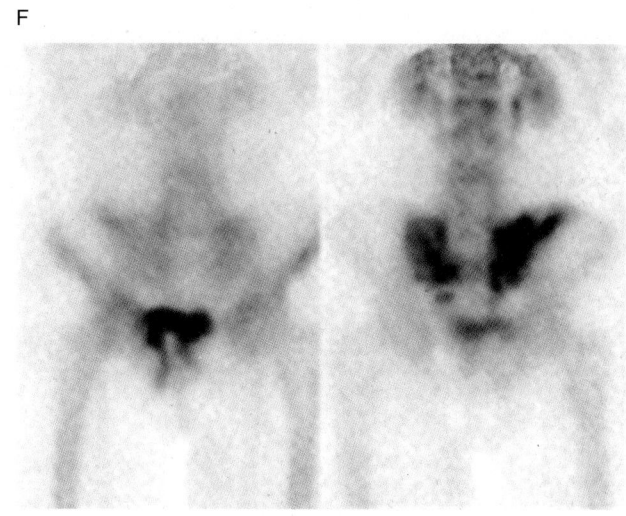

FIGURE 8.6 *(Cont'd)* **E:** T1-weighted and fat-suppression image with contrast enhancement of MRI, **F:** Bone scintigraphy. Reconstructed CT images show symmetric longitudinal fracture lines parallel to the sacroiliac joints and coexistence of parasymphyseal fractures of the right pubic bone *(arrow heads)*. MRI indicates surrounding marrow edema and abnormal enhancement that are undetectable on CT images. Bone scintigraphy shows increased radionuclide uptake on the sacroiliac joints and upper limbs of pubic bones. CT, Computed tomography; MRI, magnetic resonance imaging. (From Ikushima H, Osaki K, Furutani S, et al. Pelvic bone complications following radiation therapy of gynecologic malignancies: Clinical evaluation of radiation-induced pelvic insufficiency fractures. *Gynecol Oncol.* 2006;103(3):1100–1104. Copyright 2006, with permission from Elsevier)

MRI and/or demonstration of fracture lines or sclerotic changes without osteolytic lesion on CT and no evidence of bone metastases during the clinical course (Fig 8.7).

Although insufficiency fracture is often misdiagnosed as a bone metastasis, biopsy of the lesion is not recommended because of a high probability of osteonecrosis and the low diagnostic efficiency. Typically, patients present with groin, low back, or buttock pain. Pain complaints may be in more than one location. Many patients have pain intense enough to render the patient nonambulatory. Physical examination may reveal low back or groin tenderness with restricted hip movement. Diagnosis is usually made radiologically in patients with a previous history of pelvic radiation therapy. The use of a multibeam arrangement for pelvic radiation therapy to reduce the volume and dose of irradiated pelvic bone can be helpful to minimize the risk of fracture, especially in elderly women with low body weight.[48]

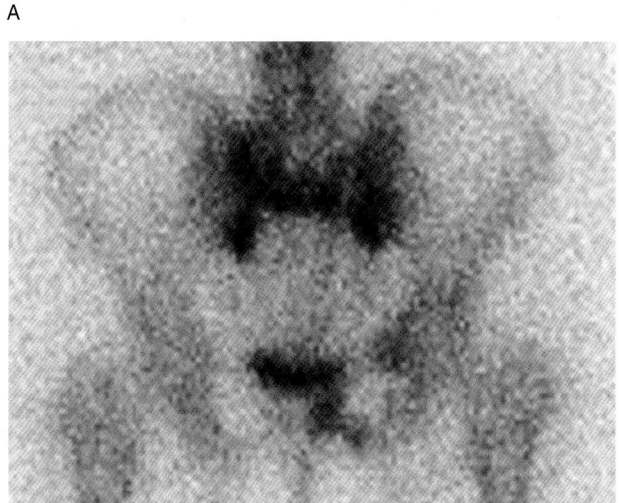 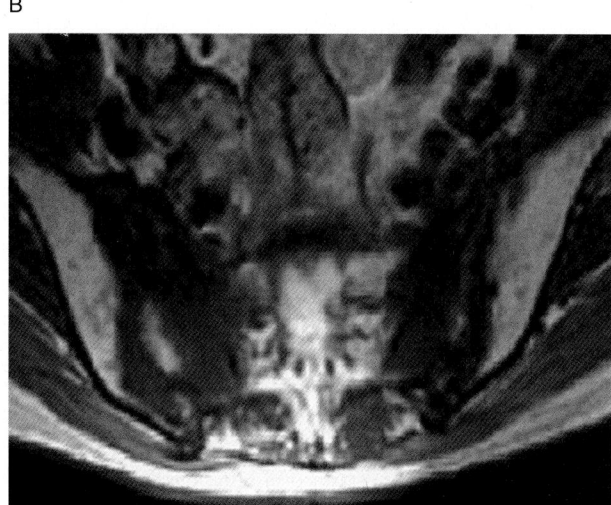

FIGURE 8.7 Bone scintigraphy shows **(A)** "H" sign: hot uptake in bilateral SI joints and the sacral body. Magnetic resonance imaging shows **(B)** low signal intensity in both SI joints on T1-weighted image and *(Continued on next page)*

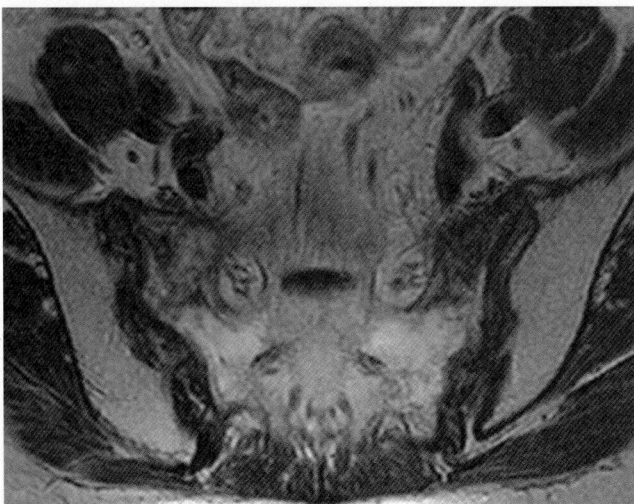
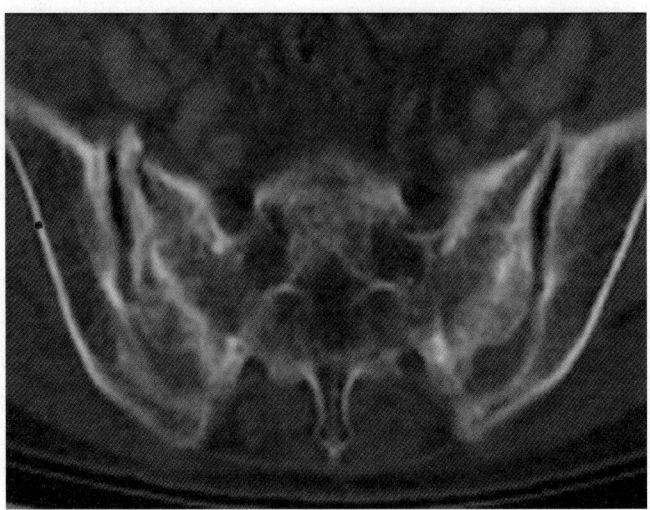

FIGURE 8.7 *(Cont'd)* (C) high signal intensity on T2-weighted image. Bone window CT shows (D) sclerotic changes and cortical fracture in both sacroiliac alae. SI, sacroiliac; CT, computed tomography. (Oh D, Huh SJ, Nam H, et al. Pelvic insufficiency fracture after pelvic radiotherapy for cervical cancer: analysis of risk factors. *Int J Radiat Oncol Biol Phys.* 2008;70(4):1183–1188. With permission from Elsevier.)

References

1. Tubiana-Hulin M. Incidence, prevalence and distribution of bone metastases. *Bone.* 1991;12(Suppl 1):S9-S10.
2. Wagner G. Frequency of pain in patients with cancer. *Recent Results Cancer Res.* 1984;89:64–71.
3. Nielsen OS, Munro AJ, Tannock IF. Bone metastases: pathophysiology and management policy. *J Clin Oncol.* 1991;9:509–524.
4. Brescia FJ, Adler D, Gray G, et al. Hospitalized advanced cancer patients: a profile. *J Pain Symptom Manage.* 1990;5:221–227.
5. Morris JN, Mor V, Goldberg RJ, et al. The effect of treatment setting and patient characteristics on pain in terminal cancer patients: a report from the National Hospice Study. *J Chronic Dis.* 1986;39:27–35.
6. Twycross RG, Fairfield S. Pain in far-advanced cancer. *Pain.* 1982;14:303–310.
7. Banning A, Sjogren P, Henriksen H. Pain causes in 200 patients referred to a multidisciplinary cancer pain clinic. *Pain.* 1991;45:45–48.
8. Paterson AH, Ernst DS, Powles TJ, et al. Treatment of skeletal disease in breast cancer with clodronate. *Bone.* 1991;12 Suppl 1:S25-30.
9. Kanis JA, McCloskey EV. Bone turnover and biochemical markers in malignancy. *Cancer.* 1997;80:1538–1545.
10. Kanis JA, McCloskey EV, Taube T, et al. Rationale for the use of bisphosphonates in bone metastases. *Bone.* 1991;12 Suppl 1:S13-8.
11. Koutsilieris M, Rabbani SA, Bennett HP, et al. Characteristics of prostate-derived growth factors for cells of the osteoblast phenotype. *J Clin Invest.* 1987;80:941–946.
12. Clavel M. Management of breast cancer with bone metastases. *Bone.* 1991;12 Suppl 1:S11-2.
13. Fisher MS. Lumbar spine metastasis in cervical carcinoma: a characteristic pattern. *Radiology.* 1980;134:631–634.
14. Choong PF. The molecular basis of skeletal metastases. *Clin Orthop Relat Res.* 2003:S19-31.
15. Thomas RJ, Guise TA, Yin JJ, et al. Breast cancer cells interact with osteoblasts to support osteoclast formation. *Endocrinology.* 1999;140:4451–4458.
16. Kozlow W, Guise TA. Breast cancer metastasis to bone: mechanisms of osteolysis and implications for therapy. *J Mammary Gland Biol Neoplasia.* 2005;10:169–180.
17. Liao J, McCauley LK. Skeletal metastasis: Established and emerging roles of parathyroid hormone related protein (PTHrP). *Cancer Metastasis Rev.* 2006;25:559–571.
18. Jonsson OG, Sartain P, Ducore JM, et al. Bone pain as an initial symptom of childhood acute lymphoblastic leukemia: association with nearly normal hematologic indexes. *J Pediatr.* 1990;117:233–237.
19. Coleman RE. Clinical features of metastatic bone disease and risk of skeletal morbidity. *Clin Cancer Res.* 2006;12:6243s-6249s.
20. DeWald RL, Bridwell KH, Prodromas C, et al. Reconstructive spinal surgery as palliation for metastatic malignancies of the spine. *Spine.* 1985;10:21–26.
21. Body JJ, Coleman RE, Piccart M. Use of bisphosphonates in cancer patients. *Cancer Treat Rev.* 1996;22:265–287.
22. Mercadante S. Malignant bone pain: pathophysiology and treatment. *Pain.* 1997;69:1–18.
23. Sabino MA, Mantyh PW. Pathophysiology of bone cancer pain. *J Support Oncol.* 2005;3:15–24.
24. Oster MW, Vizel M, Turgeon LR. Pain of terminal cancer patients. *Arch Intern Med.* 1978;138:1801–1802.
25. Front D, Schneck SO, Frankel A, et al. Bone metastases and bone pain in breast cancer. Are they closely associated? *JAMA.* 1979;242:1747–1748.
26. Ralston SH. Pathogenesis and management of cancer associated hypercalcaemia. *Cancer Surv.* 1994;21:179–196.
27. Mundy GR. Mechanisms of osteolytic bone destruction. *Bone.* 1991;12(Suppl 1):S1-6.
28. Lecouvet FE, Malghem J, Michaux L, et al. Skeletal survey in advanced multiple myeloma: radiographic versus MR imaging survey. *Br J Haematol.* 1999;106:35–39.
29. Ghanem N, Uhl M, Brink I, et al. Diagnostic value of MRI in comparison to scintigraphy, PET, MS-CT and PET/CT for the detection of metastases of bone. *Eur J Radiol.* 2005;55:41–55.
30. Walker R, Kessar P, Blanchard R, et al. Turbo STIR magnetic resonance imaging as a whole-body screening tool for metastases in patients with breast carcinoma: preliminary clinical experience. *J Magn Reson Imaging.* 2000;11:343–350.
31. Ghanem N, Lohrmann C, Engelhardt M, et al. Whole-body MRI in the detection of bone marrow infiltration in patients with plasma cell neoplasms in comparison to the radiological skeletal survey. *Eur Radiol.* 2006;16:1005–1014.
32. Koenders PG, Beex LV, Kloppenborg PW, et al. Human breast cancer: survival from first metastasis. Breast Cancer Study Group. *Breast Cancer Res Treat.* 1992;21:173–180.
33. Jones PW, Bogardus CR, Anderson DW. Significance of initial "performance status" in patients receiving halfbody radiation. *Int J Radiat Oncol Biol Phys.* 1984;10:1947–1950.
34. Blitzer PH. Reanalysis of the RTOG study of the palliation of symptomatic osseous metastasis. *Cancer.* 1985;55:1468–1472.
35. Fielding LP, Henson DE. Multiple prognostic factors and outcome analysis in patients with cancer. Communication from the American Joint Committee on Cancer. *Cancer.* 1993;71:2426–2429.
36. Lai PP, Perez CA, Lockett MA. Prognostic significance of pelvic recurrence and distant metastasis in prostate carcinoma following definitive radiotherapy. *Int J Radiat Oncol Biol Phys.* 1992;24:423–430.

37. Reuben DB, Mor V, Hiris J. Clinical symptoms and length of survival in patients with terminal cancer. *Arch Intern Med.* 1988;148:1586–1591.
38. Sherry MM, Greco FA, Johnson DH, et al. Breast cancer with skeletal metastases at initial diagnosis. Distinctive clinical characteristics and favorable prognosis. *Cancer.* 1986;58:178–182.
39. Yamashita K, Denno K, Ueda T, et al. Prognostic significance of bone metastases in patients with metastatic prostate cancer. *Cancer.* 1993;71:1297–1302.
40. Kant AK, Glover C, Horm J, et al. Does cancer survival differ for older patients? *Cancer.* 1992;70:2734–2740.
41. Sherry MM, Greco FA, Johnson DH, et al. Metastatic breast cancer confined to the skeletal system. An indolent disease. *Am J Med.* 1986;81:381–386.
42. Saraux A, Valls I, Guedes C, et al. Insufficiency fractures of the sacrum in elderly subjects. *Rev Rhum Engl Ed.* 1995;62:582–586.
43. Howland WJ, Loeffler RK, Starchman DE, et al. Postirradiation atrophic changes of bone and related complications. *Radiology.* 1975;117:677–685.
44. Baxter NN, Habermann EB, Tepper JE, et al. Risk of pelvic fractures in older women following pelvic irradiation. *JAMA.* 2005;294:2587–2593.
45. Ikushima H, Osaki K, Furutani S, et al. Pelvic bone complications following radiation therapy of gynecologic malignancies: clinical evaluation of radiation-induced pelvic insufficiency fractures. *Gynecol Oncol.* 2006;103:1100–1104.
46. Ogino I, Okamoto N, Ono Y, et al. Pelvic insufficiency fractures in postmenopausal woman with advanced cervical cancer treated by radiotherapy. *Radiother Oncol.* 2003;68:61–67.
47. Blake SP, Connors AM. Sacral insufficiency fracture. *Br J Radiol.* 2004;77:891–896.
48. Oh D, Huh SJ, Nam H, et al. Pelvic insufficiency fracture after pelvic radiotherapy for cervical cancer: analysis of risk factors. *Int J Radiat Oncol Biol Phys.* 2008;70:1183–1188.

CHAPTER 9 ■ VISCERAL PAIN

Malignant infiltration of the viscera is a common cause of pain in cancer patients. Often, ascites and pleural effusions are associated with advanced visceral disease and can present significant pain management problems. Almost 75% of all malignant pleural effusions arise from malignancies of the breasts, lungs, ovaries, and lymphomas. Malignant pleural effusions are mostly recurrent and often resistant to systemic treatment. Patients with pleural effusions often complain of dyspnea, cough, thoracic discomfort, and pain. Ascites results from multiple mechanisms, including vascular permeability changes, peritoneal carcinomatosis, lymph drainage obstruction, hepatic congestion due to tumor infiltration, or neoplastic production of exudative fluid. Significant issues may arise, such as respiratory restriction and respiratory distress because of diaphragmatic compression, bacterial peritonitis (either spontaneous or iatrogenic from drainage), electrolyte and hemodynamic disturbances, hepatorenal syndrome, and physical discomfort with limitation of movement, leading to reduction of quality of life. Malignant ascites can lead to dyspnea, nausea, diminished appetite, early satiety, fatigue, lower extremity edema, and limited mobility. Additional issues associated with tumor infiltration of viscera, including malignant bowel obstruction, may also occur, presenting a difficult management dilemma, particularly in the patient who is a poor surgical candidate. Table 9.1 lists the common pain syndromes associated with tumor infiltration.

MECHANISM

Pain that emanates from organs in the thorax, abdomen, or pelvis is labeled *visceral*. The factors thought to be capable of inducing pain in visceral structures include abnormal distention and contraction of hollow visceral walls, rapid stretching of the capsules of solid visceral organs, ischemia of visceral musculature, formation and accumulation of algogenic substances, direct action of chemical stimuli on compromised mucosa, and traction or compression of ligaments, vessels, or mesentery.[1–3] Mechanical insult to normal mucosa causes no pain, implying that preceding inflammation is necessary for pain to occur.

There are two distinct classes of nociceptive sensory receptors in viscera.[4] The first class is composed of "high-threshold" receptors that respond to mechanical stimuli within the noxious range. These have been identified within many viscera, including the heart, lungs, gastrointestinal tract, ureters, and urinary bladder. The second class is composed of receptors that have a low threshold to natural stimuli and encode the stimulus intensity in the magnitude of their discharges, the so-called "intensity-encoding" receptors. Both receptor types are mainly concerned with mechanical stimuli, such as stretch, and are involved in the peripheral encoding of noxious stimuli in viscera. In the presence of local inflammation or tissue injury, these afferents become sensitized and respond to previously innocuous natural stimuli. High-threshold afferents signal acute visceral pain. Local ischemia, hypoxia, and inflammation cause pain by sensitizing high-threshold receptors and these previously "silent" or unresponsive receptors. Apart from innervating the gut wall, afferents also have endings located in the mesentery and serosa.[5–6]

Pain in visceral structures is not necessarily linked to tissue injury, but is more dependent on the nature of the provoking stimulus. Adequate stimuli that induce pain are distension, ischemia, and inflammation. Hollow organs such as the colon are very sensitive to luminal distension or inflammation but are totally insensitive to cutting or burning stimuli. Nociceptive afferents from thoracic and abdominal viscera travel along the path of visceral sympathetic efferent fibers. Abdominal nociceptive afferents travel to the celiac plexus and the thoracic splanchnics before entering the sympathetic trunks and dorsal horn. Spinal visceral afferents represent 10%–20% of nerve fibers in splanchnic nerves, and project to all layers of the gut wall including the serosa and mesenteric attachments where they terminate as bare nerve endings.[7] By contrast, the pelvic visceral nociceptor afferents converge on the pelvic splanchnic nerves, which are primarily parasympathetic efferent fibers. Some pelvic afferents also pass through the lumbar sympathetic splanchnic nerves. Poorly localized visceral pain may be explained by the low

TABLE 9.1

PAINS RELATED TO VISCERAL INFILTRATION BY TUMOR

Pain Location	Organ Involvement
Chest/retrosternum	Esophagus
Shoulder	Diaphragm (referred pain)
Upper abdomen	Pancreas
Right upper abdomen/lower chest	Liver capsule
Left upper abdomen/flank	Spleen
Diffuse abdomen	Peritoneum or mesentery
Localized or diffuse abdomen	Bowel obstruction or perforation
Unilateral chest	Pleura
Right upper abdomen	Biliary
Flank	Ureter
Suprapubic or pelvic	Bladder
Perianal	Perineum

density of visceral nociceptors, the functional divergence of visceral input with the central nervous system, and viscerovisceral convergence in the spinal cord.

Localization of visceral pain is difficult. Afferent nerves from viscera to the spinal cord are relatively few in number and comprise only 2% to 15% of all afferents to the spinal cord.[8-9] Unlike autonomic efferents that synapse in celiac, hypogastric plexuses, or sympathetic ganglia, first-order spinal afferents traverse paravertebral and prevertebral ganglia to synapse like somatic afferents in the dorsal horn. Visceral afferents have a widespread distribution in laminae I, II, V, and X.[9-10] Viscerosomatic convergence at the level of the dorsal horn of the spinal cord accounts for the referral experienced with visceral pain. These visceral nociceptive afferents can excite many second-order neurons in the spinal cord which in turn generate extensive divergence within the CNS, sometimes involving supraspinal loops. Such a divergent input activates several systems—sensory, motor and autonomic—and, thus, triggers the general reactions that are characteristic of visceral nociception: diffuse and referred pain, and prolonged autonomic and motor activity.[1] Second-order neurons project to the brain through the spinoreticular, spinomesencephalic, spinohypothalamic, and spinothalamic tracts,[11] all of which lie in the anterolateral quadrant of the spinal cord.

The dorsal column in the spinal cord contains an ascending excitatory pathway that plays a role in the perception of visceral pain, especially under the conditions of peripheral inflammation.[12] This pathway has been established in the dorsal columns of animals[13-14] which passes via ipsilateral dorsal column nuclei to the contralateral ventroposterolateral nucleus of the thalamus.[13] In humans, the role of this pathway is unclear. Activation of thalamic neurons by the dorsal column pathway, through a relay in the dorsal column nuclei, may be an important element in this mechanism. The dorsal column pathway may contain an ascending part of an amplification loop that enhances the responsiveness of spinal cord neurons through a descending facilitating pathway, possibly originating in the rostroventral medulla.[15] This amplification circuit could lead to potentiation of the responses of different projection neurons, including viscerosensitive spinothalamic and postsynaptic dorsal column neurons. The effectiveness of the midline myelotomy in visceral pain patients could thus be explained by a direct reduction in the activation of thalamic neurons mediated by postsynaptic dorsal column neurons, as well as by an interruption of the amplification loop, thereby preventing the potentiation of the visceral responses of other projection neurons, such as spinothalamic tract cells.

Visceral pain is either true, referred, nonreferred parietal, or referred parietal. True parietal abdominal pain is dull and poorly localized; it occurs in the region of the epigastric, periumbilical, or lower midabdominal region. Patients may describe the pain as gnawing or cramping, and it is often associated with nausea, sweating, pallor, and, occasionally, vomiting. Referred visceral pain is more precisely localized, usually in the dermatomal or myosomal regions of the same segments of the spinal cord involved. Parietal pain may localize directly over the organ without referral. Patients locate referred parietal pain in a body region distant from the nociceptive site. For example, patients complain of pain in the shoulder area when the cause is inflammation of the middle diaphragm.

Nociception can be generated by tumor invasion of adjacent blood vessels. Mechanisms include perivascular lymphangitis causing vasospasm, occlusion with resultant ischemia, venous engorgement, and edema.

Obstruction of hollow viscera from tumor leading to viscus distention may cause pain. Distention causes intense contraction of smooth muscle that generates nociception. Patients experience visceral pain that is poorly localized and diffuse but usually localized in the same dermatomal area of the cord segments of the viscera.

Pain from tumor involvement of parenchymal viscera such as liver, spleen, pancreas, and kidney typically results from acute distention of the pain-sensitive fascia. These fascia contain many mechanical receptors, and nociception occurs when they are acutely stretched or placed under tension. This type of pain is poorly defined, dull, and generally located in the dermatomal region of the involved organ.

VISCERAL PAIN DESCRIPTIONS BY SITE

Esophageal cancer frequently produces a history of heartburn: a burning or gnawing substernal discomfort. Patients usually describe the pain as being located in the epigastric or retrosternal areas, which often radiates to the back or interscapular region. The pain occurs soon after eating, and may be influenced by body position changes such as reclining or bending forward.

Gastric pain has a colicky quality associated with delayed emptying and slowed motility and digestive symptoms. The pain also localizes in the epigastrium, is usually sharply focused, and may radiate into the back.

Small intestine pain is usually crampy or colicky and localized in the periumbilical area. The cause of pain is usually a lesion causing distention with resultant abnormal mobility. Eating usually precipitates the pain, and defecation or fasting may afford relief. *Colon* pain tends to occur in the lower abdomen, varying according to which portion of the colon is affected. Change in bowel habits and occult blood in the stool often accompanies symptoms of discomfort. *Peritoneal* carcinomatosis is frequently found with abdominal tumors and advanced ovarian cancer. Pain may result from peritoneal irritation, mesenteric involvement, and abdominal distention with ascites. Bowel obstruction often complicates peritoneal carcinomatosis.

Liver parenchyma is insensitive to tumor distention and associated chemical changes. Right upper quadrant pain from liver pathology occurs only when there is acute distention of the liver capsule. It is usually a dull aching sensation in the right upper abdominal quadrant and flank, and is often referred to the right scapula and shoulder.

Perineal pain, often worse when sitting and described as aching and pressure-like, is the first and, for a long time, can be the only symptom of pelvic tumors. The pain may be associated with visceral problems such as tenesmus. Complications from cancer and its treatment such as fistulas and recurrent infections can aggravate the pain complaint in this area. Ureteral obstruction is not uncommon. Direct invasion of the sacrum, sacral roots, plexus, or cauda equina are additional frequent complications exacerbating the pain complaint. Pain from the *fundus of the uterus* typically occurs in the hypogastrium. Pain originating from the *uterine cervix* is commonly referred to the low back and sacral area as well as to the hypogastrium. *Ovarian* pain results from stretching of the surrounding peritoneum to which the ovaries adhere.

Ureteral pain and obstruction is usually due to metastatic disease by direct tumor compression of the ureters, extrinsic compression from a retroperitoneal mass, or encasement of the ureters with metastatic lymph nodes. Progressive obstructive uropathy with electrolyte imbalances and persistent urinary tract infections may result. Pain due to acute ureteral obstruction is generally caused by pressure or stretch in the lumen and nociceptive signals are subsequently transmitted by renal afferent nerves to the dorsal horn neurons and suprasegmental modulatory areas, including the midbrain paraventricular gray and periaqueductal gray.[16]

References

1. Cervero F. Mechanisms of acute visceral pain. *Br Med Bull.* 1991;47:549–560.
2. Cervero F. Visceral pain: mechanisms of peripheral and central sensitization. *Ann Med.* 1995;27:235–239.
3. Gebhart GF, Ness TJ. Central mechanisms of visceral pain. *Can J Physiol Pharmacol.* 1991;69:627–634.
4. Cervero F. Sensory innervation of the viscera: peripheral basis of visceral pain. *Physiol Rev.* 1994;74:95–138.
5. Brunsden AM, Brookes SJ, Bardhan KD, et al. Mechanisms underlying mechanosensitivity of mesenteric afferent fibers to vascular flow. *Am J Physiol Gastrointest Liver Physiol.* 2007;293:G422–G428.
6. Tassicker BC, Hennig GW, Costa M, et al. Rapid anterograde and retrograde tracing from mesenteric nerve trunks to the guinea-pig small intestine in vitro. *Cell Tissue Res.* 1999;295:437–452.
7. Blackshaw LA, Gebhart GF. The pharmacology of gastrointestinal nociceptive pathways. *Curr Opin Pharmacol.* 2002;2:642–649.
8. Cervero F, Connell LA. Distribution of somatic and visceral primary afferent fibres within the thoracic spinal cord of the cat. *J Comp Neurol.* 1984;230:88–98.
9. Ness TJ, Gebhart GF. Visceral pain: a review of experimental studies. *Pain.* 1990;41:167–234.
10. Grundy D, Al-Chaer ED, Aziz Q, et al. Fundamentals of neurogastroenterology: basic science. *Gastroenterology.* 2006;130:1391–1411.
11. Almeida TF, Roizenblatt S, Tufik S. Afferent pain pathways: a neuroanatomical review. *Brain Res.* 2004;1000:40–56.
12. Palecek J, Willis WD. The dorsal column pathway facilitates visceromotor responses to colorectal distention after colon inflammation in rats. *Pain.* 2003;104:501–507.
13. Al-Chaer ED, Feng Y, Willis WD. Comparative study of viscerosomatic input onto postsynaptic dorsal column and spinothalamic tract neurons in the primate. *J Neurophysiol.* 1999;82:1876–1882.
14. Al-Chaer ED, Kawasaki M, Pasricha PJ. A new model of chronic visceral hypersensitivity in adult rats induced by colon irritation during postnatal development. *Gastroenterology.* 2000;119:1276–1285.
15. Palecek J. The role of dorsal columns pathway in visceral pain. *Physiol Res.* 2004;53 Suppl 1:S125–S130.
16. Roza C, Laird JM. Pressor responses to distension of the ureter in anaesthetised rats: characterisation of a model of acute visceral pain. *Neurosci Lett.* 1995;198:9–12.

CHAPTER 10 ■ NEUROPATHIC PAIN

Neuropathic pain is a result of dysfunction, either in peripheral nerves or in the central processing within the spinal cord and brain. It is possible to categorize neuropathic pains on the basis of underlying pathology, the region of the nervous system that is affected, and the individual patient's responses to the pain syndrome. It is common to find alterations in sensation in the sensory territory of damaged nerves or their central projection pathways. Neuropathic pains have many etiologies, including tumors compressing or invading nerves, surgical trauma of nerves, inflammation of nerves, neurotoxins, endocrinological disorders affecting nerve function, vascular compromise of peripheral (PNS) or central (CNS) nervous system structures, and viral infection of the nervous system. Neuropathic pains are often characterized by the paradoxical combination of sensory loss, perversions of sensation, and pain in a defined region of the body. Common causes of neuropathic pain in the cancer patient include compression or infiltration of nerves by tumor, nerve trauma secondary to diagnostic or surgical procedures, and nervous system (including spinal cord) injury following treatments such as chemotherapy or radiation.[1]

Neuropathic pain is characterized by both positive and negative symptoms.[2] Positive symptoms include spontaneous pain, paresthesia, dysesthesia, after-sensations, and abnormal temporal and spatial summation, as well as a pain evoked by normally innocuous stimuli (allodynia) and an exaggerated or prolonged pain to noxious stimuli (hyperalgesia or hyperpathia). The negative symptoms reflect either the loss of sensation due to axonal or neuronal death or, alternatively, central inhibition. The positive symptoms reflect abnormal excitability within the nervous system. Neuropathic pain may be reported as burning or lancinating. These abnormal sensory phenomena can be further characterized as elicited by static or dynamic stimuli. A distinction should be made between stimulus-evoked pain and spontaneous (stimulus-independent) pain, which may have different underlying mechanisms. Spontaneous pain can be either constant or intermittent (even paroxysmal), and most patients describe having both (eg, constant "burning" pain plus intermittent pain that is "shooting" or "electric shock–like"). In addition, spontaneous paresthesias and dysesthesias may manifest as abnormal sensations, including crawling, numbness, itching, and tingling.

Patients may have sensory deficits with one modality, such as pinprick sensitivity, and hyperalgesia to another, such as light touch, both in the same nerve distribution.[3] Dynamic mechanical allodynia can be elicited by lightly rubbing or brushing the skin with a cotton swab or brush; static mechanical allodynia can be provoked by blunt pressure with a finger; and thermal allodynia can be assessed with a warm or cool tuning fork. An increased sensation of pain in response to a normally painful stimulus is termed *hyperalgesia*, which can be assessed using painful thermal (cold or heat) or punctate (eg, pinprick) stimuli. Painful summation and wind-up to repeated stimuli, especially when the initial sensation is reduced, is important evidence of abnormal sensory processing. Diagnosing neuropathic pain can be difficult, as it may occur in conjunction with pains of other etiology, as seen in the patient with low back and leg pain secondary to spondylolisthesis. Furthermore, there may be a significant neuropathic component from nerve root injury, but mechanical instability or secondary myofascial pain can mask this component.

The majority of research into neuropathic pain mechanisms has concentrated on changes in the peripheral nerve or spinal cord after peripheral nerve injury and, therefore, most available evidence relates to changes in these parts of the nervous system.[4] Nevertheless, it is important to recognize that alterations in the brain have also been demonstrated following peripheral nerve injury, but much less is known about the significance of these changes. For example, phantom limb pain has been shown to be associated with reorganization of the cortex of humans.[5] Also, lesions exclusively in the CNS, such as a stroke involving the lateral thalamus, can produce a neuropathic pain syndrome.

Nerve fibers can develop abnormal ectopic excitability at or near a site of injury. The mechanisms include unusual distributions of Na^+ channels, as well as abnormal responses to endogenous algogenic substances and cytokines such as tumor necrosis factor α (TNF-α).[6] Injury anywhere in a peripheral nerve produces changes in the associated dorsal root ganglion cells and the dorsal horn neurons which the peripheral axons project upon. The spread of pathophysiology includes upregulation of nitric oxide synthase in axotomized neurons, deafferentation hypersensitivity of spinal neurons following afferent cell death, long-term potentiation of spinal synaptic transmission, and attenuation of central pain inhibitory mechanisms. Repeated or prolonged noxious stimulation and the persistent abnormal input following nerve injury activate a number of intracellular second messenger systems. Although these processes of increasing nervous system excitability may be considered a strategy to compensate for functional deficits following nerve injury, the result is widespread nervous system sensitization resulting in pain and hyperalgesia.

Another sequel of nerve injury or disease such as virus attack is apoptosis of neurons in the PNS and CNS. Apoptosis appears to induce neuronal sensitization and loss of inhibitory systems, and these potentially irreversible processes might underlie both nervous system damage by brain trauma or ischemia as well as neuropathic pain.[6] Factors contributing to central sensitization and disinhibition of pain pathways (and thus, central pain) include gain in neuronal excitability, loss of inhibition, and increased facilitation.[7] Activated microglia (usually as a consequence of an inflammatory process) appear to maintain neuronal hyperexcitability in the spinal cord dorsal horn through an extracellular signal-regulated kinase-regulated PGE2 signaling mechanism.[8]

The CNS adapts to both PNS and CNS injury, sometimes in beneficial ways, but also with reorganization that can be maladaptive.[9] Advances in functional imaging techniques have resulted in significant improvements in our knowledge of brain function. Modern neuroimaging methods include positron-emission tomography (PET), functional magnetic resonance imaging (fMRI) and magnetoencephalography (MEG). The primary use of MEG is the measurement of time courses of activity of neuronal function and to pinpoint sources in primary auditory, somatosensory, and motor areas in creating functional maps. PET and fMRI have been used to determine whether different neuropathic pain symptoms involve similar brain structures and whether these structures are related to the physiological "pain matrix."[10] PET can be used as a measure of local brain activity by using radionuclides to produce maps representing changes in cerebral blood flow. PET has been applied to investigate the neural substrates involved in pain processing and perception in human subjects.[11]

PET studies have suggested that spontaneous neuropathic pain is associated principally with changes in thalamic activity and the medial pain system, which is preferentially involved in the emotional dimension of pain.[12] Also, in patients with neuropathic pain, PET imaging of regional blood flow demonstrated that activity in the cortical network involved in the sensory-discriminative processing of nociceptive pain is increased in neuropathic pain, whereas decreased activity occurs in the orbitofrontal and insular cortices.[13] fMRI has demonstrated new regions of the brain involved in pain processing such as the nucleus of the solitary tract.[14] In patients with neuropathic pain, fMRI was used to determine different brain regions involved in response to allodynic stimuli.[15] Both PET and fMRI have been used to investigate the basis of allodynia. The results obtained have been very variable, probably reflecting the heterogeneity of patients in terms of etiology, lesion topography, symptoms and stimulation procedures. Functional neuroimaging may someday play a role in the diagnosis and evaluation of chronic pain. Today, they are used more in research than in our clinical practice.

The neuropathic pain scale (NPS) was developed to assess distinct qualities associated with neuropathic pain and is sensitive to measuring outcomes for a variety of therapeutic interventions.[16] The NPS is valid and reliable in the assessment of central pain associated with multiple sclerosis[17] and is currently considered the most valid as a measure of therapeutic outcome of eight available tools used in the assessment of neuropathic pain.[18] The NPS appears to be able to discriminate between neuropathic and nonneuropathic pain,[19] although some authors question this ability.[20] The Pain Quality Assessment Scale is a tool that includes the NPS items and may prove to be even more useful in the assessment of neuropathic pain because it includes pain descriptors common to people with neuropathic and other chronic pain conditions not included on the NPS.[18] Appendix M lists the Neuropathic Pain Scale.

Bedside examination of the patient should include quantification and mapping of motor, sensory, and autonomic abnormalities, if present. Touch (Aβ fibers) may be assessed using cotton wool and a tuning fork may be used for vibration sense (Aβ fibers). A wooden cocktail stick may be used for assessment of pinprick and sharp pain (Aδ fibers). Thermal sense (C fibers) may be evaluated by metal thermorollers or by using a tuning fork that can be heated or cooled using tap water. Quantitative sensory testing (QST) is helpful to quantify the effects of treatments on allodynia and hyperalgesia and may reveal a differential efficacy of treatments on different pain components. However, QST is time consuming and difficult to use in clinical practice. Standard neurophysiologic responses to electrical stimuli, such as nerve conduction studies and somatosensory-evoked potentials, are useful to demonstrate, locate, and quantify damage along the peripheral or central sensory pathways. These measures do not assess function of nociceptive pathways and have no bearing upon the presence or absence of pain.

The following common cancer pain syndromes present with a major neuropathic component.

NEUROPATHIC PAIN SECONDARY TO CRANIAL NEUROPATHIES

Painful cranial neuralgias can arise from base of skull metastases, leptomeningeal metastases, or head and neck cancers.[21] Several well-described pain syndromes are seen with skull base metastases[22] and most often occur with primary tumors of the breast, lung, and prostate. Constant aching pain in the region of the bone destruction and progressive cranial nerve palsies are the principal manifestations.

The cavernous sinus consists of a venous plexus, the carotid artery, cranial nerves, and sympathetic axons. Cavernous sinus syndrome (CSS) is caused by multiple etiologies, and MRI is the most sensitive tool for diagnosis.[23] The syndrome is characterized by multiple cranial neuropathies. The clinical presentation includes impairment of ocular motor nerves, Horner syndrome, and sensory loss of the 1st or 2nd divisions of the trigeminal nerve in various combinations. The pupil may be involved or spared. Various degrees of pain including painful opthalmoplegia may occur dependent on the particular cranial nerve involved. Tumors are a frequent cause of CSS and include pituitary adenomas, meningiomas, nasopharyngeal carcinoma, lymphoma, and metastases. CSS typically involves cranial nerves III, IV, V (V1, V2), and VI. Patients may complain of periocular pain, paresthesia, and diplopia.

The middle cranial fossa syndrome is characterized by facial numbness, paresthesias, or dysesthetic neuropathic pain in the distribution of the second or third divisions of the trigeminal nerve, and by associated motor deficits such as weakness in the masseter or temporalis muscles or abducens palsy.

Glossopharyngeal neuralgia may be the presenting symptom of the jugular foramen syndrome.[22] Pain is perceived over the ear or the mastoid region and may radiate into the neck or shoulder. Neurologic deficits can include a Horner-syndrome as well as paresis of the palate, vocal cords, sternocleidomastoid muscle, or trapezius muscle. Syncopal attacks have also been reported.[24] This syndrome has also been ascribed to leptomeningeal metastases[25] and to local extension of head and neck malignancies.[26] It is sometimes associated with syncope.

Tumors in the middle or posterior fossa rarely can produce a syndrome which resembles classical trigeminal neuralgia.[27–30] Leptomeningeal metastases in the posterior fossa can also generate this type of pain.[31] A small fraction (between 1% and 6%) of patients with pain in the trigeminal distribution is discovered to have tumors affecting the trigeminal nerve.[27–28,30] The most common tumors are meningiomas, acoustic neuromas, and epidermoid tumors. Other tumors that have been reported to cause facial pain include trigeminal schwannomas, carcinomas of the cranial base, brainstem gliomas, arachnoid cysts, and lymphomas.[32] Tumors affecting the trigeminal nerve root are typically associated with trigeminal neuralgia or tic douloureux, whereas tumors involving either the trigeminal ganglion or divisions are more likely to cause painful trigeminal neuropathy (atypical facial pain).[27] New onset of trigeminal neuralgia in a patient with cancer should lead to careful imaging of the base of skull with computed tomography (CT) or MRI.[28] Trigeminal neuralgia that is secondary to tumor usually presents as a constant, dull, well-localized pain related to the underlying pathology involving bone and other somatic structures, associated with paroxysmal episodes of lancinating or throbbing pain.[33]

Perineural spread of head and neck tumors may also be associated with significant pain. Squamous cell carcinomas of the face commonly extend by perineural spread, and are an important cause of facial pain syndromes.[34] Other head and neck cancers spreading perineurally may also cause pain in a trigeminal distribution.[35] Perineural spread, when present, typically involves cranial nerves V and VII because of their extensive subcutaneous distributions.[36] Glossopharyngeal neuralgia usually is caused by local nerve infiltration in the neck or base of skull. It typically produces throat and neck pain, radiating to the ear and mastoid, and may be aggravated by swallowing. Occasionally, syncope accompanies severe pain.[37–38] Malignant mental neuropathy is a neurologic manifestation of cancer characterized by numbness in the region innervated by the mental nerve (skin of the chin, oral mucosa, and lower lip). Distally, mandibular bone tumors, with direct nerve infiltration, were the most frequent original neoplasm, being found in 50% of cases. Proximally, the most frequent were tumors located at the base of the skull; these lesions may cause bone destruction or infiltration of the leptomeninges close to the gasserian ganglion region.[39] Although the lesion can be painful, it is relatively infrequent. The syndrome may be associated with breast cancer, lymphomas, prostate cancer, and leukemia. The appearance of the syndrome may be a warning sign of a systemic cancer or of its recurrence.

TUMOR-RELATED MONONEUROPATHY

Intercostal nerve injury secondary to rib metastases with local extension is the most commonly described tumor-related painful mononeuropathy. Patients with tumor invasion of the sciatic notch may present with symptoms resembling sciatica. Other nerves may be involved as well, but this is not a common clinical issue.

RADICULAR PAIN/ RADICULOPATHY

Radicular pain is described as corresponding to the dermatomal territory innervated by the dorsal spinal roots. Cancer-related radiculopathy may be unilateral or bilateral, but it tends to be unilateral in the cervical and lumbosacral regions and bilateral in the thorax. Radiculopathy in cancer patients typically is caused by epidural tumor mass or leptomeningeal metastases. Coughing, sneezing, positional change, and physical strain exacerbate the pain, which often has dysesthetic qualities. Leptomeningeal metastases are also capable of generating radicular pain and are characterized by multifocal neurological signs and symptoms at a variety of levels, including cranial neuralgias. Generalized headache with radicular pain in the low back and buttocks is a common presentation of this disease.[40]

LEPTOMENINGEAL METASTASES

Leptomeningeal metastasis has been described as the detection of tumor cells in the leptomeninges or cerebrospinal fluid (CSF) remote from the site of a primary tumor. Synonyms include carcinomatous meningitis, neoplastic meningitis, neoplastic meningosis, leukemic meningitis (for leukemia), lymphomatous meningitis (for lymphoma), and meningeal carcinomatosis (for carcinoma). Oncologists and neurologists have increasingly reported diffuse leptomeningeal metastases of extracranial malignant tumors, most commonly with adenocarcinoma of the lung and breast, lymphomas, and melanomas.[40–42]

Leptomeningeal spread has been reported in 5% to 8% of solid tumors, 5% to 29% of non-Hodgkin lymphomas (NHL), and 11% to 70% of leukemias.[43] Although the incidence of metastatic lesions in the brain is high in patients with small-cell lung carcinoma (SCLC), clinical problems from metastases to the spinal cord or leptomeninges have been rare.[44] Meningeal involvement was once a common complication of acute lymphoblastic leukemia before the advent of CNS prophylaxis, but it now occurs in fewer than 5% of patients. Leptomeningeal metastases develop in 1% to 8% of patients with systemic cancer[45]; median survival is 3 to 6 months.[46] Without treatment, the prognosis is dismal: survival averages 6 weeks.[47]

Several mechanisms may be responsible for leptomeningeal spread, including hematogenous, direct extension, (transport through the valveless venous plexus, extension along nerves, perineural/perivascular lymphatics, escape from choroid plexus or subependymal metastases, and from surgical manipulation. Leptomeningeal tumors can encase spinal and cranial nerves or directly invade them and lead to demyelination and axon destruction. Dissemination, once tumor cells reach the leptomeninges, is by exfoliation into the CSF space. Leptomeningeal metastases can cause symptoms by direct compression of brain structures (by meningeal nodules causing focal symptoms), irritation of adjacent brain (seizures), blocking of CSF pathways (leading to hydrocephalus and increased intracranial pressure), ischemia, or stroke (by constriction of pial arteries), cranial and peripheral nerve palsies (by direct nerve involvement), metabolic derangements (by decreasing available glucose for brain by rapidly growing tumor cells), and by causing meningeal fibrosis.

The characteristic clinical presentation of leptomeningeal metastases is the simultaneous occurrence of symptoms and signs related to more than one area of the neuraxis. The clinical presentation of leptomeningeal metastasis is pleomorphic and commonly affects the cerebral hemispheres, cranial nerves, or spinal cord and its roots. Symptoms are usually multifocal and more diffuse than one discrete lesion could present. They include headache, back and radicular pain, multiple cranial and spinal nerve involvement, and alterations in mental status. Pain is present in 30% to 76% of cases.[40,48] Table 10.1 lists the frequency of spinal cord symptoms and signs in patients with leptomeningeal metastases. Pain is by far the most common symptom (80%); 25% of patients report diffuse headache; and pain in a spinal, radicular, or meningeal pattern is reported by 50%. Focal neurologic findings include cranial neuropathies, mononeuritis, radiculopathy, urinary incontinence, and visual disturbance.

The diagnosis is dependent upon identifying malignant cells with CSF examination or upon characteristic gadolinium-enhanced MRI findings. T1-weighted gadolinium-enhanced sequence of the entire neuraxis (brain and spine) plays an important role in supporting the diagnosis, demonstrating the involved sites and guiding treatment (Fig. 10.1). MRI images typically show enhancing nodular lesions. The combination of CSF studies and neuroimaging is the optimal diagnostic strategy. Neurologic examination will reveal multifocal involvement of the CNS, cranial nerves, and spinal roots, which are the clinical hallmark of this disease. Although CSF analysis is almost always abnormal, only a positive CSF cytology

TABLE 10.1

FREQUENCY OF SPINAL CORD SYMPTOMS AND SIGNS IN PATIENTS WITH CARCINOMATOUS MENINGITIS

Symptoms or Signs	Percentage
Weakness	33
Paresthesia	31
Back pain	25
Radicular pain	19
Bowel/bladder dysfunction	13
Reflex asymmetry	67
Weakness	4
Cauda equina syndrome	33
Sensory loss	31
Positive straight leg raise	13
Decreased tone of anal sphincter	12
Nuchal rigidity	11

(With permission from Zachariah B, Zachariah SB, Varghese R, et al. Carcinomatous meningitis: Clinical manifestations and management. *Int J Clin Pharmacol Ther.* 1995;33:7–12. Copyright 1995, Drusti Verlag, Publisher.)

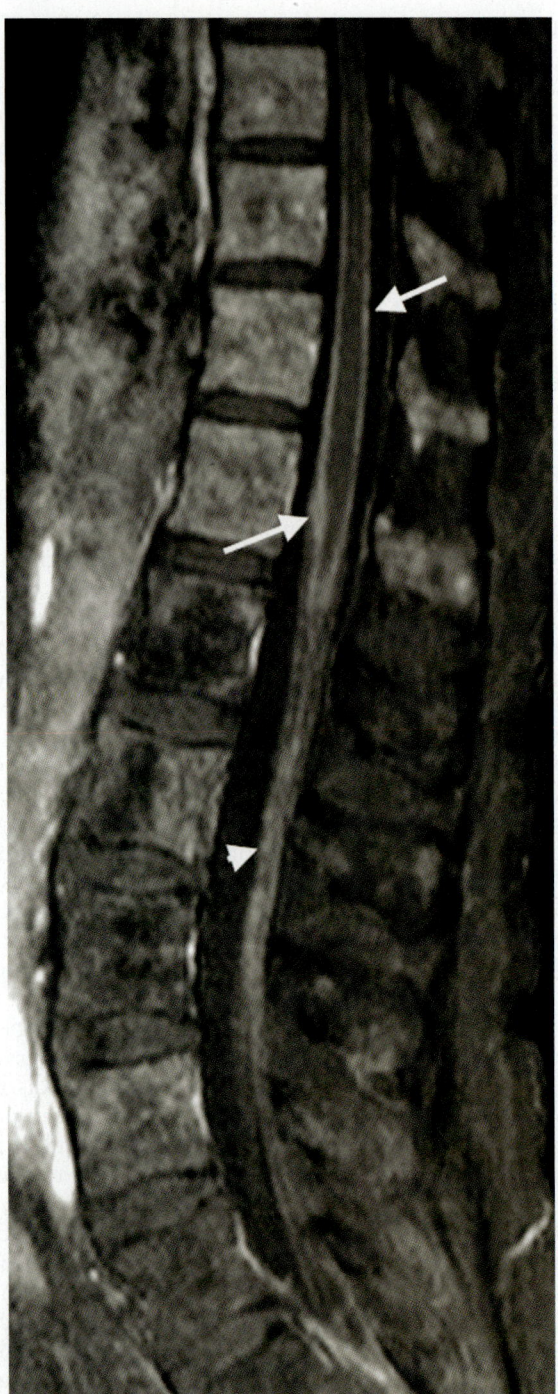

FIGURE 10.1 A 60-year-old woman with metastatic breast cancer who presented with increasing confusion and unsteadiness with walking. Sagittal lumbar spine MRI (T1, fat suppressed, postgadolinium) shows leptomeningeal enhancement in the thoracolumbar canal *(arrows)* with nodular meningeal enhancement in the lower lumbar region *(arrow head)*. MRI, Magnetic resonance imaging.

or demonstration of intrathecal synthesis of tumor markers is pathognomonic.

CERVICAL PLEXOPATHY

Pain syndromes can arise from infiltration of the cervical plexus.[49] The upper four cervical ventral rami join to form the cervical plexus, which lies adjacent to C1-C4 vertebrae. The four cutaneous branches can be found at the posterior border of the sternocleidomastoid muscle as they enter the posterior triangle of the neck. Nociceptive referral patterns from the face and neck overlap because sensory afferents from the cervical plexus terminate in the spinal tract of the trigeminal along with the sensory afferents from cranial nerves V, VII, IX, and X. Local pain accompanied by lancinating or dysesthetic components referred to the retroauricular and nuchal areas (lesser and greater auricular nerves), preauricular area (greater auricular nerve), anterior neck and shoulder (transverse cutaneous and supraclavicular nerves), and the jaw (marginomandibular nerve) characterize cervical plexopathy.[21] Ipsilateral Horner syndrome or hemidiaphragmatic paralysis may also occur. CT or MRI evaluation may be necessary to determine the location of the tumor in soft tissues or within the epidural space. Local extension of a head and neck tumor or cervical lymph node metastasis is the common predisposing diagnosis. In patients with head and neck tumors who have previously had radical neck dissection and radiation therapy, new onset or worsening pain includes a differential diagnosis of post–radical neck dissection syndrome or tumor recurrence. Infections often complicate and exacerbate pain in this region.

BRACHIAL PLEXOPATHY

Lung or breast cancers are the most likely to invade the brachial plexus (Fig. 10.2). The lower plexus is usually the first portion to be involved. Tumor infiltration of the brachial plexus commonly stems from lymph node metastases from breast carcinoma or lymphoma, or by direct extension from lung carcinoma (ie, Pancoast tumor). The designation of "Pancoast" tumor is described in "Neoplastic Processes and Pain, Lung Cancer." Both compression of the plexus or invasion of the nerves of the plexus by tumor cells can lead to severe, neuropathic pain.

Brachial plexopathy commences with pain in 85% of patients. Neurologic deficits usually develop well after the pain has become an issue.[50–51] The pain is then associated with numbness, paresthesias, allodynia, and hyperesthesias in the entire upper extremity (Fig. 10.3). Typically, the pain begins in the shoulder girdle, where it is often described as pressure or aching, and radiates to the elbow,

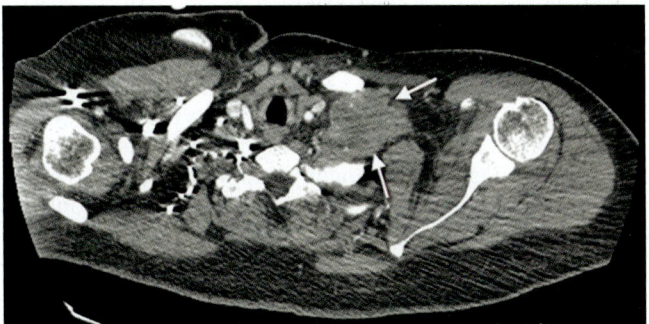

FIGURE 10.2 Chest CT scan of 53-year-old woman with inflammatory breast cancer. Patient had moderate-to-severe intensity pain in the left upper extremity and in the left upper posterior chest wall area. CT shows extensive left supraclavicular fossa mass involving the first rib and brachial plexus (arrows). CT, Computed tomography.

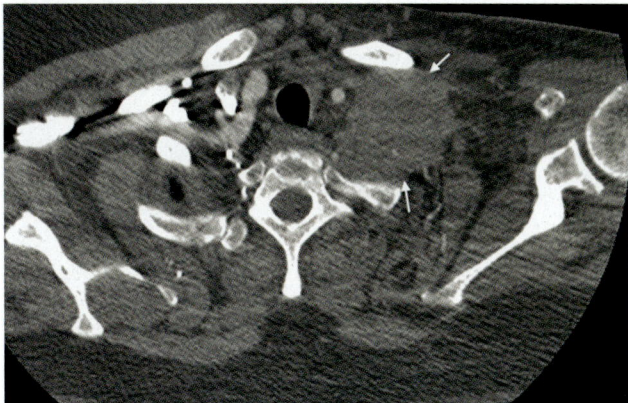

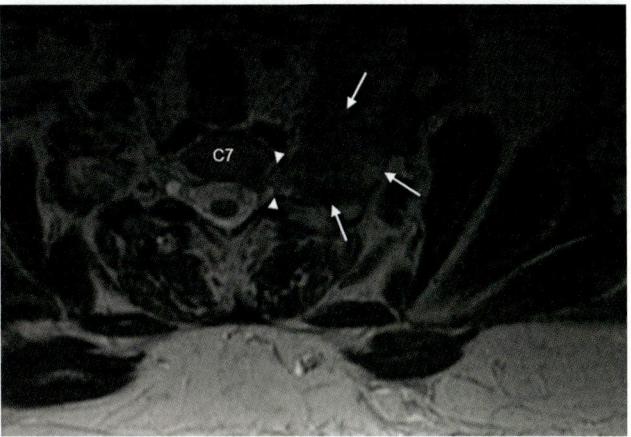

FIGURE 10.3 A 54-year-old woman with metastatic breast cancer to the left supra- and infraclavicular fossa involving the brachial plexus. Patient had severe pain, predominantly in the left shoulder region. Her left upper extremity was not functional, with evidence of diffuse lymphedema. Axial CT scan (**A**) shows an extensive mass below the clavicle *(arrows)*. Axial MRI (**B**) shows a large mass in the left supraclavicular region *(arrows)* with abnormal contrast enhancement extending into the left C7-T1 neural foramen *(arrow heads)*. The mass diffusely invades the brachial plexus. No mass is identified within the spinal canal. CT, Computed tomography; MRI, magnetic resonance imaging.

medial forearm, and fourth and fifth fingers. This is related to the observation that initially the lower plexus is more likely to be involved than the upper portion. The triceps reflex is often absent. Eventually, the patient is likely to report a burning quality to the pain. Hyperesthesia along the ulnar aspect of the forearm and the hand is a frequent finding. Both motor and sensory changes usually imply C7, C8, and T1 involvement.[51]

Upper plexus (C5, C6) involvement frequently leads to pain in the shoulder girdle, with burning pain in the tips of both the index finger and thumb. Upper plexus involvement usually progresses into panplexopathy. Lung tumors can present with pain in the distribution of the intercostobrachial nerve (axilla and upper chest wall).[52]

Horner syndrome and tumor invasion of adjacent vertebrae may accompany plexus invasion; there is a high risk of concurrent epidural extension.[48,53] We advise that when a patient with tumor-based brachial plexopathy is imaged (usually with an MRI), the adjacent epidural space be included in the imaging. With this information, the

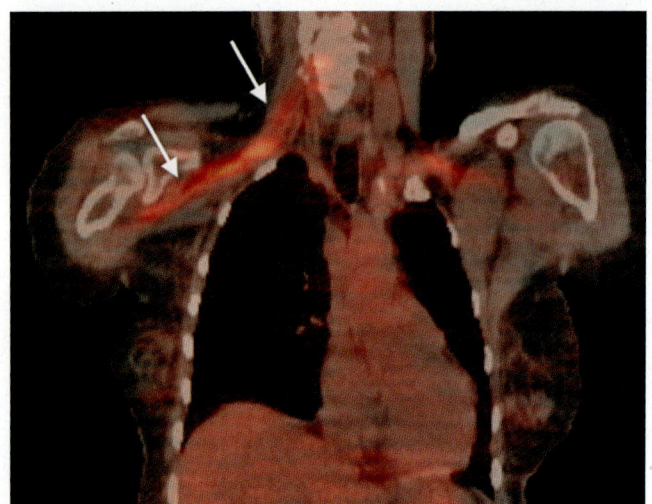 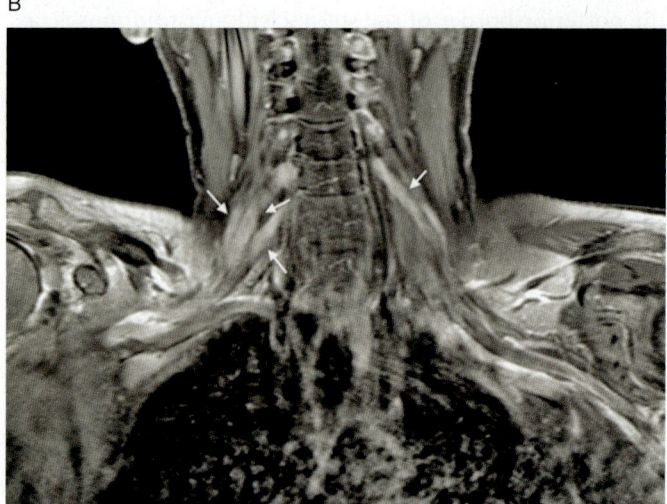

FIGURE 10.4 A 54-year-old woman with B-cell lymphoma. Complaining of diffuse weakness in the right upper extremity. No symptoms in left upper extremity. **A:** Coronal PET-CT shows FDG uptake extending from neural foramina C5, C6, and C7 extending along the entire brachial plexus (*arrows*). Coronal T1 MRI of the same patient shows markedly enhanced and enlarged nerve roots and trunks (*arrows*) on the right side. There is also evidence of enhancement on the left (*arrow*). PET-CT, Positron-emission tomography-computed tomography; MRI, magnetic resonance imaging.

radiation oncologist can plan the treatment field so as to include the entire tumor. Clinical examination findings can also imply tumor extension into the spinal foramina. A Spurling maneuver can help to identify the spinal canal as the site of pathology.[54] The Spurling maneuver requires the examiner to produce oblique extension of the neck on the affected side with axial compression to the head. By narrowing the affected foramen, pain may be produced in the upper extremity. Any patient with paraspinal or foraminal disease should be suspected to harbor epidural extension of tumor.

Neuroradiologic evaluation for brachial plexopathy has been the CT and the MRI. Fluorodeoxyglucose (FDG)-PET scanning is a very useful tool for the assessment of patients with suspected metastatic plexopathy, particularly if other imaging studies are normal (Fig. 10.4).[55] FDG-PET can also distinguish *radiation-induced* from *metastatic* plexopathy. Another useful tool to make this distinction is electromyography (EMG) (Table 10.2). In patients with metastatic brachial plexopathy, the EMG usually shows fibrillation potentials and positive waves (evidence of denervation) in affected muscles. Radiation-induced brachial plexopathy tends to have slowed nerve conduction velocity in both motor and sensory nerves.

LUMBOSACRAL PLEXOPATHY

The lumbosacral plexus can be damaged by direct tumor infiltration from adjacent soft tissues or lymph nodes or by compression from metastases in the adjacent bony pelvis. Local extension or nodal metastases from colorectal and other pelvic tumors (cervix, uterus, bladder, prostate), sarcomas (Fig. 10.5), and lymphomas are the common causes of lumbosacral plexopathy, but rarer causative neoplasms include metastases from breast or lung cancer or melanoma[49] (Table 10.3). The most common neurologic complication in patients with advanced cervical cancer has been lumbosacral plexopathy caused by retroperitoneal lymph node metastases.[56]

Carcinomatous lumbosacral plexopathy is manifested by severe, aching, pressure-like, unrelenting pain localized varyingly in the pelvis, low back, or hip, or referred into the leg in a radicular or nonradicular pattern.[57] The sites of referred pain are dependent upon the components of the plexus that are involved. The pain can be described as burning, cramping, or lancinating. Sensory symptoms of numbness and paresthesias, as well as weakness and leg edema, commonly develop weeks to months later. Lumbosacral plexopathy may lead to "hot and dry foot" syndrome that suggests sympathetic fiber dysfunction.[58] Clinical signs of lumbosacral plexopathy are leg weakness (86%), sensory loss (73%), reflex loss (64%), and leg edema (47%). Associated findings commonly include positive straight-leg raising tests and sciatic notch tenderness.[59]

The specific clinical syndrome produced by tumor invasion of the lumbosacral plexus depends on the levels of nerve involvement. Approximately one third of patients will present with infiltration of the upper plexus and present with pain in the back, lower abdomen, flank, iliac crest, or anterolateral thigh as well as neurological findings suggesting L1-L4 involvement. Involvement of the lower plexus occurs in approximately one half of patients and presents with pain in the buttocks and perineum with referral to the posterolateral leg and thigh. L4-S1 neurological deficits, leg edema, and bowel or bladder dysfunction (Fig. 10.6) frequently accompany the pain. Sacral plexopathy may arise directly from a bony sacral lesion or a presacral mass. Involvement of the lumbosacral trunk is characterized by numbness of the dorsal medial foot and sole with associated weakness of knee flexion, ankle dorsiflexion, and inversion. Sphincter dysfunction and perineal sensory loss are caused by coccygeal plexus invasion. One fifth of patients manifest panplexopathy; their pain may refer anywhere in the territory of the lumbosacral plexus. Associated leg edema frequently accompanies lumbosacral plexopathy.[58]

Jaeckle et al.[57] reported on 85 patients with lumbosacral plexopathy and pelvic tumor documented by CT

TABLE 10.2

DIFFERENTIATING FEATURES OF BRACHIAL PLEXOPATHY INDUCED BY TUMOR INFILTRATION, RADIATION FIBROSIS, AND REVERSIBLE RADIATION INJURY

	Tumor Infiltration	Radiation Fibrosis	Reversible Radiation Injury
Incidence of pain	89%	18%	40%
Typical location of pain	Shoulder upper arm, elbow, radiating to 4th and 5th fingers	Shoulder wrist, hand	Hand, forearm
Nature of pain	Dull aching in shoulder, Lancinating pain in elbow and ulnar aspect of hand; Occasional dysesthesias, burning, or freezing sensations	Aching shoulder pain; Paresthesias in C5, C6 distribution in hand	Aching shoulder pain; Paresthesias in hand and forearm
Severity of pain	Moderate to severe (severe in 98% of patients)	Mild to moderate (severe in 35% of patients)	Mild
Course	Progressive neurologic dysfunction; atrophy and weakness with C7-T1 distribution; persistent pain; Horner syndrome	Progressive weakness with C5, C6 distribution; stabilizing pain with appearance of weakness	Transient weakness and atrophy affecting C6-C7, T1; complete resolution of motor findings
CT scan findings	Circumscribed mass with diffuse infiltration of tissue planes	Diffuse infiltration of tissue planes	Normal
EMG findings	Segmental slowing; no myokymia	Myokymia	Segmental slowing; no myokymia

CT, Computed tomography; EMG, electromyography. (Modified from Foley KM. Brachial plexopathy in patients with breast cancer. In: Harris JR, Hellman S, Henderson IC, Kinne DW, eds. *Breast diseases*. Philadelphia: JB Lippincott Co, 1987:537.)

or biopsy. They described three clinical syndromes: lower (L4-S1), 51%; upper (L1-L4), 31%; and panplexopathy (L1-S3), 18%. Three fourths of the patients reported the insidious onset of pelvic or radicular leg pain, followed by sensory symptoms and weakness that began weeks to months later. The combination of leg pain, weakness, edema, rectal mass, and hydronephrosis suggests plexopathy due to cancer. CT showed pelvic tumor in 96% of such patients. Roughly, one half of such patients will have epidural extension seen on an imaging study.

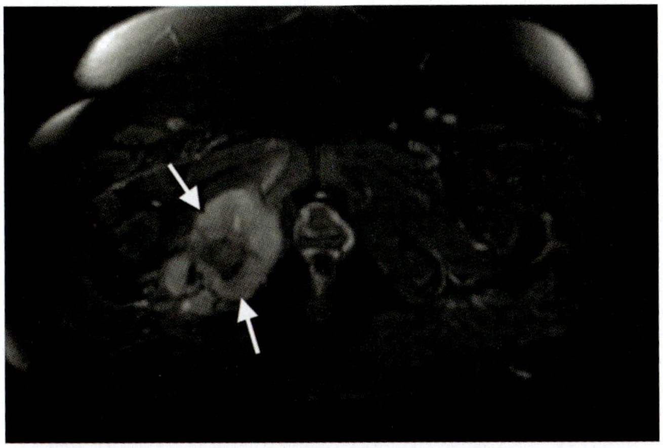

Patients who have been previously treated with radiation therapy present a difficult distinction between tumor or radiation plexopathy. MRI has been found to be more sensitive than CT for diagnosing cancer-induced lumbosacral plexopathy.[60] MRI is, therefore, the best choice for the evaluation of patients with clinical and electrophysiologic evidence of plexopathy who are suspected to have a systemic cancer. Imaging must include the L1 vertebral body through to the true pelvis. The common neurologic findings include leg weakness, sensory loss, reflex asymmetry, focal tenderness to palpation (in the lumbar region in an upper plexopathy, sciatic notch and sacrum in a lower plexopathy, and lumbosacral region in

FIGURE 10.5 Axial Fat-suppressed MRI scan of pelvis. Patient is a 34-year-old woman with extensive tumor infiltration from a recurrent high-grade pelvic sarcoma on the right side extending toward the right hip joint and soft tissues adjacent to the right ischial tuberosity and greater and lesser sciatic foramen *(arrows)*. Patient complained of severe right hip and lower extremity pain, necessitating placement of an externalized intrathecal catheter for pain control. MRI, Magnetic resonance imaging.

TABLE 10.3

COMMON NEOPLASMS CAUSING LUMBOSACRAL PLEXOPATHY

Tumor	% of Lumbosacral Plexopathy
Colorectal	20
Sarcoma	16
Breast	11
Lymphoma	9
Cervix	7
All Others	7

(From Jaeckle KA. Neurological manifestations of neoplastic and radiation-induced plexopathies. *Semin Neurol*. 2004;24(4):385–393. Reprinted with permission from Thieme, Inc.)

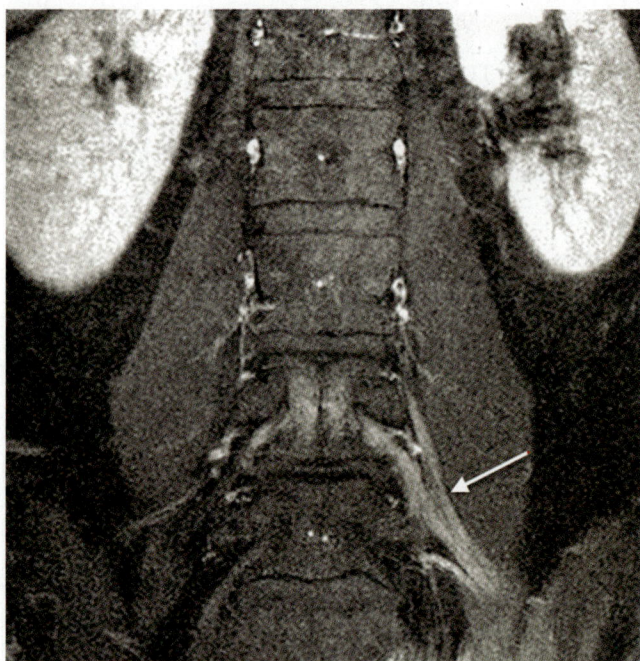

FIGURE 10.6 Coronal T1 MRI showing enlarged left L4 nerve root *(arrow)*. Patient is a 36-year-old man with peripheral nerve sheath tumor. MRI, Magnetic resonance imaging.

pan-plexopathy), rectal mass, decreased sphincter tone, and positive direct and reverse straight leg raising signs.

TUMOR INFILTRATION OF THE SACRUM AND SACRAL NERVES

Pain over the sacrum is usually the result of the spread of cancer of the bladder, pelvic organs, or colon. Such tumors lead to a dull, aching midline pain as well as burning or throbbing pain in the soft tissues of the rectal and/or perineal region. The pain is exacerbated by sitting or lying. With bilateral involvement, sphincter incontinence and impotence in the male are commonly seen. The sacrum and the sciatic notches may be tender to palpation. Both direct and reverse straight leg raising tests may be positive. Compromise of the S1 and S2 roots can lead to weakness of ankle plantar flexion and the absence of ankle jerk reflexes (Fig. 10.7). There is usually sensory loss in both the perianal and genital regions; pain and sensory loss as well as distortions of sensation are common.

SPINAL AND RADICULAR PAIN

Radicular pain is reported as radiating into a limb or around the trunk wall. The pain is sharp and lancinating in quality and travels in a restricted zone from central to peripheral. It may be described as episodic, recurrent, or paroxysmal. Although radicular pain may be described by some patients as a deep tissue pain, it almost always has a cutaneous component in proportion to the number of cutaneous afferent fibers that are ectopically activated. Nociceptive pain is induced by activity at the peripheral terminals of Aδ and C fibers, whereas radicular pain is caused by the ectopic firing of axons and does not originate in nerve terminals. Ectopic activation of axons may occur as a result of mechanical deformation of a dorsal root ganglion, mechanical stimulation of previously damaged axons in peripheral nerve or nerve roots, inflammation of a dorsal root ganglion, and possibly by ischemic damage to the dorsal root ganglia. Acute or chronic spine pain may be described as cramping or knifelike, but may also be just dull or aching. Chronic spine pain without a radicular component is generally aching, dull, or burning, or any combination of these three features. Movement or change in position often exacerbates spinal pain.

CENTRAL PAIN CAUSED BY CANCER

Central pain is defined as pain due to disease or dysfunction in the CNS and includes pathology in the spinal cord, brain stem, or cerebral hemispheres. Central pain mechanisms are complex. Gain in neuronal excitability, loss of

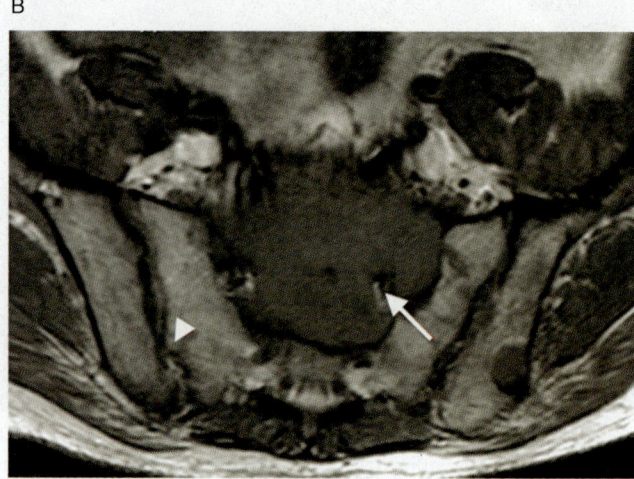

FIGURE 10.7 A: CT of pelvis in 61-year-old man who presented with extensive lytic lesion completely replacing the sacrum *(arrows)* and involving the sacral foramina from a tumor of unknown origin. **B:** Axial T1 MRI of sacrum of same patient showing left S2 nerve root encroachment of tumor *(arrow)*. The sacrum is essentially replaced with tumor. *Arrow head* shows normal bone. CT, Computed tomography; MRI, magnetic resonance imaging.

inhibition, and increased facilitation may contribute to a central sensitization and disinhibition of pain pathways.[7] Central pain problems due to spinal cord injury and stroke are well described.[61-62] Damage to spinothalamic sensory pathways, although not the only mechanism, is thought to be important in the pathogenesis of both of these sources of neuropathic pain. In addition, damage to the pain and temperature pathways is an important contributor to the development of central pain in traumatic brain injury patients.[63] The occurrence of hyperexcitability and hyperreactivity within the nervous system is also an important mechanism in the pathogenesis of central pain. Clinically, this may be manifested by the presence of allodynia, hyperpathia, and exaggerated wind-up sensations. Electrophysiologic studies and brain scans confirm that deafferented neurons in the thalamus and somatosensory cortex of patients with central pain may undergo plastic changes and become hyperexcitable.[64-66] At a cellular level, the glia play a crucial role in the maintenance of neuronal homeostasis in the CNS.[67-68] Glial cells represent 70% of the cells in the CNS under normal conditions, and microglia represent 5% to 10% of glia.[69] Microglia are rapidly activated in the CNS in response to pathological events, including trauma, ischemia, inflammation, hypoxia, neurodegeneration, and viral or bacterial infection, releasing proinflammatory cytokines and causing pathological pain.[70] Microglia also repair injured cells by releasing neurotrophic factors and appear to dynamically modulate neuronal function under both normal and pathological conditions.[68] Microglial cells secrete a large variety of substances, including growth factors, cytokines, complement components, lipid mediators, extracellular matrix components, enzymes, free radicals, neurotoxins, nitric oxide, and prostaglandins.[71] Microglial activation appears to have an important role in neuropathic pain.[72]

Central pain syndromes are not commonly ascribed to cancer. Gonzales et al.[73] reported on the prevalence and characteristics of central pain states in hospitalized patients with cancer. The prevalence of central pain was 4%. Primary and metastatic tumors and their treatment, including surgery, radiation, and chemotherapy, were all potential causes. Furthermore, the occurrence of central pain in patients with primary CNS tumors was higher in patients with spinal tumors compared to patients with brain tumors ($P < .0001$). Of the 27 patients reported with cancer or cancer treatment–related central pain, nearly all levels of the CNS were involved in central pain, except for the brainstem. Including leptomeningeal-related pain, 78% of patients had a spinal cord site of injury. Seventeen patients had thoracic spinal cord injury pain, two had cervical cord injury pain, and three parietal injury pain. The primary CNS tumor types included spinal cord ependymoma,[4] astrocytoma,[1] melanocytoma,[1] glioblastoma,[1] neuroectodermal,[1] melanocytoma;[1] thalamic oligodendroglioma,[1] lymphoma,[1] or astrocytoma.[1] The onset of central pain after CNS injury was delayed in one patient for 6 years. Altered temperature sensation was also observed frequently in patients with central pain states.

Although spinal cord compression from an epidural mass is frequently painful, central pain is not likely to be the predominant symptom. Rather, nociceptive input secondary to bony destruction by metastasis is the usual cause of the pain in this condition. There may be, of course, associated radicular pain due to nerve root compression and spinal instability. Intrinsic neoplasms such as gliomas can lead to central pain, but this is rare. It can be seen infrequently with neoplasms originating in the spinal cord; pain is usually perceived in the portions of the body that have disturbed sensory function (Fig. 10.8). Neoplasms within the brain itself do not usually produce central pains, in contrast to sudden infarction from embolus or hemorrhage. If pain is associated with brain neoplasms, this is usually predominantly nociceptive in origin because of nociceptor activation within the dura and blood vessels. Consequently, most of the central pain states seen in cancer patients are side effects of cancer treatment, most often related to radiation therapy. Radiation myelopathy is principally a white-matter injury of the spinal cord induced by ionizing radiation after a variable latent period. It involves myelinated fibers and blood vessels, and the lateral funiculi are most preferentially affected. Delayed-onset radiation myelopathy results in nontransverse myelopathy symptoms, such as dissociated sensory disturbance, unilateral leg weakness, and gait disturbance with asymmetric steps. Spinal MRI shows initial cord swelling and a long T1/T2 intramedullary lesion with enhancement; later cord atrophy is observed.

Chemotherapy and surgical treatment, especially amputation, can also lead to central pain states. Chemotherapeutic agents can cause central neurotoxicity. Intrathecal methotrexate can cause aseptic meningitis, transverse myelopathy, stroke-like syndrome, and leukoencephalopathy.[74] Patients can also report back pain, sometimes radiating into the legs, followed by sensory loss, and paraplegia.[75] Intrathecal cytarabine may cause aseptic meningitis and rarely myelopathy.[76] The amputation of a limb or another significant portion of the body can be associated with phantom sensations, including pain. Phantom pain is discussed in "Postsurgical Neuropathic Pain."

PERIPHERAL NEUROPATHY IN CANCER PATIENTS

Peripheral neuropathy can arise in a wide range of situations in malignancy (Table 10.4). Neuropathy may result from direct tumor infiltration, either from solid tumor or lymphoma. Neuropathy may also occur indirectly as a consequence of an immune mechanism, for example in the case of lymphomas associated with antimyelin-associated glycoprotein IgM production, or in patients with vasculitis or paraneoplastic neuropathies. Although significant peripheral neuropathy is common in cancer patients, only a small minority are paraneoplastic. Chemotherapy accounts for a large group of cancer-associated neuropathies as discussed on page 103. In patients who are not known to harbor a malignancy, unexplained neuropathies should prompt further investigation of an occult cancer.

Axonal neuropathy may result from vasculitides and cancer should be carefully eliminated whenever the vasculitic mechanism is confirmed. Zivkovic et al.[77] reported an association of histopathologically proven vasculitic axonal neuropathies with cancer in 15% of cases. In a

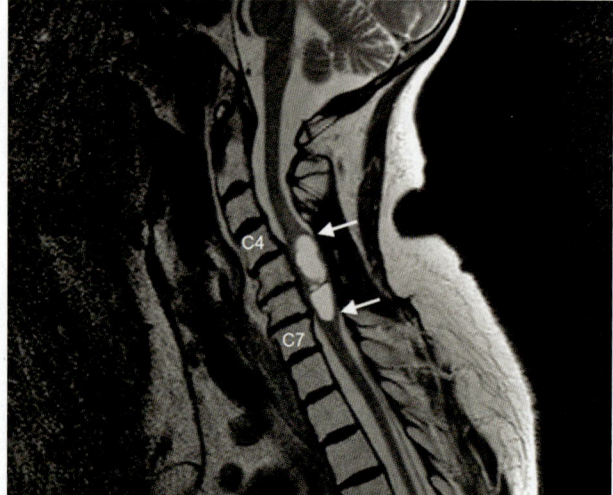
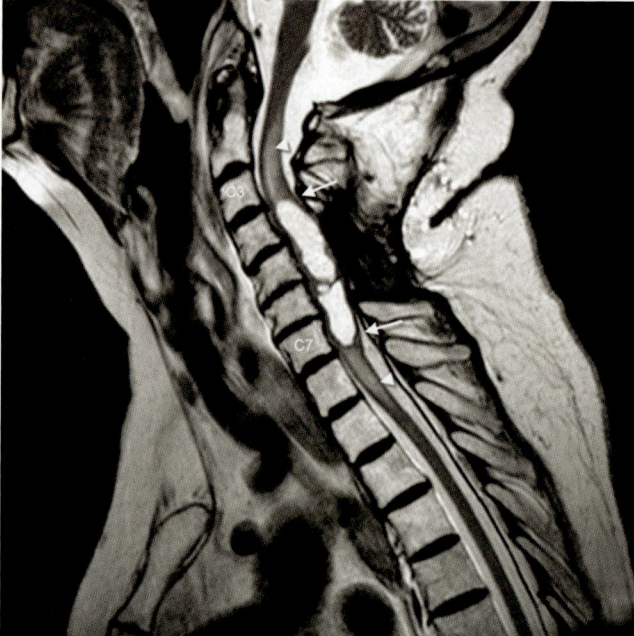
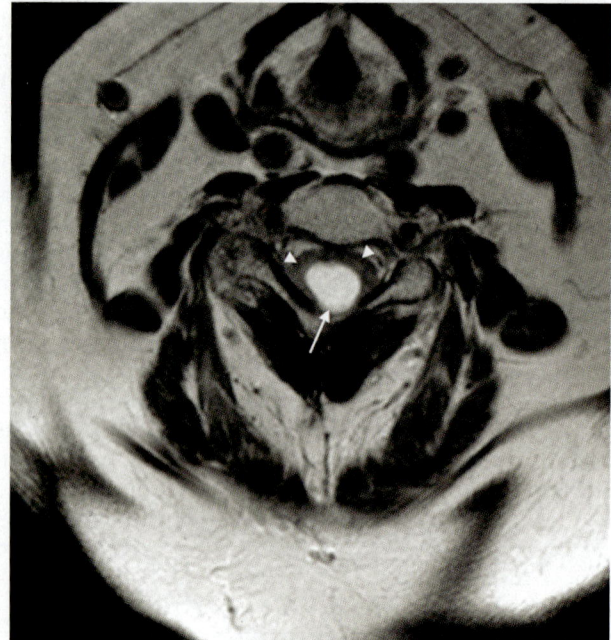

FIGURE 10.8 A 63-year-old woman with known cervical spinal cord pilocytic astrocytoma. Patient was treated with cervical decompression and radiation treatment to a total dose of 4500 cGy 2 years before presentation at the Pain Clinic. At presentation (**A**), she complained of persistent pain radiating throughout her upper extremity. Sagittal T2 MRI shows a stable cystic lesion extending from C4-C7 *(arrows)*. Her pain was initially well controlled on a combination of methadone, transmucosal fentanyl, amitriptyline, and gabapentin. Two months later (**B**), she was admitted with increasing left upper extremity pain and localized back pain. Sagittal T2 MRI shows an increase in size of her cystic lesion *(arrows)* with cord edema cephalad and caudad to the lesion *(arrow heads)* suggestive of progressive tumor growth. Axial T2 MRI (**C**). A large cystic lesion *(arrow)* is seen within the spinal cord. Normal cord is seen peripherally *(arrow head)*.

multicenter review of 60 patients who developed vasculitides associated with malignancies (with the exception of vasculitis due to immunosuppressants). Fain et al.[78] described an overall 32% rate of peripheral neuropathy. The complication was more frequent in patients with solid tumors (48%) or lymphoid malignancies (35%) than in patients with myelodysplastic syndromes (14%). Neuropathy is a challenging complication when chemotherapy is being administered, especially in multitreated patients who may present with several potential etiologies for peripheral nerve involvement. Cancer treatment should have priority over remediation of the neuropathy, especially in cases in which complete remission is possible. In other cases, the decision to taper the doses or to stop a chemotherapy agent should be based upon on the experience of the oncology team prescribing the drug, on the impairment induced by its prescription and on the choices of the patients.

PARANEOPLASTIC NEUROLOGICAL SYNDROMES

Paraneoplastic syndrome describes a group of disorders (caused by, or associated with, cancers) that are neither direct effects of the primary tumor mass nor metastasis to other organs. Any portion of the nervous system may be affected. Among the most well-known syndromes are paraneoplastic encephalomyelitis, cerebellar degeneration, sensory neuronopathy, and Lambert-Eaton myastenic syndrome. There are various associated tumors, in particular small cell lung cancer, cancers of the breast and ovary, and thymoma. The onset of neurological symptoms often precedes the cancer diagnosis, and the recognition of a paraneoplastic syndrome should lead to an immediate search for cancer.

TABLE 10.4

PERIPHERAL NEUROPATHY IN CANCER PATIENTS

Causes	Examples
Metastatic	Spinal cord compression
	Leptomeningeal metastases
	Metastases to peripheral nerves
Nonmetastatic	Metabolic nutritional
	Therapy side effects
Paraneoplastic	Subacute or chronic sensorimotor peripheral neuropathy
	Acute polyradiculopathy (Guillain-Barré syndrome)
	Mononeuritis multiplex and microvasculitis of peripheral nerve
	Acute brachial neuritis
	Autonomic neuropathy
	Peripheral neuropathy associated with paraproteinemia
Unrelated to cancer	Diabetes mellitus
	Vitamin B12 deficiency
Chemotherapy	Bortezomib, taxanes, lenalidomide
Cancer-associated vasculitides	Solid tumor, lymphoma, myelodysplastic syndromes

(Modified from Darnell RB, Posner JB. Paraneoplastic syndromes affecting the nervous system. Semin Oncol. 2006;33(3):270–298. Copyright 2006, with permission from Elsevier.)

Paraneoplastic syndromes usually stem from an autoimmune reaction to an *onconeural* antigen shared by the cancer and the nervous system.[79] Antibodies to onconeural antigens, expressed in the tumor of the affected individual and in normal neurons, are found in many of the patients. These antibodies are useful markers for paraneoplastic etiology.[80] Examination of the CSF frequently demonstrates pleocytosis, intrathecal synthesis of IgG, and oligoclonal bands, supporting an inflammatory or immune-mediated etiology. Examination of the CSF is generally not required for detection of antibodies; these can almost always be detected in serum as well.[81]

The incidence varies with the neurological syndrome and with the tumor type. Approximately 10% of patients with plasma cell disorders accompanied by malignant monoclonal gammopathies are affected by a paraneoplastic peripheral neuropathy. More than half of the patients with the rare osteosclerotic form of myeloma develop a severe, predominantly motor, paraneoplastic peripheral neuropathy. In other hematological malignancies, the incidence of paraneoplastic syndromes is very low, with the exception of Hodgkin disease. However, the incidence of the syndrome even in Hodgkin disease is below 1%. In solid tumors, the more common neurological syndromes are myasthenia gravis, which occurs in 15% of patients with a thymoma, and Lambert-Eaton myasthenic syndrome, which affects 3% of patients with SCLC. For other solid tumors, the incidence of paraneoplastic syndrome is less than 1%.

Antibodies and T-cell responses against nervous system antigens have been defined for many of these disorders. The immunologic response is elicited by the ectopic expression of neuronal antigens by the tumor. Expression of these onconeural antigens is limited to the tumor and the nervous system, and sometimes also the testis. Most paraneoplastic antigens are located in the cytoplasm (eg, the Yo antigen) or nucleus (eg, the Hu and Ri antigens). Although the immune reaction may retard growth of the cancer, it also damages the nervous system. Autoantibodies found in individual patients with paraneoplastic syndromes are usually associated with specific tumors. Neurologic disorders that are clinically and pathologically identical to paraneoplastic syndromes are known to occur in some patients without cancer, but such patients do not have paraneoplastic antibodies. The diagnosis of a paraneoplastic syndrome depends on its increased incidence in patients with cancer, the occasional response of the neurologic syndrome to treatment of the underlying cancer, and the presence of specific autoantibodies.

Antibodies that serve as clinical markers of a paraneoplastic etiology have been available for over 20 years, originating with the description of anti-Hu in 1985.[82] About 500 patients in four series have been reported.[83–86] The most common (or classical) symptoms have been sensory neuronopathy, paraneoplastic limbic encephalitis, and paraneoplastic cerebellar degeneration. Cancers were found in 80% to 90% of these patients. The neurological symptoms preceded discovery of the cancer in 70% to 100%. The associated cancers were often small and showed no metastases (other than to mediastinal lymph nodes). Low titer Anti-Hu is also present in about 16% of patients with SCLC who do not have neurological symptoms.[87]

Limbic encephalitis and subacute cerebellar degeneration are usually associated with cancer. These are called "classical" paraneoplastic neurological syndromes. Other neuropathic syndromes, such as sensorimotor polyneuropathy, are much more prevalent, and their association with cancer may be by chance. Detection of paraneoplastic antibodies can help diagnose the neurological syndrome as paraneoplastic and may direct the search for an underlying neoplasm. Patients with a possible paraneoplastic neurological syndrome include those with:

1. A classical syndrome without paraneoplastic antibodies and no cancer but at high risk to have an underlying tumor (eg, smoking habit).
2. A neurological syndrome (classical or not) without cancer but with partially characterized paraneoplastic antibodies.
3. A nonclassical neurological syndrome, no paraneoplastic antibodies, and cancer that presents within 2 years of the neurologic syndrome.

Four types of paraneoplastic polyneuropathy have been described: sensory, motor, autonomic, and sensorimotor. Most paraneoplastic peripheral neuropathies are sensorimotor and axonal. Pure sensory neuronopathy, suggesting pathology in the dorsal root ganglion, is likely to be a paraneoplastic syndrome associated with the anti-Hu antibody. A pure motor neuropathy subacutely developing could be the Guillain-Barré syndrome associated with Hodgkin disease or a multifocal motor neuropathy with conduction block associated with plasma cell dyscrasias. It could also be unrelated to a neoplasm. An autonomic neuropathy can also be associated with the anti-Hu syndrome. Autonomic paraneoplastic disorders commonly arise in the setting of encephalomyelitis. In some patients the autonomic symptoms are much more prominent or even rarely the only evidence for a paraneoplastic neuropathy. The most common sign of autonomic involvement is pseudo-obstruction of the bowel, but anhydrosis, orthostatic hypotension, hypoventilation, sleep apnea, and cardiac arrhythmias can also present either alone or, more commonly, as part of a more widespread autonomic neuropathy. Most autonomic polyneuropathies are associated with SCLC and the anti-Hu syndrome. The presence of mononeuritis multiplex usually is the hallmark of a vasculitis which could possibly be paraneoplastic in origin.

The classic paraneoplastic polyneuropathy is sensory neuronopathy, including subacute pan-sensory neuropathy and a predominantly distal sensory neuropathy. Subacute sensory neuronopathy is the most common,[88] occurring mostly in SCLC (70% to 80% of cases) and sometimes in breast or ovarian cancer, Hodgkin disease, or sarcomas. Patients describe an asymmetrical and painful sensory neuropathy, which evolves into complete loss of proprioception. Pseudoathetotic movement of the hands and sensory ataxia are very severe in most cases.

Paraneoplastic motor neuropathies may be acute or chronic, progressive or remitting, demyelinating, axonal or neuronal. They cannot be distinguished from the more common nonparaneoplastic motor neuropathies, unless they resolve after treatment of the cancer or are associated with a paraneoplastic antibody. Nonparaneoplastic motor neuropathies include the Guillain-Barré syndrome, which occurs more frequently in patients with Hodgkin disease than in the general population; a remitting and relapsing polyneuropathy resembling relapsing chronic inflammatory demyelinating polyneuropathy; and a subacute motor neuronopathy affecting patients with Hodgkin disease or other lymphomas.

Paraneoplastic peripheral neuropathies are important because they may be the first sign of an otherwise occult cancer. In addition, they may disable the patient and impair quality of life even when the cancer itself is asymptomatic. Patients with paraneoplastic neurological disorders present to the neurologist without a known tumor in at least two thirds of cases. A thorough assessment of a patient with possible paraneoplastic neuropathy is required, including searching for anti-Hu or anti-CV2/CRMP5 antibodies, CT scan of the chest, abdomen, and pelvis and PET scan in case of negative workup. These investigations should be repeated in case of initial negative results at 3- to 6-month intervals for 2 to 3 years.

THERAPY-INDUCED NEUROPATHIC PAIN

Pain syndromes can occur during or after the treatment of cancer with surgery, chemotherapy, or radiation. Injury to the peripheral nerves or spinal cord is the basis for this type of neuropathic pain. These syndromes can occur long after the therapy is implemented. Differential diagnosis between recurrent disease and a complication of therapy may be a difficult undertaking.

Neuropathic Pains After Surgery

Postmastectomy

Pain is common after surgery in breast cancer patients; prevalence has been estimated between 20% and 56%.[89–91] Pain can appear in the immediate postmastectomy period as a consequence of the disruption of normal neural pathways, or it may follow the development of lymphedema or the presence of metastases. The nature of the surgical procedure can influence the development of pain. Compared to radical mastectomy, patients treated with breast-conserving surgery had significantly less arm and shoulder problems including lymphedema.[92] In addition, the experience of the surgeon performing the surgery may also influence the incidence of pain.[93] In a study of patients undergoing breast surgery (mastectomy with reconstruction, simple mastectomy), 47% of patients with simple mastectomy showed slight hypoesthesia-paresthesia in the breast, armpit and arm zones, 39% slight hypoesthesia in the same locations, and 18% severe hypoesthesia. In patients with mastectomy and reconstruction, 75% showed slight hypesthesia-paresthesia, 16% a slight hypoesthesia, and 9% severe hypesthesia.[94] Pain often is the result of persistent restrictions in the range of motion of the shoulder girdle, with tender or trigger points in the pectoral and shoulder muscle groups. Axillary dissection is a major contributor to chronic neuropathic pain after mastectomy.[95] However, chronic pain can occur in women who have undergone any surgical procedure on the breast from lumpectomy to radical mastectomy.[96] Post–axillary dissection pain is probably a more appropriate name than the usual postmastectomy pain for this syndrome.[97] Patients commonly describe paroxysms of lancinating pain superimposed upon a background of burning, aching, and tight constriction in the axilla, medial upper arm, and/or chest. This problem can persist for prolonged periods.[98] Sensory perversions including hyperesthesia, dysesthesia, hyperalgesia, allodynia, or hypoesthesia in the intercostobrachial nerve distribution may occur. The intercostobrachial nerve is a cutaneous sensory branch of T1 and T2. It is highly variable in size and distribution, rendering it vulnerable in surgical procedures.

The exact cause of postmastectomy pain is unclear; various theories have included dissection of the intercostobrachial nerve, intraoperative damage to the axillary nerve or its branches, and pain caused by neuroma formation. Gottrup et al.[99] demonstrated increased evoked pain intensity after repetitive pinprick stimulation in the area near the scar suggested the possibility of central sensitization in patients with chronic pain after breast cancer surgery with axillary lymph node dissection. Steegers et al.[100] studied the effect of axillary lymph node dissection on the prevalence and intensity of chronic and phantom pain in 495 patients and noted a prevalence of 32% with a mean follow-up period of 22 months. The authors noted that chronic pain prevalence doubles with axillary lymph node dissection. Chemotherapy and radiation also increase chronic pain prevalence. Although pain usually develops shortly after surgery, its onset can also be months after surgery. Other causes such as recurrent chest wall disease or bone metastases must always be considered in late-onset pain. The postmastectomy pain syndrome can be distinguished from metastatic or radiation-induced brachial plexopathy on the basis of a different pattern of sensory loss, lymphedema, and usually, more severe pain with either metastasis or radiation injury. Phantom breast pain has been described after mastectomy with a broad range of reported prevalences from 1% to 53%.[101–103] Bjorkman et al.[104] noted that phantom breast pain can be difficult to describe and position spatially. Dijkstra et al.[101] noted that 2 years after modified radical mastectomy, phantom breast pain was present in only 1% of patients. The mechanisms responsible for phantom pain remain unclear at this time. The origin cannot be just the loss of the body part, as most of those who sustain such an injury do not develop this form of pain. Predisposing factors include the presence of pain before amputation.

Neck Dissection

Surgical procedures are plentiful for the treatment of cancer in cervical lymph nodes.[105] These have been classified as radical neck dissection (RND), extended RND, modified RND, and selective neck dissection. When RND is utilized for head and neck cancers, an iatrogenic syndrome characterized by ipsilateral face and neck pain with associated paresthesiae can develop. Pain usually emerges weeks to months after surgery. It is believed that this is due to injury to the cervical plexus or individual cervical nerves.[21] RND routinely leads to impairment of shoulder function due to transection of the spinal accessory nerve that denervates the upper trapezius muscle. Although most anatomists consider the spinal accessory nerve to be the only motor nerve supply to the trapezius, the cervical plexus (C2-4) may also contribute to the motor supply.[106] The spinal accessory nerve enters the posterior triangle of the neck at the lateral border of the sternocleiodmastoid muscle, on average 8.2 cm cranial to the clavicle. One to three branches of the cervical plexus run into the trapezius muscle and contribute to its innervation.[107] Modified radical and selective neck dissections are intended to reduce the prevalence of spinal accessory nerve injury commonly seen after radical neck dissection. However, subclinical spinal accessory nerve impairment can be observed even after selective neck dissections.[105] Tsuji et al.[108] compared EMG findings of the upper trapezius muscle in patients after different selective neck dissections. Complete or incomplete denervation of the upper trapezius was caused by axonal injury of the spinal accessory nerve, even though it was spared, probably because of traction in the nerve during neck dissection. In addition, the excision of the C2 to C4 rami of the cervical plexus led to more damage to the upper trapezius. Early detection of spinal accessory nerve palsy can be challenging and the condition is often misdiagnosed. Nahum et al.[109] coined the term *shoulder syndrome* to describe the clinical picture, consisting of pain and limited abduction of the shoulder combined with full passive range of motion, as well as anatomic deformities such as scapular flaring, droop, and protraction. Pain has been attributed to strain placed on other supporting muscles, including the rhomboids and levator scapulae, as a consequence of shoulder drooping due to trapezius paralysis. The shoulder syndrome can be accompanied by sternoclavicular joint hypertrophy, probably related to the abnormal torque-like forces applied to the medial head of the clavicle. This can lead to stress fracture of the middle third of the clavicle. Kelley et al.[110] reported on the signs and symptoms of spinal accessory nerve palsy in 20 patients who presented with pain and decreased shoulder function following head and neck surgery or trauma to the neck region. All patients presented with a cluster of signs and symptoms including trapezius atrophy, shoulder girdle depression, limited active shoulder abduction to less than 90 degrees, shoulder pain, and shoulder weakness. A positive scapular flip sign was present in all cases. This test is performed with the patient standing and the examiner standing behind the patient. The patient holds his or her arms adducted at the side of the body, with the arm in neutral rotation and with elbow flexed 90 degrees. The patient is asked to externally rotate and this motion is resisted by the examiner. A positive test is observed when the medial border of the scapula of the affected extremity becomes more prominent medially than the other extremity (implying medial border winging of the scapula). With the flip sign, the scapula has more of a rotational component than is seen during winging. Recovery in function of the trapezius muscle after spinal accessory nerve injury may be predicted by sequential EMG examination. In patients with permanent denervation of the upper trapezius, there are very limited treatment options and these patients are at risk for subsequent shoulder injury because of a significant restriction in range of motion of the shoulder girdle. Finally, it should be remembered that recurrent tumor can also be a source of pain after neck dissection.

Thoracotomy

Common symptoms after thoracotomy include pain, dyspnea, and fatigue. Pain may persist 6 months to 1 year after surgery.[111–112] Neuropathic pain can develop in the distribution of one or several intercostal nerves adjacent to the thoracotomy scar (post-thoracotomy pain). The pain may remain stable after onset or then gradually increase or decrease over a period of months or years. Dajczman et al.[113] reviewed both the prevalence and functional significance of long-term post-thoracotomy pain in 56 patients who were at least 2 months after surgery. Thirty patients (54%) with a median follow-up of 19.5 months had persistent pain; 26 others were pain free at a median of 30.5 months post-thoracotomy. Pain was reported by 24 of 44 patients (55%) at more than 1 year after surgery, 13 of 29 patients (45%) more than 2 years, six of 16 (38%) more than 3 years, and three of ten patients (30%) greater than 4 years post-thoracotomy (Table 10.5). Pain intensity was low, but 13 patients stated that pain "slightly" or "moderately" interfered with their lives. Five of 56 patients (9%) reported sufficiently severe chronic pain to justify daily analgesic use, nerve blocks, relaxation therapy, acupuncture, or referral to a pain clinic. Thoracic pain that increases with time, or which first appears more than 3 months after surgery, may signal recurrent tumor and should prompt further investigation.

Maguire et al.[114] found two distinct patterns of nerve injury after thoracotomy and also demonstrated that differences between surgical techniques might influence the presence of pain. Thoracotomy with rib resection resulted in more clinically detectable nerve damage than cautery along the top of the rib and pericostal closure. However, intercostal nerve damage at the time of operation was not

TABLE 10.5

FREQUENCY OF POSTTHORACOTOMY PAIN AT VARIOUS INTERVALS FOLLOWING SURGERY

Time Postthoracotomy	No. of Patients with Pain	Total Number of Patients Evaluable	% of Evaluable Patients with Pain
1 yr*	6	12	50
1-2 yrs	11	15	73
2-3 yrs	7	13	54
3-4 yrs	3	6	50
4-5 yrs	3	10	30
Total	30	56	

*Patients at least 2 months post-thoracotomy.
(From Dajczman E, Gordon A, et al. Long-term postthoracotomy pain. *Chest*. 1991;99(2): 270–274. Reproduced with permission of Am College of Chest Physicians)

associated with chronic pain or altered cutaneous sensation at 3 months postoperative, suggesting that either the amount of intraoperative nerve damage is not indicative of long-term nerve damage or that there is a more significant cause for chronic pain than intercostal nerve injury. Video-assisted thoracoscopic surgery (VATS) is accepted as reducing acute postoperative pain and analgesic requirements compared to both muscle-sparing and standard thoracotomy.[115–116] Comparative studies have shown no difference in chronic pain occurrence between VATS and open thoracotomy.[117–118] In our experience, pain in the shoulder girdle region following thoracic surgical procedures is frequently not from intercostal nerve damage but is the result of a persistent inability to normally range the shoulder girdle region. This was confirmed by Steegers et al.[119] who reported that only half of patients who experience chronic pain after thoracic surgery have pain associated with a neuropathic component. Similar issues may also be involved in sternal-splitting cardiovascular procedures. Many of these patients demonstrate persistent myofascial tenderness in the muscles of the shoulder girdle region (pectorals, trapezius, rhomboids, and deltoid) rather than a neuropathic pain, although brachial plexus compression can also be a factor after sternum-splitting operations.

Phantom Pains

Phantom limb sensation may be defined as any nonpainful sensation in the absent limb, whereas phantom pain is any painful sensation referred to the absent limb (where the patient is not). Stump pain is pain localized to the stump (where the patient is). Nonpainful sensations may include a specific position, shape, or movement of the phantom, feelings of warmth or cold, itching, and tingling. Phantom pain is often reported as if the limb is in a distorted position. Phantom pain may be exacerbated and ameliorated by a range of physical factors (eg, changes in weather) and psychological factors (eg, emotional stress). It may be more intense in the distal portions of the phantom and can have several different qualities, such as stabbing, throbbing, burning, or cramping. Phantom pain is a major problem for many who undergo amputation of a body part for malignancy.[120] The majority of patients report that phantom pain and sensations begin immediately after surgery.[121] Phantom limb pain is said to be more likely to occur in patients who experienced pain in the body part before amputation. Although phantom pain is most common after the amputation of an extremity (arm or leg), it can also occur after the surgical removal of other body parts such as breast, rectum, penis, testicles, eye, tongue, or teeth. Phantom breast pain occurs in 13% of patients up to 1 year following mastectomy.[122] Phantom rectal pain occurs in up to 18% of patients after surgery for rectal carcinoma.[123] Only a fraction of patients who lose a limb or other body part report chronic pain, casting doubt upon the different theories for the causation of post amputation pain. The long-term course of phantom limb pain is unclear. There are reports of a slight decline in the proportion of patients affected over the course of several years after surgery,[124] but others have described high rates also in long-term amputees.[125] The clinician should carefully distinguish nonpainful phantom sensations from phantom pain, and neuropathic stump pain from nonneuropathic stump pain. The latter can be a sign of local disease such as infection or tumor recurrence.

Radiation Myelopathy, Plexopathy, and Neuropathy

Tolerance of the nervous system to radiation depends on several factors such as volume of tissue irradiated, total dose, dose per fraction, duration of irradiation, and patient age. Radiation therapy may cause pain by damage to peripheral nerves, spinal cord, or brain by altering the microvascular connective tissues surrounding peripheral nerve, via fibrosis and chronic inflammation in connective tissues, or bringing about demyelination and focal necrosis of the white and gray matter in the spinal cord. These changes usually occur late in the course of a patient's illness. The differential diagnosis should always include recurrent tumor. In most instances, pain is a component of the clinical picture, but it is rarely as severe as that associated with recurrent tumor. The pathological findings of radiation-induced progressive myelopathy may include demyelination, focal necrosis and axonal loss, and vascular abnormalities such as telangiectasias, endothelial swelling with fibrin exudates, hyaline degeneration, thickening and fibrinoid necrosis of vessel walls with perivascular fibrosis, and sometimes vasculitis.[126]

Early-delayed radiation myelopathy occurs from 6 weeks to 6 months after RT, and improvement follows in most cases within 2 to 9 months, although in some instances symptoms may persist for a long period of time. The cervical and thoracic spinal cord is the most commonly involved. Clinical signs are generally limited to a Lhermitte sign (brief, unpleasant sensation of numbness, tingling, and often electric-like discharge going from the neck to the spine and extremities, triggered by neck flexion). The spinal cord MRI is usually normal. Transient demyelination, probably resulting from radiation injury of oligodendrocytes, is felt to be the main pathogenic mechanism of early-delayed myelopathy.[127] Late-delayed radiation-induced spinal cord complications include progressive myelopathy and spinal hemorrhage. Progressive myelopathy or delayed radiation myelopathy may follow radiation therapy by 6 months to approximately 10 years. Risk factors include older age, previous irradiation (incidental or medical) particularly during childhood, large radiation port involving the dorsal or lumbar spinal cord, and large radiation dose and fractions. The clinical onset of delayed radiation myelopathy may be acute but it is more often progressive. Patients present with para- or tetraparesis with rapid development of sensory and/or motor deficits. The development of a Brown-Séquard syndrome is a classic presentation. Brown-Séquard syndrome consists of ipsilateral pyramidal tract and posterior column signs and contralateral loss of spinothalamic function. Light touch is usually unaffected.

Another possible presentation is a transverse myelopathy with bilateral leg weakness and sensory loss up to the level of irradiation. Patients may develop bladder or bowel dysfunction; pain has been occasionally reported. The involvement of the upper cervical spinal cord can cause diaphragm dysfunction. The course of symptoms is difficult to predict; some patients improve and others deteriorate. Despite its lack of specificity, MRI findings are important. Other potential causes of myelopathy should be carefully investigated.

Neuropathic syndromes that are associated with chest wall or axillary radiation therapy include brachial plexopathy, malignant peripheral nerve tumors, nerve entrapment in a lymphedematous shoulder and ischemia. Both early- and late-onset brachial plexopathy occur. Clinically, the plexopathy involves mixed sensory and motor deficits, with or without pain.

Olsen et al.[128] described the incidence and latency period of radiation-induced brachial plexopathy (RBP) in 79 patients with breast cancer. Thirty-five percent of patients developed RBP. Fifty percent had involvement of the entire plexus, 18% of the upper plexus alone, 4% of the lower plexus alone, and a definite level of involvement could not be determined in 28% of patients. RBP began in most patients either during or immediately after radiation therapy. RBP was more common in patients who received combination treatment with chemotherapy and radiation than with radiation alone. The risk of radiation induced brachial plexopathy was smaller than 1% after administrating doses per fraction between 2.2 and 2.5 Gy with the total dose between 34 and 40 Gy. The use of doses per fraction in the range 2.2 Gy and 4.58 Gy with the total doses between 43.5 Gy and 60 Gy causes a significant increase of the risk of brachial plexus injury from 1.7% up to 73%.[129] Although some authors suggest that pain is rarely a prominent symptom in radiation-induced plexopathy,[130–132] several studies[133–137] suggest the opposite. Zeidman et al.[137] estimate that up to 20% of cases may report severe pain. Typically, however, patients with radiation-induced injury of the brachial plexus present with sensory (paresthesias or dysesthesias) or motor (weakness, paresis) dysfunction in the upper extremity. Mondrup at al.[135] noted that the most prominent symptoms for RBP were numbness or paresthesia (71%) and pain (41%), and the most prominent objective signs were decreased or absent muscle stretch reflexes (93%) closely followed by sensory loss (82%) and weakness (71%). The neurological deficits are relentlessly progressive and ultimately result in a useless yet painful limb. In contrast to malignant infiltration, patients with radiation injury to the plexus tend to have abnormal sensory and normal motor nerve conduction studies and characteristically manifest more fasciculations or myokymia on EMG than patients with neoplastic disease.[138]

Radiation fibrosis of the lumbosacral plexus is relatively rare. The most common cause sems to be intracavitary radium implants for carcinoma of the cervix.[139] Paresthesias, distal weakness progressing proximally, and, on occasion, pain, occur in the lower extremities 2 to 3 months after radiation affects the sacral plexus.[140] The pathogenesis of this is probably reversible demyelination. The symptoms and signs are usually bilateral upon presentation. The weakness commences distally in the L5-S1 segments and slowly progresses.[141] Painless, indolent leg weakness occurs early in radiation disease, whereas pain with or without unilateral weakness usually characterizes plexopathy due to neoplastic invasion. Radiation disease often results in serious neurologic disability.

Diagnostic studies can confirm the diagnosis of radiation plexopathy. Approximately 60% of patients with radiation-induced plexopathy will show myokymia on EMG. MRI imaging of the plexus is also helpful. Enhancement of nerve roots and T2-weighted hyperintensity usually suggests tumor; radiation plexopathy does not usually produce nerve enhancement, although increase in T2 signal may be present.[142] In general, RBP-associated fibrosis appears as a diffusely thickened plexus with signal intensity similar to skeletal muscle on T1- and T2-weighted images. However, isolated reports exist of variable intensity of the fibrosis associated with RBP, with signal enhancement with gadolinium as long as 21 years after radiation. PET/CT scanning is also helpful in distinguishing tumor from radiation changes.[143]

Features distinguishing radiation plexopathy from neoplastic plexopathy are summarized in Table 10.6.

Peripheral Neuropathy from Chemotherapy

Peripheral neuropathy is a common dose-limiting toxicity of chemotherapy. It is a toxic neuropathy resulting from the direct injury of the PNS by the chemotherapeutic agent. Chemotherapy-induced peripheral neuropathy (CIPN) causes numerous debilitating symptoms, impairs functional capacity, and results in dose reductions or even cessation of chemotherapy. The incidence of CIPN ranges from 30% to 40% of patients receiving chemotherapy.[144]

TABLE 10.6

CLINICAL DISTINCTION OF RADIATION PLEXOPATHY FROM NEOPLASTIC PLEXOPATHY

Feature	Neoplastic	Radiation
Presentation	Pain	Paresthesia, weakness
Pain	Early, severe	Later in course
Edema	Occasional	Common
Plexus involvement:		
Brachial	Often lower plexus	Usually whole plexus
Lumbosacral	Lower, usually unilateral	Commonly bilateral
Horner syndrome	Common	Unusual
Local tissue necrosis	Not present	Common
Rectal mass (LSP)	Common	Not a feature
Myokymia (EMG)	Unusual	Present
Nerve enhancement (MRI)	Present	Usually absent
PET scan	Positive	Usually negative

LSP, lumbosacral plexopathy; EMG, electromyography; PET, positron-emission tomography. (From Jaeckle KA. Neurological manifestations of neoplastic and radiation-induced plexopathies. *Semin Neurol*. 2004; 24(4):385–393. Reprinted with permission from Thieme, Inc.)

A number of factors influence the incidence of CIPN in patients receiving neurotoxic chemotherapy, including patient age, dose intensity, cumulative dose, therapy duration, coadministration of other neurotoxic chemotherapy agents, and pre-existing conditions such as diabetes and alcohol abuse.

The drugs most commonly reported to cause CIPN include taxanes, platinum agents, vinca alkaloids, thalidomide, and bortezomib. The diagnosis of CIPN must be approached cautiously, particularly in patients with potential coexisting or previous conditions that involve or predispose to peripheral neuropathy. In these patients, diagnostic efforts should be directed at the differentiation of CIPN from other causes of peripheral neuropathy. The clinical manifestations of CIPN are subjective and predominantly manifest as pure sensory symptoms. They are most commonly reported as progressive distal symmetrically distributed symptoms of numbness, tingling, pins and needles, burning, decreased or altered sensation, or increased sensitivity that may be painful in the feet and hands. The primary clinical objective in assessing patients is to determine the presence and severity of CIPN-associated symptoms that result in interference with activities of daily living, because this finding is critical for treatment decisions. Symptoms of motor weakness from CIPN are less commonly reported, and when present, are observed in patients with more persistent and severe sensory findings. Motor weakness is typically manifest as distal weakness such as a foot drop.

Isolated motor weakness due to CIPN without sensory involvement has not been reported. If such findings are observed in a patient, consideration should be given to other diagnoses that may produce pure motor weakness including steroid myopathy (proximal), Eaton-Lambert myasthenic syndrome, diabetic neuropathy, cachexia with decreased activity level, paraneoplastic motor neuropathy, and unmasked Charcot-Marie-Tooth disease. If the patient has coexisting diabetes, it can be quite difficult to differentiate the onset or progression of diabetic neuropathy from CIPN. This emphasizes the importance of careful evaluation and recording of the patient's baseline neurologic findings and symptoms before initiation of the neurotoxic chemotherapy. Diabetic neuropathy can be asymmetrical or symmetrical, focal or diffuse, or manifest as mononeuritis multiplex in its involvement and has many different clinical forms. The most common form of diabetic neuropathy, the distal symmetrical polyneuropathic form, has clinical symptoms similar to CIPN. Cancer patients also may have neuropathy from a paraneoplastic syndrome. Patients with leukemia or lymphoma may have lymphomatous infiltration of the peripheral nerves, which also presents as a neuropathy.

The onset of CIPN is usually gradually progressive, but some patients have rapid onset following administration of neurotoxic chemotherapy. The most commonly observed clinical findings of CIPN are symmetrical progressive onset of the following sensory symptoms and findings in a stocking-glove distribution: paresthesias, hyperesthesias, hypoesthesias, and dysesthesias, which more commonly appear earlier and with more pronounced symptoms in the toes and feet, with later involvement of the fingers and hands. Concurrent loss of deep tendon reflexes (distal usually earlier than proximal) in the affected extremities is an important diagnostic sign associated with greater neurosensory damage. Sensory findings, including diminished or absent proprioception, vibration, touch, two-point discrimination, sharp/dull discrimination, temperature, and touch/pain are typically observed in a stocking-glove distribution in symptomatic patients. Autonomic neuropathy is often more difficult to diagnose. Orthostatic hypotension may be the only autonomic manifestation of vincristine neuropathy.

Different chemotherapeutic agents lead to CIPN, which is similar: the length-dependent, symmetrical stocking-glove distribution with predominantly sensory symptoms noted by the patient (Table 10.7). CIPN generally arises as

TABLE 10.7

AGENTS REPORTED TO CAUSE PERIPHERAL NEUROPATHY

Sensory	Sensory and Motor	Demyelinating and Axonopathy	Autonomic	Cranial Nerves
Bortezomib	Ara-C, Ara-A, Ara-G	Suramin	Docetaxel	Vincristine
Carboplatin	Docetaxel		Vincristine	
Cisplatin	Epothilones			
Etoposide	Hexamethylmelamine			
Gemcitabine	Paclitaxel (all formulations)			
Ifosfamide	Vincristine			
Interferon	Vinblastine			
Misonidazole	Vinorelbine			
Oxaliplatin	Vindesine			
Procarbazine				
Suramin				
Thalidomide				

(Modified from Hausheer FH, Schilsky RL, et al. Diagnosis, management, and evaluation of chemotherapy-induced peripheral neuropathy. *Semin Oncol*. 2006;33(1):15-49. Copyright 2006 with permission from Elsevier.)

a consequence of the disruption of axoplasmic microtubule-mediated transport, distal axonal (Wallerian) degeneration, and direct damage to the sensory nerve cell bodies of the dorsal root ganglia (DRG). Demyelination (diffuse or segmental) secondary to chemotherapy is an uncommon finding (but occasionally observed with cisplatin), and when observed, it is typically a secondary and isolated finding relative to the extent of axonal and DRG pathological findings. It is important to recognize that CIPN commonly follows the administration of chemotherapeutic agents that cannot appreciably distribute across the blood-brain barrier (eg, taxanes, platinum agents, vinca alkaloids, thalidomide, and bortezomib. CIPN is most commonly characterized as a distal axonopathy, less commonly as a neuronopathy, and may simultaneously manifest with both forms in some patients. Some agents may cause subclinical nerve injury that only becomes apparent when combined with other neurotoxic agents or in patients with comorbid conditions that predispose to neuropathy.

The most sensitive and reliable method of detecting CIPN is by history and physical examination. Nerve conduction studies and EMG are not necessary for initial evaluation and should only be used if other sources of neuropathy are in question. Typically, the sensory examination consists of testing light touch, pinprick, vibration, and joint position sense, and Romberg testing. Motor examination will usually involve assessment of distal muscles. Foot dorsiflexion and wrist extension should be tested in patients receiving vincristine. Deep tendon reflexes, especially ankle jerks should also be examined, because reflex loss may be an early sign of CIPN. The clinical evaluation of CIPN is listed in Figure 10.9.

To improve accurate and reliable reporting of chemotherapy-induced neuropathy, various grading systems have been developed.[145] Of the grading scales in use, the National Cancer Institute-Common Toxicity Criteria (NCI-CTC), Eastern Cooperative Oncology Group (ECOG), and World Health Organization (WHO) are the most commonly used. Grading scales for chemotherapy-induced peripheral neuropathy are listed in Table 10.8.

Platinum Agents (Cisplatin, Carboplatin, Oxaliplatin)

All platinum agents are associated with CIPN that is dose-dependent, cumulative, and predominantly sensory in nature. Cisplatin is a widely used agent; the reported incidence of CIPN for single-agent cisplatin ranges from 49% to 100% depending on dose, schedule, and combination of other agents used.[146–148] Symptoms and signs of cisplatin neuropathy usually occur during treatment. However, it is important to recognize that the cisplatin-induced neuropathy may occur up to several weeks after the last administered dose of cisplatin and the patient's symptoms may continue to progress even after cisplatin therapy has been discontinued. The CIPN symptoms associated with cisplatin may be irreversible and may be more frequent and severe when the drug is used in combination with other neurotoxic drugs. Carboplatin is associated with the development of CIPN that is clinically indistinguishable from cisplatin with an incidence of CIPN ranging from 13% to 42%. Oxaliplatin is used in the treatment of advanced colorectal cancer. Acute oxaliplatin neuropathy is usually transient and predominantly sensory. This may regress during treatment cycles but frequently recurs with further treatment. Persistent sensory CIPN is gradually progressive in onset and is related to the cumulative dose. Some patients develop delayed onset or worsening of CIPN even after treatment is discontinued.[149] The persistent form of oxaliplatin-induced neuropathy commonly results in treatment delays, and in severe cases, discontinuation of treatment.

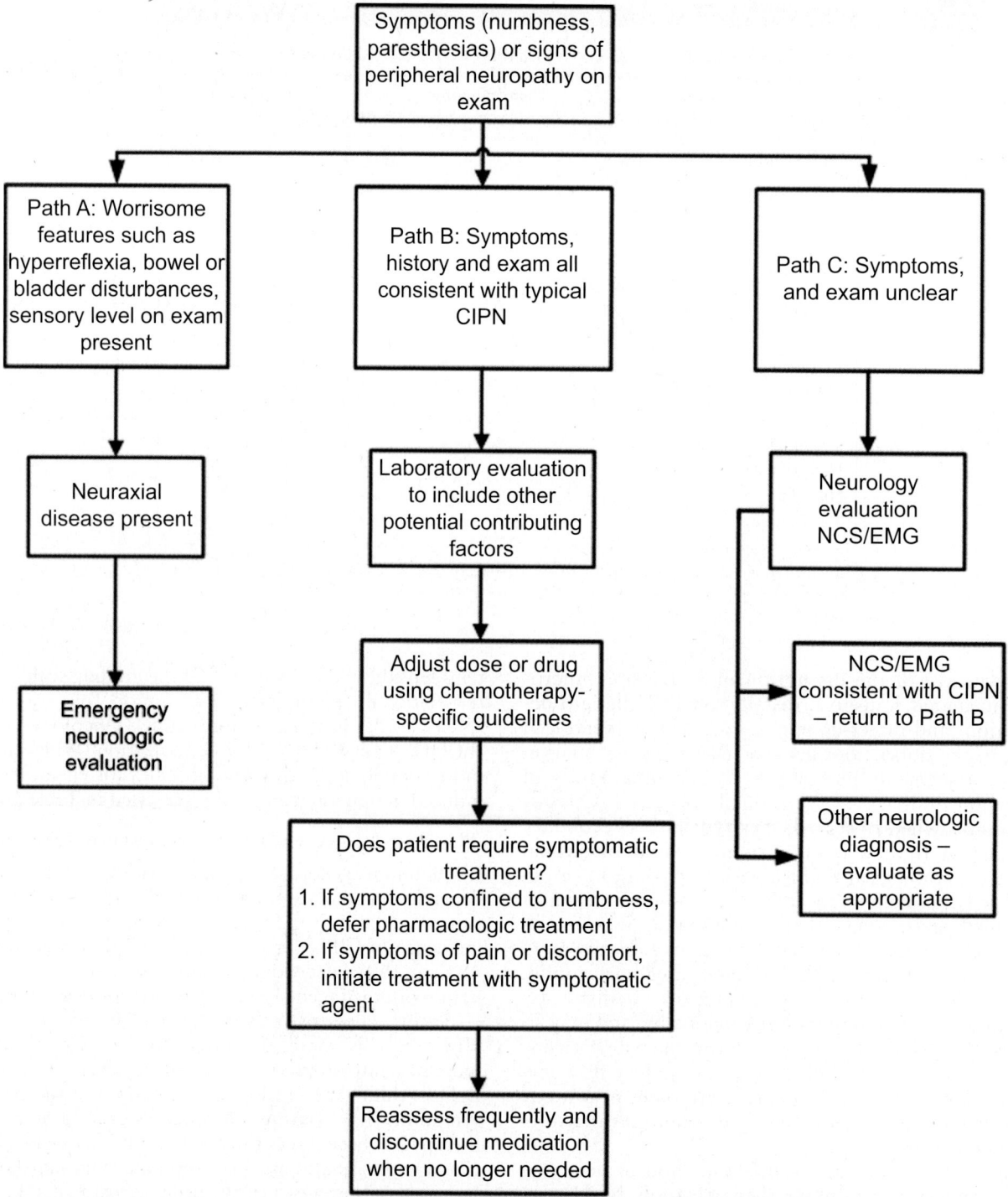

FIGURE 10.9 Clinical evaluation of suspected CIPN. Laboratory tests include glycosylated hemoglobin, thyroid testing, vitamin B12 level, folate level etc. CIPN, Chemotherapy-induced peripheral neuropathy; NCS, nerve conduction study; EMG, electromyography. (Modified from Kaley TJ, and eangelis LM. Therapy of chemotherapy-induced peripheral neuropathy. *Br J Haematol.* 2009;145(1): 3–14. Reprinted by permission from Wiley-Blackwell.)

Taxanes (Paclitaxel, Docetaxel)

Taxanes are widely used against various types of malignancy. Paclitaxel (Taxol) is used in patients with metastatic carcinoma of the ovary after failure of first-line therapy and in patients with metastatic breast cancer or AIDS-related Kaposi sarcoma. Paclitaxel-induced neuropathy, manifested primarily by peripheral sensory neuropathy with relative sparing of motor function, is a common side effect that can be dose-limiting. Similar to platinum-induced CIPN, paclitaxel neuropathy manifests as a symmetrical progressive, length-dependent stocking-glove distribution of paresthesias, numbness, tingling, burning pain, dysesthesias, and decreased vibration and proprioception, which in more advanced stages is accompanied by the symmetrical loss of deep tendon reflexes with initial involvement of distal reflexes and later involving proximal reflexes. Docetaxel (Taxotere) is well established

TABLE 10.8

GRADING SCALES FOR CHEMOTHERAPY-INDUCED PERIPHERAL NEUROPATHY

Scale	Grade 0	Grade 1	Grade 2	Grade 3	Grade 4
WHO	None	Paresthesia and/or decreased tendon reflexes	Severe paresthesias and/or mild weakness	Intolerable paresthesias and/or marked motor loss	Paralysis
ECOG	None	Decreased deep tendon reflexes, mild paresthesias, mild constipation	Absent deep tendon reflexes, severe paresthesias, severe constipation, mild weakness	Disabling sensory loss, severe peripheral neuropathic pain, obstipation, severe weakness, bladder dysfunction	Respiratory dysfunction secondary to weakness, obstipation requiring surgery, paralysis confining patient to bed/wheelchair
NCIC-CTC (revised 1999)					
Neuropathy Sensory	Normal	Loss of deep tendon reflexes or paresthesia (including tingling) but not interfering with function	Objective sensory loss or paresthesia (including tingling) interfering with function, but not interfering with activities of daily living	Sensory loss or paresthesia interfering with activities of daily living	Permanent sensory loss that interferes with function
Neuropathy Motor	Normal	Subjective weakness but no objective findings	Mild objective weakness interfering with function, but not interfering with activities of daily living	Objective weakness interfering with activities of daily living	Paralysis

WHO, World Health Organization; ECOG, Eastern Cooperative Oncology Group; NCI-CTC, National Cancer Institute-Common Toxicity Criteria. (Modified from Postma TJ, Heimans JJ. Grading of chemotherapy-induced peripheral neuropathy. *Ann Oncol.* 2000; 11(5):509–513. Copyright 2000 by the European Society for Medical Oncology and Oxford University Press.)

in the treatment of breast, ovarian, and non–small cell lung cancer. Docetaxel-induced neuropathy is clinically indistinguishable from paclitaxel-induced neuropathy, and manifests as a symmetrical progressive, length-dependent sensory neuropathy often accompanied by paresthesia, pain, numbness, loss of dexterity, unsteady gait, sensory loss motor weakness, and loss of the distal deep tendon reflexes.[150]

Paclitaxel Acute Pain Syndrome

Paclitaxel-induced toxicity is a syndrome of subacute aches and pains, commonly referred to as arthralgias and myalgias. It may occur in up to 58% of patients receiving paclitaxel.[151] Symptoms begin 1 to 3 days after drug administration and often resolve within 7 days.[144] Patients often complain of pain in the back, hips, shoulders, thighs, legs, and feet. The pain may be described as aching or deep. The pathophysiology of this syndrome is unknown and has not been demonstrated to be associated with any alteration of muscle or joints.[152]

Vinca Alkaloids (Vincristine, Vinblastine, Vinorelbine, Vindesine)

Vincristine commonly produces sensory CIPN, but autonomic neuropathy and demyelination may also occur. The development of severe motor neurotoxicity accompanied by neurosensory impairment due to vincristine is rare. Common symptoms experienced by patients on vincristine include symmetrical length-dependent paresthesias, pain in the hands and feet, muscle cramps, numbness and tingling in the hands and feet, loss of deep tendon reflexes, postural hypotension, and distal hyperesthesia. Loss of ankle stretch reflexes is an early and almost universal sign, and with continued therapy all reflexes may diminish or disappear. Weakness in the form of a length dependent symmetrical, progressive distal axonopathy is the most common clinical presentation. Motor weakness from vincristine can become severe enough to render patients immobile. Although vinblastine and vinorelbine are all reported to cause CIPN that is clinically similar to that of vincristine, the incidence appears to be lower than for vincristine.

Thalidomide. Thalidomide is used in the treatment of multiple myeloma. The mechanism of action may be related to both immunomodulation and antiangiogenesis. CIPN is a common and potentially severe side effect that may be permanent. It causes length-dependent, predominantly sensory axonal neuropathy that affects large and small fibers. CIPN generally occurs following chronic use over a period of months. The clinical signs and symptoms of thalidomide-induced neuropathy include numbness and tingling, which can be painful and occur in a symmetrical distribution in the hands and feet. The combination of bortezomib and thalidomide induces a reversible length-dependent, sensorimotor, predominantly axonal, large fiber/small fiber poyneuropathy.[153]

Bortezomib. Bortezomib (Velcade) is an intravenous agent used for the treatment of multiple myeloma. The most commonly reported symptoms of bortezomib-induced CIPN include burning sensation, hyperesthesias, hypoesthesias, paresthesias, and discomfort from neuropathic pain. Although the incidence of more severe peripheral neuropathy with bortezomib is low, up to one third of patients require a dose reduction or discontinuation due to peripheral neuropathy.[154] In the majority of patients, dose reduction results in improvement of symptoms.

Procarbazine, Cytarabine, Etoposide, α-Interferon. Procarbazine-induced neuropathy is manifested by neurosensory features similar to those produced by other chemotherapeutic agents. Cytarabine-induced neuropathy is characterized by a symmetrical, length-dependent sensory and motor involvement, which may be permanent. Peripheral neuropathy associated with cytarabine has been characterized in both upper and lower extremities as muscle weakness, gait disturbances, walking difficulties, paresthesias, numbness, hypoalgesia, hypoesthesia, and myalgia. Etoposide is occasionally reported to cause peripheral neuropathy. α-interferon is associated with a very low incidence of peripheral neuropathy.

Hematopoietic Growth Factors

Although these agents do not typically cause neuropathic pain in cancer patients, they are a significant source of pain and a brief account is included for completeness. Current options for hematopoietic growth factors include erythropoietin, which stimulates red cell production; Granulocyte Colony Stimulating Factor (GCSF) or filgrastim, which stimulates white blood cell production; and GM-CSF, which has similar effects. Erythropoietin seldom produces systemic side effects, but the granulocyte CSFs cause low-grade fever, myalgias, and a "flu-like syndrome," which rapidly resolves. Filgrastim is generally well tolerated. The most frequent adverse reaction is mild to moderate medullary bone pain, reported by approximately 20% of patients.[155]

Aromatase Inhibitors. Aromatase inhibitors (AIs) are hormonal drugs used as both treatment and preventative agents for estrogen-positive breast cancer (early- and late-stage). Three AIs are approved by the FDA: anastrazole (Arimidex), exemestane (Aromasin), and letrozole (Femara). These agents do not cause neuropathic pain but are a frequent source of pain, particularly in breast cancer patients. They typically are prescribed for prolonged periods of time (often 5 years and more) and pain complaints often persist. Increased survival in breast cancer patients is largely due to the benefits of hormonal therapy, such as tamoxifen and AIs, for the treatment of hormone-sensitive breast cancer. Breast cancer patients taking AIs have a higher incidence of osteoporosis, bone fractures, and musculoskeletal symptoms, particularly joint pain and stiffness.[156] Joint pain is frequent (30% to 40%) and quite often disabling (5% to 10%).[157] In one study, 16% of metastatic breast cancer patients complained of joint pain within 2 months of starting anastrozole and 5% had to discontinue therapy because of severe arthralgia.[158] The problem may be exacerbated in patients who received previous chemotherapy. Crew et al.[156] reported a greater than fourfold increased risk of AI-related joint symptoms in patients who received previous taxane therapy. The exact mechanism of AI-related arthralgia is unclear, but is believed to be related to estrogen deprivation. Two estrogen receptors α and β in human articular chondrocytes provided additional evidence that cartilage is sensitive to estrogens.[159] Furthermore, estrogen has well-described antinociceptive effects.[160] Estrogen receptors are present in opioid-containing neurons in the spinal cord and brain.[161–162] Morales et al.[163] showed that the functional impairment of hands in the AI-associated arthralgia syndrome is characterized by tenosynovial changes on MRI. With the increasing use of long-term AI therapy in the adjuvant setting, AI-induced arthralgia is a major issue for cancer survivors and treating physicians. The majority of women who experience arthralgias continue with their treatment given the profound benefits associated with these medications.[164]

The side effects of chemotherapeutic agents frequently involve a peripheral neuropathy that may lead to both chronic pain and loss of function. These side effects can force the reduction of dose or even cessation of the agent, thereby reducing treatment efficacy. Accurate diagnosis of the cause of the neuropathy is therefore critical in patient management.

HERPES ZOSTER AND POSTHERPETIC NEURALGIA

The natural history of varicella zoster virus (VZV) infection and the molecular mechanisms of viral pathogenesis are incompletely understood. During viraemia, T-cells transport VZV to the skin, where cell-free viral replication facilitates person-to-person spread, and transmission to the neurons where latency is established.[165] VZV causes chickenpox, usually in childhood, and most children manifest only mild neurologic sequelae. Herpes zoster is caused by reactivation of VZV in dorsal root ganglion neurons. The incidence of zoster is increased substantially in persons with hematologic malignancies and solid tumors.[166]

Herpes zoster episodes usually commence with a prodromal period of about 4 days. The rash is preceded by a prodrome of dermatomal pain that is accompanied by burning, numbness or tingling sensations, and systemic symptoms such as malaise, headache and myalgia, but rarely fever. This is followed by a rash lasting approximately 2 to 4 weeks, with possible subacute herpetic neuralgia for up to 3 months, followed, in some patients, by a period of postherpetic neuralgia (PHN) lasting months or possibly years. The erythematous maculopapular rash progresses to clusters of clear vesicles which continue to form for 3 to 5 days and evolve through stages of pustulation, ulceration, and crusting (Fig. 10.10). The cutaneous eruption is almost always unilateral and does not cross the midline. Thoracic, cervical, and ophthalmic involvement are most common. Facial zoster is usually present in the ophthalmic division of the trigeminal nerve and are frequently accompanied by keratitis, which is almost always a potential cause of blindness if not recognized and treated promptly. Zoster in the maxillary and mandibular divisions of the trigeminal nerve may be associated with osteonecrosis and spontaneous exfoliation of teeth. When the seventh cranial nerve is involved, there is weakness of all facial muscles on one side, along with rash in the ipsilateral external ear (zoster oticus) or hard palate. Cervical zoster is occasionally associated with arm weakness (zoster paresis) and less often with diaphragmatic paralysis. Lumbosacral zoster can be accompanied by leg weakness as well as bladder and bowel dysfunction.

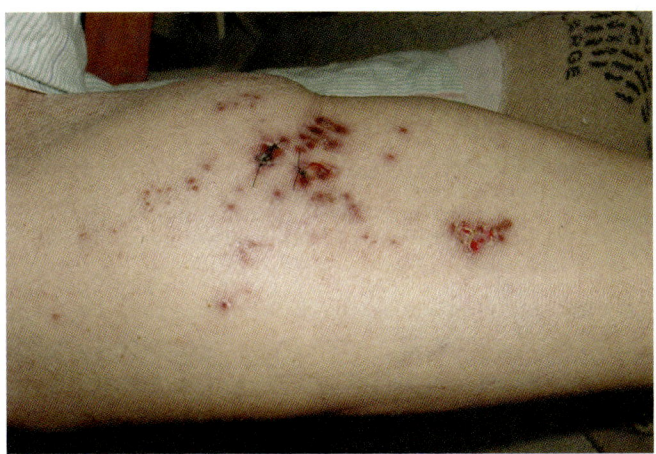

FIGURE 10.10 A 67-year-old man admitted for pain control because of intractable left lower extremity pain of recent onset. Over the course of several days, he developed a posterior left calf rash which, on biopsy (sutures), provided positive results for a herpes zoster infection. Photograph shows several crusted lesions.

The histologic hallmark of zoster is inflammation and neuronal loss in ganglia that corresponds to the segmental distribution of rash. Intense lymphocytic inflammation and vasculitis in nerves cause degeneration of motor and sensory roots and may spread into adjacent parts of the spinal cord, with localized leptomeningitis and gray-matter necrosis of varying degrees, or demyelination.[167–168]

There are three phases of pain in herpes zoster: acute herpetic neuralgia, subacute herpetic neuralgia, and PHN.[169–170] Acute herpetic neuralgia is pain from onset of the prodrome to 30 days. Subacute herpetic neuralgia is pain between 30 days from prodrome onset and 3 to 4 months. Definitions of PHN vary. Most define PHN as "presence of pain" without specifying a numerical threshold, but use different time points after rash onset or rash healing.[171] The time interval used in the definition of PHN varies from 1 to 6 months after resolution of the rash and some suggest that PHN occurs with persistence of pain of herpes zoster more than 3 months after resolution of the rash.[172] Severe acute pain is more likely in older women and those with a prodrome or severe rash. However, VZV infection may not present in the characteristic dermatomal distribution of vesicles in patients who have undergone bone marrow transplantation.[173] *Zoster sine herpete* is a rare pain syndrome in which no cutaneous rash occurs but a segmental pain syndrome is transiently present and associated with evidence of varicella infection. It may progress to postherpetic neuralgia.

The usual presentation of herpes zoster is a self-limiting painful dermatomal, unilateral, vesicular rash which may be accompanied by PHN, its most common complication. PHN is characterized by persisting pain in the affected dermatome after rash healing and which lasts for years. However, zoster can result in other complications, many of which have unusual presentations and serious sequelae. VCZ outbreaks cause significant morbidity in patient suffering from blood-related malignancies (particularly in patients with lymphoproliferative disorders) and in those undergoing hemopoietic stem-cell transplantation (HSCT).[174] In immunocompromised individuals, especially those with cancer or acquired immunodeficiency syndrome, deeper tissue penetration of the virus may occur (compared with immunocompetent individuals), with resultant myelitis, small-vessel vasculopathy, ventriculitis, and meningoencephalitis.[175] Ocular complications of ophthalmic zoster are relatively frequent. Delayed contralateral hemiparesis is a rare complication of ophthalmic zoster that may present as stroke, temporally remote from the zoster episode. Ramsay Hunt syndrome is caused by reactivation of VZV involving the facial nerve; facial paralysis, ear pain, and vesicles in the ear are diagnostic. Facial paralysis in the absence of vesicles may indicate zoster sine herpete, which can be mistaken for Bell palsy. Detection of the virus in neurons, oligodendrocytes, meningeal cells, ependymal cells, or the blood vessel wall often requires a combination of morphologic, immunohistochemical, in situ hybridization, and polymerase chain reaction (PCR) methods. The PCR analysis of CSF remains the mainstay for diagnosing the neurologic complications of VZV.[175]

Among autologous HSCT patients, the VZV reactivation rate is reported to be 15% to 45%;[176] moreover, one third of these VZV patients developed PHN.[177] In the general population, recognized predictive factors for PHN are older age, female sex, presence of a prodrome, greater rash severity, and greater acute pain severity.[178] Patients with hematological malignancies have a high risk of VZV reactivation, given the presence in this population of the most recognized predisposing factors: the underlying malignancy; older age; age-related immune decline; and waning of specific cell-mediated immunity induced by cytotoxic treatments, steroids, and HSCT.

Two separate mechanisms of PHN have been proposed: (1) that the excitability of primary afferent neurons is increased after nerve damage, causing irritable nociceptors and central sensitization, resulting in pain and allodynia; (2) that the degeneration of nociceptive neurons leads to deafferentation with central hyperactivity, causing pain but without allodynia. Both mechanisms may coexist in an individual patient. Peripheral and central demyelination as well as neuronal destruction is involved.

The risk of developing PHN in patients with zoster is approximately 10% to 18%.[179] PHN is considered as the debilitating chronic pain that persists, in some individuals, for many months or years after the herpes zoster rash has healed. It is more prevalent in the elderly and is characterized by constant or intermittent burning, itching, or aching, with or without paroxysmal or lancinating pain. Other primary characteristics, such as numbness, tingling, and allodynia, also contribute to the burden of PHN. Secondary characteristics of PHN include sleep disturbance, anorexia and weight loss, chronic fatigue and depression, accompanied by social isolation. The pain may extend beyond the margins of the original zoster eruption. The skin may be unusually sensitive to even the lightest touch (as from clothing), to the smallest breeze, and to changes in temperature (either hot or cold). This is, of course, allodynia. Both the severity and the duration of PHN increase with age.

References

1. Martin LA, Hagen NA. Neuropathic pain in cancer patients: mechanisms, syndromes, and clinical controversies. *J Pain Symptom Manage.* 1997;14:99–117.

2. Woolf CJ. Dissecting out mechanisms responsible for peripheral neuropathic pain: implications for diagnosis and therapy. *Life Sci.* 2004;74:2605–2610.
3. Rasmussen PV, Sindrup SH, Jensen TS, et al. Symptoms and signs in patients with suspected neuropathic pain. *Pain.* 2004;110:461–469.
4. Bridges D, Thompson SW, Rice AS. Mechanisms of neuropathic pain. *Br J Anaesth.* 2001;87:12–26.
5. Knecht S, Henningsen H, Elbert T, et al. Cortical reorganization in human amputees and mislocalization of painful stimuli to the phantom limb. *Neurosci Lett.* 1995;201:262–264.
6. Zimmermann M. Pathobiology of neuropathic pain. *Eur J Pharmacol.* 2001;429:23–37.
7. Finnerup NB. A review of central neuropathic pain states. *Curr Opin Anaesthesiol.* 2008;21:586–589.
8. Zhao P, Waxman SG, Hains BC. Extracellular signal-regulated kinase-regulated microglia-neuron signaling by prostaglandin E2 contributes to pain after spinal cord injury. *J Neurosci.* 2007;27:2357–2368.
9. Casey KL. Concepts of pain mechanisms: the contribution of functional imaging of the human brain. *Prog Brain Res.* 2000;129:277–287.
10. Geha PY, Apkarian AV. Brain imaging findings in neuropathic pain. *Curr Pain Headache Rep.* 2005;9:184–188.
11. Stephenson DT, Arneric SP. Neuroimaging of pain: advances and future prospects. *J Pain.* 2008;9:567–579.
12. Moisset X, Bouhassira D. Brain imaging of neuropathic pain. *Neuroimage.* 2007;37 Suppl 1:S80-8.
13. Witting N, Kupers RC, Svensson P, et al. A PET activation study of brush-evoked allodynia in patients with nerve injury pain. *Pain.* 2006;120:145–154.
14. Zambreanu L, Wise RG, Brooks JC, et al. A role for the brainstem in central sensitisation in humans. Evidence from functional magnetic resonance imaging. *Pain.* 2005;114:397–407.
15. Peyron R, Schneider F, Faillenot I, et al. An fMRI study of cortical representation of mechanical allodynia in patients with neuropathic pain. *Neurology.* 2004;63:1838–1846.
16. Galer BS, Jensen MP. Development and preliminary validation of a pain measure specific to neuropathic pain: the Neuropathic Pain Scale. *Neurology.* 1997;48:332–338.
17. Rog DJ, Nurmikko TJ, Friede T, et al. Validation and reliability of the Neuropathic Pain Scale (NPS) in multiple sclerosis. *Clin J Pain.* 2007;23:473–481.
18. Jensen MP. Review of measures of neuropathic pain. *Curr Pain Headache Rep.* 2006;10:159–166.
19. Fishbain DA, Lewis JE, Cutler R, et al. Can the neuropathic pain scale discriminate between non-neuropathic and neuropathic pain? *Pain Med.* 2008;9:149–160.
20. Jensen MP, Gammaitoni AR, Olaleye DO, et al. The pain quality assessment scale: assessment of pain quality in carpal tunnel syndrome. *J Pain.* 2006;7:823–832.
21. Vecht CJ, Hoff AM, Kansen PJ, et al. Types and causes of pain in cancer of the head and neck. *Cancer.* 1992;70:178–184.
22. Greenberg HS, Deck MD, Vikram B, et al. Metastasis to the base of the skull: clinical findings in 43 patients. *Neurology.* 1981;31:530–537.
23. Fernandez S, Godino O, Martinez-Yelamos S, et al. Cavernous sinus syndrome: a series of 126 patients. *Medicine (Baltimore).* 2007;86:278–281.
24. Metheetrairut C, Brown DH. Glossopharyngeal neuralgia and syncope secondary to neck malignancy. *J Otolaryngol.* 1993;22:18–20.
25. Sozzi G, Marotta P, Piatti L. Vagoglossopharyngeal neuralgia with syncope in the course of carcinomatous meningitis. *Ital J Neurol Sci.* 1987;8:271–275.
26. Macdonald DR, Strong E, Nielsen S, et al. Syncope from head and neck cancer. *J Neurooncol.* 1983;1:257–267.
27. Bullitt E, Tew JM, Boyd J. Intracranial tumors in patients with facial pain. *J Neurosurg.* 1986;64:865–871.
28. Cheng TM, Cascino TL, Onofrio BM. Comprehensive study of diagnosis and treatment of trigeminal neuralgia secondary to tumors. *Neurology.* 1993;43:2298–2302.
29. Nomura T, Ikezaki K, Matsushima T, et al. Trigeminal neuralgia: differentiation between intracranial mass lesions and ordinary vascular compression as causative lesions. *Neurosurg Rev.* 1994;17:51–57.
30. Puca A, Meglio M, Vari R, et al. Evaluation of fifth nerve dysfunction in 136 patients with middle and posterior cranial fossae tumors. *Eur Neurol.* 1995;35:33–37.
31. DeAngelis LM, Payne R. Lymphomatous meningitis presenting as atypical cluster headache. *Pain.* 1987;30:211–216.
32. Pollock BE, Iuliano BA, Foote RL, et al. Stereotactic radiosurgery for tumor-related trigeminal pain. *Neurosurgery.* 2000;46:576–582;discussion 582-3.
33. Barker FG, 2nd, Jannetta PJ, Babu RP, et al. Long-term outcome after operation for trigeminal neuralgia in patients with posterior fossa tumors. *J Neurosurg.* 1996;84:818–825.
34. Clouston PD, Sharpe DM, Corbett AJ, et al. Perineural spread of cutaneous head and neck cancer. Its orbital and central neurologic complications. *Arch Neurol.* 1990;47:73–77.
35. Boerman RH, Maassen EM, Joosten J, et al. Trigeminal neuropathy secondary to perineural invasion of head and neck carcinomas. *Neurology.* 1999;53:213–216.
36. Catalano PJ, Sen C, Biller HF. Cranial neuropathy secondary to perineural spread of cutaneous malignancies. *Am J Otol.* 1995;16:772–777.
37. Ferrante L, Artico M, Nardacci B, et al. Glossopharyngeal neuralgia with cardiac syncope. *Neurosurgery.* 1995;36:58–63.
38. Weinstein RE, Herec D, Friedman JH. Hypotension due to glossopharyngeal neuralgia. *Arch Neurol.* 1986;43:90–92.
39. Galan Gil S, Penarrocha Diago M, Penarrocha Diago M. Malignant mental nerve neuropathy: systematic review. *Med Oral Patol Oral Cir Bucal.* 2008;13:E616–E6121.
40. Wasserstrom WR, Glass JP, Posner JB. Diagnosis and treatment of leptomeningeal metastases from solid tumors: experience with 90 patients. *Cancer.* 1982;49:759–772.
41. Sorensen SC, Eagan RT, Scott M. Meningeal carcinomatosis in patients with primary breast or lung cancer. *Mayo Clin Proc.* 1984;59:91–94.
42. Theodore WH, Gendelman S. Meningeal carcinomatosis. *Arch Neurol.* 1981;38:696–699.
43. Kesari S, Batchelor TT. Leptomeningeal metastases. *Neurol Clin.* 2003;21:25–66.
44. Fox RM. Spinal-cord metastasis after combination chemotherapy and prophylactic whole-brain irradiation in small-cell carcinoma of lung [letter]. *Lancet.* 1977;2:136.
45. Posner JB, Chernik NL. Intracranial metastases from systemic cancer. *Adv Neurol.* 1978;19:579–592.
46. Siegal T, Lossos A, Pfeffer MR. Leptomeningeal metastases: analysis of 31 patients with sustained off-therapy response following combined-modality therapy. *Neurology.* 1994;44:1463–1469.
47. Little JR, Dale AJ, Okazaki H. Meningeal carcinomatosis. Clinical manifestations. *Arch Neurol.* 1974;30:138–143.
48. Kaplan JG, DeSouza TG, Farkash A, et al. Leptomeningeal metastases: comparison of clinical features and laboratory data of solid tumors, lymphomas and leukemias. *J Neurooncol.* 1990;9:225–229.
49. Jaeckle KA. Nerve plexus metastases. *Neurol Clin.* 1991;9:857–866.
50. de Verdier HJ, Colletti PM, Terk MR. MRI of the brachial plexus: a review of 51 cases. *Comput Med Imaging Graph.* 1993;17:45–50.
51. Kori SH, Foley KM, Posner JB. Brachial plexus lesions in patients with cancer: 100 cases. *Neurology.* 1981;31:45–50.
52. Marangoni C, Lacerenza M, Formaglio F, et al. Sensory disorder of the chest as presenting symptom of lung cancer. *J Neurol Neurosurg Psychiatry.* 1993;56:1033–1034.
53. Rodichok LD, Harper GR, Ruckdeschel JC, et al. Early diagnosis of spinal epidural metastases. *Am J Med.* 1981;70:1181–1188.
54. Yeung MC, Hagen NA. Cervical disc herniation presenting with chest wall pain. *Can J Neurol Sci.* 1993;20:59–61.
55. Ahmad A, Barrington S, Maisey M, et al. Use of positron emission tomography in evaluation of brachial plexopathy in breast cancer patients. *Br J Cancer.* 1999;79:478–482.
56. Saphner T, Gallion HH, Van Nagell JR, et al. Neurologic complications of cervical cancer. A review of 2261 cases. *Cancer.* 1989;64:1147–1151.
57. Jaeckle KA, Young DF, Foley KM. The natural history of lumbosacral plexopathy in cancer. *Neurology.* 1985;35:8–15.
58. Dalmau J, Graus F, Marco M. 'Hot and dry foot' as initial manifestation of neoplastic lumbosacral plexopathy. *Neurology.* 1989;39:871–872.
59. Jaeckle KA. Neurological manifestations of neoplastic and radiation-induced plexopathies. *Semin Neurol.* 2004;24:385–393.
60. Taylor BV, Kimmel DW, Krecke KN, et al. Magnetic resonance imaging in cancer-related lumbosacral plexopathy. *Mayo Clin Proc.* 1997;72:823–829.
61. Defrin R, Ohry A, Blumen N, et al. Characterization of chronic pain and somatosensory function in spinal cord injury subjects. *Pain.* 2001;89:253–263.

62. Hansson P. Post-stroke pain case study: clinical characteristics, therapeutic options and long-term follow-up. *Eur J Neurol.* 2004;11 Suppl 1:22–30.
63. Ofek H, Defrin R. The characteristics of chronic central pain after traumatic brain injury. *Pain.* 2007;131:330–340.
64. Lenz FA, Tasker RR, Dostrovsky JO, et al. Abnormal single-unit activity recorded in the somatosensory thalamus of a quadriplegic patient with central pain. *Pain.* 1987;31:225–236.
65. Pattany PM, Yezierski RP, Widerstrom-Noga EG, et al. Proton magnetic resonance spectroscopy of the thalamus in patients with chronic neuropathic pain after spinal cord injury. *AJNR Am J Neuroradiol.* 2002;23:901–905.
66. Peyron R, Garcia-Larrea L, Gregoire MC, et al. Parietal and cingulate processes in central pain. A combined positron emission tomography (PET) and functional magnetic resonance imaging (fMRI) study of an unusual case. *Pain.* 2000;84:77–87.
67. Kreutzberg GW. Microglia: a sensor for pathological events in the CNS. *Trends Neurosci.* 1996;19:312–318.
68. Nakajima K, Kohsaka S. Microglia: activation and their significance in the central nervous system. *J Biochem.* 2001;130:169–175.
69. Watkins LR, Milligan ED, Maier SF. Spinal cord glia: new players in pain. *Pain.* 2001;93:201–205.
70. Watkins LR, Milligan ED, Maier SF. Glial activation: a driving force for pathological pain. *Trends Neurosci.* 2001;24:450–455.
71. Minghetti L, Levi G. Microglia as effector cells in brain damage and repair: focus on prostanoids and nitric oxide. *Prog Neurobiol.* 1998;54:99–125.
72. Colburn RW, Rickman AJ, DeLeo JA. The effect of site and type of nerve injury on spinal glial activation and neuropathic pain behavior. *Exp Neurol.* 1999;157:289–304.
73. Gonzales GR, Tuttle SL, Thaler HT, et al. Central pain in cancer patients. *J Pain.* 2003;4:351–354.
74. Mott MG, Stevenson P, Wood CB. Methotrexate meningitis. *Lancet.* 1972;2:656.
75. Bates S, McKeever P, Masur H, et al. Myelopathy following intrathecal chemotherapy in a patient with extensive Burkitt's lymphoma and altered immune status. *Am J Med.* 1985;78:697–702.
76. Dunton SF, Nitschke R, Spruce WE, et al. Progressive ascending paralysis following administration of intrathecal and intravenous cytosine arabinoside. A Pediatric Oncology Group study. *Cancer.* 1986;57:1083–1088.
77. Zivkovic SA, Ascherman D, Lacomis D. Vasculitic neuropathy—electrodiagnostic findings and association with malignancies. *Acta Neurol Scand.* 2007;115:432–436.
78. Fain O, Hamidou M, Cacoub P, et al. Vasculitides associated with malignancies: analysis of sixty patients. *Arthritis Rheum.* 2007;57:1473–1480.
79. Dalmau JO, Posner JB. Paraneoplastic syndromes affecting the nervous system. *Semin Oncol.* 1997;24:318–328.
80. Storstein A, Vedeler CA. Paraneoplastic neurological syndromes and onconeural antibodies: clinical and immunological aspects. *Adv Clin Chem.* 2007;44:143–185.
81. Inuzuka T. Autoantibodies in paraneoplastic neurological syndrome. *Am J Med Sci.* 2000;319:217–226.
82. Graus F, Cordon-Cardo C, Posner JB. Neuronal antinuclear antibody in sensory neuronopathy from lung cancer. *Neurology.* 1985;35:538–543.
83. Dalmau J, Graus F, Rosenblum MK, et al. Anti-Hu–associated paraneoplastic encephalomyelitis/sensory neuronopathy. A clinical study of 71 patients. *Medicine (Baltimore).* 1992;71:59–72.
84. Graus F, Keime-Guibert F, Rene R, et al. Anti-Hu-associated paraneoplastic encephalomyelitis: analysis of 200 patients. *Brain.* 2001;124:1138–1148.
85. Lucchinetti CF, Kimmel DW, Lennon VA. Paraneoplastic and oncologic profiles of patients seropositive for type 1 antineuronal nuclear autoantibodies. *Neurology.* 1998;50:652–657.
86. Sillevis Smitt P, Grefkens J, de Leeuw B, et al. Survival and outcome in 73 anti-Hu positive patients with paraneoplastic encephalomyelitis/sensory neuronopathy. *J Neurol.* 2002;249:745–753.
87. Dalmau J, Furneaux HM, Gralla RJ, et al. Detection of the anti-Hu antibody in the serum of patients with small cell lung cancer—a quantitative western blot analysis. *Ann Neurol.* 1990;27:544–552.
88. Graus F, Delattre JY, Antoine JC, et al. Recommended diagnostic criteria for paraneoplastic neurological syndromes. *J Neurol Neurosurg Psychiatry.* 2004;75:1135–1140.
89. Caffo O, Amichetti M, Ferro A, et al. Pain and quality of life after surgery for breast cancer. *Breast Cancer Res Treat.* 2003;80:39–48.
90. Carpenter JS, Andrykowski MA, Sloan P, et al. Postmastectomy/postlumpectomy pain in breast cancer survivors. *J Clin Epidemiol.* 1998;51:1285–1292.
91. Poleshuck EL, Katz J, Andrus CH, et al. Risk factors for chronic pain following breast cancer surgery: a prospective study. *J Pain.* 2006;7:626–634.
92. Nesvold IL, Dahl AA, Lokkevik E, et al. Arm and shoulder morbidity in breast cancer patients after breast-conserving therapy versus mastectomy. *Acta Oncol.* 2008;47:835–842.
93. Tasmuth T, Blomqvist C, Kalso E. Chronic post-treatment symptoms in patients with breast cancer operated in different surgical units. *Eur J Surg Oncol.* 1999;25:38–43.
94. Passavanti MB, Pace MC, Barbarisi A, et al. Pain and sensory dysfunction after breast cancer surgery: neurometer CPT evaluation. *Anticancer Res.* 2006;26:3839–3844.
95. Vecht CJ. Arm pain in the patient with breast cancer. *J Pain Symptom Manage.* 1990;5:109–117.
96. Stevens PE, Dibble SL, Miaskowski C. Prevalence, characteristics, and impact of postmastectomy pain syndrome: an investigation of women's experiences. *Pain.* 1995;61:61–68.
97. Vecht CJ, Van de Brand HJ, Wajer OJ. Post-axillary dissection pain in breast cancer due to a lesion of the intercostobrachial nerve. *Pain.* 1989;38:171–176.
98. Macdonald L, Bruce J, Scott NW, et al. Long-term follow-up of breast cancer survivors with post-mastectomy pain syndrome. *Br J Cancer.* 2005;92:225–230.
99. Gottrup H, Andersen J, Arendt-Nielsen L, et al. Psychophysical examination in patients with post-mastectomy pain. *Pain.* 2000;87:275–284.
100. Steegers MA, Wolters B, Evers AW, et al. Effect of axillary lymph node dissection on prevalence and intensity of chronic and phantom pain after breast cancer surgery. *J Pain.* 2008;9:813–822.
101. Dijkstra PU, Rietman JS, Geertzen JH. Phantom breast sensations and phantom breast pain: a 2-year prospective study and a methodological analysis of literature. *Eur J Pain.* 2007;11:99–108.
102. Kroner K, Knudsen UB, Lundby L, et al. Long-term phantom breast syndrome after mastectomy. *Clin J Pain.* 1992;8:346–350.
103. Rothemund Y, Grusser SM, Liebeskind U, et al. Phantom phenomena in mastectomized patients and their relation to chronic and acute pre-mastectomy pain. *Pain.* 2004;107:140–146.
104. Bjorkman B, Arner S, Hyden LC. Phantom breast and other syndromes after mastectomy: Eight breast cancer patients describe their experiences over time: A 2-year follow-up study. *J Pain.* 2008;9(11):1018-1025..
105. Cappiello J, Piazza C, Nicolai P. The spinal accessory nerve in head and neck surgery. *Curr Opin Otolaryngol Head Neck Surg.* 2007;15:107–111.
106. Pu YM, Tang EY, Yang XD. Trapezius muscle innervation from the spinal accessory nerve and branches of the cervical plexus. *Int J Oral Maxillofac Surg.* 2008;37:567–572.
107. Kierner AC, Zelenka I, Heller S, et al. Surgical anatomy of the spinal accessory nerve and the trapezius branches of the cervical plexus. *Arch Surg.* 2000;135:1428–1431.
108. Tsuji T, Tanuma A, Onitsuka T, et al. Electromyographic findings after different selective neck dissections. *Laryngoscope.* 2007;117:319–322.
109. Nahum AM, Mullally W, Marmor L. A syndrome resulting from radical neck dissection. *Arch Otolaryngol.* 1961;74:424–428.
110. Kelley MJ, Kane TE, Leggin BG. Spinal accessory nerve palsy: associated signs and symptoms. *J Orthop Sports Phys Ther.* 2008;38:78–86.
111. Gotoda Y, Kambara N, Sakai T, et al. The morbidity, time course and predictive factors for persistent post-thoracotomy pain. *Eur J Pain.* 2001;5:89–96.
112. Handy JR, Jr., Asaph JW, Skokan L, et al. What happens to patients undergoing lung cancer surgery? Outcomes and quality of life before and after surgery. *Chest.* 2002;122:21–30.
113. Dajczman E, Gordon A, Kreisman H, et al. Long-term postthoracotomy pain. *Chest.* 1991;99:270–274.
114. Maguire MF, Latter JA, Mahajan R, et al. A study exploring the role of intercostal nerve damage in chronic pain after thoracic surgery. *Eur J Cardiothorac Surg.* 2006;29:873–879.
115. Landreneau RJ, Hazelrigg SR, Mack MJ, et al. Postoperative pain-related morbidity: video-assisted thoracic surgery versus thoracotomy. *Ann Thorac Surg.* 1993;56:1285–1289.
116. Landreneau RJ, Wiechmann RJ, Hazelrigg SR, et al. Effect of minimally invasive thoracic surgical approaches on acute and chronic postoperative pain. *Chest Surg Clin N Am.* 1998;8:891–906.

117. Kirby TJ, Mack MJ, Landreneau RJ, et al. Lobectomy–video-assisted thoracic surgery versus muscle-sparing thoracotomy. A randomized trial. *J.Thorac Cardiovasc Surg.* 1995;109: 997–1001;discussion 1001-2.
118. Landreneau RJ, Mack MJ, Hazelrigg SR, et al. Prevalence of chronic pain after pulmonary resection by thoracotomy or video-assisted thoracic surgery. *J Thorac Cardiovasc Surg.* 1994;107:1079–1085;discussion 1085-6.
119. Steegers MA, Snik DM, Verhagen AF, et al. Only half of the chronic pain after thoracic surgery shows a neuropathic component. *J Pain.* 2008.
120. Weinstein SM. Phantom pain. *Oncology (Huntingt).* 1994;8: 65–70.
121. Woodhouse A. Phantom limb sensation. *Clin Exp Pharmacol Physiol.* 2005;32:132–134.
122. Kroner K, Krebs B, Skov J, et al. Immediate and long-term phantom breast syndrome after mastectomy: incidence, clinical characteristics and relationship to pre-mastectomy breast pain. *Pain.* 1989;36:327–334.
123. Ovesen P, Kroner K, Ornsholt J, et al. Phantom-related phenomena after rectal amputation: prevalence and clinical characteristics. *Pain.* 1991;44:289–291.
124. Jensen TS, Krebs B, Nielsen J, et al. Immediate and long-term phantom limb pain in amputees: incidence, clinical characteristics and relationship to pre-amputation limb pain. *Pain.* 1985;21: 267–278.
125. Kooijman CM, Dijkstra PU, Geertzen JH, et al. Phantom pain and phantom sensations in upper limb amputees: an epidemiological study. *Pain.* 2000;87:33–41.
126. Behin A, Delattre JY. Complications of radiation therapy on the brain and spinal cord. *Semin Neurol.* 2004;24:405–417.
127. Li YQ, Jay V, Wong CS. Oligodendrocytes in the adult rat spinal cord undergo radiation-induced apoptosis. *Cancer Res.* 1996; 56:5417–5422.
128. Olsen NK, Pfeiffer P, Mondrup K, et al. Radiation-induced brachial plexus neuropathy in breast cancer patients. *Acta Oncol.* 1990;29:885–890.
129. Galecki J, Hicer-Grzenkowicz J, Grudzien-Kowalska M, et al. Radiation-induced brachial plexopathy and hypofractionated regimens in adjuvant irradiation of patients with breast cancer—a review. *Acta Oncol.* 2006;45:280–284.
130. Gerard JM, Franck N, Moussa Z, Hildebrand J. Acute ischemic brachial plexus neuropathy following radiation therapy. *Neurology.* 1989;39:450–451.
131. Harper CM, Jr., Thomas JE, Cascino TL, et al. Distinction between neoplastic and radiation-induced brachial plexopathy, with emphasis on the role of EMG. *Neurology.* 1989;39:502–506.
132. Salner AL, Botnick LE, Herzog AG, et al. Reversible brachial plexopathy following primary radiation therapy for breast cancer. *Cancer Treat Rep.* 1981;65:797–802.
133. Fardin P, Lelli S, Negrin P, et al. Radiation-induced brachial plexopathy: clinical and electromyographical (EMG) considerations in 13 cases. *Electromyogr Clin Neurophysiol.* 1990;30:277–282.
134. Killer HE, Hess K. Natural history of radiation-induced brachial plexopathy compared with surgically treated patients. *J Neurol.* 1990;237:247–250.
135. Mondrup K, Olsen NK, Pfeiffer P, et al. Clinical and electrodiagnostic findings in breast cancer patients with radiation-induced brachial plexus neuropathy. *Acta Neurol Scand.* 1990;81:153–158.
136. Olsen NK, Pfeiffer P, Johannsen L, et al. Radiation-induced brachial plexopathy: neurological follow-up in 161 recurrence-free breast cancer patients. *Int J Radiat Oncol Biol Phys.* 1993;26: 43–49.
137. Zeidman SM, Rossitch EJ, Nashold BS Jr. Dorsal root entry zone lesions in the treatment of pain related to radiation-induced brachial plexopathy. *J Spinal Disord.* 1993;6:44–47.
138. Lederman RJ, Wilbourn AJ. Brachial plexopathy: recurrent cancer or radiation? *Neurology.* 1984;34:1331–1335.
139. Stryker JA, Sommerville K, Perez R, et al. Sacral plexus injury after radiotherapy for carcinoma of cervix. *Cancer.* 1990;66: 1488–1492.
140. Schiodt AV, Kristensen O. Neurologic complications after irradiation of malignant tumors of the testis. *Acta Radiol Oncol Radiat Phys Biol.* 1978;17:369–378.
141. Thomas JE, Cascino TL, Earle JD. Differential diagnosis between radiation and tumor plexopathy of the pelvis. *Neurology.* 1985; 35:1–7.
142. Qayyum A, MacVicar AD, Padhani AR, et al. Symptomatic brachial plexopathy following treatment for breast cancer: utility of MR imaging with surface-coil techniques. *Radiology.* 2000;214: 837–842.
143. Luthra K, Shah S, Purandare N, et al. F-18 FDG PET-CT appearance of metastatic brachial plexopathy in a case of carcinoma of the breast. *Clin Nucl Med.* 2006;31:432–434.
144. Wolf S, Barton D, Kottschade L, et al. Chemotherapy-induced peripheral neuropathy: prevention and treatment strategies. *Eur J Cancer.* 2008;44:1507–1515.
145. Postma TJ, Heimans JJ. Grading of chemotherapy-induced peripheral neuropathy. *Ann Oncol.* 2000;11:509–513.
146. Cersosimo RJ. Cisplatin neurotoxicity. *Cancer Treat Rev.* 1989;16:195–211.
147. Hol EM, Bar PR. Cisplatin neuropathy. *Neurology.* 1995;45:596; author reply 596-7.
148. Mollman JE, Glover DJ, Hogan WM, et al. Cisplatin neuropathy. Risk factors, prognosis, and protection by WR-2721. *Cancer.* 1988;61:2192–2195.
149. Cassidy J, Misset JL. Oxaliplatin-related side effects: characteristics and management. *Semin Oncol.* 2002;29:11–20.
150. Lee JJ, Swain SM. Peripheral neuropathy induced by microtubule-stabilizing agents. *J Clin Oncol.* 2006;24:1633–1642.
151. Kunitoh H, Saijo N, Furuse K, et al. Neuromuscular toxicities of paclitaxel 210 mg m(-2) by 3-hour infusion. *Br J Cancer.* 1998;77:1686–1688.
152. Loprinzi CL, Maddocks-Christianson K, Wolf SL, et al. The Paclitaxel acute pain syndrome: sensitization of nociceptors as the putative mechanism. *Cancer J.* 2007;13:399–403.
153. Chaudhry V, Cornblath DR, Polydefkis M, et al. Characteristics of bortezomib- and thalidomide-induced peripheral neuropathy. *J Peripher Nerv Syst.* 2008;13:275–282.
154. Badros A, Goloubeva O, Dalal JS, et al. Neurotoxicity of bortezomib therapy in multiple myeloma: a single-center experience and review of the literature. *Cancer.* 2007;110:1042–1049.
155. Frampton JE, Lee CR, Faulds D. Filgrastim. A review of its pharmacological properties and therapeutic efficacy in neutropenia. *Drugs.* 1994;48:731–760.
156. Crew KD, Greenlee H, Capodice J, et al. Prevalence of joint symptoms in postmenopausal women taking aromatase inhibitors for early-stage breast cancer. *J Clin Oncol.* 2007;25:3877–3883.
157. Laroche M, Borg S, Lassoued S, et al. Joint pain with aromatase inhibitors: abnormal frequency of Sjogren's syndrome. *J Rheumatol.* 2007;34:2259–2263.
158. Donnellan PP, Douglas SL, Cameron DA, et al. Aromatase inhibitors and arthralgia. *J Clin Oncol.* 2001;19:2767.
159. Claassen H, Hassenpflug J, Schunke M, et al. Immunohistochemical detection of estrogen receptor alpha in articular chondrocytes from cows, pigs and humans: in situ and in vitro results. *Ann Anat.* 2001;183:223–227.
160. Felson DT, Cummings SR. Aromatase inhibitors and the syndrome of arthralgias with estrogen deprivation. *Arthritis Rheum.* 2005;52:2594–2598.
161. Eckersell CB, Popper P, Micevych PE. Estrogen-induced alteration of mu-opioid receptor immunoreactivity in the medial preoptic nucleus and medial amygdala. *J Neurosci.* 1998;18:3967–3976.
162. Flores CA, Shughrue P, Petersen SL, et al. Sex-related differences in the distribution of opioid receptor-like 1 receptor mRNA and colocalization with estrogen receptor mRNA in neurons of the spinal trigeminal nucleus caudalis in the rat. *Neuroscience.* 2003;118: 769–778.
163. Morales L, Pans S, Verschueren K, et al. Prospective study to assess short-term intra-articular and tenosynovial changes in the aromatase inhibitor-associated arthralgia syndrome. *J Clin Oncol.* 2008;26:3147–3152.
164. Hershman DL. Getting a grip on aromatase inhibitor-associated arthralgias. *J Clin Oncol.* 2008;26:3120–3121.
165. Breuer J, Whitley R. Varicella zoster virus: natural history and current therapies of varicella and herpes zoster. *Herpes.* 2007;14 Suppl 2:25–29.
166. Rusthoven JJ, Ahlgren P, Elhakim T, et al. Varicella-zoster infection in adult cancer patients. A population study. *Arch Intern Med.* 1988;148:1561–1566.
167. Nagashima K, Nakazawa M, Endo H. Pathology of the human spinal ganglia in varicella-zoster virus infection. *Acta Neuropathol.* 1975;33:105–117.

168. Oaklander AL. The pathology of shingles: Head and Campbell's 1900 monograph. *Arch Neurol.* 1999;56:1292–1294.
169. Desmond RA, Weiss HL, Arani RB, et al. Clinical applications for change-point analysis of herpes zoster pain. *J Pain Symptom Manage.* 2002;23:510–516.
170. Jung BF, Johnson RW, Griffin DR, et al. Risk factors for postherpetic neuralgia in patients with herpes zoster. *Neurology.* 2004;62:1545–1551.
171. Dworkin RH, Portenoy RK. Pain and its persistence in herpes zoster. *Pain.* 1996;67:241–251.
172. Dubinsky RM, Kabbani H, El-Chami Z, et al. Practice parameter: treatment of postherpetic neuralgia: an evidence-based report of the Quality Standards Subcommittee of the American Academy of Neurology. *Neurology.* 2004;63:959–965.
173. Hyland JM, Butterworth J. Severe acute visceral pain from varicella zoster virus. *Anesth Analg.* 2003;97:1117–1118, table of contents.
174. Niscola P, Perrotti AP, del Poeta G, et al. Case reports: zoster pain in haematological malignancies: effective pain relief with oxycodone in patients unresponsive to other analgesic measures. *Herpes.* 2007;14:45–47.
175. Kleinschmidt-DeMasters BK, Gilden DH. Varicella-Zoster virus infections of the nervous system: clinical and pathologic correlates. *Arch Pathol Lab Med.* 2001;125:770–780.
176. Bilgrami S, Chakraborty NG, Rodriguez-Pinero F, et al. Varicella zoster virus infection associated with high-dose chemotherapy and autologous stem-cell rescue. *Bone Marrow Transplant.* 1999;23:469–474.
177. Offidani M, Corvatta L, Olivieri A, et al. A predictive model of varicella-zoster virus infection after autologous peripheral blood progenitor cell transplantation. *Clin Infect Dis.* 2001;32:1414–1422.
178. Volpi A, Gatti A, Pica F, et al. Clinical and psychosocial correlates of post-herpetic neuralgia. *J Med Virol.* 2008;80:1646–1652.
179. Harpaz R, Ortega-Sanchez IR, Seward JF. Prevention of herpes zoster: recommendations of the Advisory Committee on Immunization Practices (ACIP). *MMWR Recomm Rep.* 2008;57:1–30;quiz CE2-4.

CHAPTER 11 ■ METASTATIC EPIDURAL SPINAL CORD COMPRESSION

Spinal metastases can be classified according to anatomic location and are considered to be either intradural (intramedullary or extramedullary) or extradural (epidural). Extradural lesions account for up to 95% of spinal lesions and may be divided into pure epidural lesions and those originating from the vertebra and subsequently impinging on the thecal sac. Pure epidural lesions are relatively rare. Metastatic epidural spinal cord compression (MESCC) is, thus, caused by a tumor extrinsic to the dura that compresses the spinal cord or cauda equina nerve roots. After the lungs and liver, bone (including the spine) is the system most often involved by metastases. MESCC is the most common neurological complication of cancer after brain metastases. MESCC usually occurs in patients with disseminated disease but may present as an isolated finding in patients not diagnosed with cancer. The progression of nearly all types of malignancies can be complicated by the occurrence of spinal cord compression. Different incidence rates are reported with different tumor types, but both breast and lung cancer each account for 15% to 20% of cases of MESCC[1-2] and prostate cancer approximately 14%.[3] If left untreated, virtually 100% of patients will become paraplegic. Although most patients with MESCC have limited survival, up to one third will survive beyond 1 year.[4]

MECHANISM

Most epidural spinal cord compression comes from a solid tumor metastasis to the vertebral body, which spreads posteriorly to the epidural space (observed in 85% to 90% of cases), and presents as an osteolytic bony lesion in 70% of patients resulting in anterior compression of the spinal cord (Fig. 11.1). Other tumors such as lymphoma, paragangliomas, and neuroblastomas, which invade the epidural space through the intervertebral foramina, account for 10% to 15% of cases. The frequency of metastasis appears to correlate with the volume of bone in that region of the spine, which is presumably related to blood flow and blood-borne metastasis. As such, the thoracic spine is most likely to have a metastatic lesion, owing to its 12 vertebral bodies; the lumbosacral spine is the next most likely to have involvement, owing to the large size of the vertebral bodies; and the small cervical vertebral bodies are the least likely to be affected. The most significant damage caused by MESCC appears to be vascular in nature. The epidural tumor causes epidural venous plexus compression, which leads to spinal cord edema (Fig. 11.2). The increased vascular permeability and edema lead to increased pressure on the small arterioles. Capillary blood flow diminishes as the disease progresses, leading to white matter ischemia. Prolonged ischemia eventually results in infarction and permanent cord damage.[5-6] The early mechanism of injury is vasogenic edema of white matter with direct involvement of cytokines, inflammatory mediators, and neurotransmitters.[7] Production of vascular endothelial growth factor (VEGF) is associated with spinal-cord hypoxia and has been implicated as a potential mechanism of damage after spinal-cord injury.[8] The beneficial effects of dexamethasone in the central nervous system (CNS) are at least partly mediated by its downregulation of VEGF expression.[9] In the later stages of MESCC, vasogenic edema is replaced by ischemic-hypoxic neuronal injury and by onset of cytotoxic edema, a transition associated with the glutamate system that is characterized by release of presynaptic glutamate, influx of calcium through NMDA-linked ion channels, excitotoxic neuronal injury, and neuronal disintegration.[10] Noncompetitive NMDA antagonists have been shown to delay the onset of paraplegia after onset of MESCC[7] (Fig.11.3).

The segment of spine involved (approximately 10% cervical, 70% thoracic, 20% lumbosacral) reflects the number and volume of vertebral bodies in each anatomic segment.[11-13] MESCC at one site is often accompanied by spinal involvement elsewhere, particularly in the case of widely disseminated breast or prostate cancer or myeloma. Reported frequencies of second asymptomatic epidural metastases range from 8% to 37%. Multiple sites of metastatic epidural spinal cord compression occur in 17% to 30% of all patients.[14] This is particularly common in breast cancer and is uncommon in lung cancer.[12]

Severe, local back pain that gradually increases in intensity over time is the earliest and most common symptom (Fig 11.4). In general, pain occurs an average of 7 weeks before other neurological deficits. As the bone marrow does not contain pain receptors, discomfort usually occurs only when the enlarging mass invades the periosteum, paravertebral soft tissues, or nerves. Pain may also be caused by the mass effect of the spinal cord compression itself, spinal instability, pathological fracture, and the inflammatory and nociceptor stimulating substances that malignant cells secrete. Progressive pain practically always occurs in patients with MESCC. Weakness is the second most common symptom, which develops in approximately 80% of patients. As the thoracic cord is the most common site of epidural metastases, weakness usually involves the lower limbs, causing gait disorders. Gait difficulties may also be caused by sensory ataxia, presumably from posterior column compression.

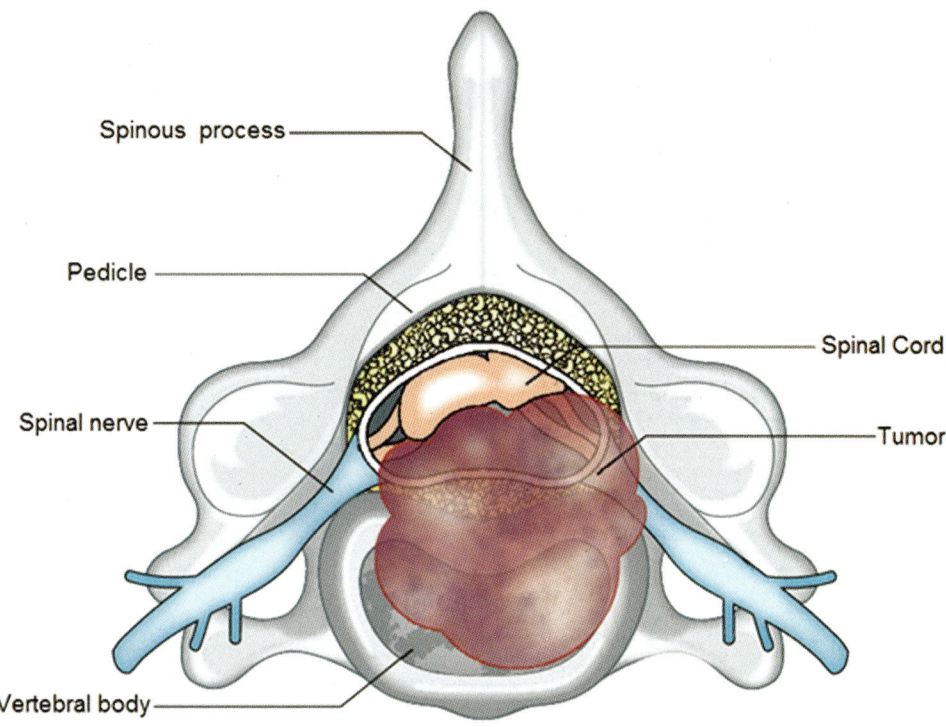

FIGURE 11.1 Tumor in the vertebral body. (From Cole JS and Patchell RA. Metastatic epidural spinal cord compression. *Lancet Neurol* 2008 7(5):459–466. Copyright 2008, with permission from Elsevier.)

Certain spinal tracts appear to be more vulnerable to compression than others.[15] The corticospinal tracts and posterior columns are particularly vulnerable, the spinothalamic tracts and descending autonomic fibers less so. As a result, weakness, spasticity, and reflex hyperactivity tend to be the earliest signs of spinal cord compression, with paresthesias and vibratory and position sense loss occurring soon thereafter. Loss of pain and temperature sensation and of bladder and bowel function usually occurs late in the course of spinal cord compression. The spinocerebellar pathways are also sensitive to compression, and at times ataxia may be the only sign of spinal cord compression.

PATTERN OF PAIN

Four patterns of pain have been associated with epidural metastases. The majority of patients have *local* pain over the involved vertebral body, which results from involvement of the vertebral periosteum, is dull and exacerbated by recumbency. The worsening of pain on recumbency is the most distinctive feature of the pain of epidural spinal cord compression. Many patients with cord compression find they must sleep in a sitting position. Even if pain is absent in the lying position, turning over in bed or rising from a lying position may be particularly painful.

Radicular pain from compressed or damaged nerve roots is usually unilateral in the cervical and lumbosacral regions and may be bilateral in the thorax, where patients often describe it as a tight band across the chest or abdomen. The pain is experienced in the overlying spine, deep in certain muscles supplied by the compressed root, and in the cutaneous distribution of the injured root. The pain is usually least severe when the patient is in a position that minimizes compression of the root and most severe in positions that compress or stretch the root. Pain

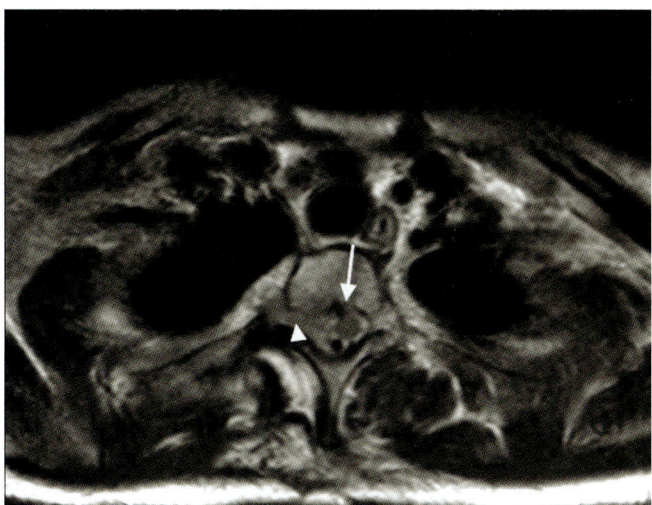

FIGURE 11.2 Axial T2 MRI image of thoracic spine in a 26-year-old woman with metastatic sarcoma. She presented with intractable back and upper extremity pain. Image shows abnormal epidural soft tissue within the right portion of the spinal canal *(arrow head)* extending from the lower C7 level to the upper T5 level. The dural sac is deviated to the left and compressed *(arrow)* without evidence of cord compression or cord signal abnormality. The patient's pain was completely relieved by surgical decompression. MRI, Magnetic resonance imaging.

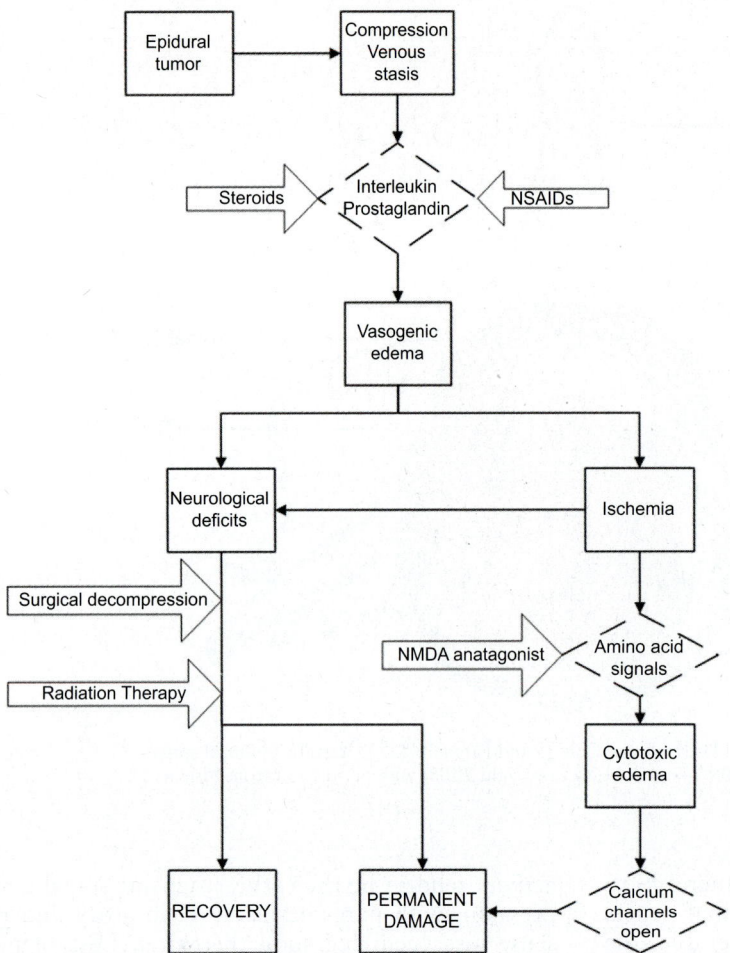

FIGURE 11.3 Pathophysiology of spinal cord compression. (Modified from Prasad D, Schiff D. Malignant spinal-cord compression. *Lancet Oncol.* 2005;6(1):15–24. Copyright 2005, with permission from Elsevier.)

is also increased by increasing intraspinal pressure, eg, coughing, sneezing, and straining. Radicular pain is present in 90% of patients with lumbosacral, 79% with cervical and 55% with thoracic metastatic spinal cord compression.[11]

Referred pain in the midscapular region or in both shoulders may accompany cervicothoracic epidural disease. Bilateral sacroiliac and iliac crest pain may occur with L1 vertebral compression. The pain has a deep aching quality and is often associated with tenderness of subcutaneous tissues and muscles at the site of referral. Maneuvers that affect local pain usually have the same effect on referred pain. When pain is referred from pathologic processes in the low back it is usually appreciated in the buttocks and posterior thighs. Pain from the upper lumbar spine is often referred to the flank, groin, and anterior thigh.

Funicular pain may be an early complaint in patients with cord compression and presumably results from compression of the ascending sensory tracts in the spinal cord. It usually occurs some distance below the site of compression and it has hot or cold qualities in a poorly localized nondermatomal distribution. The pain is less sharp than radicular pain but like root pain is usually exacerbated by movements that stretch the compressed structure (neck flexion, straight leg raising) or that increase intraspinal pressure (coughing, sneezing, straining).

PRESENTATION AND PHYSICAL FINDINGS

The vast majority of patients have a known cancer diagnosis. Even without a previous cancer diagnosis, MESCC should be suspected in anyone who presents with progressively worsening back pain, incontinence, or paraplegia, especially in the high-risk population such as long-time smokers or women with a strong family history of breast cancer. The clinical picture of metastatic epidural spinal cord compression is uniformly reported as various combinations of pain, weakness, sensory loss and autonomic dysfunction.[16-18] Table 11.1 summarizes the incidences of these features.

Although severe back pain is the initial symptom in greater than 80% of patients with epidural spinal cord compression, it may be the only neurologic symptom despite a complete or nearly complete block in 10% of patients.[19] The intensity of pain and the extent of neurological deficit depend upon the size of the epidural metastasis and its growth rate. Patients with small epidural lesions may have no pain and no neurological deficit.[20] After weeks of progressive pain, the patient may develop weakness, sensory loss, autonomic dysfunction, and reflex abnormalities. Weakness may be segmental owing to nerve root damage or regional in distribution if the spinal cord is injured. Once weakness is present, progression is

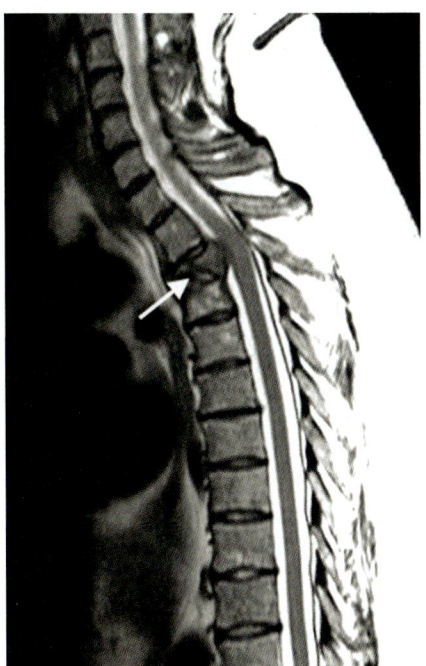
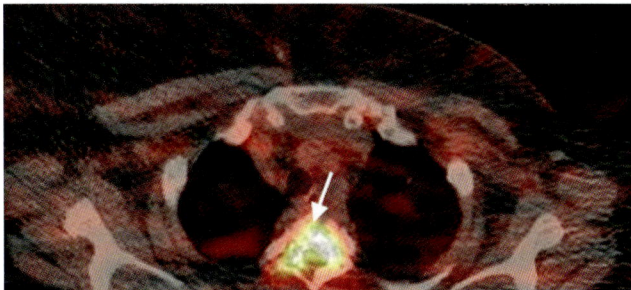

FIGURE 11.4 A 45-year-old woman with metastatic breast cancer. Presented complaining of severe upper back pain. Sagittal T2 MRI (A) shows pathologic fracture of the T2 vertebral body with loss of height and soft tissue epidural extension causing moderate dural compression *(arrow)*. Epidural soft tissue extends cranially to T1 and caudally to T3 involving bilateral T1/2 and T2/3 neural foramen bilaterally. Axial PET-CT (B) shows hypermetabolic activity at T2 vertebral level *(arrow)*. MRI, Magnetic resonance imaging; PET-CT, positron-emission tomography-computer tomography.

often rapid and urgent investigations with treatment are essential. Survival time is relatively short, especially in nonambulatory patients, and can only be improved by restoration of gait function in nonambulatory patients by immediate treatment.[21] Sensory abnormalities include ascending paresthesias, a sensory level, or complete loss of all sensory modalities below the dermatomal level in paraplegic patients. The upper level of sensory findings may correspond to the location of the epidural tumor or be below it by many segments. Bladder and bowel dysfunction is rarely a presenting symptom, but may appear after sensory symptoms have developed. The exception to this generalization occurs with compression of the conus medullaris, which can present as acute urinary retention and constipation without preceding motor or sensory symptoms.

Helweg-Larsen and Sorensen[22] reported on the frequency and the progression of symptoms in 153 patients with metastatic spinal cord compression. At the time of diagnosis, 88% of patients complained of low back pain. Radicular pain was more frequent in tumors localized in the lumbosacral area (91%) than in tumors localized in the thoracic region (69%), whereas the severity of paresis was more pronounced in patients with metastases in the thoracic region. Reflex abnormalities from spinal cord involvement include loss of superficial cutaneous reflexes, increase in deep cutaneous and deep tendon reflexes at or below the level of compression, and extensor plantar responses. Asymmetric flaccid motor weakness and sensory loss, with absent lower limb reflexes, characterize cauda equina compression. Conus medullaris lesions typically cause a rapidly progressive symmetric perineal pain followed by early autonomic dysfunction, saddle sensory loss, and motor weakness. Limited straight leg raising usually points to an epidural or intradural extramedullary lesion causing root compression, whereas segmental pain and sacral sparing suggests intramedullary disease (Table 11.2).

Ataxia without pain has been the presenting complaint in about 1% of patients with epidural compression of the spinal cord. In patients with back pain and a normal neurological examination, the presence of greater-than-50%

TABLE 11.1

CLINICAL PRESENTATION OF MALIGNANT EPIDURAL SPINAL CORD COMPRESSION

Number of Patients	Pain, %	Weakness, %	Sensory Deficit, %	Autonomic Dysfunction, %
398	83	67	90	48
153	88	61	78	40
130	96	76	51	57
79	70	91	46	44
77	94	85	57	52

(From Prasad D, Schiff D. Malignant spinal-cord compression. *Lancet Oncol.* 2005;6(1):15–24. Copyright 2005, with permission from Elsevier.)

TABLE 11.2			
SIGNS OF ACUTE SPINAL COMPRESSION			
SIGN/DEFICIT	SPINAL CORD	CONUS MEDULLARIS	CAUDA EQUINA
Limb weakness	Symmetrical, profound	Lower extremity—symmetrical, variable	Lower extremity only—less profound
Deep tendon reflexes	Absent	Absent	Present
Plantar response	Absent	Absent	Plantar
Sensory	Symmetric sensory level	Saddle area only	Asymmetric, radicular
Sphincters	Flaccid	Flaccid	Variable (root dependent)
Progression	Rapid	Rapid	Variable

collapse of the vertebral body on plain radiographs is associated with an 86% chance of epidural spinal cord compression.[20] Back pain in patients with normal radiographs requires further work-up, including bone scan and magnetic resonance imaging (MRI) scan.

The diagnosis of epidural spinal cord compression is all too often delayed 1 week or more,[23] even after the onset of other neurological symptoms. Ventafridda et al.[24] reported an association between Lhermitte sign (shocking sensation radiating from the back of the head down the spine and into the extremities as the neck is bent forward) and epidural spinal cord compression. In their series, the sign appeared at an early stage of compression, particularly with thoracic lesions but may also be seen with cervical MESCC. Lhermitte sign, however, lacks specificity and also occurs in patients with radiation myelopathy,[25] following cisplatin chemotherapy,[26] and in noncancer-related problems such as multiple sclerosis[27] and subacute combined degeneration of the cord.[28] Differential diagnosis for a patient with back pain includes intramedullary metastases, herniated disks, epidural hematoma or abscess, transverse myelopathy, and subluxation of the spine from pathological fractures.

INVESTIGATIONS

Bone scan is the most effective screening procedure of vertebral involvement, and MRI effectively shows epidural involvement. Currently, MRI is the most sensitive diagnostic tool. Diagnosis is on an emergency basis, because, once neurological signs develop, they usually progress rapidly. When definitive imaging of the epidural space is required, the best approach is MRI. MRI is noninvasive, effectively demonstrates metastatic epidural spinal cord compression, and gives a positive image of the spinal cord to better diagnose intramedullary disease. Sagittal MRI is superior to myelography in demonstrating multiple epidural metastases, which occur in 25% to 40% of cases (70% of these involving more than region of the spine).[29] Fluorodeoxyglucose (FDG) positron-emission tomography (PET-CT) provides better specificity for detection of malignant involvement of the spine than does FDG PET, allowing for precise localization of lesions and identifies accompanying soft-tissue involvement, which is of potential neurologic significance.[30] Patients with suspected malignant spinal cord compression may present with a misleading sensory level or have multiple levels of compression that are not apparent clinically or on imaging of a limited area of the spine. Cook et al.[31] recommend MRI imaging of the whole spine in cases of suspected MESCC. In 85 of 127 scans, there was evidence of compression or impingement upon the spinal cord. A sensory level was present in 47 of these 85 patients, but in 12 of the 47 patients (26%) the sensory level was four or more segments below or three or more segments above the actual lesion. Multiple levels of compression or impingement were found in 33 of the 85 (39%) patients; in 24 of these, more than one region (cervical/thoracic/lumbar) of the cord was involved.

PROGNOSIS

Metastatic spinal cord compression is a severely disabling complication of malignant disease and mandates prompt intervention.[32] Effective therapy is necessary to maintain functional integrity for the remainder of the patient's life. The two most potent factors affecting survival are the nature of the primary tumor, and the degree of the neurological deficit. Thus, patients with breast carcinoma have the longest survival, patients with lung cancer have the shortest survival, and patients with prostatic carcinoma have an intermediate expected length of survival. The mean survival time from the diagnosis of MESCC is 14 months in breast cancer (range: 0.6 to 49 months), 12 months in prostate cancer (range: 0.2 to 61 months), 6 months (range: 3 weeks to 7 months) in malignant melanoma, and 3 months (range: 0 to 18 months) in lung cancer.[33–34] Overall median survival time in patients with epidural compression is approximately 7 months, with a 36% probability of 1-year survival. Prasad and Schiff[10] reported that median survival in patients undergoing radiation therapy for MESCC varies between 3 months and 6 months according to historical series with survival being higher in patients who are ambulatory either before or after radiation. Survival is also related to the systemic spread of the neoplastic disease. The presence of multiple spinal epidural metastases (around 25% to 40% of patients) has been reported as an independent prognostic factor for poorer survival.[29] The nature of the primary tumor and neurological status are important factors determining outcome of treatment.[32] Once a neurological deficit appears, most patients do not recover. However, the majority of patients with Hodgkin and non-Hodgkin lymphoma became ambulatory after radiation/chemotherapy, even if paretic at presentation.[35]

References

1. Nelson KA, Walsh D, Abdullah O, et al. Common complications of advanced cancer. *Semin Oncol.* 2000;27:34–44.
2. Quinn JA, DeAngelis LM. Neurologic emergencies in the cancer patient. *Semin Oncol.* 2000;27:311–321.
3. Mut M, Schiff D, Shaffrey ME. Metastasis to nervous system: Spinal epidural and intramedullary metastases. *J Neurooncol.* 2005;75:43–56.
4. Maranzano E, Latini P, Checcaglini F, et al. Radiation therapy in metastatic spinal cord compression. A prospective analysis of 105 consecutive patients. *Cancer.* 1991;67:1311–1317.
5. Ikeda H, Ushio Y, Hayakawa T, et al. Edema and circulatory disturbance in the spinal cord compressed by epidural neoplasms in rabbits. *J Neurosurg.* 1980;52:203–209.
6. Kato A, Ushio Y, Hayakawa T, et al. Circulatory disturbance of the spinal cord with epidural neoplasm in rats. *J Neurosurg.* 1985;63:260–265.
7. Siegal T. Spinal cord compression: From laboratory to clinic. *Eur J Cancer.* 1995;31A:1748-1753.
8. Benton RL, Whittemore SR. VEGF165 therapy exacerbates secondary damage following spinal cord injury. *Neurochem Res.* 2003;28:1693–1703.
9. Heiss JD, Papavassiliou E, Merrill MJ, et al. Mechanism of dexamethasone suppression of brain tumor-associated vascular permeability in rats. Involvement of the glucocorticoid receptor and vascular permeability factor. *J Clin Invest.* 1996;98:1400–1408.
10. Prasad D, Schiff D. Malignant spinal-cord compression. *Lancet Oncol.* 2005;6:15–24.
11. Gilbert RW, Kim JH, Posner JB. Epidural spinal cord compression from metastatic tumor: Diagnosis and treatment. *Ann Neurol.* 1978;3:40–51.
12. Stark RJ, Henson RA, Evans SJ. Spinal metastases. A retrospective survey from a general hospital. *Brain.* 1982;105:189–213.
13. Torma T. Malignant tumors of the spine and the spinal epidural space. *Acta Clin Scand.* 1957;225:1.
14. van der Sande JJ, Kroger R, Boogerd W. Multiple spinal epidural metastases;an unexpectedly frequent finding. *J Neurol Neurosurg Psychiatry.* 1990;53:1001–1003.
15. Tarlov IM. Acute spinal cord compression paralysis. *J Neurosurg.* 1972;36:10–20.
16. Bach F, Larsen BH, Rohde K, et al. Metastatic spinal cord compression. Occurrence, symptoms, clinical presentations and prognosis in 398 patients with spinal cord compression. *Acta Neurochir (Wien).* 1990;107:37–43.
17. Barron KD, Hirano A, Araki S, et al. Experiences with metastatic neoplasms involving the spinal cord. *Neurology.* 1959;9:91–106.
18. Constans JP, de Divitiis E, Donzelli R, et al. Spinal metastases with neurological manifestations. Review of 600 cases. *J Neurosurg.* 1983;59:111–8.
19. Greenberg HS, Deck MD, Vikram B, et al. Metastasis to the base of the skull: Clinical findings in 43 patients. *Neurology.* 1981;31:530–537.
20. Portenoy RK, Galer BS, Salamon O, et al. Identification of epidural neoplasm. Radiography and bone scintigraphy in the symptomatic and asymptomatic spine. *Cancer.* 1989;64:2207–2213.
21. Helweg-Larsen S, Sorensen PS, Kreiner S. Prognostic factors in metastatic spinal cord compression: A prospective study using multivariate analysis of variables influencing survival and gait function in 153 patients. *Int J Radiat Oncol Biol Phys.* 2000;46:1163–1169.
22. Helweg-Larsen S, Sorensen PS. Symptoms and signs in metastatic spinal cord compression: A study of progression from first symptom until diagnosis in 153 patients. *Eur J Cancer.* 1994;30A:396-398.
23. Shaw MD, Rose JE, Paterson A. Metastatic extradural malignancy of the spine. *Acta Neurochir (Wien).* 1980;52:113–120.
24. Ventafridda V, Caraceni A, Martini C, et al. On the significance of Lhermitte's sign in oncology. *J Neurooncol.* 1991;10:133–137.
25. Jones A. Transient radiation myelopathy (with reference to Lhermitte's sign of electrical paraesthesia). *Br J Radiol.* 1964;37:727–744.
26. Eeles R, Tait DM, Peckham MJ. Lhermitte's sign as a complication of cisplatin-containing chemotherapy for testicular cancer. *Cancer Treat Rep.* 1986;70:905–907.
27. Kanchandani R, Howe JG. Lhermitte's sign in multiple sclerosis: A clinical survey and review of the literature. *J Neurol Neurosurg Psychiatry.* 1982;45:308–312.
28. Gautier-Smith PC. Lhermitte's sign in subacute combined degeneration of the cord. *J Neurol Neurosurg Psychiatry.* 1973;36:861–863.
29. Schiff D, O'Neill BP, Wang CH, et al. Neuroimaging and treatment implications of patients with multiple epidural spinal metastases. *Cancer.* 1998;83:1593–1601.
30. Metser U, Lerman H, Blank A, et al. Malignant involvement of the spine: Assessment by 18F-FDG PET/CT. *J Nucl Med.* 2004;45:279–284.
31. Cook AM, Lau TN, Tomlinson MJ, et al. Magnetic resonance imaging of the whole spine in suspected malignant spinal cord compression: Impact on management. *Clin Oncol (R Coll Radiol).* 1998;10:39–43.
32. Solberg A, Bremnes RM. Metastatic spinal cord compression: Diagnostic delay, treatment, and outcome. *Anticancer Res.* 1999;19:677–684.
33. Donaldson WFd, Peppelman WC, Jr., Yaw KM. Symptomatic metastatic malignant melanoma to the spine. *J Spinal Disord.* 1993;6:360–363.
34. Grant R, Papadopoulos SM, Greenberg HS. Metastatic epidural spinal cord compression. *Neurol Clin.* 1991;9:825–841.
35. Turner S, Marosszeky B, Timms I, et al. Malignant spinal cord compression: A prospective evaluation. *Int J Radiat Oncol Biol Phys.* 1993;26:141–146.

CHAPTER 12 ■ SYSTEMATIC PAIN ASSESSMENT

A comprehensive and rational strategy for cancer pain assessment begins with data collection and terminates with a correct and clinically relevant diagnosis. This outcome requires a thorough evaluation of the multiple factors that contribute to the complaint of pain. Certainly, this evaluation involves discovery of the etiology of the pain and predicting its future evolution. Each of the sites from which pain originates may have a different mechanism and prognosis and treatment strategy. Pain is likely to affect sleep, functional capability, activity level, and psychological well-being; all must be considered. Another key factor is the impact of the cancer itself on the patient. A comprehensive evaluation will allow the clinician to evaluate possible therapeutic interventions and establish long-term goals with the collaboration of the patient and the patient's family.

Table 12.1 describes the goals of a comprehensive pain-related history. Such goals must be specified and the pain syndrome and its underlying mechanisms evaluated in a comprehensive assessment.

COMPONENTS OF PAIN HISTORY

Table 12.2 itemizes the essential components of the assessment of the pain complaint in a patient with cancer.

Location

Multiple pains at different sites characterize many patients with advanced disease. This is particularly true in patients with breast, lung, and prostate cancer, compared with those harboring gastrointestinal cancers.[1] A tumor usually produces pain in the region in which it is growing. Somatic pain from bone metastases is usually well localized. However, a tumor involving viscera tends to produce diffuse pain and is often referred to remote regions, based upon the embryologic developmental patterns. Neuropathic pain is typically in the sensory distribution of a nerve or nerve root. For example, prostate cancer may initially present with localized pelvic pain, because of localized tumor growth within the prostate or adjacent organs such as the bladder. With tumor progression, infiltration of the adjacent lumbosacral plexus can produce radicular lower extremity symptoms suggestive of neuropathic pain. Remote metastasis to bone can produce localized somatic pain. The location of pain is obviously the first step in its characterization and often determines subsequent diagnostic investigations.

Intensity

The published guidelines promulgated by the Agency for Health Care Policy and Research,[2] the American Pain Society,[3] and the American Society of Anesthesiologists[4] all have advocated the routine use of pain rating scales. Rating scales are particularly important when initiating therapy for pain or when changing treatment regimens. All of these guidelines suggest that clinicians teach patients and families to use assessment tools at home so that consistency of pain management can be established and maintained. Standard pain intensity assessment tools for determining the intensity of pain are discussed in Chapter 6, "Characteristics of Cancer Pain."

Quality

The descriptors utilized by patients can be helpful in identifying the origin of the pain. Cancer can be nociceptive (somatic or visceral structures) or neuropathic. Patients tend to describe pain that is neuropathic in origin as burning, shock-like, or shooting in quality, whereas they often describe pain originating from somatic structures as aching, nagging, throbbing, or sharp. Pain qualities are the cornerstone of the McGill Pain Questionnaire and often permit diagnosis by themselves.

TABLE 12.1

USES OF THE PATIENT'S HISTORY

Define extent of disease
Characterize the pain(s)
Assess impact of pain on functional capacities
Determine previous treatments and their efficacy
Delineate associated symptoms

TABLE 12.2

ASPECTS OF PAIN COMPLAINT

Onset
Location
Duration
Character
Aggravating factors
Relieving factors
Temporal
Severity (intensity)

Timing and Duration

Pain intensity may fluctuate with time of day or activities. The first criterion is whether the pain is constant or intermittent. Constant pain is present continuously but usually varies in intensity. Intermittent pain implies that pain is present for definite periods of time and absent between episodes. One type of intermittent pain is *breakthrough pain*: a sudden and brief flare of pain associated with activity or change of position occurring in a patient who has chronic pain and is receiving opioids. It is essential that patients and their caregivers understand the concept of breakthrough pain and its management. Breakthrough pain is discussed in Chapter 6, "Patterns of Cancer Pain."

Acute and chronic pains have traditionally been distinguished solely by the duration of the complaint. This distinction may have some validity for short-term complaints but does not take into account the multidimensional nature of chronic pain. Von Korff and Dunn[5] compared duration-based and prospective approaches to defining chronic pain in terms of their ability to predict future pain course and outcomes for primary care patients with chronic pain and determined that long-term pain outcomes were highly variable and uncertain, with less dependence on pain duration alone. Chronic pain always leads to changes in the nervous system that may not be present in acute pain; this, rather than duration alone, is probably the discriminating factor that separates acute from chronic pain.

Modulating Factors

Knowledge of the issues that make pain worse or better helps clinicians to design an appropriate pain treatment plan. Activities, position changes, or eating, for example, may produce pain increases in a wide array of cancers. Patients with metastatic disease to weight-bearing bones may report more pain when they stand or sit. Breast cancer metastatic to the axillary nodes may produce severe pain with abduction of the upper extremity during positioning for external beam radiation therapy. Recognition of such positional and activity-related changes in pain levels is required for the implementation of optimal pain management.

Responses to Previous Analgesic and Disease-Modifying Therapies

Past history and, in particular, past exposure to medications must be ascertained. Understanding of previous opioid use and its benefits or side effects is essential for treatment planning. Side effects with a particular opioid may limit successful future titration with the same opioid. This is also true for other medications commonly used for pain and symptom management. A positive response to chemotherapy or radiation therapy with decrease in tumor bulk may alleviate pain. The recurrence of pain at a later date mandates reevaluation for the possibility of tumor recurrence.

Pain Impact

Information about changes in activities of daily living, such as work and recreational activities, mood, appetite, mobility, sleep patterns, and sexual functioning, must be part of pain assessment. Symptom checklists and quality of life measures are useful in this evaluation. A discussion of some of the instruments we routinely use for the assessment of pain impact and other variables follows.

Pain intensity, pain relief, and mood are assessed by the Memorial Pain Assessment Card (MPAC), a brief, validated measure that uses visual analog scale (VAS) scores. It also contains a mood scale that has been correlated with other measures of global psychological distress, depression, and anxiety. It is considered to be a very useful but brief measure of global symptom distress. The MPAC does not provide detailed descriptors of pain, but its brevity and simplicity facilitate the collection of essential data while minimizing patient burden. Compliance is definitely enhanced when the assessment tool is less cumbersome.

The Brief Pain Inventory (BPI) measures both the pain intensity (sensory dimension) and pain interference in the life of the patient (reactive dimension). Pain relief, pain quality, and patient perception of the cause of pain are also assessed. Pain *in general, at its worst, at its least,* and *right now* are determined via numerical scales. A pain diagram is used to localize the regions of pain. Interference with daily functions, mood, and enjoyment of life are also quantified. This questionnaire is self-administered, easy to understand, and available in many languages. The BPI has been validated in many languages, including Chinese, Filipino, French, Hindi, Italian, Spanish, Greek, Turkish, and Vietnamese, and has been shown to produce similar data from patients in these countries and from many different cultures. BPI has several applications, including studies of the epidemiology of cancer pain, the routine clinical assessment of pain, efforts to assure the quality of pain management, and the conduct of clinical trials examining the effectiveness of cancer pain treatments.

Pain and the Activities of Daily Living

Mild pain may not impair function or distract some patients.[6] However, as severity of pain increases, a threshold may be crossed; the pain can no longer be ignored. Now the pain disrupts the patient's life. Constant, daily pain usually adversely impacts activities of daily living. As pain increases over time, restriction in activity occurs and depression is likely to ensue.[7] We strongly believe that indicators of physical, psychological, and social functional status must be included in the comprehensive assessment of functioning. These include interference with general activities, mood, walking, ability to work, relations with others, and sleep. A reliable, valid and brief measure of pain-related disability, The Pain Disability Index (PDI), was developed as a self-report measure of general and domain-specific, pain-related disability[8] (Appendix A).

Many factors in addition to pain intensity play a role in disability.[9] Pain site, patient age, how much of the time pain is experienced, use of pain medication, and the number of pain locations have all been found to be associated with disability.[10] The Pain Disability Questionnaire (PDQ) is designed to evaluate chronic disabling musculoskeletal disorders (Appendix L). Patients are scored on total functional disability from 0 (optimal function) to 150 (total disability). The focus, like other health inventories, is primarily on disability and activities of daily living. However, unlike most other measures, this instrument is designed for the full array of chronic disabling painful musculoskeletal disorders, including upper extremity and lower extremity disorders, rather than just low back pain, or spinal disorders. In addition, psychosocial variables also form a core in the PDQ. Gatchel et al.[11] reported on the validity of the PDQ in patients with chronic disabling musculoskeletal disorders.

Maltoni et al.[12] identified selected clinical parameters as prognostic indicators for terminal cancer patients, including clinical experiences, physical capabilities, and clinical symptoms both relating to and unrelated to nutritional state. We believe that Performance Status Tables are useful adjuncts to the assessment of physical activity levels (see Table 8.3 and Table 12.3). It must be recognized, however, that the palliative treatment of advanced cancer and the terminally ill is based upon a concept of well-being that extends beyond physical functioning alone.[13]

Psychological State

Assessment of the cancer patient must reflect awareness of the many relevant psychological factors. Distress in the cancer patient is modulated by psychological factors such as personality, coping skills, past experiences, and environmental interactions. Knowing that the patient has received outpatient or inpatient psychiatric care in the past helps to clarify psychological risks. Information on how the patient handled previous stressful or painful events may provide insight into whether the patient is likely to manifest chronic illness behaviors. Past experiences as well as anticipated consequences influence the present psychological state and must be considered in formulating a diagnosis and plan for management.

Familial and Professional Function

The prudent clinician wants to learn about the patient's familial and social resources, financial situation, as well as his or her physical environment. Insights into the responses to previous physical illness or the genesis of psychological symptoms may be gleaned from knowledge of the patient's and family's previous experience with cancer or other diseases. The influence of social factors on treatment preferences and desire for aggressive cancer therapy is still poorly defined. Patient willingness to accept aggressive treatment has been reported to be based upon positive social well-being, as well as upon having children living at home.[14] Patient preferences for alternative and complementary medical therapies are also an important factor to consider when evaluating treatment options.

QUALITY OF LIFE (QOL) ASSESSMENT

Cancer patients may suffer from a number of psychosocial problems related to disease progression as well as to standard medical interventions. Two essential features are prolongation of survival and maintenance or improvement of health-related QoL. In an end-of-life care setting, patients reported that receiving adequate pain and symptom management, avoiding inappropriate prolongation of dying, achieving a sense of control, relieving burden, and strengthening relationships with loved ones were focal points of care.[15] The use of health-related QoL assessments in daily clinical practice may aid detection of physical or psychosocial problems that might be overlooked, monitor disease and treatment, and improve delivery of care.[16-17] Velikova et al.[18] noted that measuring quality of life in routine oncology practices improved communication and patient well-being. The severity of symptoms and the potential toxicities of treatments make QoL a major area of concern when treating cancer patients, particularly the elderly. QoL has been defined as the person's evaluation of his or her well-being and functioning in different life domains. It is a subjective, phenomenological, multidimensional, dynamic, evaluative, and yet quantifiable, construct. For complete assessment of the benefits of an intervention it is essential to provide evidence of the impact on the patient in terms of health status and health-related quality of life (HRQoL). These terms refer

TABLE 12.3

EASTERN COOPERATIVE ONCOLOGY GROUP

	Performance Status
Grade	Performance Level
0	Fully active, able to carry on all predisease performance without restriction
1	Restricted in physically strenuous activity but ambulatory and able to carry out work of a light or sedentary nature (eg, light house work, office work)
2	Ambulatory and capable of all self-care but unable to carry out any work activities. Up and about more than 50% of waking hours
3	Capable of only limited self-care, confined to bed or chair more than 50% of waking hours
4	Completely disabled. Cannot carry on any self-care. Totally confined to bed or chair
5	Dead

(From Oken M, Creech R, Tormey D, et al. Toxicity and Response Criteria of the Eastern Cooperative Oncology Group. *Am J Clin Oncol*. 1982;5:649–655. Eastern Cooperative Oncology Group. Robert Comis, MD, Group Chair.)

to experiences of illness such as pain, fatigue, and disability as well as broader aspects of the individual's physical, emotional, and social well-being. The application of patient assessed measures of health outcome is important to the evaluation of health care. Types of measures used for this purpose have included generic, disease- or population-specific, dimension-specific, and utility measures (developed for economic evaluation and incorporate preferences for health states).[19]

The routine assessment of QoL facilitates patient care by fostering patient-provider communication, identifying frequently overlooked problems, prioritizing problems, and evaluating the impact of palliative and rehabilitative efforts. QoL is sensitive to the treatment of pain and treatment modalities. Significant pain is not synonymous with poor QoL, as it is only one of the important factors that affect QoL. Pain reduction is not necessarily accompanied by improvement in QoL. Among the commonly used assessment tools in oncology are the European Organization for Research and Treatment of Cancer (EORTC) Quality of Life Questionnaire Core 30 Items (QLQ-C30) scale and the Functional Assessment of Cancer Therapy–General (FACT-G).[20] QLQ-C30 is a 30-item measure developed to assess multiple dimensions of quality of life in patients with cancer. In addition to assessing 6 domains of quality of life, the QLQ-C30 assesses seven symptom domains, including pain. FACT-G is self-reported, uses a five-point Likert-type scale, and includes questions on physical, functional, emotional, and social/family well-being (Appendix B). We use the FACT-G questionnaire routinely during our outpatient visits.

GENERAL ASSESSMENT

A complete medical history that reviews the cancer diagnosis, the chronology of significant cancer-related events, previous therapies, and all relevant medical, surgical, and psychiatric problems is the initial step in the assessment of a symptomatic cancer patient (Table 12.4). Medication assessment should include current and previous use of prescription and nonprescription drugs, drug allergies, and previous adverse drug reactions and side effects. Information is required for the treatment of each symptom. The interviewer must document the patient's understanding of his or her current disease status so that other providers will be able to effectively interact with the patient and the family. Other providers involved with the patient's care can help determine disease status and they must be consulted. Table 12.5 lists the different possible categories for a patient's clinical status. This table represents what the known current disease status of the patient is (known disease or disease is unknown) and correlates this with the predicted treatment course (active treatment, palliative care, surveillance for progression or recurrence). By doing this, the clinician can make decisions on pain management based on predicted course of disease or treatment.

The initial pain assessment must include a thorough physical examination, with particular emphasis on neurologic status. Previously performed laboratory and imaging studies must be reviewed, because they can provide information about the causes of pain and the extent of the underlying disease. The selection of additional tests and imaging studies is also based upon what has already been undertaken, although additional investigations are often needed to clarify uncertainties in the provisional assessment. The extent of these investigations must be appropriate to the patient's general status and the overall goals of care (Fig. 12.1).

All of the patient's symptoms and associated psychosocial issues need to be incorporated in the initial diagnosis and management plan. Our experience has taught us that the initial assessment is a major determinant of the success of the patient's management plan. We cannot overemphasize how important it is that all relevant issues be considered.

ASSOCIATED SYMPTOMS

The degree to which each symptom induces or exacerbates other physical or psychological symptoms should be quantified, because there may be significant interaction among symptoms. It is important to ascertain whether the patient's symptoms are concurrent but of unrelated etiology, concurrent and related to one underlying disease,

TABLE 12.4

COMPONENTS OF MEDICAL HISTORY: CANCER HISTORY, MEDICATIONS, PAST MEDICAL HISTORY, AND PSYCHOSOCIAL FACTORS

Cancer History	Current Medications and Past History	Psychosocial and Family History
Tumor diagnosis	Past medical and surgical issues	Family history (disease/addiction)
Chronology of disease including recurrences	Concurrent medical conditions	Social resources and financial constraints
Therapeutic interventions including surgeries, chemotherapy, radiation treatments	Drug reactions and responses	Impact of disease and symptoms on patient and family
Explore patient's knowledge of extent of disease	Other pain treatment responses	Patient's and family's goals of care
Determine clinical status (see Table 12.6)		Personal history of addiction

TABLE 12.5
AUTHORS' CLASSIFICATION OF CLINICAL STATUS

Category	Characteristics of Disease and Treatment
I	Active disease; care is palliative and supportive only
II	Active disease; treatment (eg, chemotherapy, radiation therapy) in progress
III	Active disease, no current treatment, surveillance of tumor status
IV	No active disease; treatment of tumor in progress
V	No active disease; no current treatment, surveillance of tumor status
VI	No active disease; no current treatment, specialized care (eg, medical oncology) not required

concurrent with the one symptom directly, or an indirect consequence of a pathologic process that has initiated another symptom, or concurrent with one symptom appearing as a consequence or side effect of therapy directed against the other. Progression of the cancer increases the number of factors that can diminish quality of life and add to the prevalence and severity of physical and psychological symptoms. In addition to pain, patients with advanced cancer often have fatigue, generalized weakness, dyspnea, delirium, nausea, and vomiting. The most prevalent symptom reported by cancer patients is fatigue.[21] Multiple symptoms have a major impact on both pain reporting and the quality of life.

The Memorial Symptom Assessment Scale (MSAS) is a self-assessment tool that provides multidimensional information relevant to the common symptoms reported by cancer patients. The MSAS is a reliable and valid instrument for the assessment of symptom prevalence, characteristics, and magnitude of distress. Comprehensive symptom assessment is useful in clinical trials and studies that incorporate quality of life measures or symptom epidemiology.[22] Portenoy et al.[23] studied using the MSAS and other measures of psychological condition, performance status, symptom distress, and overall quality of life with prostate, colon, breast, or ovarian cancer patients. In 50% of these patients, the Karnofsky Performance Status (KPS) score was 80 or below. In the population he studied, 40% to 80% experienced lack of energy, pain, feeling drowsy, dry mouth, insomnia, or other symptoms suggesting psychological distress. The mean (SD; range) number of symptoms per patient was 11.5 (6.0; 0-25).

LABORATORY AND IMAGING DATA

Previous laboratory and imaging studies can provide important additional information and deserve careful review by the clinician. Additional radiologic or laboratory tests can be ordered to clarify ambiguities that remain after the history, physical examination, and review of previous studies. This information can provide the basis for a provisional pain diagnosis that clarifies both the status of the underlying disease and the nature of other concurrent concerns that may require treatment.

Multiple studies that clarify extent of disease, assess the pain problem, or evaluate other symptoms may be needed in some patients. Other members of the health care team can provide assistance that is required to evaluate related physical or psychosocial problems that have been identified during the initial assessment. When the diagnostic evaluation is completed, it is essential to discuss the findings with the patient, family and other essential parties so that all can participate in the health care decisions that must now be made. Eventual outcomes that would benefit from contingency planning, including the need for advanced medical directives, the evaluation of home care resources, and prebereavement interventions with the family should be discussed at this time.

PHYSICAL EXAMINATION

The initial pain assessment must include a physical examination, particularly focusing on a neurologic and musculoskeletal examination. The physical examination should clarify the underlying causes of the pain problem, detail the extent of the underlying disease, and discern the relation of the pain complaint to the disease. The need for a thorough neurologic assessment is justified by the high prevalence of painful neurologic conditions in the cancer population.[24] Before a directed examination, the patient's posture while seated and sitting tolerance should be noted. Neurologic examination in suspected neuropathic pain should include quantification and mapping of motor, sensory, and autonomic phenomena in order to identify all signs of neurologic dysfunction. With experience, the territory of each sensory deficit or pain can be mapped separately to reflect different areas of impairment. Tactile sense may be assessed by a piece of cotton wool, pinprick sense by a wooden cocktail-stick, thermal sense by warm and cold objects, and vibration sense by a 128-Hz tuning fork. The intensity, quality, and spatial–temporal aspects of the evoked sensations should be noted, as there may be aberrations in all of them. Often, the diagnosis of

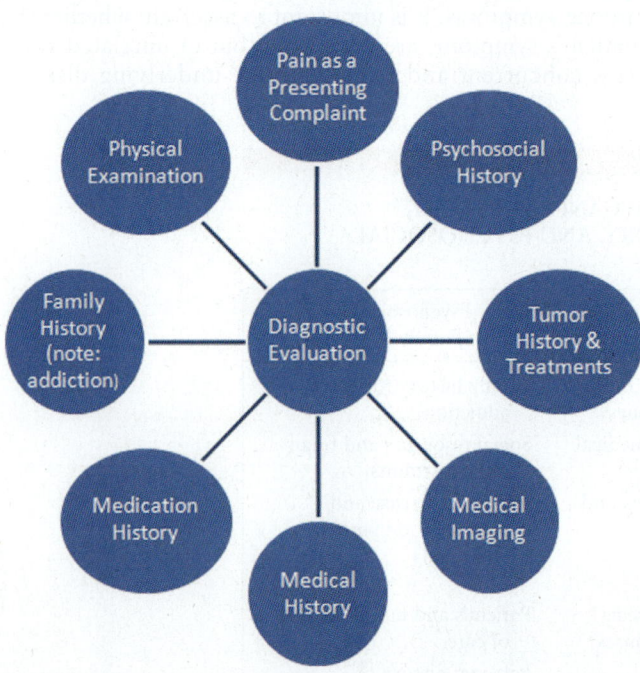

FIGURE 12.1 Components of diagnosis in cancer patients.

radicular and pseudoradicular low back pain in patients complaining of back and/or lower extremity pain can be difficult. Efforts should be made to identify and fine-tune clinical tests that specifically try to evoke nerve-root tension signs or dural irritation, through combinations of manipulations. Cervical flexion by itself provokes a displacement of lumbar roots[25] and an additional flexion of the hip increases this effect.[26] Van Boxem et al.[27] proposed a triad of clinical tests to facilitate this process: active flexion in standing position with a passive cervical flexion, a straight-leg raising test with a passive dorsiflexion of the foot and a straight-leg raising test with a passive cervical flexion. Routine motor examination of the upper and lower extremity nerve roots are listed in Table 12.6. Sensory examination of the various dermatomes is shown in Figure 12.2. Table 12.7 summarizes radicular innervation patterns. Cranial nerve function should also be assessed.

For pain complaints suggestive of a myofascial source, a detailed musculoskeletal examination should be

TABLE 12.6

MOTOR EXAMINATION OF UPPER AND LOWER EXTREMITY NERVE ROOTS

Area	Root	Muscle Movement
Upper Extremity	C5	Elbow flexion
	C6	Wrist extension
	C7	Elbow extension
	C8	Finger flexion (distal phalanx of middle finger)
	T1	Finger abduction (little finger)
Lower Extremity	L2	Hip flexion
	L3	Knee extension
	L4	Ankle dorsiflexion
	L5	Long toe extension (may also be ankle dorsiflexion)
	S1	Ankle plantar flexion

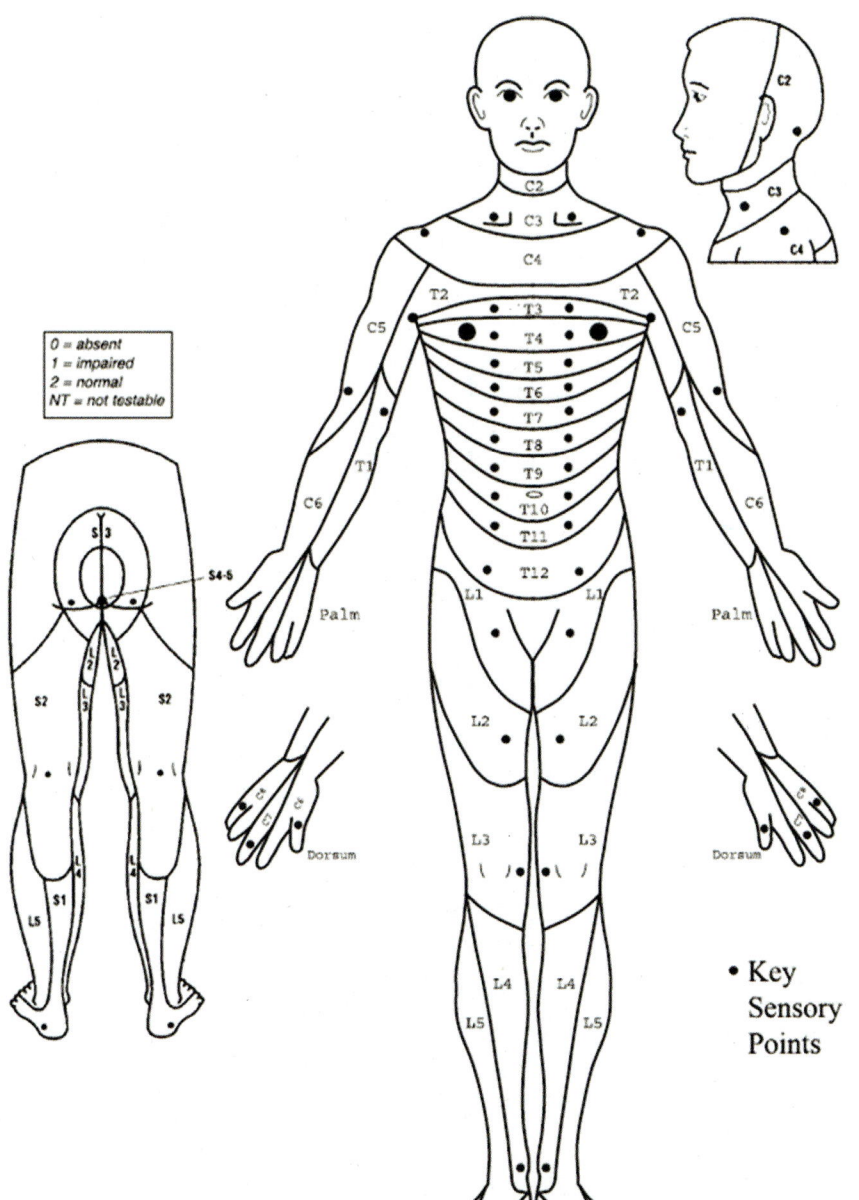

FIGURE 12.2 Sensory examination of dermatomes. The patient is examined with a safety pin at various key sensory points. Sensation is either normal, impaired, absent, or not testable at these areas. (Adapted from American Spinal Injury Association. International Standards for Neurological Classification of Spinal Cord Injury. www.asia_spinalinjury.org/publications/2006_Classif_worksheet.pdf. Revised 2000; reprinted 2008.)

TABLE 12.7
RADICULAR INNERVATION PATTERNS

Extremity	Root	Pain Location	Motor Action	Sensory Distribution	Reflex
Upper	C5	Shoulder upper arm	Shoulder abduction + external rotation (deltoid / supra / infraspinatus). Elbow flexion.	Upper/lateral aspect shoulder	Biceps
	C6	Radial forearm	Elbow flexion (biceps / brachialis); supination; wrist extensors (extensor carpi radialis longus + brevis).	Radial forearm + digit 1	Thumb + brachio-radialis
	C7	Dorsal forearm	Elbow extension (triceps)	Digits 2&3	Triceps
	C8	Ulnar forearm hand digits 4&5	Middle finger distal flexion	Digits 4&5	None
	T1	Ulnar forearm hand	Finger abduction / adduction (intrinsics)	Ulnar forearm + hand	
Lower	L3	Anterior thigh	Knee extension (quadriceps)	Anteromedial thigh	Patellar
	L4	Lower back, hip, posterolateral thigh, ant leg	Ankle dorsiflexion (tibialis anterior)	Anteromedial thigh + knee	Patellar
	L5	SI joint, hip, lat thigh, lat leg	Big toe dorsiflexion (ext hallucis longus)	Lateral leg, 1st 3 toes	None
	S1	SI joint, hip, post/lat thigh, leg to heel	Ankle plantarflexion (gastrocnemius / soleus)	Back of calf, lat heel, lat foot, toe	Achilles tendon

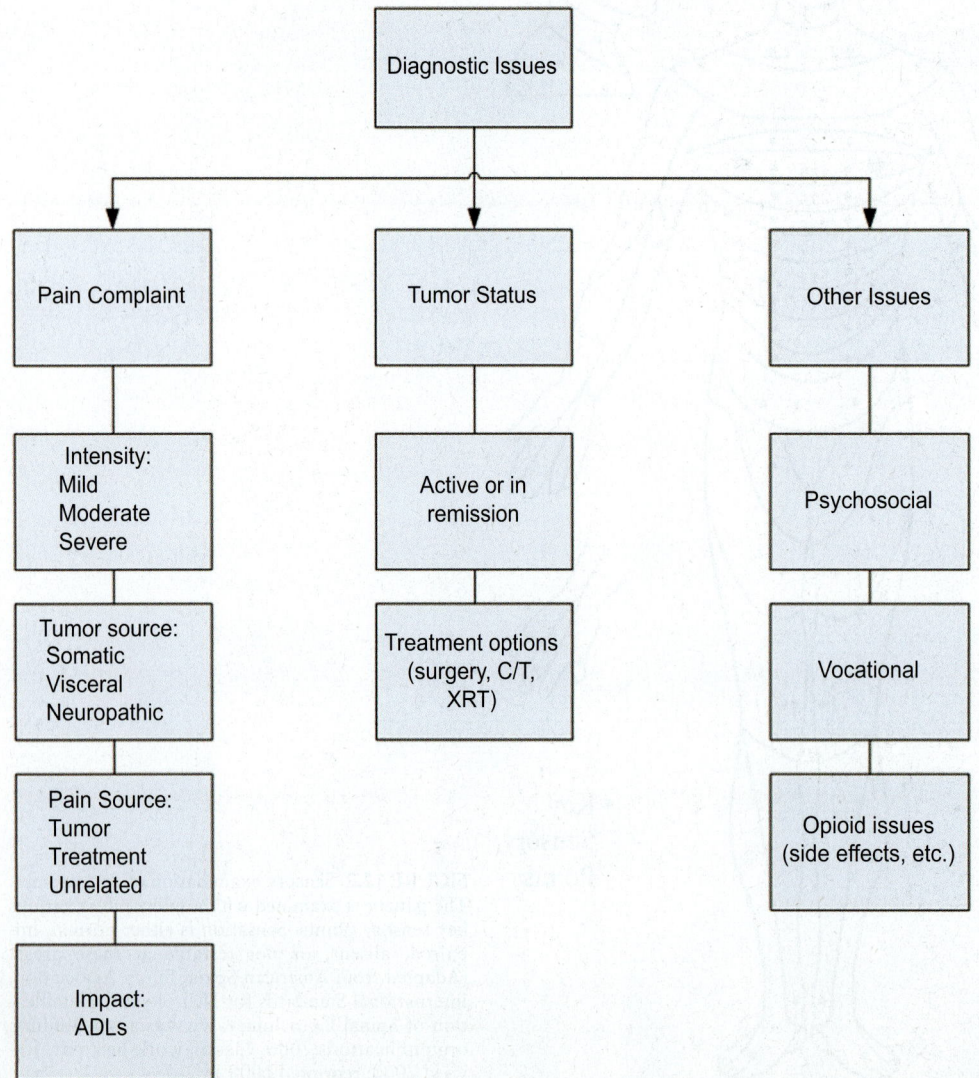

FIGURE 12.3 Final assessment summary. ADLs, Activities of daily living.

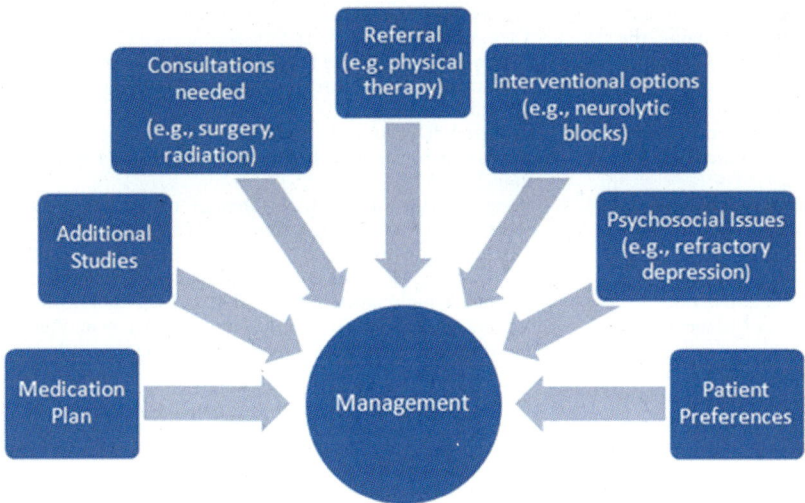

FIGURE 12.4 Management strategy.

performed. When a clinician evaluates a patient with a history of diffuse body pain, the examination should include a careful assessment both of joints for evidence of arthritis and of the soft tissues around the joints for sites of tenderness. In many patients with myofascial pain, there will be evidence of diffuse tender points, particularly in the thoracolumbar paraspinal region. Examination should include assessment of mechanical limitations in the range of motion of the spine (cervical, thoracic, and lumbosacral) and of upper and lower extremities. The patient's gait should be observed, particularly for any unusual postures and movements. The patient should be closely observed when moving from lying or sitting to the standing position, because this may reveal problems with lower-extremity strength or pelvic issues. Furthermore, the patient should be observed while removing upper body clothing, particularly if the pain complaint involves the shoulder girdle. Myofascial examination entails palpating soft tissues for evidence of tightness and trigger points, focal areas of tightness and tenderness that, when palpated, reproduce the patient's original pain complaint and other symptoms. Cervical spine range of motion should be determined, when relevant. Cervical paraspinal and shoulder girdle muscle tenderness should be elicited.

DIAGNOSIS AND MANAGEMENT

Careful, comprehensive pain assessment and diagnosis is the key to successful pain management in the cancer patient with pain (Fig. 12.3). Clinical decision making will be based upon the diagnoses of the issues contributing to the pain complaint (Fig. 12.4). Each issue outlined must be addressed as appropriate to the overall management of the patient. Because of the large amount of information that needs to be collected and reviewed for each patient, we have developed templates in our practice for both new patient evaluations and for return visits. These templates are shown in Appendices L1 and L2. We have found that the use of templates increases the likelihood that a complete assessment has been accomplished. Inferences about the pathophysiology of the pain and an assessment of all aspects of the pain syndrome are essential. Other symptoms and associated psychosocial issues must also be assessed. When necessary, additional in depth analysis of unresolved problems should be carried out before treatment implementation.

References

1. Twycross R, Harcourt J, Bergl S. A survey of pain in patients with advanced cancer. *J Pain Symptom Manage*. 1996;12:273–282.
2. AHCPR. Management of cancer pain guideline overview. Agency for Health Care Policy and Research Rockville, Maryland. *J Natl Med Assoc*. 1994;86:571–573, 634.
3. Society AP. Quality improvement guidelines for the treatment of acute pain and cancer pain. American Pain Society Quality of Care Committee. *JAMA*. 1995;274:1874–1880.
4. ASA. Practice guidelines for cancer pain management. A report by the American Society of Anesthesiologists Task Force on Pain Management, Cancer Pain Section. *Anesthesiology*. 1996;84:1243–1257.
5. Von Korff M, Dunn KM. Chronic pain reconsidered. *Pain*. 2008;138:267–276.
6. Serlin RC, Mendoza TR, Nakamura Y, et al. When is cancer pain mild, moderate or severe? Grading pain severity by its interference with function. *Pain*. 1995;61:277–284.
7. Williamson GM, Schulz R. Activity restriction mediates the association between pain and depressed affect: A study of younger and older adult cancer patients. *Psychol Aging*. 1995;10:369–378.
8. Tait RC, Chibnall JT, Krause S. The Pain Disability Index: Psychometric properties. *Pain*. 1990;40:171–182.
9. Turner JA, Franklin G, Heagerty PJ, et al. The association between pain and disability. *Pain*. 2004;112:307–314.
10. Scudds RJ, Robertson JM. Pain factors associated with physical disability in a sample of community-dwelling senior citizens. *J Gerontol A Biol Sci Med Sci*. 2000;55:M393-9.
11. Gatchel RJ, Mayer TG, Theodore BR. The pain disability questionnaire: Relationship to one-year functional and psychosocial rehabilitation outcomes. *J Occup Rehabil*. 2006;16:75–94.
12. Maltoni M, Pirovano M, Scarpi E, et al. Prediction of survival of patients terminally ill with cancer. Results of an Italian prospective multicentric study. *Cancer*. 1995;75:2613–2622.
13. Schaafsma J, Osoba D. The Karnofsky Performance Status Scale re-examined: A cross-validation with the EORTC-C30. *Qual Life Res*. 1994;3:413–424.
14. Yellen SB, Cella DF. Someone to live for: Social well-being, parenthood status, and decision-making in oncology. *J Clin Oncol*. 1995;13:1255–1264.
15. Singer PA, Martin DK, Kelner M. Quality end-of-life care: Patients' perspectives. *JAMA*. 1999;281:163–168.
16. Espallargues M, Valderas JM, Alonso J. Provision of feedback on perceived health status to health care professionals: A systematic review of its impact. *Med Care*. 2000;38:175–186.

17. Greenhalgh J, Meadows K. The effectiveness of the use of patient-based measures of health in routine practice in improving the process and outcomes of patient care: A literature review. *J Eval Clin Pract.* 1999;5:401–416.
18. Velikova G, Booth L, Smith AB, et al. Measuring quality of life in routine oncology practice improves communication and patient well-being: A randomized controlled trial. *J Clin Oncol.* 2004;22:714–724.
19. Garratt A, Schmidt L, Mackintosh A, et al. Quality of life measurement: Bibliographic study of patient assessed health outcome measures. *BMJ.* 2002;324:1417.
20. Cella D, Chang CH, Lai JS, et al. Advances in quality of life measurements in oncology patients. Semin Oncol. 2002;29:60–68.
21. Smets EM, Garssen B, Schuster-Uitterhoeve AL, et al Fatigue in cancer patients. *Br J Cancer.* 1993;68:220–224.
22. Portenoy RK, Thaler HT, Kornblith AB, et al. The Memorial Symptom Assessment Scale: An instrument for the evaluation of symptom prevalence, characteristics and distress. *Eur J Cancer.* 1994;30A:1326-1336.
23. Portenoy RK, Thaler HT, Kornblith AB, et al. Symptom prevalence, characteristics and distress in a cancer population. *Qual Life Res.* 1994;3:183–189.
24. Clouston PD, DeAngelis LM, Posner JB. The spectrum of neurologic disease in patients with systemic cancer. *Ann Neurol.* 1992;31:268–273.
25. Breig A, Marions O. Biomechanics of the Lumbosacral Nerve Roots. *Acta Radiol Diagn (Stockh).* 1963;1:1141–1160.
26. Lew PC, Morrow CJ, Lew AM. The effect of neck and leg flexion and their sequence on the lumbar spinal cord. Implications in low back pain and sciatica. *Spine.* 1994;19:2421–2424.
27. Van Boxem K, Van Zundert J, Van Zundert J, et al. Pseudoradicular and radicular low-back pain: How to diagnose clinically? *Pain.* 2008;135:311–312; author reply 313–315.

SECTION II ■ MANAGEMENT

CHAPTER 13 ■ OVERVIEW OF MANAGEMENT

Pain has been inadequately addressed and managed for a variety of cultural, educational, political, religious, and logistical reasons.[1] Persisting pain has major physiologic, psychological, economic, and social ramifications for patients and their families, as well as for society. All of the developed and many developing countries have the ability to significantly improve the treatment of pain of all types; it is not just cancer pain management that is deficient. Furthermore, global disparities in incidence of certain preventable cancers (eg, cervical), as well as in survival from several that are treatable (eg, lymphoma, leukemia, testicular carcinoma), are a demonstration of a lack of equity in the provision of health care, apparently determined solely by the hazard of what country one resides in.[2]

Worldwide, a total of 10.9 million new cases of cancer were reported in 2002. In the same year, there were 6.7 million deaths ascribed to cancer and 24.6 million persons within 3 years of diagnosis alive with their cancers.[2] At least 70% of patients suffered from pain caused by their cancer or its treatment.[1] Approximately 25% of cancer patients die without adequate pain relief in spite of the availability of appropriate tools for adequate pain control.[3-4] Adequate pain treatment is more often found in patients on palliative anticancer treatment than those receiving curative anticancer treatment.[5] It has also been shown that patients with better performance status[6] or without metastases[7] are likely to receive less-than-adequate pain treatment. Cancer patients are exposed to the well-known barriers that impede adequate pain relief, such as fear of opioid and other medications and the completely inappropriate fear of starting opioids too early so that pain relief will not be available because of tolerance when the disease enters its terminal phase.

It is unfortunately true that the majority of the world's cancer patients do not present until their disease has reached advanced status. For such patients, the currently available treatment options consist of pain management and palliative care. However, the course of disease leads to varying levels of pain, both acute and chronic, yet some cancer patients need pain relief throughout the entire course of their illness. It has been suggested that pain occurs in approximately one third of patients who are receiving ongoing active anticancer treatment. Treatment of the cancer and pain relief efforts must both remain the focus of the clinician. A recent NIH Consensus Conference on symptom management in cancer estimated that 5-year survival will occur in at least 60% of patients.[8] This will mean that the need to address the effect of symptoms of cancer and its treatments on individuals' lives will become progressively more important in the effort to reduce the pain, suffering, and disability, as well as the health care costs, of cancer.

The methods of measuring the adequacy of pain management have been the subject of numerous studies. The Pain Management Index (PMI) is a validated method of assessing the adequacy of pain control based on several widely accepted guidelines.[9] This instrument examines the congruence between the patient's self-reported level of pain and the appropriateness of the analgesic therapy. The PMI is a composite measure that is computed by subtracting a patient's worst pain intensity from the rating of the most potent analgesic prescribed. The PMI is a conservative estimate; it does not take into consideration the doses of the analgesics used or the schedule at which they are prescribed. Even when the PMI is utilized, one half of patients with cancer pain seem to be undertreated.[10] We strongly recommend the use of this or another validated instrument to assess the adequacy of cancer pain treatment.

The causes of inadequate pain management are certainly multifactorial and, often, exceedingly complex. Some of the factors that contribute to under-treatment of pain are itemized in Table 13.1. The inadequate prescription of opioids is a major component of the undertreatment of cancer pain. There are also patient characteristics, such as age, minority status, or lower educational achievement, that have been associated with an increased likelihood of inadequate pain treatment.[6,11-13] Gender also appears to play a role in the adequacy of cancer pain management; women were significantly less likely to have been prescribed high-potency opioids by their primary oncology team and significantly more likely to report inadequate pain management in a study of 131 cancer patients.[14]

More than 90% of oncology care occurs on an outpatient basis, and consists predominantly of prescriptions for medications. Clinicians should be aware of the factors that contribute to the likelihood that prescribed medications will be taken as ordered. Adherence to prescriptions implies the active, voluntary collaboration by the patient in a mutually acceptable course of behavior that leads to the desired preventive or therapeutic result.[15] Undertreatment can result from failure to adhere to prescriptions. Adherence rates are difficult to determine because of differences in the parameters chosen for defining variability. For example, Du Pen et al.[16] reported that 62% to 72% of oncology patients adhered to their prescribed opioid therapy. By contrast, Miaskowski et al.[17] reported that overall adherence rates for PRN analgesics ranged from 22.2% to 26.6%. Enting et al.[18] found that 65% of 915 cancer patients receiving outpatient care were undertreated, as indicated by a negative PMI. Both physicians and patients contributed to ineffective pain management, characterized both by poor analgesic prescriptions and by poor adherence to those prescriptions. Valeberg et al.[19] reported that only 41% of oncology outpatients were adherent to their

TABLE 13.1

FACTORS CONTRIBUTING TO UNDERTREATMENT OF CANCER PAIN IN THE UNITED STATES

Factor	Reason
Patient-related	Underreporting of pain complaint/intensity:
	concerns about disease progression
	perceived lack of time or inadequate amount of time spent discussing pain problems with physician
	stoicism
	ethnic and cultural factors
	Poor compliance with prescribed medications:
	misunderstanding of prescription instructions
	inability to follow instructions (eg, cognitive issues)
	pseudoaddiction
	intentional nonmedical use of medications
Physician-related	Opioid-related:
	inadequate/limited knowledge of opioid use
	concerns about opioid addiction and diversion
	censure/legal issues regarding overprescription or perceived overprescription of opioids
	Pain complaints not accurately assessed
	Outdated strategies for cancer pain management
	Limited available resources to manage complex patients and complex pain problems

analgesic regimen—women less so than men. Higher adherence scores occurred in patients with higher average pain intensity scores, higher pain relief scores, and with those receiving strong opioid analgesics.

The persistence of undermedication despite the availability in developed countries of opioids and other analgesics for the treatment of cancer pain points either to limitations in current pain management guidelines or failure of those caring for cancer patients to utilize the existing guidelines. Even with the implementation of routine documentation of pain intensity in the United States, the quality of pain management did not appear to improve significantly.[20] Some of the issues identified include the health care professionals' knowledge and attitudes about opioid prescribing;[21-22] patient reluctance to use opioids for pain relief (including the family's reaction to such treatment);[23] and practitioner concern about regulatory scrutiny.[24] There are also a variety of restrictive drug control and health care policies governing the medical use of prescription medications for pain management in the form of laws, regulations, and guidelines. Some of these policies may establish parameters for legitimate medicine that impinge on patient care decisions about pain management, palliative care, and end-of-life care. Medical professionals' comfort when treating pain often is influenced by what their state policies say about this practice or, often more importantly, by what medical professionals believe the policies to say.[25] Many states continue to have policies that create barriers to patients getting their pain treated adequately or are silent about recognizing pain relief as part of quality health care practice.[26]

Although most state medical boards have adopted regulations, guidelines, or policy statements relating to controlled substances and pain management, some state medical boards actually have rejected prescribing practices that are considered acceptable by today's standards.[26] In 1998, the Federation of State Medical Boards of the United States attempted to address physicians' concerns about regulatory scrutiny of opioid prescription which can negatively affect patient care. Professional licensure is regulated at the state level, with medical boards overseeing professional practice to determine violations of laws and regulations related to professional practice and controlled substances. Usually questions of professional judgment regarding prescribing are matters for medical boards to investigate. Federal, state, or local law enforcement interventions are reasonable when a practitioner's conduct is knowingly and intentionally outside legitimate professional practice. However, many have expressed the belief that regulatory state and federal agencies were intruding upon the legitimate practice of medicine.

As a result of physician concerns, the Federation published *"Model Guidelines for the Use of Controlled Substances for the Treatment of Pain,"* which was disseminated to all medical boards for consideration and adoption.[27] The basic principle of these guidelines asserts that efforts to prevent misuse of controlled drugs such as opioid analgesics should not interfere with relieving pain and suffering, and that drug regulatory policy should not contradict medical and scientific knowledge about pain management. By 2004, 25 state boards had adopted the guidelines either in whole or in part, and many communicated these new guidelines to their licensees. In 2004, the Federation updated its guidelines and also recognized undertreatment of pain as a significant departure from acceptable medical standards. At the state level in the United States, there have also been efforts to reform prescription monitoring, to make education in pain management mandatory, and to affirm the appropriateness of using opioids to treat intractable pain.[28]

Internationally, there are many reasons why patients receive inadequate cancer pain control.[29] Table 13.2 lists some of these reasons. In response to these issues, the World Health Organization (WHO) advocated a strategy which included the development of national or state policies that supported cancer pain relief through government endorsement of education and drug availability, educational programs for the public, health care personnel, regulators, etc., and modification of laws and regulations to improve the availability of drugs, especially opioid analgesics. The WHO has been involved with pain in three overlapping areas: the promotion and dissemination of guidelines on pain management, advocacy of improved access to opioid analgesics, and national programs of palliative care and pain relief. For over two decades, the WHO Cancer Unit has led a global initiative in pain management.

TABLE 13.2

INTERNATIONAL REASONS FOR INADEQUATE CANCER PAIN CONTROL

Absence of national policies on cancer pain relief and palliative care

Lack of awareness on the part of health care workers, policymakers, administrators, and the public that most cancer pain can be relieved

Shortage of financial resources and limitations of health care delivery systems and personnel

Concern that medical use of opioids will produce psychological dependence and drug abuse

Legal restrictions on the use and availability of opioid analgesics

(From *Cancer pain relief and palliative care*. Technical Report Series 804, Geneva, Switzerland: World Health Organization, 1990.)

TABLE 13.3

STRATEGIES FOR ADDRESSING UNDERTREATMENT OF PAIN

World Health Organization programs in collaboration with international pain relief organizations

International promotion of pain control programs in all countries

Education for health undergraduate and graduate students

Continuing medical education programs

Promulgation of pain management strategies by professional societies at state and national level

Rationalization of governmental policies on opioid availability and prescription

Establishment of reasonable pricing for pain medications

Appropriate reimbursement for pain management activities

Correction of the under-treatment of cancer pain requires an integrated approach such as that outlined in Table 13.3.

High quality pain management begins with an adequate patient evaluation. This includes: screening for the presence of pain, a comprehensive initial assessment when pain is present, and appropriate reassessments of the patient's responses to treatment. To accomplish these, an interdisciplinary, collaborative plan for care that includes patient and family input is required. Treatment should be efficacious, cost conscious, culturally and developmentally appropriate, and safe. Access to specialty care as needed must be provided.[30] The American Pain Society (APS) Quality of Care Committee prepared guidelines for the treatment of acute pain and cancer pain;[31] these were revised in 2005.[30] The impact of implementation of the APS guidelines in a focused program at an academic cancer hospital was studied by Bookbinder et al.[32] Their program looked for organizational obstacles to effective pain management and included routine monitoring of pain, staff education, and focus groups. After the first year of the program, patient satisfaction was improved, but the self-reported "worst pain levels over the past 24 hours" were unchanged. Pain intensity on the targeted hospital units improved further in the second and third years of the program. Pain assessment did not become routine until the outcomes data had been presented to the staff and the physicians were convinced to participate in the programs. The revision of the APS guidelines recommended that all health care organizations establish structured, multilevel systems approaches, sensitive to the type of pain, population served, and setting of care. Essentials to be included were: prompt recognition and treatment of pain, involvement of patients and families in the pain management plan, improved treatment patterns, regular reassessment and adjustment of the pain management plan, and measurement of processes and outcomes of pain management. The essentials of the revised APS guidelines on pain management are contained in Table 13.4.

There are many paths to effective pain relief in the cancer patient. (Table 13.5). Treatment must be tailored to the individual patient: matching drug treatment,

TABLE 13.4

AMERICAN PAIN SOCIETY 2005 KEY RECOMMENDATIONS

Recommendation	Reason
Recognize and treat pain promptly	Emphasis on comprehensive assessment and importance of preventive and prompt treatment based on evidence for neuroplasticity
Involve patients and families in pain management plan	Emphasis on customization of care and participation of patient in treatment plan
Improve treatment patterns	Eliminate inappropriate practices, provide multimodal therapy
Reassess and adjust pain management plan as needed	Respond not only to pain intensity but to functional status and side effects
Monitor processes and outcomes of pain management	New standardized QI indicators

QI, Quality improvement.
(Modified from Gordon DB, Dahl JL, Miaskowski C, et al. American Pain Society recommendations for improving the quality of acute and cancer pain management: American Pain Society Quality of Care Task Force. *Arch Intern Med*. 2005;165:1574–1580.)

TABLE 13.5

APPROACHES TO PAIN MANAGEMENT IN CANCER PATIENTS

Psychological Approaches	Understanding
	Companionship
	Cognitive behavioral therapies
Modification of Pathological Process	Radiation therapy
	Hormone therapy
	Chemotherapy
	Surgery
Drugs	Analgesics
	Antidepressants
	Anxiolytics
	Neuroleptics
Interruption of Pain Pathways	Local anesthetics
	Neurolytics
	Ablation (radiofrequency, cryoablation)
	Neurosurgery
Modification of Daily Activities	Use of ambulatory devices (eg, walker)
Immobilization	Rest
	Cervical collar or corset
	Plastic splints or slings
	Orthopedic surgery

(Modified from *Cancer pain relief with a guide to opioid availability*. Geneva, Switzerland: World Health Organization, 1996.)

anesthetic, neurosurgical, psychological, as well as behavioral approaches to the patient's needs. Successful management of the patient's chronic pain can only be achieved when those responsible for pain management are familiar with all these aspects of care and are integrated into the overall oncology treatment plans.

It is widely believed by leading pain clinician–educators that the traditional medical model for providing health care to cancer patients requires the addition of supplemental interventions in health care systems to influence the routine behaviors of both clinicians and patients.[32–37] This viewpoint is consonant with the quality improvement (QI) movement.[38–39] It appears that although clinicians may be concerned with patient comfort, their daily habits and clinical modus operandi often do not lead to effective pain relief. Some experts have stated that many symptoms of medical illness, especially pain, have been neglected because medical practices and accountability for outcomes have evolved from a focus on structural disease rather than on patient complaints.[40–41] For this reason, quality improvement programs that have been designed to facilitate the treatment of cancer pain should focus upon the elements as outlined in Table 13-4.[30] These key elements are: recognition and treatment of pain promptly, involvement of patients and families in the pain management plan, improvement of treatment patterns, reassessment and adjustment of the pain management plan as needed, and prospective monitoring of processes and outcomes of pain management.

Algorithmic approaches to cancer pain management are a means of implementing guidelines or standards for care.[42–43] The transfer of guideline-based knowledge into clinical practice focuses on training physicians and nurses to use the guideline and, subsequently, evaluate any change in practice outcomes. Implementation of a clinical guideline in a health care setting is a complex process involving many different issues. These include incorporation of the guideline into institution-specific policies and procedures, standardized documentation, and education on the use of interventions throughout the system and across disciplines. However, educational efforts with health care providers do not always produce positive results. Du Pen et al.[44] noted a clear deterioration in the impact of training over time. Physicians and nurses were randomized to either "training" or "no training" for a previously tested algorithm for cancer pain management. Role model physician/nurse teams were the core faculty for a day-long seminar. Although patients of trained providers had a significant reduction in usual pain over a 4-month period compared to patients of untrained providers, these improvements deteriorated over time with a gradual return to baseline practice. Although treatment algorithms are beneficial, methods need to be developed to improve retention of knowledge and maintain improved outcomes.

High-quality pain management is achievable in cancer pain, but a scientific and systems-oriented approach is crucial. Quality improvement activities, evidence-based standards of care, patient involvement in decision-making, and disease management models for care delivery all can improve the quality of pain management. Barriers to the implementation of pain quality improvement goals should be identified and addressed to reduce the risk of inadequate pain management. The integration of new knowledge and favorable behaviors into everyday pain management practice is a challenging but essential component of the goal of improving the delivery of high-quality pain management.

References

1. Brennan F, Carr DB, Cousins M. Pain management: A fundamental human right. *Anesth Analg.* 2007;105:205–221.
2. Parkin DM, Bray F, Ferlay J, et al. Global cancer statistics, 2002. *CA Cancer J Clin.* 2005;55:74–108.
3. McCaffery M. Pain control. Barriers to the use of available information. World Health Organization Expert Committee on Cancer Pain Relief and Active Supportive Care. *Cancer.* 1992;70:1438–1449.
4. Zech DF, Grond S, Lynch J, et al. Validation of World Health Organization Guidelines for cancer pain relief: A 10-year prospective study. *Pain.* 1995;63:65–76.
5. Van den Beuken-van Everdingen MH, de Rijke JM, Kessels AG, et al. High prevalence of pain in patients with cancer in a large population-based study in The Netherlands. *Pain.* 2007;132:312–320.
6. Cleeland CS, Gonin R, Baez L, et al. Pain and treatment of pain in minority patients with cancer. The Eastern Cooperative Oncology Group Minority Outpatient Pain Study. *Ann Intern Med.* 1997;127:813–816.
7. Okuyama T, Wang XS, Akechi T, et al. Adequacy of cancer pain management in a Japanese Cancer Hospital. *Jpn J Clin Oncol.* 2004;34:37–42.
8. NIH State-of-the-Science Statement on symptom management in cancer: Pain, depression, and fatigue. 2002;19:1–29.
9. Cleeland CS, Gonin R, Hatfield AK, et al. Pain and its treatment in outpatients with metastatic cancer. *N Engl J Med.* 1994;330:592–596.

10. Deandrea S, Montanari M, Moja L, et al. Prevalence of undertreatment in cancer pain. A review of published literature. *Ann Oncol.* 2008;19:1985–1991.
11. Anderson KO, Mendoza TR, Payne R, et al. Pain education for underserved minority cancer patients: A randomized controlled trial. *J Clin Oncol.* 2004;22:4918–4925.
12. Anderson KO, Mendoza TR, Valero V, et al. Minority cancer patients and their providers: Pain management attitudes and practice. *Cancer.* 2000;88:1929–1938.
13. Anderson KO, Richman SP, Hurley J, et al. Cancer pain management among underserved minority outpatients: Perceived needs and barriers to optimal control. *Cancer.* 2002;94:2295–2304.
14. Donovan KA, Taliaferro LA, Brock CW, et al. Sex differences in the adequacy of pain management among patients referred to a multidisciplinary cancer pain clinic. *J Pain Symptom Manage.* 2008;36:167–172.
15. Turk DC, Meichenbaum D. Adherence to self-care regimens: The patient's perspective. In: Sweet JJ, Rozensky RH, Tovian SM, eds. *Handbook of clinical psychology in medical settings.* New York: Plenum Press, 1991:249–266.
16. Du Pen SL, Du Pen AR, Polissar N, et al. Implementing guidelines for cancer pain management: Results of a randomized controlled clinical trial. *J Clin Oncol.* 1999;17:361–370.
17. Miaskowski C, Dodd MJ, West C, et al. Lack of adherence with the analgesic regimen: A significant barrier to effective cancer pain management. *J Clin Oncol.* 2001;19:4275–4279.
18. Enting RH, Oldenmenger WH, Van Gool AR, et al. The effects of analgesic prescription and patient adherence on pain in a dutch outpatient cancer population. *J Pain Symptom Manage.* 2007;34:523–531.
19. Valeberg BT, Miaskowski C, Hanestad BR, et al. Prevalence rates for and predictors of self-reported adherence of oncology outpatients with analgesic medications. *Clin J Pain.* 2008;24:627–636.
20. Mularski RA, White-Chu F, Overbay D, et al. Measuring pain as the 5th vital sign does not improve quality of pain management. *J Gen Intern Med.* 2006;21:607–612.
21. Joranson DE, Gilson AM. Pharmacists' knowledge of and attitudes toward opioid pain medications in relation to federal and state policies. *J Am Pharm Assoc (Wash).* 2001;41:213–220.
22. Lebovits AH, Florence I, Bathina R, et al. Pain knowledge and attitudes of healthcare providers: Practice characteristic differences. *Clin J Pain.* 1997;13:237–243.
23. Breitbart W, Passik S, McDonald MV, et al. Patient-related barriers to pain management in ambulatory AIDS patients. *Pain.* 1998;76:9–16.
24. Chan KT, Fishman SM. Legal aspects of chronic opioid therapy. *Curr Pain Headache Rep.* 2006;10:426–430.
25. Gilson AM, Joranson DE, Maurer MA. Improving state pain policies: Recent progress and continuing opportunities. *CA Cancer J Clin.* 2007;57:341–353.
26. Joranson DE, Gilson AM, Dahl JL, et al. Pain management, controlled substances, and state medical board policy: A decade of change. *J Pain Symptom Manage.* 2002;23:138–147.
27. Model policy for the use of controlled substances for the treatment of pain. *J. Pain Palliative Care Pharmacother.* 2005;19:73–78.
28. Dahl JL. Pain: Impediments and suggestions for solutions. *J Natl Cancer Inst Monogr.* 2004:124–126.
29. *Cancer pain relief and palliative care.* Geneva, Switzerland: World Health Organization, 1990.
30. Gordon DB, Dahl JL, Miaskowski C, et al. American pain society recommendations for improving the quality of acute and cancer pain management: American Pain Society Quality of Care Task Force. *Arch Intern Med.* 2005;165:1574–1580.
31. Society AP. Quality improvement guidelines for the treatment of acute pain and cancer pain. American Pain Society Quality of Care Committee. *JAMA.* 1995;274:1874–1880.
32. Bookbinder M, Coyle N, Kiss M, et al. Implementing national standards for cancer pain management: Program model and evaluation. *J Pain Symptom Manage.* 1996;12:334–347.
33. Weissman DE, Dahl JL. Update on the cancer pain role model education program. *J Pain Symptom Manage.* 1995;10:292–297.
34. Weissman DE, Griffie J, Gordon DB, et al. A role model program to promote institutional changes for management of acute and cancer pain. *J Pain Symptom Manage.* 1997;14:274–279.
35. Moote CA. Postoperative pain management—back to basics [editorial]. *Can J Anaesth.* 1995;42:453–457.
36. Janjan NA, Martin CG, Payne R, et al. Teaching cancer pain management: Durability of educational effects of a role model program. *Cancer.* 1996;77:996–1001.
37. Dahl JL. State cancer pain initiatives. *J Pain Symptom Manage.* 1993;8:372–375.
38. Donabedian A. Quality and cost: Choices and responsibilities. *J Occup Med.* 1990;32:1167–1172.
39. Kritchevsky SB, Simmons BP. Continuous quality improvement. Concepts and applications for physician care. *JAMA.* 1991;266:1817–1823.
40. Max MB. Improving outcomes of analgesic treatment: Is education enough? *Ann Intern Med.* 1990;113:885–889.
41. Portenoy RK, Thaler HT, Kornblith AB, et al. Symptom prevalence, characteristics and distress in a cancer population. *Qual Life Res.* 1994;3:183–189.
42. Cohen MZ, Easley MK, Ellis C, et al. Cancer pain management and the JCAHO's pain standards: An institutional challenge. *J Pain Symptom Manage.* 2003;25:519–527.
43. National Cancer Care Network, Fort Washington, PA. NCCN. Adult Cancer Pain, 2008.
44. Du Pen AR, Du Pen S, Hansberry J, et al. An educational implementation of a cancer pain algorithm for ambulatory care. *Pain Manag Nurs.* 2000;1:116–128.

CHAPTER 14 ■ COMPREHENSIVE CARE OF THE CANCER PATIENT WITH PAIN

Comprehensive cancer care encompasses a continuum that progresses from disease-oriented, curative, life-prolonging treatment through symptom-oriented, supportive, and palliative care extending to terminal hospice care. This continuum requires that care is both of high quality and comprehensive in nature. Elements of high-quality care include the use of evidence-based treatment, where evidence is gained from high-quality clinical trials; doing what is done often and, hopefully, done well; recognizing the need to treat the whole patient and not just the disease; and treating the patient with compassion. Comprehensive care implies coordinated, integrated care that involves providers and patients working together to address each of the varied issues that impact the cancer patient and family.

Traditional cancer care systems have frequently not offered cancer patients a prospective and comprehensive plan for treatment and symptom management, with provisions for updating and evaluating such a plan with the assistance of a health care professional, and a follow-up plan for monitoring and treating possible late effects of cancer and its treatment. Cancer survivors commonly experience the underdiagnosis and undertreatment of the symptoms of cancer, a problem that begins at the time of diagnosis and often becomes more severe at the end of life. The failure to treat the symptoms, side effects, and late effects of cancer and its treatment has a serious adverse impact on the health, well-being, and the quality of life of cancer survivors. Patients with cancer are sometimes put in the untenable position of choosing between potentially curative therapies and palliative care instead of being assured access to comprehensive care that includes appropriate treatment and symptom management.

Comprehensive cancer care should incorporate access to psychosocial services and management of the symptoms of cancer (and the symptoms of its treatment), including pain, nausea and vomiting, fatigue, and depression. Pain management is, and should be, an integral component of comprehensive cancer care.[1] Designing an effective pain control strategy for the individual patient requires knowledge of the ways in which a patient's cancer, cancer therapy, and pain therapy can interact. Collaboration with different health care providers (such as medical oncologists and radiation oncologists) is essential to successful pain management. The National Cancer Institute (NCI)–designated cancer centers are characterized by scientific excellence and the capability to integrate a diversity of research approaches to focus on cancer. Many organizations that are dedicated exclusively to health care designate themselves comprehensive cancer centers based on their self-assessment of their prevention, diagnostic, and treatment services. However, the term "comprehensive" as used by the NCI requires more than state-of-the-art care and services and includes a strong research base interactive with a wide spectrum of prevention, care, education, information and dissemination activities that broadly serve communities and regions of the country. From a pure clinical perspective, the goals of patient care in oncology are often complex, but they broadly comprise prolonged survival, as well as optimizing comfort and function. Adoption of these goals logically leads to a multimodality treatment approach targeted to specific problems (Fig. 14.1).

Treatment of the whole patient requires that the clinician not only attempts to treat the tumor and to increase survival, but also relieves the side effects of both the cancer and the treatment, and improves quality of life.[2] Rapid progress in the fields of molecular biology, oncology, and supportive care requires clinicians to make individualized judgments on the best available treatment of the most relevant health outcomes, while respecting patient preferences. Clinical practice guidelines are one approach to improved quality of care and cost control. Guidelines are important tools for encouraging a comprehensive approach to cancer care, and they contribute to bridging the gap between research results and clinical practice so as to improve the management and the outcomes of patients with cancer. These are usually systemically developed statements by experts to assist both practitioner and patient with decisions about appropriate health care for specific clinical circumstances. Such guidelines usually include clinical pathways and care maps and should clearly define the intended function of the guideline, for whom it is intended, and in which circumstances it is applicable. With the introduction of clinical guidelines, costs and length of stay can be reduced, practice variations minimized, and patient quality of care and satisfaction maintained.[3] However, the various guidelines used in cancer care have considerable heterogeneity in development, structure, user, and end points.[4] If guidelines are to improve the quality of health care they must be credible, and inspire confidence in prospective users; their quality is an important contribution to their credibility.

Many different specialties have attempted to coordinate care through multidisciplinary management conferences and multidisciplinary clinics. In the latter, physicians from several specialties conduct clinics in the same location at the same time. In addition to streamlining workup and treatment planning, multidisciplinary conferences and clinics provide a forum for collegial exchange of professional opinions. Team approach and consensus development enables the managing clinician to convey a clear and consistent management opinion to the patient. Different factors affect the feasibility of multiple specialty

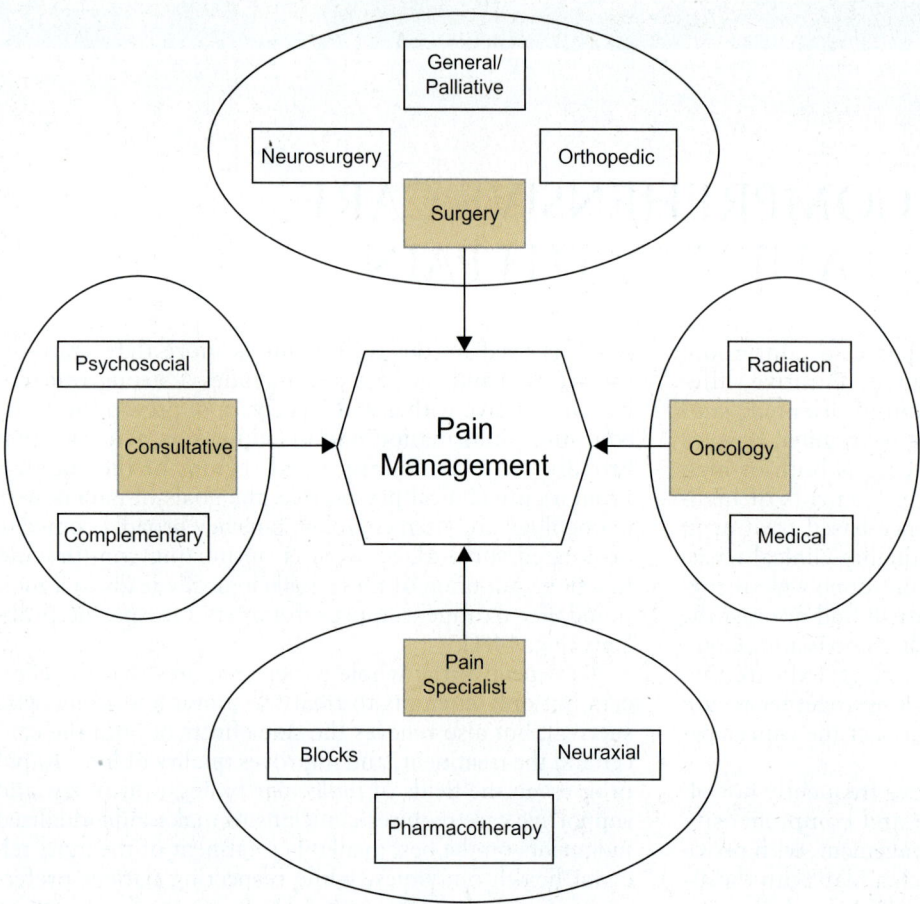

FIGURE 14.1 Multimodality therapeutic management of cancer pain.

evaluations. The availability of physicians with appropriate expertise and willingness to interact in this manner is critical. Economic factors often have broad impact, affecting motivation of patients, participating physicians, and referring physicians. Compensation for the time spent by multiple physicians in a single encounter may prove to be an obstacle in some settings. These issues need to be considered when forming multidisciplinary teams, because the durability of the program will often hinge on how effectively these issues are addressed and managed. Comprehensive oncology pain care requires many of these elements. Successful management of the cancer patient with pain depends on the ability of the involved providers to accurately assess problems, delineate current and future status of oncology care, identify and evaluate the components that contribute to the pain complaint, and formulate a plan for continuing care that is responsible for the evolving goals and needs of the patient and the patient's family.

Management decisions emanating from multidisciplinary conferences should be guided by locally agreed-on adaptations of clinical practice guidelines or other evidence. The use of clinical practice guidelines modified to fit local practice patterns improves both the process and the outcome of care.[3] Where appropriate, all patients should be evaluated as potential candidates for clinical trials, and patient enrollment should be encouraged. Ideally, these trials should include opportunities to evaluate the full range of approaches, including interventions with curative and palliative intent, as well as studies of comfort care near the end of life. At every stage of treatment, patients and their families should be offered clear, full, and prompt information in both verbal and written form. It is very important that all members of the treatment team have clear and efficient channels of communication. Patients should have clear instructions regarding who to contact for urgent problems.

The ability to treat cancer modifies the need for pain management (successful treatment reduces the likelihood of pain) and the appropriateness of invasive pain procedures. Cancer nonpain pathophysiology can interfere with the oral administration of medications, narrow the patient's therapeutic window for analgesic drugs, limit the effectiveness of psychological pain therapies, and complicate or preclude invasive pain-reducing procedures. In addition, cancer therapy can interfere with, or enhance, pain therapy and vice versa. Antineoplastic treatment can interfere with pain therapy by causing pain or by producing other adverse effects such as fatigue. Pain therapy can sometimes interfere with cancer therapy by increasing or complicating the adverse effects of cancer therapy. It can enhance cancer therapy by improving patient function or sense of wellbeing, and certain palliative surgical procedures may have the ancillary effect of improving organ function.

Patient life expectancy always influences treatment decisions. For example, if life expectancy exceeds several weeks then treatment may focus on how to enable the patient to function at the highest possible level. One goal should be to relieve pain and prevent therapy from interfering with normal activities. On the other hand, those likely to die within a few days or weeks require less emphasis on maintaining an active lifestyle and more on tolerance of the side effects associated with pain therapies. The emphasis for these patients should be on treatments that provide immediate relief, rather than those that require a long period of time to become effective. Because maintenance of mental clarity and alertness is almost always valued, even in the last days or hours of life, patients may be willing to undergo more interventional methods of pain management to achieve better pain control without alteration of consciousness common with high dose opioids. The guiding principle in developing pain management goals is to individualize the approach to the patient's needs. Part of the process of developing treatment goals is to take into consideration the risks and benefits of different treatment options and the "price" that the patient and family is willing to "pay" for pain relief. Clinicians may find that patient treatment goals differ from their own, either because patients feel that pain is inevitable, or because patients expect pain to be relieved with minimal effort on their part.

The basic principles of tumor-directed pain control include:

1. Modification of the source of pain by cancer treatment (eg, chemotherapy, surgery, radiation therapy)
2. Alteration of central pain perception, for example, by the use of analgesics, psychotropics, antidepressants, anxiolytics, and cognitive-behavioral therapies
3. Interruption of nociceptive transmission (central or peripheral), for example, with anesthetic techniques (eg, neuraxial analgesia, spinal/plexus neurolysis), specialized neurosurgery procedures (eg, cordotomy, myelotomy), tumor ablation (thermal/chemical ablation)

References

1. Levy MH. Supportive oncology: Forward. *Semin Oncol.* 1994;21 699–700.
2. Tannock IF. Treating the patient, not just the cancer. *N Engl J Med.* 1987;317:1534–1535.
3. Smith TJ, Hillner BE. Ensuring quality cancer care by the use of clinical practice guidelines and critical pathways. *J Clin Oncol.* 2001;19:2886–2897.
4. Pentheroudakis G, Stahel R, Hansen H, et al. Heterogeneity in cancer guidelines: Should we eradicate or tolerate? *Ann Oncol.* 2008;19: 2067–2078.

CHAPTER 15 ■ PRIMARY ANTICANCER TREATMENTS

There is no national cancer care program or system of care in the United States. Efforts to diagnose cancer and coordinate care are left to individual physicians, health plans, and cancer care centers. Health care concerns are magnified with a cancer diagnosis because of the nature of the disease, the complexity of management, the frequent reliance upon new and experimental interventions, and the high costs of care. The continuum of care spans prevention, early detection and screening, diagnosis and treatment of new cases, care of survivors, palliative care, and finally, support for terminally ill patients and their families.

Upon diagnosis of cancer, patients and their families have to cope not only with the diagnosis and an uncertain outcome but also with unfamiliar procedures and the presentation of treatment options. Patients are often asked to make choices between different therapeutic options, and many wish to be involved in the decision-making process of their care. Detailed information on treatment options has a number of beneficial effects, including the ability of the patient to gain control, to reduce anxiety, to improve compliance, to create realistic expectations, to promote self-care and participation, and to generate feelings of safety and security. Increasingly, patients are health consumers and want to be active participants in medical decision-making. As communities have become better educated and information about health care has become more accessible, a fundamental shift in society's expectations of clinicians has occurred. There is increased accountability of clinicians to standardize medical care according to best medical practices and to improve health care outcome. The quality of information available to patients on health care treatment options has improved, particularly with access to the internet, and with pressure from various consumer advocacy groups, patients now more frequently participate in treatment decisions. For example, the decision making regarding early-stage breast cancer is complex, and the decision-making process is problematic for many patients, especially minority patients.[1] Katz et al.[2] examined the relationship between patient involvement in decision making and type of surgical treatment for women with breast cancer. The authors surveyed a population-based sample of women diagnosed in 2002 with early-stage breast cancer from Detroit and Los Angeles, which are two areas that have previously demonstrated differing practice patterns with respect to breast-conserving surgery. Among these women, approximately 70% underwent breast conserving surgery, and 30% received mastectomy. Thirty-seven percent of the women perceived the surgeon to recommend neither surgical procedure over the other. However, when a specific recommendation was perceived by women, breast-conserving surgery was reported as being recommended by the surgeon more often (49% of women) than mastectomy (15% of women). Almost 80% of the women reported making their own decision or sharing the decision with their surgeon. Greater patient involvement in decision-making was associated with greater use of mastectomy rather than greater use of breast-conserving surgery.

There are often many therapeutic options for treating different cancers. Traditionally, most cancers have been treated with surgery, radiation, chemotherapy, or some combination of the three. Surgery is the mainstay of treatment for solid tumors (ie, most cancers except lymphoma or leukemia). For most nonmetastatic cancers, and locally confined tumors, surgery can be curative. Radiation is the primary treatment for some cancers (notably Hodgkin disease and other lymphomas), but is most often used in conjunction with surgery. Chemotherapy (including hormone therapy) may be used alone to treat some cancers (lymphomas or leukemia) but it is used more often in combination with surgery and radiation. In many cases, patients begin a protracted course of chemotherapy after surgery. Surgery and radiation therapy generally attempt to cure localized malignancies, whereas chemotherapy treats disseminated neoplasms. Recently, the advantages of combined therapy have become evident, and an increasing number of patients receive combinations of these three therapeutic approaches.[3] The rationale for such combination therapy comes from observations that surgery is most likely to fail locally at the edges of tumor resection (*positive surgical margins*), radiation therapy is most likely to fail in the center of tumors, and chemotherapy is most likely to fail in the presence of bulk disease.

Other types of treatments use the body's own immune system to resist disease. Biologic response modifiers modeled on the body's own natural products (eg, interferon, the interleukins, and tumor necrosis factor) are commonly used in conjunction with other treatments. Much of cancer treatment involves managing cancer symptoms such as pain or the effects of treatment. Some effects of treatment are short-lived (eg, nausea or hair loss) but others may be permanent (eg, infertility). Frequently, cancer patients also consider complementary or alternative options to conventional treatment. However, the majority of patients use complementary and alternative medicine to supplement their cancer treatment or help them cope with the treatment and/or its side effects. The more popular therapies appear to be dietary treatments, herbalism, homeopathy, hypnotherapy, and imagery/visualization.[4] A European study indicated that 36% of cancer patients reported using some form of complementary therapy,[4] and most U.S. studies report a higher use, often above 40%.[5-6] This form of treatment is discussed further in "Complementary and Alternative Treatment." The more traditional primary treatments of radiation therapy, chemotherapy and biotherapy, and surgery are discussed further.

RADIATION THERAPY

Radiation therapy is the most widely and frequently used treatment for cancer[7] and is primarily delivered utilizing three different modalities: external beam radiation therapy (EBRT), brachytherapy, or radioimmunotherapy. EBRT delivered via a linear accelerator is the most commonly used therapeutic radiation. Radiation is produced in the form of high-energy x-rays by a device that uses high-frequency electromagnetic waves to accelerate charged particles, such as photons and electrons, through a linear tube. Linear accelerators have the ability to treat with shallow depth penetration (electrons) or deep depth penetration (photons). Research suggests that DNA is the target of the cytotoxic effects of radiation.[8] The unit of radiation is the Gray (Gy), which is equal to 100 rads. EBRT can be administered with high-energy photons or electrons. Dosage is specified by the number of Grays for a number of fractions, eg, 3 Gy for ten fractions. Radiation tolerance is inversely proportional to the daily radiation dose and volume irradiated. Conformal and intensity modulated radiation therapies (IMRTs) are newer external techniques that improve the ability to localize the radiation dose and minimize side effects in adjacent normal tissue. Conformal therapy localizes the radiation dose with multiple fields and can be adapted to targets with irregular contours. IMRT is a refinement of conformal therapy whereby different doses of radiation are delivered to different areas in the same radiation fraction. Intraoperative radiation therapy (IORT) is the delivery of irradiation at the time of surgery and is performed by different techniques, including intraoperative electron beam techniques and high-dose-rate brachytherapy. IORT is usually given in combination with EBRT with or without chemotherapy and surgical resection. The addition of IORT to conventional treatment methods has improved local control as well as survival in many disease sites in both the primary and locally recurrent disease settings.

Brachytherapy involves the temporary or permanent placement of selected radioactive sources directly into a body cavity (intracavitary), into tissue (interstitial), into a passageway (intraluminal), or onto a tissue surface (plaque) (Fig 15.1). Brachytherapy delivers a prescribed treatment dose to a specified tumor volume with a rapid fall-off in radiation dose to adjacent normal tissues. High- or low-dose-rate brachytherapy can be used to treat a number of malignancies, including gynecologic, breast, lung, esophageal, and head and neck cancers, brain and prostate tumors, choroidal melanoma, and others. Brachytherapy can be used as primary treatment or in combination with EBRT to cure or palliate malignancies. By irradiating a small volume of tissue, complications are minimized and organ function can be preserved. Brachytherapy is most often performed using reactor-produced radionuclides such as cesium-137, iridium-192, iodine-125, palladium-103, and gold-198.

With palliative radiation, shorter EBRT schedules that include administering a higher radiation dose with each radiation fraction are generally used. This is called *hypofractionation*. It is believed that relief can occur more rapidly due to greater tumor cell kill per fraction. Furthermore, as patient survival is generally shorter, there is less concern about late-onset tissue toxicity. Longer courses with smaller fractions provide more durable pain relief due to larger absolute numbers of tumor cell kill without the increased risk of increased normal tissue toxicity. Table 15.1 lists cancers commonly treated by conventional radiation.

Radiosurgery is an EBRT technique that uses multiple convergent beams to deliver a high single dose of radiation to a small volume. In radiosurgery, multiple, highly collimated beams of radiation are stereotactically directed toward a radiographically discrete treatment site. The hallmark of all stereotactic radiation techniques is the rapid dose fall-off at the target edges. The most common use is for intracranial lesions, in which a stereotactic frame is applied to the head; high-resolution neurodiagnostic imaging is performed to define the target; image-integrated three-dimensional (3D) dose planning is performed by high-speed computers; and an accurate and

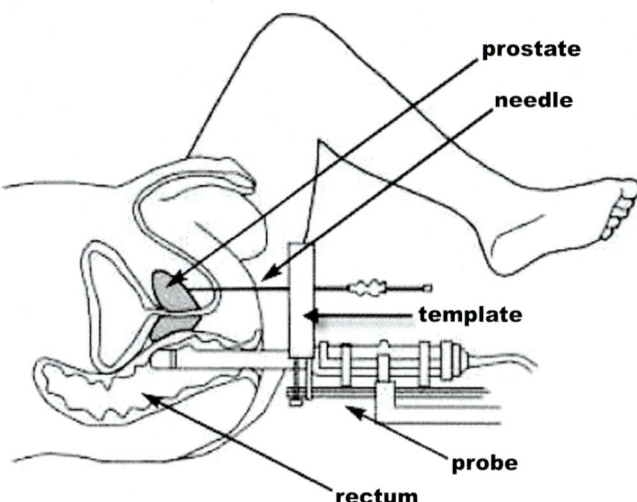

FIGURE 15.1 Prostate brachytherapy. An ultrasound probe is placed in the rectum for needle placement. The template is used to aid accurate placement of the needles delivering the seeds.

TABLE 15.1

DISEASES COMMONLY TREATED BY PRIMARY RADIATION THERAPY

Hodgkin disease
Non-Hodgkin lymphoma
Cervical carcinoma (stage dependent)
Prostate carcinoma (stage dependent)
Head and neck cancers
Breast cancer (stage dependent)
Multiple metastatic tumors of the central nervous system
Retinoblastoma
Choroidal melanoma
Unresectable lung carcinoma
Unresectable pancreatic carcinoma
Unresectable sarcoma

dependable technology is used to deliver photon energy to the target volume to achieve the desired clinical effect.

Radiosurgery is currently performed with one of two types of high-energy radiation technologies: x-rays, produced by linear accelerators, and the Gamma Knife, producing γ rays. Radiosurgery is used to treat malignant tumors, such as selected cases of brain metastases and malignant gliomas (for which stereotactic radiosurgical boosts are used in conjunction with fractionated radiation therapy), as well as benign tumors (eg, meningiomas, acoustic neuromas, and pituitary adenomas). It has become an important treatment alternative to surgery for a variety of intracranial lesions.

Linear accelerator–based stereotactic radiosurgery techniques have traditionally been used to treat central nervous system CNS tumors. The process combines stereotactic localization techniques, 3D planning imagery, and a sharply focused beam of radiation aimed at a specific, well-defined intracranial lesion. When treating intracranial CNS tumors, patients are positioned in a halo device used for immobilization or noninvasive system with image guidance, primarily to ensure accuracy and reproducibility of the treatment set-up. The CyberKnife is a compact 6-MV linear accelerator (LINAC) that is mounted on a computer-controlled robotic arm and can deliver multiple, nonisocentric, noncoplanar radiation beams. It is essentially a robotic, frameless, image-guided stereotactic radiosurgery system (Fig 15.2). By using bone landmarks or implanted fiducial markers, stereotactic radiosurgery has been used to treat lesions of the spine, pancreas, prostate, and lung. Because this type of radiosurgery does not require the application of a head frame, staged radiosurgery (ie, fractionation) is feasible. Two standard diagnostic x-ray tubes are rigidly fixed to the CyberKnife treatment room and are set up so that two orthogonal (90-degree offset) images of the target can be obtained. The images are gathered using two amorphous silicon x-ray screens capable of generating high-resolution digital images. For initial coarse alignment, identical features from anatomy are visually identified by the operator, and the position of the patient is adjusted by use of a five-axis support table. When the patient's position is adjusted so that the offset is less than 10 mm, the CyberKnife tracking system automatically compensates for alignment offset and patient motion by adjusting the location of the treatment "isocenter." In addition, tracking of the position of either a radiopaque (skeletal) target directly or of radiopaque fiducials with known

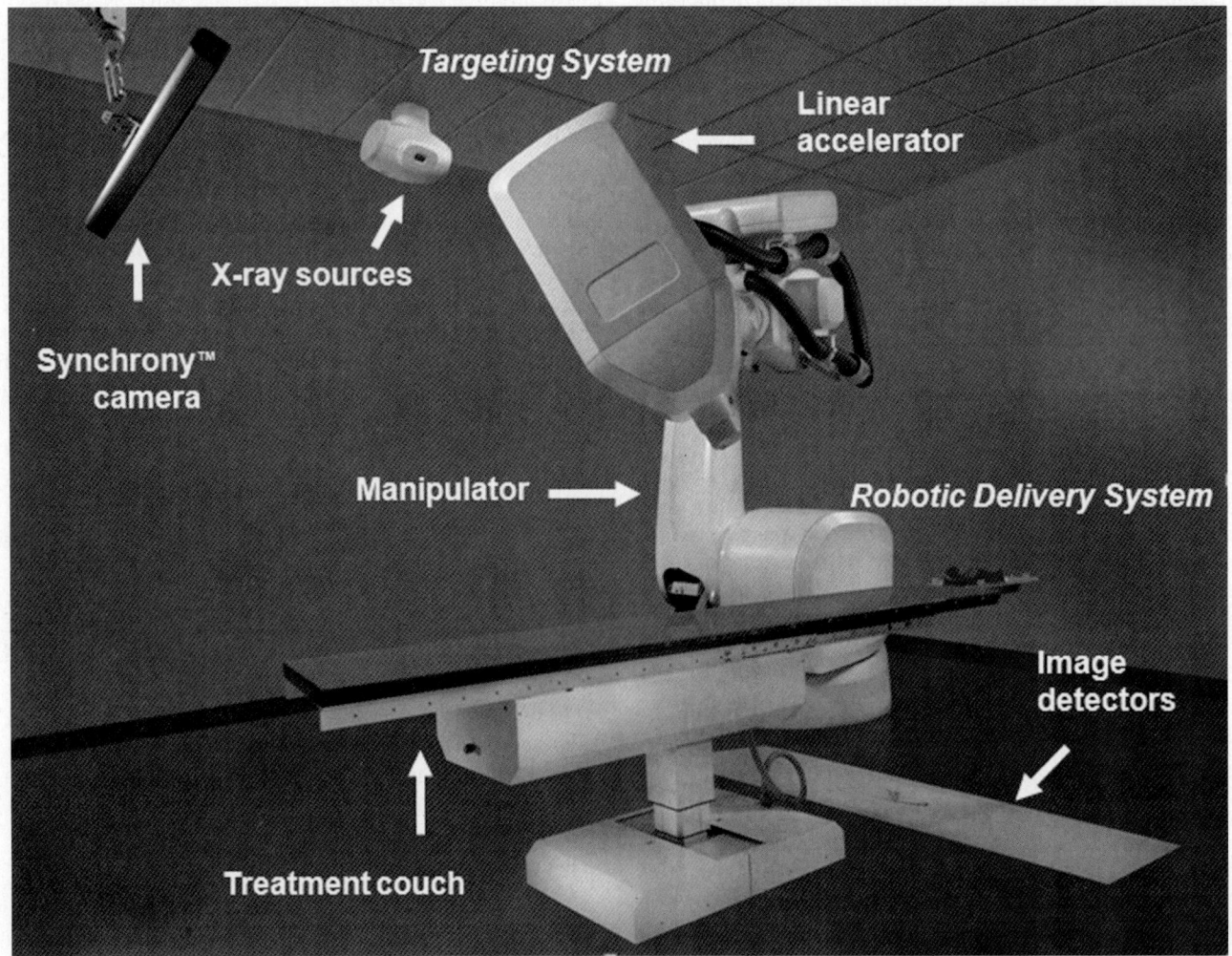

FIGURE 15.2 Cyberknife Robotic Radiosurgery system. The Synchrony camera incorporates fiber optic sensing technology that tracks respiratory motion so that intrathoracic lesions can be tracked accurately throughout treatment.

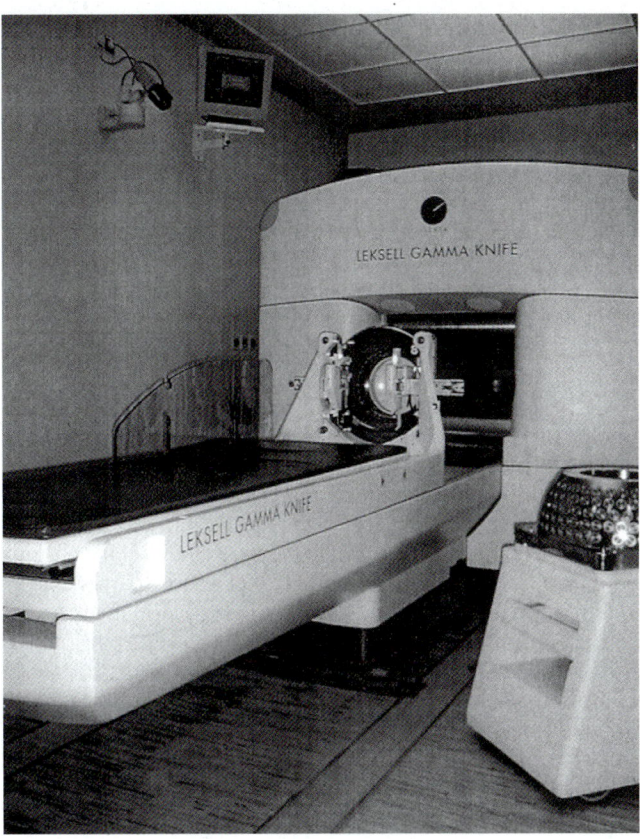

FIGURE 15.3 Gamma knife radiosurgery.

geometric distances from an x-ray radiolucent target can be performed.[9]

The Gamma Knife is a self-contained unit with 201 cobalt-60 sources arranged in a hemispheric array such that the emitted beams of radiation reach a common point of intersection (Fig 15.3). It was designed only to treat intracranial and skull base lesions. The overall time of radiation delivery varies depending on the prescribed dose, but it generally ranges from 15 to 45 minutes. The mechanical accuracy of radiation delivery with use of the Gamma Knife is less than 0.3 mm of variation, due to use of a stereotactic head frame.

High-quality radiation therapy can provide excellent local tumor control for either definitive treatment or palliation. The hallmark of good-quality radiation therapy is adequate tumor coverage while minimizing the risk of injury to normal tissue. This can be achieved by a team of physicians, physicists, nurses, dosimetrists, and therapists who can work as a team to deliver the correct dose to the tumor in the appropriate dose per fraction.

The role of radiation therapy in the management of painful conditions will be discussed further under "Radiation Strategies" in Chapter 21.

Complications of Radiation Therapy

Damage to normal tissues remains the most important limiting factor in the treatment of cancer by radiation therapy. Patients may experience symptoms associated with damage to normal tissue during the course of therapy for a few weeks after therapy or months or years later (Tables 15.2 and 15.3). Delayed progression of late effects for 20 to 34 years after therapy has been described.[10] The pathological processes of radiation injury begin immediately after radiation exposure, but the clinical and histologic features may not become apparent for some time. Symptoms may be caused by cell death or wound healing initiated within irradiated tissue, and may be precipitated by exposure to further injury or trauma. Radiation injury is commonly classified as acute, consequential, or late effects, according to the time before appearance of symptoms. Acute (early) effects are those that are observed during the course of treatment or within a few weeks after treatment. Consequential effects (sometimes called consequential late effects) appear later, and are caused by persistent acute damage. Late effects emerge months to years after radiation exposure. Acute radiation damage is most prominent in tissues with rapidly proliferating cells, such as in epithelial surfaces of the skin or gastrointestinal tract. Symptoms develop when functional cells are lost as part of normal tissue turnover and are not replaced because of damage to the stem-cell compartment. Late effects may occur in tissues with a slow turnover of cells, such as subcutaneous tissue, fatty tissue, muscle, brain, kidney, and liver, and in sites of slow turnover within tissues that contain rapidly-proliferating cells, such as the wall of the intestine.

TABLE 15.2

EARLY EFFECTS ASSOCIATED WITH RADIATION THERAPY

System	Effects
Hematological	Anemia, leucopenia, thrombocytopenia
Gastrointestinal	Gastritis, enteritis, proctitis, esophagitis, oral mucositis
Respiratory	Radiation pneumonitis
Urologic	Cystitis
Dermatologic	Erythema, pruritus, desquamation
Other (constitutional)	Fatigue

TABLE 15.3

LATE EFFECTS ASSOCIATED WITH RADIATION TREATMENT

System	Effects
Hematological	Myelofibrosis
Gastrointestinal	Mucosal stricture and fistula; xerostomia; loss of taste
Respiratory	Radiation pneumonitis
Urologic	Radiation nephritis, sterility
Dermatologic	Fibrosis, late ulceration, pigmentation
Musculoskeletal	Osteoradionecrosis (mandible, femoral head); muscle contractures
Neurologic	Plexopathy, myelitis, cognitive impairment
Other	Secondary tumors
Other (constitutional)	Fatigue

Significant musculoskeletal complications can result from radiation therapy and include muscle fibrosis and atrophy, fractures, and limb length discrepancy. Higher radiation doses (>60 Gy) can result in more pain and larger doses per fraction may lead to more muscle and soft tissue damage. Progression of injury may continue for as long as 10 years.[11] Hormone therapy, chemotherapy, radiation therapy, and castration all directly or indirectly damage bone and lead to loss of bone mass. Bone mineral density is usually measured by dual energy x-ray absorptiometry (DEXA) and this is considered the "gold standard" when performed at the femoral neck or total hip.[12] Bone densimetry results are often reported as t-scores, which represent the difference in the number of standard deviations (SD) between the individual's bone mineral density (BMD) and the mean value for a group of young adults of the same sex. Normal bone mass is defined by the World Health Organization as BMD within 1 SD of young adult mean (t-score ≥1); osteopenia as increased bone loss, with bone mass between 1 and 2.5 SD below normal (t-score,); and osteoporosis as bone mass >2.5 SD below normal (t-score >2.5).[13] For every SD by which BMD is below peak bone mass, fracture risk approximately doubles.[14]

Xerostomia is a common side effect encountered by patients receiving radiation to the oral cavity because of the proximity to the salivary glands. It can be transient or permanent, depending on the radiation dose. Evidence shows that mean doses of less than 26 Gy to the parotid glands may avoid permanent xerostomia.[15] Radiation mucositis (radiation-induced mucosal injury) usually occurs 2 to 4 weeks into treatment and abates 3 weeks to 2 months after the completion of radiation. Acute mucositis can be painful, and pain issues need to be addressed immediately to allow the patient to continue to eat. To minimize the chance of secondary infection, most radiation oncologists recommend baking soda mouthwash. If secondary infections (most often thrush) occur, appropriate antibiotic treatment is initiated. Topical anesthetic mouthwashes provide pain relief for 10 to 30 minutes and may help with eating. Many patients require narcotic analgesia for adequate pain control. Mucositis often causes significant swelling, which may be managed by nonsteroidal anti-inflammatory drugs (NSAIDs) or steroids. Usually, mucositis resolves 4 to 6 weeks after radiation is completed, but occasionally it can last for several months, necessitating close surveillance. Late complications of EBRT for base of tongue cancers include soft-tissue necrosis/ulceration, osteoradionecrosis (ORN), and xerostomia.[16] The mandible is among the bones most frequently affected by irradiation. ORN of the mandible is a serious late complication of high-dose radiation therapy for tumors of the oropharynx and oral cavity. The diagnosis of ORN is principally based on the clinical picture of chronically exposed bone. Radiological symptoms include decreased bone density with fractures, cortical destruction, and loss of spongiosa trabeculation. Numerous factors that may be associated with the risk of ORN include treatment-related variables (for example, total radiotherapy dose, biologically effective dose, photon energy, brachytherapy dose rate, combination of external beam irradiation and interstitial brachytherapy, field size, fraction size, volume of the mandible irradiated with a high dose), patient-related variables (eg, deep parodontitis, preirradiation bone surgery, poor oral hygiene, alcohol and tobacco abuse, bone inflammation, dental extraction after radiotherapy) and tumor-related factors (tumor size or stage, proximity of the tumor to bone, anatomic tumor site).[17] Primary management of postradiation bone lesions include conservative modalities such as saline irrigations, antibiotics during infectious episodes, topically applied antiseptics, gentle sequestrectomy and removal of visibly loosened bone elements as well as treatment with hyperbaric oxygen. Surgery is reserved for persistent ORN and includes radical resection of the lesion (sequestrectomy, hemi-mandibulectomy, and so on) with reconstruction.

The risk of injury to the intestine is dose limiting during abdominal and pelvic radiation therapy. Delayed bowel toxicity is difficult to manage and adversely impacts the quality of life of cancer survivors. The rectum is the area most often affected by pelvic radiation for treatment of prostate and cervical cancer. The acute symptoms are diarrhea from loss of integrity of the epithelium and increased secretion of mucus. The most frequent but relatively uncommon late effects include increased stool frequency, urgency, spotting of blood, and partial incontinence. Much less common are ulceration, severe bleeding, pain, stricture, severe incontinence, and fistula. Treatments for rectal complications include: oral anti-inflammatory agents, pain management, stool softeners, intrarectal steroids, transfusions (for bleeding), and dilatation of strictures. For serious or refractory complications, hyperbaric oxygen or surgical intervention with temporary or permanent colostomy may be required. Hyperbaric oxygen therapy significantly improved the healing responses in patients with refractory radiation proctitis.[18]

Pelvic radiation causes chronic fibrosis and progressive endarteritis in poorly oxygenated bladder submucosal and muscular tissues, with eventual tissue scarring.[19] This can lead to bladder mucosal sloughing and symptomatic hemorrhagic cystitis. Delayed radiation-induced hemorrhagic cystitis may appear more than ten years after pelvic radiotherapy. Traditional treatment methods include bladder irrigation, cauterization, oral or intravenous agents, intravesical chemical instillation, iliac artery embolization, urinary diversion, and cystectomy. However, no single treatment has resulted in satisfactory symptom control in most patients. Hyperbaric oxygen therapy may be a good primary option for the management of hemorrhagic cystitis.[20] One hundred forty-five (76%) of 190 reported patients demonstrated complete or partial symptomatic improvement with hyperbaric oxygen therapy, even among those who had failed multiple previous medical, cystoscopic, or intravesical therapies.[21] Chong et al.[19] reported that delivery of hyperbaric oxygen therapy within 6 months of the onset of hematuria was associated with an increased therapeutic response rate, even in patients with a history of clot retention. In patients with persistent pelvic radiation-induced toxicity (proctitis/cystitis, long-standing vaginal ulcers and fistulas, long-standing skin injuries), hyperbaric oxygen was both safe and effective.[22]

CHEMOTHERAPY AND BIOTHERAPY

Chemotherapy consists of drugs that may be given with curative or palliative intent. Adjuvant therapy refers to additional treatment, usually given after surgery.

Adjuvant chemotherapy is given after surgery or radiation therapy in an attempt to prevent tumor recurrence. Its goal is to treat residual micrometastatic disease. Adjuvant chemoradiation is intended to prevent local or regional recurrence. It may be used in patients with positive surgical margins. Adjuvant chemotherapy reduces the rate of recurrence of some tumors, especially ovarian, breast, osteogenic sarcoma, colon cancer, and Wilms tumor. Neoadjuvant therapy, by contrast, is given before surgical resection and/or in addition to radiation therapy specifically for tumor reduction. The most common reason for neoadjuvant therapy is to reduce tumor size before surgical resection.

The majority of chemotherapy is delivered systemically, but regional therapy can also be used. The purpose of regional chemotherapy is to deliver higher concentrations of chemotherapy while minimizing systemic toxicity. Examples of regional administration include intraperitoneal and neuraxial. Chemotherapy is given neuraxially either by lumbar puncture or through an Ommaya reservoir attached to a ventricular catheter. Common intrathecal agents are methotrexate and cytarabine. Hepatic artery delivery of floxuridine (FUDR) via an implanted system in the treatment of colorectal liver metastases represents the largest application of hepatic artery therapy. Most trials have suggested an improvement in both overall and progression-free survival with hepatic artery infusion therapy.[23] Dose-limiting toxicity associated with hepatic artery infusion is related to hepatobiliary sclerosis, which has been reduced with the addition of dexamethasone as part of the treatment.

Chemotherapy for responsive tumors such as lymphoma, small–cell lung cancer, germ cell tumors, and possibly breast cancer may achieve pain relief. Chemotherapy regimens utilizing a combination of agents having different modes of action and exhibiting different forms of toxicity are more likely to cure than single-agent therapy. This is believed to be related to the low probability of double resistance to two drugs which is much less than the risk of single-drug resistance. Since the fraction of cells killed is proportional to the dose employed, maximally tolerated drug doses are indicated. The development of resistant tumor cell clones is related to single drugs, low doses, and long intervals between chemotherapy cycles. High-dose chemotherapy accompanied by autologous hematopoietic stem cell transplants is indicated for the treatment of high-grade non-Hodgkin lymphoma (relapsed) and acute myelocytic leukemia when an allogeneic donor is not available. Some have employed this approach for stage IV breast cancer in remission and to complete the adjunctive therapy of high-risk primary breast cancer.

Emerging evidence has suggested that the capability of a tumor to grow and propagate may be dependent on a small subset of cells within the tumor, termed *cancer stem cells*.[24] In an animal model, cancer stem cells have the capacity for unlimited self-renewal, as well as the ability to initiate and drive tumor progression. Thus, they would seem the most probable candidates responsible for tumor chemoresistance and recurrence. Before the recognition of cancer stem cells, cancer treatment was traditionally based on the assumption that human cancer cell populations were homogeneous. It was thought that resistance to treatment occurred because malignant cells survived chemotherapy and radiation or avoided immune surveillance of endogenous cytotoxic T cells and natural killer cells.[25] The concept of cancer stem cells may have profound implications for our understanding of tumor biology and for the design of novel treatments targeted toward these cells. Current therapeutic strategies now include targeting the cancer stem cell.[25]

Patients with metastatic solid tumors have typically been treated with palliative chemotherapy. However, there are situations where metastatic disease is potentially curable. Metastatic testicular cancer, gestational choriocarcinoma, Hodgkin disease, and high-grade lymphomas are potentially curable with chemotherapy.[26] A common feature of such curable tumors is that they arise from cells that undergo major genetic rearrangements or recombination as part of their normal physiology. The absence of further genetic and epigenetic changes in genes that regulate apoptosis, DNA repair, and senescence allows these cells to maintain their intrinsic sensitivity to chemotherapy. This process allows the cells, when challenged with chemotherapy, to undergo the natural apoptotic pathways that contribute to their intrinsic qualities of chemosensitivity and high curability.

Traditional chemotherapeutic agents are cytotoxic drugs that are either cell cycle-specific or cell cycle-nonspecific. Antimetabolites such as 5-fluorouracil (5-FU), gemcitabine, and methotrexate are more active on the S phase of the cell cycle. Vinca alkaloids and taxanes work on the M phase of the cell cycle. Cell cycle nonspecific agents such as the anthracyclines (doxorubicin, idarubicin) form free radicals that result in DNA strand breaks. However, these agents are known to have cumulative cardiotoxicity. The camptothecins (irinotecan, topotecan) inhibit topoisomerase I and cause single-strand DNA breaks. The platinums (cisplatin, carboplatin, oxaliplatin) crosslink DNA and inhibit DNA synthesis and transcription. Of note, some agents such as 5-FU can exacerbate symptoms of systemic lupus erythematosus.[27-28]

With advances in molecular and cellular biology, antineoplastic therapy has become more refined. Imatinib (Gleevec) is a tyrosine kinase inhibitor that targets an oncogene and platelet derived growth factor. It has been used successfully in the treatment of chronic myelogenous leukemia (CML) and gastrointestinal stromal tumor (GIST). Other tyrosine kinase inhibitors include erlotinib (Tarceva) which is used for lung and pancreas cancer, and sunitinib (Sutent) which is used for renal cell carcinoma and GIST. Bortezomib (Velcade), a proteosome inhibitor, is used for multiple myeloma.

Biotherapy utilizes biologicals and biologic response modifiers in the treatment of cancer. Tumors express a wide variety of proteins that can be recognized by the immune system. The immune system of the human organism comprises the innate system cells and the adaptive immune cells. The innate system includes hematopoietic cells, mast cells, basophils, monocytes, dendritic cells, and macrophages. Adaptive cells include $CD4^+$ T cells, $CD8^+$ T regulatory cells, and B cells. Biotherapy approaches to cancer treatment aim to protect and reactivate patients' adaptive immunity against tumor cells.[29] In healthy individuals there is a T helper 1 (Th1) and T helper 2 (Th2) balance, but during microbial-induced inflammation, pathogens induce an overproduction of Th2 cytokines that inhibit adaptive responses against a pathogen.[30] Tumor cells may induce increased Th2 cytokine levels that

TABLE 15.4

IMMUNE THERAPIES FOR CANCER

Established Therapies	Indication
Monoclonal Antibodies	
Rituximab (Rituxan)	Non-Hodgkin lymphoma, chronic lymphocytic leukemia
Ibritumomab tiuxetan (Zevalin)	Non-Hodgkin lymphoma
Tositumomab (Bexxar)	Non-Hodgkin lymphoma
Alemtuzumab (Campath)	Chronic lymphocytic leukemia
Gemtuzumab (Mylotarg)	Acute myelogenous leukemia
Trastuzumab (Herceptin)	Breast cancer
Cetuximab (Erbitux)	Colorectal cancer
Panitumumab (Vectibix)	Colorectal cancer
Bevacizumab (Avastin)	Colorectal, lung
Immune Adjuvants	
Bacilli Calmette-Guerin	Superficial bladder cancer
Imiquimod (Aldara)	Basal cell carcinoma, vulvar intraepithelial neoplasia, actinic keratosis
Cytokines	
Interferon-α, interleukin-2	Melanoma, renal cell carcinoma
TNF-α	Soft-tissue sarcoma, melanoma
Supportive Therapy	
G(M)-CSF (filgrastim)	Myelosuppressive chemotherapy
Leucovorin	Methotrexate rescue
Prophylactic Immune Therapy	
Hepatitis B virus vaccine	Hepatocellular carcinoma
Human papillomavirus vaccine	Cervical cancer

(Adapted from Dougan M, Dranoff G. Immune therapy for cancer. *Annu Rev Immunol.* 2009;27:83–117.)

can serve as indicators for the existence of tumors.[31] Polarized Th1 cells produce interleukin (IL)-2, IL-12, and interferon-γ. Polarized Th2 cells and hematopoietic cells produce IL-4, IL-5, IL-6, IL-10, and IL-13.[29]

Established therapies employ a variety of manipulations to activate antitumor immunity including passive immunization with monoclonal antibodies, the introduction of adjuvants into the tumor microenvironment, and the systemic delivery of cytokines (Table 15.4).[32] These various immunotherapeutic strategies include cytokines, therapeutic vaccines based on tumor cells or dendritic cells, monoclonal antibodies, and adoptive immunotherapy (T cell transfer or allogeneic hematopoietic cell transplantation). Biologic response modifiers have an established role in the treatment of certain cancers (eg, IL-2 in renal carcinoma, interferon as adjunctive therapy in melanoma, bacillus Calmette-Guérin [BCG] as local therapy for bladder tumors). The majority of biological agents in clinical use are cytokines. Examples of these agents include interferons, interleukins, hematopoietic growth factors, and tumor necrosis factor. Hematopoietic growth factors in use include granulocity colony stimulating factor (GCSF or filgrastim) and granulocyte macrophage colony stimulating factor (GMCSF or sargramostim), which stimulate the production of white blood cells. These agents facilitate host recovery from severe chemotherapy-induced myelosuppression, and permit an increase in the dose intensity of standard chemotherapeutic agents.

Monoclonal antibodies can be used as carriers to deliver drugs or toxins to tumor cells. Antibody structures are manipulated to facilitate selective interaction with host immune effectors. Monoclonal antibodies targeting non-Hodgkin lymphoma, *HER-2/neu* highly expressing metastatic breast cancer, colorectal cancer, acute myelogenous leukemia, and B-cell chronic lymphocytic leukemia are currently in use. For example, rituximab (Rituxan) is used in the treatment of non-Hodgkin lymphoma and trastuzumab (Herceptin) for metastatic breast cancer whose tumors express *HER-2*. There is also interest in the use of vaccines as active-specific immunotherapy for cancer treatment. Human papillomavirus vaccine is used as a prophylactic cervical cancer vaccine. Many strategies for generating therapeutic responses to cancer have been attempted. Of these the most promising include antigen-specific vaccines, dendritic cell vaccines, and whole tumor cell vaccines.[32] However, in spite of advances in the understanding of tumor immunology, the realization of effective therapeutic cancer vaccines to date has been below expectations.[33]

Oral Mucositis

Treatment of cancer is increasingly more effective but is associated with short- and long-term side effects. Oral side effects remain a major source of illness despite the use of a variety of agents to prevent them. One of these side effects is oral mucositis. Oral mucositis may produce oral discomfort and pain, poor nutrition, delays in drug administration, increased hospital stays and costs and, in some patients, life threatening infection.

Patients receiving chemotherapy and/or radiation therapy often develop oral mucositis, which can significantly complicate cancer treatment. The risk of oral mucositis increases as a function of the type of cancer therapy used, with the lowest risk occurring with "gentler" chemotherapeutics such as gemcitabine (Gemzar) and the higher risk occurring with more aggressive agents such as 5-FU and cisplatin and/or radiation therapy.[34] Mucositis is commonly encountered with drugs affecting DNA synthesis (S-phase-specific agents such as fluorouracil, methotrexate, and cytarabine). Mucositis may limit the patient's ability to tolerate chemotherapy or radiation therapy, and nutritional status can be compromised. It may drastically affect cancer treatment as well as the patient's quality of life. The incidence and severity of mucositis will vary from patient to patient. It will also vary from treatment to treatment. It is estimated that there is 40% incidence of mucositis in patients treated with standard chemotherapy and this will not only increase with the number of treatment cycles but also with previous episodes.[35] Similarly, patients who undergo bone marrow transplantation and who receive high doses of chemotherapy have a 76% chance of getting mucositis. The overall incidence of oral mucositis and xerostomia is approximately 80% in patients with squamous cell carcinoma of the head and neck who are treated with radiation therapy directed at the oral and pharyngeal regions.[36] The exact pathophysiology of mucositis is not known, but it is thought to be divided into direct and indirect mucositis. Chemotherapy and/or radiation therapy will interfere with the normal turnover of epithelial cells leading to mucosal injury; subsequently, it can also occur due to indirect invasion of gram-negative bacteria and fungal species because many chemotherapeutic agents will cause changes in infection resistance.

Oral mucositis is typically diagnosed based on the clinical appearance, location, timing of oral lesions, and use of certain types of therapy known to be associated with mucositis. Other common conditions can have a similar clinical presentation to oral mucositis and may confuse the differential diagnosis. They include oral candidiasis, herpes simplex virus, and graft-versus-host disease in transplant patients. Chemoradiation-induced mucosal injury (mucositis) is the result of a complex series of biological and cellular events that take place predominantly in the submucosa with the epithelium being the target tissue.[37] Radiation and chemotherapy create both DNA and non-DNA damage. Clonogenic cell death of the basal epithelial cells occurs as a consequence of DNA strand breaks. The products of this stage then set in motion a cascade of biological and cellular occurrences in the submucosa that ultimately results in death of basal epithelial cells.

Several scoring systems have been devised to assess the severity of oral mucositis and its treatment, but no one scale is uniformly employed. The two most common scales are those proposed by the World Health Organization and the National Cancer Institute Common Toxicity Criteria (Tables 15.5 and 15.6).

Topical drugs such as local anesthetics, analgesics, and coating drugs have been used in cancer patients to manage mucosal pain. Epstein et al. reported that the use of an oral rinse of doxepin in the management of pain from oral mucositis produced a reduction in oral pain by more than 50% with an extended duration of action.[38] In a follow-up study in oncology patients only, 90% of 51 patients reported a reduction in pain after rinsing with doxepin.[39] Pain reduction was highly statistically significant in the first 15 minutes after rinsing with doxepin ($P < .0001$) and at the height of pain reduction, the average patient reported 70% less pain compared to baseline ($P < .0001$). Four hours after rinsing, 19 patients (37%) still reported continuing pain reduction on the visual Analog Scale (VAS) ($P = .012$). Doxepin suspension (5 mg/mL) was prepared in an oral rinse containing 0.1% alcohol and sorbitol. Patients rinsed with 5 mL of the solution in their mouth for 1 minute and expectorated.

Worthington et al. reported on interventions used for preventing oral mucositis in cancer patients receiving treatment.[40] Four interventions were identified where there was more than one trial contributing to a meta-analysis finding a significant difference: amifostine, Chinese medicine, hydrolytic enzyme, and ice chips. Three of these, amifostine, hydrolytic enzymes ad Chinese medicine were assessed in patients with head and neck cancer, and ice chips in two studies were used on patients having chemotherapy treatment with bolus dose 5-FU, and in a third study patients received the single-agent melphalan. Clarkson et al.[41] reported on interventions used for treating oral mucositis. The evidence was weak and unreliable that allopurinol mouthwash, granulocyte macrophage-colony stimulating factor, immunoglobulin, or human placental extract improved or eradicated mucositis. There was no evidence that opioids administered by patient-controlled analgesia (PCA) were better than continuous infusion for controlling pain; however, less opioid was used per hour, and duration of pain was shorter with PCA only.

Graft Versus Host Disease

The hallmark of bone marrow transplantation is the reinfusion of marrow-derived hematopoietic stem cells to reconstitute hematopoiesis following conditioning with high-dose chemotherapy and/or radiation. Allogeneic hematopoietic stem-cell transplantation (HSCT) is a curative therapy for hematological malignancies and inherited disorders of blood cells, such as sickle cell anemia. Mature $\alpha\beta$ T cells that are contained in the allografts reconstitute T-cell immunity and can eradicate malignant cells in the recipient. Unfortunately, these T cells recognize the recipient as "nonself" and employ a wide range of immune mechanisms to attack recipient tissues in a process known as graft-versus-host disease (GVHD). Despite advances in the procedure and post-transplantation immunosuppressive therapy, more than half of HSCT recipients develop GVHD which remains a major cause of morbidity and mortality.[42] GVHD is characterized by the development

TABLE 15.6

NATIONAL CANCER INSTITUTE COMMON TOXICITY CRITERIA VERSION 3 SCORING CRITERIA FOR ORAL MUCOSITIS

Mucositis Functional/Symptomatic Score	
Grade 0	No mucositis
Grade 1	Able to eat solids
Grade 2	Requires liquid diet
Grade 3	Alimentation not possible
Grade 4	Symptoms associated with life-threatening consequences
Mucositis/Stomatitis Clinical Score	
Grade 0	No mucositis
Grade 1	Erythema of the mucosa
Grade 2	Patchy ulceration or pseudomembrane
Grade 3	Confluent ulcerations or pseudomembranes
Grade 4	Tissue necrosis

TABLE 15.5

WORLD HEALTH ORGANIZATION SCORING CRITERIA FOR ORAL MUCOSITIS

Grade	Observation
0	Normal
1	Soreness with or without erythema; no ulceration
2	Ulceration and erythema; patient can swallow a solid diet
3	Ulceration and erythema; patient cannot swallow a solid diet
4	Ulceration and pseudomembrane formation of such severity that alimentation not possible

of features reminiscent of various autoimmune or immunologic disorders, such as scleroderma, Sjogren syndrome, chronic immunodeficiency, and bronchiolitis obliterans. GVHD usually involves the skin, eyes, oral cavity, gastrointestinal tract, liver, and lungs. Symptoms typically present within 2 years following HSCT and are historically identified as limited or extensive.

Acute GVHD occurs within the first 100 days posttransplant and is clinically graded according to skin, liver, and gastrointestinal involvement. Manifestations can include more inflammatory and acute-type features such as erythematous rash, mucositis, diarrhea, transaminitis, and bronchiolitis obliterans with organizing pneumonia (BOOP), or can be more fibrotic and chronic in nature such as sclerotic or lichen planus-type skin changes, fasciitis, sicca syndrome, esophageal strictures, and bronchiolitis obliterans. In addition to these more commonly involved systems listed above, many other organ systems can be affected. Factors such as thrombocytopenia, extensive skin involvement, weight loss and chronic diarrhea have previously been established as risk factors for and prognostic indicators of GVHD. Standard GVHD frontline therapy typically consists of cyclosporine with corticosteroids but only approximately 70% of patients respond.[43] Current treatment options for GVHD include intense immunosuppression, which in turn has associated side effects, an increased risk of infective complications, and a potential for increased relapse of hematological malignancy. Strategies to prevent GVHD include T-cell depletion, immunosuppression, gut decontamination, and appropriate donor selection.[44] Cyclosporin and/or methotrexate have formed the basis of many GVHD prophylaxis strategies.

Postdural Puncture Headache and Chemotherapy

In oncology, dural puncture is a commonly performed invasive procedure for diagnostic lumbar puncture and intrathecal chemotherapy. The overall incidence of postdural puncture headache (PDPH) after intentional dural puncture varies from 0.1 to 36%; the highest incidence of 36% is found after ambulatory diagnostic lumbar puncture using a 20- or 22-gauge standard Quincke spinal needle.[45] Unintentional dural puncture with large Tuohy needle (16 and 18 gauge) is typically associated with a 75% to 85% incidence of PDPH.[46] In this study, 48% were classified "severe" and, in 49%, the headache presented within 24 hours of dural puncture.[46] Headaches appear to occur more frequently in women than in men and more commonly in young adults and in patients prone to headaches. Spinal needle tip and design play a significant role in the development in PDPH. Apan et al.[47] demonstrated in an in vitro model in situations of varying pressures that the least amount of leak occurred with small diameter (25-gauge and 26-gauge) pencil point needles, such as the Whitacre needle.

The classic description of PDPH is that of a frontal or occipital headache that is present or aggravated by assuming the upright position and essentially disappears when returning to the supine position. The pain may be throbbing in nature, often radiates to the neck, and is extremely variable in severity. Other symptoms include nausea, vomiting, neck stiffness, and ocular and auditory disturbances (photophobia, diplopia, hypoacusia, tinnitus), and, rarely cranial nerve palsies. The onset and duration of PDPH can be extremely variable. Most occur within 48 hours of dural puncture and are self-limited, lasting only days.

Although not universally accepted, most investigators favor the "leakage theory" as an explanation for PDPH. Theoretically, leakage of cerebrospinal fluid (CSF) through the dural rent causes decreased CSF pressure and volume, followed by gravity-dependent downward sagging of the brain resulting in traction on the pain-sensitive vascular structures around the brain. However, the amount of CSF leak, as demonstrated on magnetic resonance imaging (MRI), has not been shown to correlate with the incidence of headache[48] and some patients with typical features of PDPH may also have normal CSF pressures.[49] The other major mechanism thought to be responsible for PDPH is cerebral vasodilatation due to loss of CSF.[50] The successful use of epidural blood patch for the treatment of PDPH is based on the assumption that the injection of autologous blood at the site of the lumbar puncture seals the leaking rent. However, because of the relatively rapid effect of the patch in relieving the headache (often within 1 hour), the injected blood also may affect pressure dynamics within the CSF and effectively reverse cerebral vasodilation associated with CSF leak rather than stop additional CSF flow. On the basis of these findings, Boezaart et al.[50] proposed that PDPH is probably a vascular-type headache and that epidural blood patch relieves the headache by its vasoconstrictive action.

Current treatment strategies (which do not have good-quality outcome evidence) for PDPH include oral or intravenous caffeine, theophylline, sumatriptan, adrenocorticotrophic hormone, epidural saline, and epidural blood patch. The gold standard for treatment of PDPH in symptomatic patients is epidural blood patch. Persistent symptomatic relief can be expected in 61% to 75% of patients with the initial epidural blood patch.[51] Patching with nonblood solutions, although initially effective, seems to be associated with a higher incidence of headache recurrence.

Several techniques have been tried in an attempt to reduce the incidence of PDPH. The maintenance of the supine position after dural puncture is ineffective. The use of prophylactic epidural blood patches is controversial. Scavone et al.[52] noted no difference in either a decreased incidence of PDPH or the need for therapeutic epidural patch when a prophylactic epidural blood patch was administered to parturients after inadvertent dural puncture with an epidural needle. However, in this study of 64 parturients who incurred an accidental dural puncture, prophylactic epidural blood patch did shorten the duration of PDPH symptoms.

In our practice, patients who present with PDPH with functional limitations typically receive an epidural blood patch after we ascertain that there is neither neutropenia nor thrombocytopenia. If a patient's headache recurs, a second blood patch is done, preferably under fluoroscopic guidance to ensure accuracy of placement of the blood. In patients with refractory headaches, a short course of steroids may then be considered if medical circumstances allow. With truly refractory headaches, it is important to eliminate the possibility of intracranial subdural hematoma with a computed tomography (CT) scan.[53]

SURGERY

Surgery plays an important role in diagnosis, staging, and treatment of cancer. It also contributes to cancer prevention, structural and functional reconstruction with rehabilitation, and palliation of symptoms. The surgeon responsible for treating a patient with newly-diagnosed cancer has four tasks: (1) obtaining a biopsy for tissue diagnosis, (2) being involved in adequate staging of disease, (3) obtaining consultation with medical and radiation oncologists for adjuvant therapy, and (4) the appropriate timing of the surgical resection. Surgeons are also involved with the treatment of relapses or recurrence and may also play a role in the relief of symptoms caused by specific problems, such as visceral obstruction, unstable bone structures, and compression of neural tissues. Various surgical disciplines (eg, general surgery, orthopedic, neurosurgical, urologic, plastic, and reconstructive) may participate in the care of the cancer patient. Surgery is and has been the main treatment modality for solid tumors. Surgeons performing radical oncologic procedures have traditionally been involved with surgeries such as pelvic exenteration, abdominoperineal resection, limb amputation, liver resection, and esophagogastric resection. The basic principles of surgical oncology involve local tumor excision, regional lymph node removal, the management of local or regional recurrence, and the possibility of surgical resection of distant metastases.

Surgery for breast, colon, and lung cancer have become more conservative in the last 30 years of the twentieth century. Mastectomy (either radical or modified radical) had been the mainstay of the treatment of stage I and stage II breast cancer until the late 1970s. Although mastectomy still may be appropriate for some patients, breast conservation has become the preferred method of treatment, particularly for appropriately selected patients with early-stage breast cancer.[54] Organ-sparing surgery, laparoscopy, robotics systems, and image-guided ablation techniques have enabled surgeons to develop specifically tailored treatments for patients with urologic cancers.

Surgery is an important factor in tumor treatment outcome. Differences in the quality of surgery are significant contributors to wide variations in outcome of local treatment of most solid tumors.[55] For example, the influence of adequate surgical margins on the risk of recurrence is well established in the treatment of osteosarcoma[56-58] and soft-tissue sarcoma.[59] Surgical treatment is preferable for sarcoma and most commonly is performed in specialized centers.[60] Local recurrence after breast preservation may be the result of inappropriate patient selection or inadequate surgery and may contribute to the increased risk of breast cancer ecurrence. Lymphatic mapping and sentinel lymph node biopsy have become a promising alternative to axillary lymph node dissection with its associated morbidity.[61] The best chance of curing esophageal cancer requires surgery that removes the entire tumor and the draining lymph nodes with adequate proximal and distal margins.[62] Integration of γ probes into surgical oncologic procedures is becoming more established. A γ probe can facilitate localization of radio-labeled parathyroid glands.[63] γ probe-guided localization of nonpalpable breast cancers is highly accurate when the radioactive tracer used for sentinel node identification is injected close to the primary tumor.[64] Surgery is the preferred treatment option for otherwise healthy patients with pancreatic cancer without metastases. Tumors of the pancreatic head and the periampullary region can be resected using pancreaticoduodenectomy (with or without preservation of the pylorus), whereas a distal pancreatectomy can be performed for tumors of the pancreatic body and tail. In most cases, a splenectomy has to be performed when tumor localization and surgical technique do not permit preservation of the splenic vessels. Primary melanomas are now excised with narrower surgical margins of 1 to 2 cm. Sentinel-node biopsy is recommended as a nodal staging procedure in patients with tumor thickness of 1 mm and more, but the prognostic impact of this procedure has not yet been demonstrated.[65] The technique of retroperitoneal lymph node dissection is routinely performed in many gynecological cancer centers as a staging procedure or as part of surgical management of cervical and endometrial cancers. This procedure can be performed laparoscopically or as an open procedure. Extensive pelvic surgical procedures such as pelvic exenteration can also be performed laparoscopically.[66] Included in the advantages for laparoscopic surgery are cost-efficiency based on the reduction of hospital stay and recovery time.[67] Minimally-invasive approaches have revolutionized surgical care, significantly reducing postoperative pain and recovery time, with marked improvements in cosmetic outcome. Surgical advances in neuro-oncology for brain tumors have centered around technological advances that enable the fusion of preoperative structural and functional imaging datasets, the use of intraoperative MRI scanning, and awake craniotomy and cortical mapping as means to maximize resection, minimize postoperative morbidity, and improve survival times.[68]

Robotic surgery has the potential to transform laparoscopic surgery by providing instruments with distal ends that mimic the intricate movements of the human hand while at the same time providing the surgeon with a high-definition, 3D view of the operative field. Advantages over laparoscopy include a 3D vision system, wristed instrumentation, and ergonomic positioning for the surgeon while performing surgical procedures. The only FDA-approved system in the United States is the Da Vinci system. Robotic-assisted laparoscopic surgeries in gynecology include benign hysterectomy, myomectomy, tubal reanastomoses, radical hysterectomy, lymph node dissections, and sacrocolpopexies.[69] Laparoscopic-assisted and robotic-assisted urological procedures have been performed for radical cystectomy[70] and cystoprostatectomy.[71]

Only 10% to 20% of patients with primary and colorectal metastatic liver tumors are candidates for curative surgical resection.[72] Even after presumptive curative treatment, tumors recur commonly in the liver. The majority of patients with primary or metastatic hepatic tumors are not candidates for resection because of tumor size, location near major intrahepatic blood vessels precluding a margin-negative resection, multifocality, or inadequate hepatic function related to coexistent cirrhosis. Radiofrequency thermal ablation (RFA) of primary, metastatic, and recurrent liver tumors can be performed under percutaneous, laparoscopic, or open intraoperative ultrasound guidance. The local recurrence rate at 2 years was statistically significant in favor of RFA over percutaneous ethanol injection for treatment of hepatocellular carcinoma.[73]

The decision to proceed with major surgery in patients with advanced cancer requires judgment of the patient's expected survival time, overall fitness for major surgery, and the anticipated morbidity of the proposed procedure. The decision to pursue a major surgical intervention is often controversial when it is not likely to be curative and has symptom relief as its only objective. This form of palliative therapy most often involves patients with later stages of disease. Although the development of metastatic cancer usually indicates incurable disease, curative surgical resection can be accomplished in rare instances: the primary lesion must be controlled; there must be the potential for complete resection of the metastases; there must be no other equally effective or better antitumor therapy available; metastases should involve only one organ; one should anticipate reasonable postoperative function; expected survival should be better than if left untreated; and the patient must be able to tolerate the surgical procedure. Rarely, excision of the primary tumor is indicated in the presence of unresectable metastatic disease. Locally advanced tumor can be very painful and unsightly, can interfere with vital functions such as breathing and swallowing, and produce complications such as bleeding and local infection. Surgical judgment is critical in such situations.

Multidisciplinary management of cancer is more effective than sequential monotherapies and results in more cures and improved organ and overall function preservation. Surgery is suitable for local and regional disease and may result in cures in early stages of cancer, especially when there is an early detection policy. In patients with localized but extensive tumors, surgery may prove valuable in improving the quality of life and potentially in prolonging life.

Surgical oncology is not recognized universally as a distinct discipline within surgery. Surgeons who regard themselves as surgical oncologists fall into two broad but distinct categories: those who regard themselves as general surgical oncologists, able to operate on most tumors and who have a minimal practice in benign pathology; and those who are anatomically specific and treat patients with complex disorders. As the treatment of patients with cancer becomes progressively more complex and multidisciplinary, various organizations have attempted to set guidelines and standards for care. For example, in 1998, three colleges (the American College of Surgeons, the American College of Radiology, and the College of American Pathologists), the American Cancer Society, and the Society of Surgical Oncology reported on standards for diagnosis and management of invasive breast cancer.[74] The American Board of Medical Specialties (ABMS) comprises 24 medical specialty member boards and is responsible for overseeing the certification of physician specialists in the United States. The primary function of ABMS is to assist its member boards in developing and implementing educational and professional standards to evaluate and certify physician specialists. Of the recognized surgical specialties, only obstetrics and gynecology has subspecialty certification in oncology care (gynecologic oncology).

As a field of distinct expertise, surgical oncology is relatively new. The Society of Surgical Oncology defines guidelines for surgical oncology fellowships and approves 19 programs across the United States. The objective of the fellowship is to expand basic surgical knowledge and experience obtained during residency to develop skilled surgeon-investigators who will become recognized experts in the field of surgical oncology. The Society has 1,927 members in 48 states and 43 foreign countries. Membership consists of surgeons, scientists, and other health care providers who are significantly involved in oncologic patient care. This specialty is not recognized by the American Board of Medical Specialties (ABMS).

The National Cancer Institute's (NCI) Surgical Oncology Fellowship Program trains surgeons committed to academic careers in surgical oncology. The program instructs surgical oncologists in a combined modality approach to the evaluation and treatment of cancer patients that includes primary surgical treatment, chemotherapy, immunotherapy, and radiation therapy, and provides a solid basis for the conduct of clinical and laboratory research. This program is a 2-year training program of which 6 months of the first year are dedicated to clinical training in surgical oncology with rotations on various clinical surgical services. Eighteen months are spent in one of the laboratories of the Surgery Branch dedicated to basic science and translational research. Surgical oncology is not recognized as a subspecialty in all European countries. A major objective of the European Society of Surgical Oncology is to promote education in cancer surgery. Worldwide, other regions are also moving towards the development of a subspecialty in surgical oncology. Advancement in this area will improve the surgical aspects of care of the oncology patient.

STENTING AND DRAINAGE PROCEDURES

Neoplastic visceral obstruction occurs because of direct tumor infiltration or compression or metastatic involvement of lymph nodes. Obstructions of the gastrointestinal, hepatobiliary, and ureteric systems are the most common in patients with advanced cancer. The signs and symptoms of visceral obstruction are organ specific and therefore bowel obstruction, pain, jaundice, and renal insufficiency or failure may occur. Relief of the obstruction takes priority over other treatments in hopes of improving symptoms and palliating the disease process. The clinical presentation of ureteral obstruction due to advanced pelvic or abdominal malignancy can be a slow process with vague and nonspecific symptoms, such as flank discomfort or lethargy, or it may present as acute obstruction with intense pain, nausea, and vomiting. Unrelieved obstructive uropathy may result in uremia, electrolyte imbalances, and persistent urinary tract infections. Treatment of ureteral obstruction is challenging. Many patients in need of stenting are poor surgical candidates. The two common methods for urinary diversion after obstructive malignancy are retrograde ureteral stenting and percutaneous nephrostomy. Both techniques can result in leaking, tube movement, and tube dislodgment, and stenting may not completely resolve the secondary problems or it may not relieve obstruction. Stent insertion is typically performed under fluoroscopic guidance. Although intrinsic ureteral obstruction is highly amenable to endoscopic ureteral stents in cases of intrinsic obstruction (stone disease, ureteral strictures, or ureteropelvic junction obstruction), the incidence of stent failure is significantly higher in cases of extrinsic compression, particularly when accompanied by hydronephrosis.[75] Percutaneous tubes are generally placed under ultrasound or CT guidance. Difficult clinical situations may require alternative procedures such as palliative cutaneous ureterostomy, percutaneous anterograde ureteric stent placement, and a combined anterograde and retrograde technique.

Common causes of malignant biliary obstruction include pancreatic cancer, cholangiocarcinoma, and metastatic disease, either intrahepatic or from lymphadenopathy. The majority of these patients will not undergo surgical resection of the obstructing tumor due to either the advanced nature of the disease or the significant morbidity associated with surgery. The insertion of internal biliary stents (plastic or metal) by endoscopic or percutaneous methods is common practice for the palliative management of obstructive jaundice caused by malignancy, and most surgeons prefer this to the use of external biliary drains.[76] For the treatment of malignant biliary obstructions in patients with pancreatic carcinoma, endoscopic biliary drainage is the option of first choice.[77] Drainage at endoscopic retrograde cholangiopancreatography (ERCP) compared to percutaneous drainage is safer and more successful than percutaneous drainage.[78] Gastrojejunostomy is the most commonly used palliative treatment modality for malignant gastric outlet obstruction. Endoscopic stent placement may be associated with more favorable results in patients with a relatively short life expectancy, whereas gastrojejunostomy is preferable in patients with a more prolonged prognosis.[79] Because gastric outlet obstruction is a frequent feature of advanced pancreatic carcinoma, self-expandable metal stents (SEMS) allow this problem to be managed relatively simply by endoscopy rather than surgical bypass.[80] Phillips et al.[81] showed that SEMS effectively palliate gastric outlet obstructions that result from upper gastrointestinal malignancies. Stents and laser treatment have a place in both upper gastrointestinal and rectal obstruction due to advanced malignancy.[82–84] Colonic stents potentially offer effective palliation for patients with malignant bowel obstruction, and a "bridge to surgery" for those in whom emergency surgery would necessitate a stoma. SEMS placement may result in the avoidance of surgical resection in patients with metastatic disease. The presence of metastases at the time of surgery is an independent predictor of operative mortality in colorectal surgery[85] and stenting also has the potential benefit of avoiding surgery and possible stoma formation, even on a temporary basis, in these patients. Preoperatively, failure of contrast to pass through an obstructive bowel lesion is a predictor of technical failure of SEMS insertion.[86] Patients with locally unresectable tumors may benefit particularly from endoscopic placement of SEMS.[87]

Malignant pleural effusion can be the first sign of cancer or of its recurrence. Approximately 50% of effusions are malignant and only a minority benefit from suitable systemic treatment. Effusions can recur rapidly and often are disabling. Most patients with malignant pleural effusion are symptomatic; common presenting complaints are shortness of breath, cough, chest pain, and a sense of fullness within the chest. Treatment is directed toward relief of these symptoms. When thoracentesis is repeated frequently over a number of months to treat dyspnea, the resulting depletion in ions, fluid, and proteins contributes to the deterioration in the patient's general condition. No more than 1500 mL of fluid should be removed by thoracentesis at a single session. Pleurodesis (adhesion of the parietal and visceral pleura) is the symptomatic treatment of choice and should be considered as early as possible in the course of chronic malignant pleural effusions. Intrapleural instillation of chemicals is done via thoroscopy in an attempt to produce pleurodesis. Various agents including tetracycline, doxycycline, minocycline, bleomycin, fluorouracil, and talc have been used for chemical pleurodesis. Talc is generally insufflated to the lung surface through a thoracoscope under general anesthesia. Safron et al.[88] described an outpatient pleurodesis with 4 grams of talc through a 14 French pigtail catheter. Once drainage had diminished to less than 100 mL/day, the patient returned for sclerotherapy. Sclerotherapy was accomplished by instillation of 50 mL of 1% lidocaine followed by 4 g of talc slurry and 20 mL of saline solution flush. It was thought to cause pleural symphysis as a result of reactive pleuritis.[89] Of the agents used for pleurodesis, talc appears to be the most effective.[90] No more than 5 grams of talc should be used for pleurodesis.[91]

Malignant ascites can lead to abdominal distention, nausea, early satiety, anorexia, and in severe cases, respiratory compromise. It is associated with a variety of tumors, especially, breast bronchus, ovary, stomach, pancreas, and colon .[92] Paracentesis and diuretics are the most commonly used measures for treatment .[93] Frequent drainage may be necessary to relieve pain and discomfort. Sonographically-guided paracentesis is commonly used for palliation of symptomatic malignant ascites. Permanent percutaneous catheters may prevent the need for repeated paracentesis, although there is potential for infection. Peritoneovenous shunts have also been recommended for the treatment of refractory ascites.[94] These shunts are designed for continuous drainage of ascites into the systemic circulation and can be placed surgically or percutaneously. Early use of this system (all placed surgically) has been discouraging, with reported morbidity rates of 60% to 70%, shunt-related mortality rates of 10% to 35%, and shunt patency rates of 20% to 40%.[95–96] However, with the development of radiological interventional techniques, a shunt system can now be placed percutaneously. Using this technique, better results have been reported, particularly if patients with a history of variceal bleeding are excluded.[94] Becker et al.[97] provided guidelines on the management of symptomatic malignant ascites in advanced cancer (Table 15.7).

ANTIBIOTICS FOR PALLIATION

The goals of antibiotic use in terminally ill patients are sometimes to prolong life, and always to relieve symptoms. Treatment for cystitis does not usually prolong life, but may relieve the patient from painful dysuria and troublesome polyuria. Antibiotics may also have pain-relieving effects when the source of pain involves

TABLE 15.7

GUIDELINES FOR THE MANAGEMENT OF SYMPTOMATIC MALIGNANT ASCITES IN ADVANCED CANCER

1. Paracentesis is indicated for those patients who have symptoms of increasing intra-abdominal pressure. Available data show good, although temporary relief of symptoms in most patients. Symptoms like discomfort, dyspnea, nausea, and vomiting seem to be significantly relieved by drainage of up to 5 L of fluid.
2. When removing up to 5 L of fluid, intravenous fluids are not routinely required.
3. If patient is hypotensive or dehydrated or known to have severe renal impairment and paracentesis is still indicated, intravenous hydration should be considered. Infusion therapy is not sufficiently studied. The only investigated therapy in malignant ascites is infusion of dextrose 5%. There is no evidence for efficacy of concurrent albumin infusions in patients with malignant ascites.
4. To avoid repeated paracenteses, peritoneovenous shunting may be considered. Major complications (pulmonary edema, pulmonary emboli, clinically relevant disseminated intravascular coagulation, and infection) have to be expected in about 6% of patients.
5. There are no randomized controlled trials assessing the efficacy of diuretic therapy in malignant ascites. The available data are controversial and there are no clear predictors to identify which patients would benefit from diuretics. The use of diuretics therefore should be considered in all patients, but has to be evaluated individually. Patients with malignant ascites due to massive hepatic metastasis seem more likely to respond - to diuretics than patients with malignant ascites caused by peritoneal carcinomatosis or chylous ascites.
6. Choice of diuretics is not evaluated. As available data suggest that the efficacy of diuretics in malignant ascites depends on plasma renin/aldosterone concentration, aldosterone antagonists like spironolactone should be used, either alone or in combination with a loop diuretic.
7. Dose regimens of diuretics are not evaluated in patients with malignant ascites. There is no evidence to diverge from standard clinical practice. Therefore dosage should be performed according to manufacturer's instructions and package inserts.

(From Becker G, Galandi D, Blum HE. Malignant ascites: Systematic review and guideline for treatment. *Eur J Cancer.* 2006;42:589–597.)

infection, as illustrated by the treatment of pyonephrosis and osteitis pubis. Delayed breast cellulitis is primarily related to a bacterial infection in the setting of impaired lymphatic drainage and may appear months after completion of radiation therapy in patients undergoing breast conserving therapy (primarily lumpectomy and radiation therapy).[98] It is characterized by the late onset of breast erythema, edema, tenderness, and warmth. Delayed breast cellulitis may be treated conservatively with antibiotics to cover β-hemolytic *Streptococci spp.* and *Staphlococcus aureus* for 10 to 14 days. Terminally ill patients are susceptible to infections during the final phases of their care.[99] Infections increase symptom burden and decrease quality of life. Urinary and respiratory infections dominate. First-line therapy in cases of urinary sepsis, trimethoprim, cephalexin, and amoxycillin are effective agents. Cotrimoxazole and amoxycillin are effective agents for respiratory infections. Head and neck cancer patients who receive radiation therapy are at risk for *Candida* colonization in the oral cavity.[100] *Candida* species are the most common fungal pathogens isolated from the oral cavity. *Candida* species are responsible for all but exceptional examples of oral fungal infection. Oral candidiasis is relatively common occurring in approximately 25% of patients receiving radiation therapy for head and neck cancer.[101] Previously *Candida albicans* was the most common pathogen, but non–albicans *Candida* (in particular *Candida glabrata*) is emerging as a relatively common cause of oropharyngeal candidiasis in head-and-neck cancer patients.[101-102] The infections can be acute or chronic, pseudomembranous ("thrush") or atrophic (erythematous). Oropharyngeal candidiasis manifests clinically as acute pseudomembranous, acute atrophic, chronic atrophic, chronic hypertrophic/hyperplastic, and angular cheilitis. Infection is marked by oral pain and/or burning and can lead to significant patient morbidity. As an opportunistic organism, *Candida albicans* is extremely responsive to any process resulting in immunosuppression. Oral nystatin, clotrimazole, and fluconazole are the usual treatments. Fluconazole in doses of 100 mg/day is predominantly used to treat oropharyngeal candidiasis. Development of resistance to fluconazole in these patients has become a growing concern and usually is correlated with the degree of immunosuppression and the total dose of drug. If resistance to fluconazole does occur, its occurrence may be due to the presence of yeasts other than *C. albicans*, which are less susceptible to fluconazole.

References

1. Sepucha KR, Belkora JK, Mutchnick S, et al. Consultation planning to help breast cancer patients prepare for medical consultations: Effect on communication and satisfaction for patients and physicians. *J Clin Oncol.* 2002;20:2695–2700.
2. Katz SJ, Lantz PM, Janz NK, et al. Patient involvement in surgery treatment decisions for breast cancer. *J Clin Oncol.* 2005;23: 5526–5533.
3. Harris TJ, Hipkiss EL, Borzillary S, et al. Radiotherapy augments the immune response to prostate cancer in a time-dependent manner. *Prostate.* 2008;68:1319–1329.
4. Molassiotis A, Fernadez-Ortega P, Pud D, et al. Use of complementary and alternative medicine in cancer patients: A European survey. *Ann Oncol.* 2005;16:655–663.
5. Bernstein BJ, Grasso T. Prevalence of complementary and alternative medicine use in cancer patients. Oncology (Williston Park). 2001;15:1267–1272;discussion 1272–1278, 1283.
6. Richardson MA, Sanders T, Palmer JL, et al. Complementary/alternative medicine use in a comprehensive cancer center and the implications for oncology. *J Clin Oncol.* 2000;18:2505–2514.
7. Owen JB, Coia LR, Hanks GE. Recent patterns of growth in radiation therapy facilities in the United States: A patterns of care study report. *Int J Radiat Oncol Biol Phys.* 1992;24:983–986.
8. Munro TR. The site of the target region for radiation-induced mitotic delay in cultured mammalian cells. *Radiat Res.* 1970;44:747–757.
9. Chang SD, Main W, Martin DP, et al. An analysis of the accuracy of the CyberKnife: A robotic frameless stereotactic radiosurgical system. *Neurosurgery.* 2003;52:140–6;discussion 146–147.
10. Johansson S, Svensson H, Denekamp J. Timescale of evolution of late radiation injury after postoperative radiotherapy of breast cancer patients. *Int J Radiat Oncol Biol Phys.* 2000;48:745–750.
11. Gillette EL, Mahler PA, Powers BE, et al. Late radiation injury to muscle and peripheral nerves. *Int J Radiat Oncol Biol Phys.* 1995;31:1309–1318.

12. Hoff AO, Gagel RF. Osteoporosis in breast and prostate cancer survivors. *Oncology (Williston Park)*. 2005;19:651–658.
13. Prevention and management of osteoporosis. *World Health Organ Tech Rep Ser*. 2003;921:1–164.
14. Kaste SC, Chesney RW, Hudson MM, et al. Bone mineral status during and after therapy of childhood cancer: An increasing population with multiple risk factors for impaired bone health. *J Bone Miner Res*. 1999;14:2010–2014.
15. Ballonoff A, Chen C, Raben D. Current radiation therapy management issues in oral cavity cancer. *Otolaryngol Clin North Am*. 2006;39:365–380.
16. Gibbs IC, Le QT, Shah RD, et al. Long-term outcomes after external beam irradiation and brachytherapy boost for base-of-tongue cancers. *Int J Radiat Oncol Biol Phys*. 2003;57:489–494.
17. Jereczek-Fossa BA, Orecchia R. Radiotherapy-induced mandibular bone complications. *Cancer Treat Rev*. 2002;28:65–74.
18. Clarke RE, Tenorio LM, Hussey JR, et al. Hyperbaric oxygen treatment of chronic refractory radiation proctitis: A randomized and controlled double-blind crossover trial with long-term follow-up. *Int J Radiat Oncol Biol Phys*. 2008;72:134–143.
19. Chong KT, Hampson NB, Corman JM. Early hyperbaric oxygen therapy improves outcome for radiation-induced hemorrhagic cystitis. *Urology*. 2005;65:649–653.
20. Yoshida T, Kawashima A, Ujike T, et al. Hyperbaric oxygen therapy for radiation-induced hemorrhagic cystitis. *Int J Urol*. 2008;15:639–641.
21. Feldmeier JJ, Hampson NB. A systematic review of the literature reporting the application of hyperbaric oxygen prevention and treatment of delayed radiation injuries: An evidence based approach. *Undersea Hyperb Med*. 2002;29:4–30.
22. Safra T, Gutman G, Fishlev G, et al. Improved quality of life with hyperbaric oxygen therapy in patients with persistent pelvic radiation-induced toxicity. *Clin Oncol (R Coll Radiol)*. 2008;20:284–287.
23. Dizon DS, Kemeny NE. Intrahepatic arterial infusion of chemotherapy: Clinical results. *Semin Oncol*. 2002;29:126–135.
24. Chumsri S, Phatak P, Edelman JM, et al. Cancer stem cells and individualized therapy. *Cancer Genomics Proteomics*. 2007;4:165–174.
25. Tang C, Ang BT, Pervaiz S. Cancer stem cell: Target for anti-cancer therapy. *Faseb J*. 2007;21:3777–3785.
26. Savage P, Stebbing J, Bower M, et al. Why does cytotoxic chemotherapy cure only some cancers? *Nat Clin Pract Oncol*. 2009;6:43–52.
27. Adachi A, Nagai H, Horikawa T. Anti-SSA/Ro antibody as a risk factor for fluorouracil-induced drug eruptions showing acral erythema and discoid-lupus-erythematosus-like lesions. *Dermatology*. 2007;214:85–88.
28. Weger W, Kranke B, Gerger A, et al. Occurrence of subacute cutaneous lupus erythematosus after treatment with fluorouracil and capecitabine. *J Am Acad Dermatol*. 2008;59:S4–S6.
29. Becker Y. Molecular immunological approaches to biotherapy of human cancers—a review, hypothesis and implications. *Anticancer Res*. 2006;26:1113–1134.
30. Kidd P. Th1/Th2 balance: The hypothesis, its limitations, and implications for health and disease. *Altern Med Rev*. 2003;8:223–246.
31. Pellegrini P, Berghella AM, Del Beato T, et al. Disregulation in TH1 and TH2 subsets of CD4+ T cells in peripheral blood of colorectal cancer patients and involvement in cancer establishment and progression. *Cancer Immunol Immunother*. 1996;42:1–8.
32. Dougan M, Dranoff G. Immune Therapy for Cancer. *Annu Rev Immunol*. 2009;27:83–117.
33. Itoh K, Yamada A, Mine T, et al. Recent advances in cancer vaccines: An overview. *Jpn J Clin Oncol*. 2009;39:73–80.
34. Peterson DE. New strategies for management of oral mucositis in cancer patients. *J Support Oncol*. 2006;4:9–13.
35. Naidu MU, Ramana GV, Rani PU, et al. Chemotherapy-induced and/or radiation therapy-induced oral mucositis—complicating the treatment of cancer. *Neoplasia*. 2004;6:423–431.
36. Trotti A, Bellm LA, Epstein JB, et al. Mucositis incidence, severity and associated outcomes in patients with head and neck cancer receiving radiotherapy with or without chemotherapy: A systematic literature review. *Radiother Oncol*. 2003;66:253–262.
37. Sonis ST. The pathobiology of mucositis. *Nat Rev Cancer*. 2004;4:277–284.
38. Epstein JB, Truelove EL, Oien H, et al. Oral topical doxepin rinse: Analgesic effect in patients with oral mucosal pain due to cancer or cancer therapy. *Oral Oncol*. 2001;37:632–637.
39. Epstein JB, Epstein JD, Epstein MS, et al. Oral doxepin rinse: The analgesic effect and duration of pain reduction in patients with oral mucositis due to cancer therapy. *Anesth Analg*. 2006;103:465–470.
40. Worthington HV, Clarkson JE, Eden OB. Interventions for preventing oral mucositis for patients with cancer receiving treatment. *Cochrane Database Syst Rev*. 2007:CD000978.
41. Clarkson JE, Worthington HV, Eden OB. Interventions for treating oral mucositis for patients with cancer receiving treatment. *Cochrane Database Syst Rev*. 2007:CD001973.
42. Schaffer JV. The changing face of graft-versus-host disease. *Semin Cutan Med Surg*. 2006;25:190–200.
43. Baird K, Pavletic SZ. Chronic graft versus host disease. *Curr Opin Hematol*. 2006;13:426–435.
44. Potter V, Moore J. Randomised trials of graft versus host disease prophylaxis in haemopoietic stem cell transplantation. *Rev Recent Clin Trials*. 2008;3:130–138.
45. Kuntz KM, Kokmen E, Stevens JC, et al. Post-lumbar puncture headaches: Experience in 501 consecutive procedures. *Neurology*. 1992;42:1884–1887.
46. Paech M, Banks S, Gurrin L. An audit of accidental dural puncture during epidural insertion of a Tuohy needle in obstetric patients. *Int J Obstet Anesth*. 2001;10:162–167.
47. Apan A, Uz A, Ugur HC, et al. The effect of changing pressures on dural puncture and leak with various spinal needles on an in vitro model. *J Clin Neurosci*. 2002;9:677–679.
48. Iqbal J, Davis LE, Orrison WW, Jr. An MRI study of lumbar puncture headaches. *Headache*. 1995;35:420–422.
49. Mokri B, Hunter SF, Atkinson JL, et al. Orthostatic headaches caused by CSF leak but with normal CSF pressures. *Neurology*. 1998;51:786–790.
50. Boezaart AP. Effects of cerebrospinal fluid loss and epidural blood patch on cerebral blood flow in swine. *Reg Anesth Pain Med*. 2001;26:401–406.
51. Duffy PJ, Crosby ET. The epidural blood patch. Resolving the controversies. *Can J Anaesth*. 1999;46:878–886.
52. Scavone BM, Wong CA, Sullivan JT, et al. Efficacy of a prophylactic epidural blood patch in preventing post dural puncture headache in parturients after inadvertent dural puncture. *Anesthesiology*. 2004;101:1422–1427.
53. Chiravuri S, Wasserman R, Chawla A, et al. Subdural hematoma following spinal cord stimulator implant. *Pain Physician*. 2008;11:97–101.
54. Jacobson JA, Danforth DN, Cowan KH, et al. Ten-year results of a comparison of conservation with mastectomy in the treatment of stage I and II breast cancer. *N Engl J Med*. 1995;332:907–911.
55. Landheer ML, Therasse P, van de Velde CJ. The importance of quality assurance in surgical oncology. *Eur J Surg Oncol*. 2002;28:571–602.
56. Bacci G, Ferrari S, Longhi A, et al. Pattern of relapse in patients with osteosarcoma of the extremities treated with neoadjuvant chemotherapy. *Eur J Cancer*. 2001;37:32–38.
57. Lindner NJ, Ramm O, Hillmann A, et al. Limb salvage and outcome of osteosarcoma. The University of Muenster experience. *Clin Orthop Relat Res*. 1999:83–89.
58. Weeden S, Grimer RJ, Cannon SR, et al. The effect of local recurrence on survival in resected osteosarcoma. *Eur J Cancer*. 2001;37:39–46.
59. Stotter AT, A'Hern RP, Fisher C, et al. The influence of local recurrence of extremity soft tissue sarcoma on metastasis and survival. *Cancer*. 1990;65:1119–1129.
60. Gustafson P, Dreinhofer KE, Rydholm A. Soft tissue sarcoma should be treated at a tumor center. A comparison of quality of surgery in 375 patients. *Acta Orthop Scand*. 1994;65:47–50.
61. Bass SS, Cox CE, Ku NN, et al. The role of sentinel lymph node biopsy in breast cancer. *J Am Coll Surg*. 1999;189:183–194.
62. Miller JD, Jain MK, de Gara CJ, et al. Effect of surgical experience on results of esophagectomy for esophageal carcinoma. *J Surg Oncol*. 1997;65:20–21.
63. Lal A, Bianco J, Chen H. Radioguided parathyroidectomy in patients with familial hyperparathyroidism. *Ann Surg Oncol*. 2007;14:739–743.
64. van Rijk MC, Tanis PJ, Nieweg OE, et al. Sentinel node biopsy and concomitant probe-guided tumor excision of nonpalpable breast cancer. *Ann Surg Oncol*. 2007;14:627–632.
65. Garbe C, Eigentler TK. Diagnosis and treatment of cutaneous melanoma: State of the art 2006. *Melanoma Res*. 2007;17:117–127.

66. Pomel C, Rouzier R, Pocard M, et al. Laparoscopic total pelvic exenteration for cervical cancer relapse. *Gynecol Oncol.* 2003;91:616–618.
67. Querleu D, Leblanc E, Ferron G, et al. Laparoscopic surgery in gynaecological oncology. *Eur J Surg Oncol.* 2006;32:853–858.
68. Whittle IR. Surgery for gliomas. *Curr Opin Neurol.* 2002;15:663–669.
69. Visco AG, Advincula AP. Robotic Gynecologic Surgery. *Obstet Gynecol.* 2008;112:1369–1384.
70. Haber GP, Crouzet S, Gill IS. Laparoscopic and robotic assisted radical cystectomy for bladder cancer: A critical analysis. *Eur Urol.* 2008;54:54–62.
71. Pruthi RS, Wallen EM. Robotic-assisted laparoscopic radical cystoprostatectomy. *Eur Urol.* 2008;53:310–322.
72. Machi J, Uchida S, Sumida K, et al. Ultrasound-guided radiofrequency thermal ablation of liver tumors: Percutaneous, laparoscopic, and open surgical approaches. *J Gastrointest Surg.* 2001;5:477–489.
73. Sutherland LM, Williams JA, Padbury RT, et al. Radiofrequency ablation of liver tumors: A systematic review. *Arch Surg.* 2006;141:181–190.
74. Winchester DP, Cox JD. Standards for diagnosis and management of invasive breast carcinoma. American College of Radiology. American College of Surgeons. College of American Pathologists. Society of Surgical Oncology. *CA Cancer J Clin.* 1998;48:83–107.
75. Kouba E, Wallen EM, Pruthi RS. Management of ureteral obstruction due to advanced malignancy: Optimizing therapeutic and palliative outcomes. *J Urol.* 2008;180:444–450.
76. Anderson ID, Manson JM, Martin DF, et al. Relief of metastatic biliary obstruction by stent placement: Is it worthwhile? *Surg Oncol.* 1993;2:113–117.
77. Bahra M, Jacob D. Surgical palliation of advanced pancreatic cancer. *Recent Results Cancer Res.* 2008;177:111–120.
78. Stern N, Sturgess R. Endoscopic therapy in the management of malignant biliary obstruction. *Eur J Surg Oncol.* 2008;34:313–317.
79. Jeurnink SM, van Eijck CH, Steyerberg EW, et al. Stent versus gastrojejunostomy for the palliation of gastric outlet obstruction: A systematic review. *BMC Gastroenterol.* 2007;7:18.
80. Morris-Stiff G, Hassn A, Young WT. Self-expanding metal stents for duodenal obstruction in advanced pancreatic adenocarcinoma. *HPB (Oxford).* 2008;10:134–137.
81. Phillips MS, Gosain S, Bonatti H, et al. Enteral stents for malignancy: A report of 46 consecutive cases over 10 years, with critical review of complications. *J Gastrointest Surg.* 2008;12:2045–2050.
82. Spinelli P, Dal Fante M, Mancini A. Self-expanding mesh stent for endoscopic palliation of rectal obstructing tumors: A preliminary report. *Surg Endosc.* 1992;6:72–74.
83. Lightdale CJ. Self-expanding metal stents for esophageal and gastric cancer: A new opening [editorial]. *Gastrointest Endosc.* 1992;38:86–88.
84. Garcia C, Collins T, Ide S, et al. Nd:YAG laser as a therapeutic option in the management of gastrointestinal cancer. *Del Med J.* 1993;65:369–373.
85. Tekkis PP, Poloniecki JD, Thompson MR, et al. Operative mortality in colorectal cancer: Prospective national study. *BMJ.* 2003;327:1196–1201.
86. Davies RJ, D'Sa IB, Lucarotti ME, et al. Bowel function following insertion of self-expanding metallic stents for palliation of colorectal cancer. *Colorectal Dis.* 2005;7:251–253.
87. Ptok H, Marusch F, Steinert R, et al. Incurable stenosing colorectal carcinoma: Endoscopic stent implantation or palliative surgery? *World J Surg.* 2006;30:1481–1487.
88. Saffran L, Ost DE, Fein AM, et al. Outpatient pleurodesis of malignant pleural effusions using a small-bore pigtail catheter. *Chest.* 2000;118:417–421.
89. Bubik JS. Preparation of sterile talc for treatment of pleural effusion. *Am J Hosp Pharm.* 1992;49:562–563.
90. Walker-Renard PB, Vaughan LM, Sahn SA. Chemical pleurodesis for malignant pleural effusions. *Ann Intern Med.* 1994;120:56–64.
91. Viallat JR, Rey F, Astoul P, Boutin C. Thoracoscopic talc poudrage pleurodesis for malignant effusions. A review of 360 cases. *Chest.* 1996;110:1387–1393.
92. Runyon BA. Care of patients with ascites. *N Engl J Med.* 1994;330:337–342.
93. Lee CW, Bociek G, Faught W. A survey of practice in management of malignant ascites. *J Pain Symptom Manage.* 1998;16:96–101.
94. Won JY, Choi SY, Ko HK, et al. Percutaneous peritoneovenous shunt for treatment of refractory ascites. *J Vasc Interv Radiol.* 2008;19:1717–1722.
95. Lund RH, Moritz MW. Complications of Denver peritoneovenous shunting. *Arch Surg.* 1982;117:924–928.
96. Scholz DG, Nagorney DM, Lindor KD. Poor outcome from peritoneovenous shunts for refractory ascites. *Am J Gastroenterol.* 1989;84:540–543.
97. Becker G, Galandi D, Blum HE. Malignant ascites: Systematic review and guideline for treatment. *Eur J Cancer.* 2006;42:589–597.
98. Indelicato DJ, Grobmyer SR, Newlin H, et al. Delayed breast cellulitis: An evolving complication of breast conservation. *Int J Radiat Oncol Biol Phys.* 2006;66:1339–1346.
99. Vitetta L, Kenner D, Sali A. Bacterial infections in terminally ill hospice patients. *J Pain Symptom Manage.* 2000;20:326–334.
100. Jham BC, Reis PM, Miranda EL, et al. Oral health status of 207 head and neck cancer patients before, during and after radiotherapy. *Clin Oral Investig.* 2008;12:19–24.
101. Redding SW, Dahiya MC, Kirkpatrick WR, et al. Candida glabrata is an emerging cause of oropharyngeal candidiasis in patients receiving radiation for head and neck cancer. *Oral Surg Oral Med Oral Pathol Oral Radiol Endod.* 2004;97:47–52.
102. Dahiya MC, Redding SW, Dahiya RS, et al. Oropharyngeal candidiasis caused by nonalbicans yeast in patients receiving external beam radiotherapy for head-and-neck cancer. *Int J Radiat Oncol Biol Phys.* 2003;57:79–83.

CHAPTER 16 ■ SYMPTOM-DIRECTED PAIN MANAGEMENT: MEDICATION

Interdisciplinary collaboration is the cornerstone of management of the cancer patient with pain. It is essential that the managing clinicians understand the cause or causes of pain and direct treatment appropriately and not simply treat the pain as an isolated symptom. Successful management strategies usually require a team approach, focusing not only on the nociceptive processes but also on the many other factors that influence the perception of pain. All options of pain management, which includes source modification, alteration of pain perception, and interruption of nociceptive transmission, should be considered continuously throughout the course of treatment. For example, it is not unusual to manage patients initially with pharmacologic options and then to consider focused therapy as isolated problems emerge (eg, neurolytic intercostal nerve block for an isolated rib metastasis). Figure 16.1 outlines tumor pain management strategies directed at the treatment of nociceptive and neuropathic pain at our institution. It is important to remember that eradication of the tumor with surgery, radiation, or chemotherapy are omitted from this illustration but should be factored into management strategies. Treatment options are highly individualized and multiple therapies may be required in the same patient. It is not unusual to continue oral pharmacotherapy in patients receiving neuraxial infusions. In addition, nerve blocks may be considered at any time during treatment. It is also important that the algorithm applies to *tumor-related* pain only. Different strategies are required for the management of treatment-related and unrelated (usually chronic) pain problems.

Pharmacologic strategies for the control of tumor pain are listed in Table 16.1. The rapidity of response is determined by the urgency for pain control. Patients with severe, unremitting tumor pain may require admission to hospital for additional imaging to determine the source of pain and for parenteral opioid therapy, neuraxial therapy, or both.[1] Patients with less-rapidly progressive pain can usually be treated on an outpatient basis. Most patients

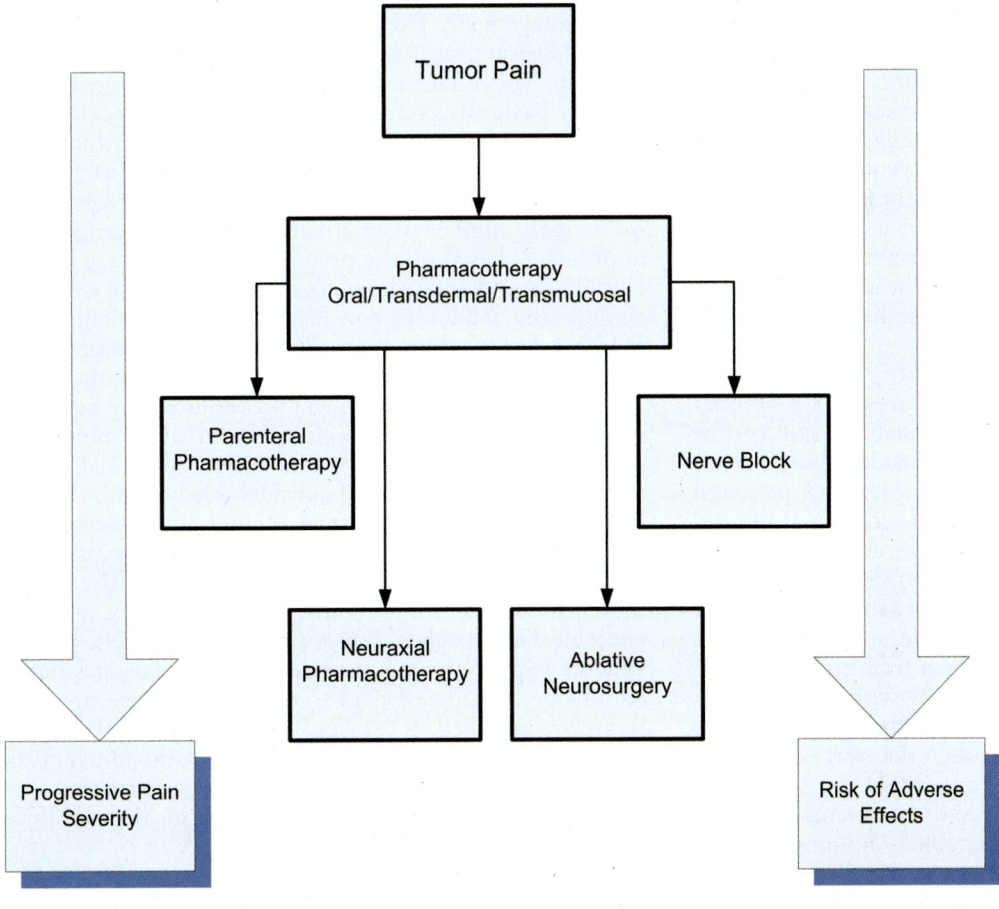

FIGURE 16.1 Tumor pain management flowchart. Strategies for pain management when direct treatment of tumor is not possible. Treatment strategy may change according to progressive pain and/or risk of adverse effects.

TABLE 16.1

PHARMACOLOGIC STRATEGIES FOR THE CONTROL OF TUMOR PAIN

Select the appropriate analgesic drug
Prescribe the appropriate dose of that drug
Administer the drug by the appropriate route
Schedule the appropriate dosing interval
Titrate the dose of drug aggressively
Anticipate and treat breakthrough pain with appropriate medications
Prevent, anticipate, and manage drug side effects

will respond satisfactorily to relatively simple oral pharmacotherapeutic strategies. Strategies should follow the principles endorsed in the World Health Organization (WHO) analgesic ladder (see "World Health Organization Recommendations for Pain Relief and Analgesic Ladder"). Unless the acuity of the clinical situation requires it, analgesics should be optimized (maximum effective doses or to the appearance of intolerable dose-limiting side effects) before considering more specialized (and usually invasive) approaches. The exception to this rule is that relatively simple ablative (chemical or thermal) procedures such as celiac and superior hypogastric plexus blocks, neurolytic subarachnoid and intercostal blocks, and selected peripheral nerve blocks or tumor ablation may be considered as an adjunct. The intent of these procedures is not to replace medication management, but rather to supplement it.

Complex interventional pain procedures may be considered for severe, uncontrolled pain, if intractable side effects occur, if patients prove refractory to conventional medication therapy, and if rapid pain control is required. These procedures include epidural analgesia and/or parenteral opioid therapy (usually intravenous or subcutaneous administration). As many of these patients have high systemic opioid requirements, it is not unusual to combine epidural and parenteral therapies. A small percentage of patients may fail even these therapies and should then be treated with intrathecal drugs, cordotomy, or myelotomy.

Some patients will have pain refractory to all the above modalities. For these patients adequate relief may only come at the cost of sedation. Controlled sedation can be accomplished through the use of benzodiazepines,[2] neuroleptics, barbiturates, and (for hospitalized patients) propofol.[3] The ethical acceptability of sedation at the end of life depends upon informed consent and an acknowledgment of the "principle of double effect," which distinguishes between the compelling primary therapeutic intent (to relieve suffering) and unavoidable, untoward consequences. Palliative sedation is distinct from euthanasia because the intent is relief from suffering without death as a required outcome.[4] In most studies on the use of palliative sedation, the period of time between the start of sedation and death is consistently in the range of 24 to 72 hours.[5–8] In one study assessing the need and effectiveness of sedation in dying patients with intractable symptoms, patients who were sedated had a longer survival when compared with patients who were not sedated.[9]

WORLD HEALTH ORGANIZATION RECOMMENDATIONS FOR PAIN RELIEF AND ANALGESIC LADDER

In the late 1970s and early 1980s, uncontrolled cancer pain was recognized as a serious health problem.[10–13] In 1986, WHO, a specialized agency of the United Nations with primary responsibility for international health matters and public health, published a monograph with the title *Cancer Pain Relief* that aimed to improve the management of cancer pain.[14] These guidelines arose from evidence of poor management of cancer pain in both the developing and the developed countries. At the time of this publication, WHO recognized that there was a lack of availability of drugs essential for the relief of cancer pain in many areas of the world. In addition, many health professionals, institutions, and governments were reluctant to use "strong" opioids because of fears of addiction and tolerance among patients, and the potential for illegal use in the wider community. Initial field testing of the WHO recommendations was encouraging.[15] This monograph has been translated into 22 languages and more than one half million copies have been sold. The WHO revised its monograph in 1990 and 1996.[16–17] We believe these three publications have been pivotal in revolutionizing cancer pain management worldwide and that they merit detailed discussion. Although the drugs recommended may have become somewhat obsolete over time, the principles of use of these classes of drugs are very important for the reader to understand and implement.

In the initial monograph, WHO emphasized the importance of a systematic approach to cancer pain assessment and management. The essence of pain management was that analgesic drugs were the mainstay in managing cancer pain. The WHO method can be applied anywhere as long as basic drugs and adequately-trained health care professionals are available. The principal contribution of this publication was a relatively simple three-step analgesic ladder approach to pain management that was based on a small number of relatively inexpensive drugs. This approach is based on the premise that health care professionals should learn how to use a few drugs well. Although the ladder is considered key to management, WHO acknowledged that not all pain complaints were equally responsive to analgesics and that alternatives such as neurolytic and neurosurgical procedures may be necessary as a supplementary approach in a small number of patients. In addition, treatments such as palliative radiation therapy may also be of considerable benefit. The first approach to care should also include anticancer treatments, if available and if appropriate. Symptomatic treatment measures should be used concurrently. These measures include drug therapy, physical therapy, and psychological approaches. Temporary local anesthetic blocks, such as trigger-point injections and regional anesthesia, should be considered if available. If pain was not adequately controlled, a "strong" opioid should be used in combination with a nonopioid analgesic and adjuvants, if necessary. When pain was localized to a dermatome or was unilateral, neurolytic and neurosurgical procedures should be considered.

In 1986, the three standard analgesics were aspirin, codeine, and morphine. Alternatives could be substituted

TABLE 16.2

BASIC DRUG LIST FOR WORLD HEALTH ORGANIZATION ANALGESIC LADDER, 1986

Category	Class	Parent Drug	Alternatives
Nonopioids		Aspirin	Paracetamol (acetaminophen)
Weak opioids		Codeine	Dextropropoxyphene
Strong opioids		Morphine	Methadone
			Pethidine (meperidine)
			Buprenorphine
			Standardized opium
			Hydromorphone
			Levorphanol
Adjuvants	Anticonvulsants	Carbamazepine	Phenytoin
	Neuroleptics	Prochlorperazine	Chlorpromazin
		Haloperidol	
	Anxiolytics	Diazepam	
		Hydroxyzine	
	Antidepressants	Amitriptyline	
	Corticosteroids	Prednisolone	Dexamethasone

Standardized opium is diluted morphine. The morphine content varies from country to country but usually represents 10% of the weight of opium powder.

as necessary (Table 16.2). In the first version of the ladder, Step 1 specifies a nonopioid for mild pain. Suggested doses of aspirin were 250 to 1000 mg every 4 to 6 hrs with a daily maximum dose of 4 g/day. Step 2 added a "weak" opioid such as codeine for moderate pain to the nonopioid. Use of the nonopioid was required in this step and adjuvant use was optional. Suggested doses of codeine were 30 to 130 mg with 500 mg of acetaminophen or 250 to 500 mg of aspirin every 4 to 6 hours. Step 3 required a "strong" opioid such as morphine to control severe cancer pain, with the option of using a nonopioid or an adjuvant drug if needed.

On the basis of considerable clinical experience and of controlled studies of analgesic use in this study, WHO proposed a series of important principles:

1. *The dose of an analgesic should be determined on an individual basis.* The right dose is that which gives adequate pain relief for a reasonable period of time, preferably 4 hours or more. Unlike the doses of nonopioids, "weak" opioids, and mixed opioid agonist-antagonists, the doses of morphine and other "strong" opioids could be increased indefinitely. WHO indicated that it was rare for a patient to need more than 200 mg of morphine by mouth every 4 hours and that most patients needed 30 mg or less.
2. *The use of oral medication is preferable.* Parenteral administration restricted a patient to either hospital or home and required additional people to perform it. Data from hospices indicated that relatively few people required injections to control pain until the last 2 or 3 days of life.
3. *Insomnia must be treated vigorously.* Pain is often worse at night and the use of a larger dose of morphine at bedtime, compared with the daytime, resulted in more prolonged relief of pain and better sleep.
4. *Side effects must be treated systemically.* Common side effects of "strong" opioids must be monitored and treated appropriately.
5. *Adjuvant drugs are necessary in certain patients.* Antidepressants are indicated for patients who remain depressed despite improved pain control and for those with deafferentation pain. Anxiolytics may be used for very anxious patients. Steroids, anticonvulsants, and neuroleptics also have a role in selected cases.
6. *The patient's progress should be monitored carefully.* Cancer patients who are prescribed analgesics need close supervision to achieve maximum comfort with minimal side effects.

One of the earliest studies subsequently validating the WHO approach was conducted by Ventafridda et al.[15] The authors reported on a 2-year experience using the WHO ladder. Correct use of the ladder reduced pain to one third of its initial intensity. Nonopioids were used on average for 19.2 days, but were discontinued in 52% because of inefficacy and in 42% because of side effects. Weak opioids were administered on average for 28 days. A shift to strong opioids was made in 92% of the cases due to inefficacy and in 8% because of side effects. Treatment with strong opioids lasted for an average of 46.6 days and was considered the mainstay of cancer pain therapy. The analgesic ladder proved efficacious in 71% of the cases; neurolytic procedures had to be used in 29%.

The successful implementation of the analgesic ladder has been verified in a number of subsequent studies. The proportion of cancer patients who received effective pain relief has varied from 75% to 90%.[18–19] According to Zech et al.,[20] 88% of patients with cancer pain should receive good pain control via the guidelines. Similarly, Schug[21] estimated that only 11% of cancer pain patients managed with WHO guidelines required alternate methods of pain management. Grond[22] found that 75% of terminally ill cancer patients received effective management with these guidelines. The largest study on the validation of WHO guidelines for cancer pain relief was conducted by Zech and Grond.[20] In this 1995 report, the course of 2,118 patients was assessed prospectively. Over the treatment period, good pain relief was reported in 76%, satisfactory in 12%, and inadequate in 12%. In the final days of life, 84% rated their pain as moderate or less.

The original WHO analgesic ladder is shown in Figure 16.2. Weak and strong opioids were recommended for the management of persisting pain at steps 2 and 3, respectively and a nonopioid analgesic was considered optional in step 2. A second edition of *Cancer Pain Relief* took into account many of the advances in understanding and practice that occurred since the mid-1980s.[16] The groundwork for this revision was started in 1989, in the context of the meeting of a WHO Expert Committee on Cancer Pain Relief and Active Supportive Care[17] which resulted in a revision in the analgesic ladder (Fig. 16.3). The major changes in the 1990 ladder essentially removed the terms "strong" and "weak" opioids. Opioids were now given for mild-to-moderate pain in step 2 and for moderate-to-severe pain in step 3. WHO also retained mandatory use of nonopioids with opioids in step 2. The distinction between "weak" and "strong" opioids was recognized as arbitrary and did not reflect pharmacologic differences; it was based on the existence of a ceiling effect and on the manner in which these drugs are usually prescribed. Whereas mixed agonist-antagonists and partial agonists have a true ceiling effect, the maximum effective dose has not been determined for most weak opioids. In the second edition, the 1996 analgesic ladder was further modified. The only change from the 1990 version was that nonopioid use was now optional in step 2 (Fig. 16.4).

The recommended basic drug list was also modified in 1996 (Table 16.3), as were the principles of pharmacotherapy (Table 16.4). The 1996 version stated that medications for pain relief should be given:

By Mouth

Analgesic medications should be taken by mouth whenever possible. The main advantage of this route is simplicity of administration. In the United States, the availability of transdermal, transmucosal, sublingual, and transnasal options for administration

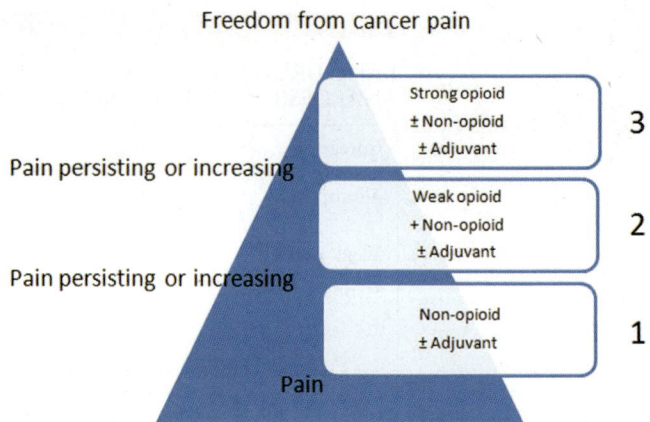

FIGURE 16.2 WHO Analgesic ladder 1986.

should also be considered and not necessarily excluded in preference to the oral route.

By the Clock

Most patients with cancer pain experience pain on a continuous basis. Unless patients take analgesic medications at fixed intervals of time, these medications have limited effectiveness. Medications should be scheduled and taken whether or not patients are experiencing pain at the time they are scheduled to take the medications. The interval between ingestion and adequate plasma level of a drug mandates that the patient must take the next dose before the effect of the previous dose has fully worn off. Some patients may need "rescue" doses for incident and breakthrough pain in addition to the regularly scheduled drug. Such medications should be taken on an as-needed basis.

By the Ladder

The 1996 ladder is essentially based on the severity of the patient's pain complaint. Patients with mild to moderate pain intensity may benefit from the use of a nonsteroidal anti-inflammatory drug (NSAID), acetaminophen, or an opioid. Any opioid may be used as long as the patient obtains benefit from it. For patients with moderate to severe pain intensity, the focus on management is primarily on opioid use and titration. Opioids used in combination (eg, combined with acetylsalicylic acid (ASA) or

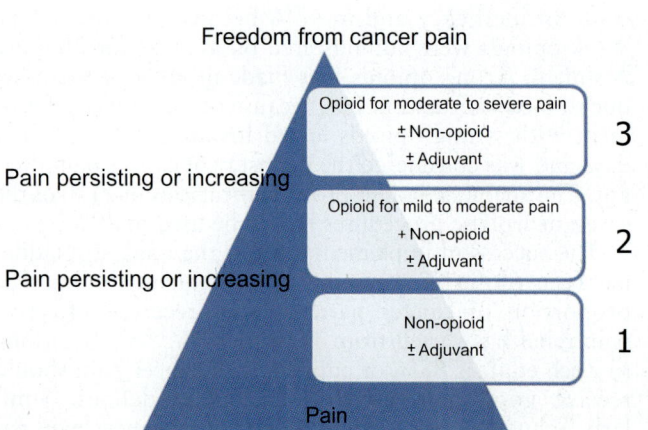

FIGURE 16.3 WHO Analgesic ladder 1990.

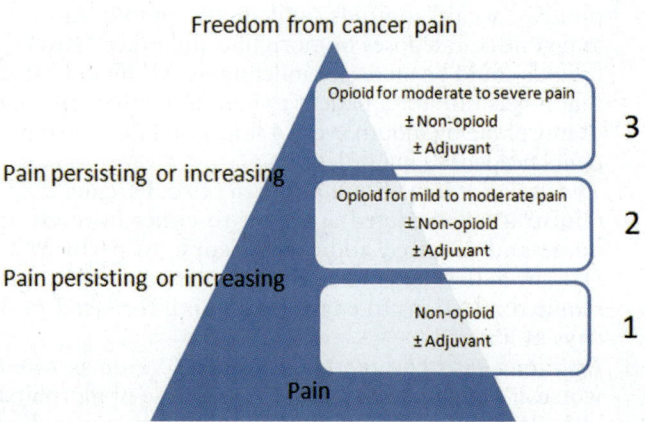

FIGURE 16.4 WHO Analgesic ladder 1996.

TABLE 16.4

THE PRINCIPLES OF DRUG THERAPY FOR CANCER PAIN

By the mouth
By the clock
By the ladder
For the individual
With attention to detail

(From *Cancer pain relief with a guide to opioid availability*. Geneva, Switzerland: World Health Organization, 1996.)

acetaminophen, which are toxic at high doses) have a dose limit in practice because of their formulation. For tumor-related pain, there is no ceiling on dosage for pure opioids as long as the patient continues to obtain benefit and can tolerate any opioid-related side effects. Adjuvant medications and NSAIDs are optional, irrespective of the source of pain. Ideally, only one drug from each of the three major categories should be used at the same time.

For the Individual

The "right" dose is the dose that which adequately relieves the patient's pain with the minimum of side effects. Do not use the same opioid if the patient had previous unsatisfactory experiences with it. If a patient reports that a particular opioid, which was appropriately used and titrated, has proven unsatisfactory for pain relief in the past, choose an alternative opioid, particularly with the increasing number of opioids now available.

With Attention to Detail

Successful implementation of the WHO Analgesic Ladder required meticuluous follow-up once a new prescription is issued. Often, medications and associated regimens are designated as failures simply because the patient did not understand the medication or its use. At each visit or on telephone follow-up, the patient's regimen should be outlined and monitored. Monitoring by a health care professional with the patient involves ascertaining compliance, drug efficacy, and side effects. At these evaluations, doses should be adjusted, if necessary, and adverse effects anticipated and treated prophylactically.

Since its introduction, the WHO analgesic ladder has received widespread approval. However, some authors have expressed concern about the validity and scientific effectiveness of published data. These concerns have focused on study design flaws such as methodologic

TABLE 16.3

A BASIC DRUG LIST FOR CANCER PAIN RELIEF

Category	Basic Drugs	Alternatives
Nonopioids	Acetylsalicylic acid (ASA)	Choline magnesium trisalicylate
	Paracetamol (acetaminophen)	Diflunisal
	Ibuprofen	Naproxen
	Indomethacin	Diclofenac
Opioids for mild to moderate pain[a]	Codeine[b]	Dihydrocodeine
		Dextropropoxyphene
		Standardized opium
		Tramadol
Opioids for moderate to severe pain[a]	Morphine	Methadone
		Hydromorphone
		Oxycodone
		Levorphanol
		Meperidine
		Buprenorphine
Opioid antagonist	Naloxone	
Antidepressants[c]	Amitriptyline	Imipramine
Anticonvulsants[c]	Carbamazepine	Valproic acid
Corticosteroids[d]	Prednisolone	Prednisone
	Dexamethasone	Betamethasone

[a]For practical purposes, the opioids are divided into those for mild to moderate pain and those for moderate to severe pain., principally on the grounds of common patterns of use.

[b]Codeine and some other opioids for mild to moderate pain are not scheduled drugs in most countries. This may make them more easily available.

[c]Antidepressants and anticonvulsants are the drugs of choice for neuropathic pain.

[d]Of value in nerve compression and spinal cord compression pain; also for headache due to raised intracranial pressure. May be used as an alternative to, or as an adjunct with, an NSAID for bone pain. If used with an NSAID, there is increased likelihood of adverse gastric events and of fluid retention.

(From *Cancer pain relief with a guide to opioid availability*. Geneva, Switzerland: World Health Organization, 1996.)

limitations including the circumstances during which assessments were made, small sample size, retrospective analyses, high rate of exclusions and dropout, inadequate follow-up, and a lack of comparison with levels of analgesia before the introduction of the analgesic ladder. Jadad et al.[23] conducted a systematic review of studies (a MEDLINE search from 1982 to 1995; a hand search of textbooks, meeting proceedings, and reference lists; and direct contact with authors) evaluating the effectiveness of the WHO ladder as an intervention for cancer pain management. Although the studies available provide valuable information on the course of cancer pain and its treatment, they fail to estimate confidently the effectiveness of the WHO analgesic ladder. A meta-analysis was not possible because the studies were essentially case series without control groups. The review also highlighted other limitations in the quality of these studies: insufficient information was provided on pain characteristics, retrospective studies were used, articles had short or variable follow-up, and a high percentage of patients were lost to follow-up. Azevedo Sao Leao Ferreira et al.[24] also conducted a systematic review from 1982 to 2004 and stated that pain relief was adequate in 45% to 100% of patients but concluded that the evidence supporting the efficacy of WHO guidelines was insufficient because of the lack of controlled clinical trials.

Treatment failures of the ladder were felt to be related to neuropathic[25] or breakthrough pain.[26] Neuropathic pains often respond poorly to nonopioid and opioid analgesics, but tricyclic antidepressants and anticonvulsants may prove more effective. Mishra et al.[27] prospectively evaluated the effectiveness of using WHO Analgesic ladder in 818 patients with neuropathic pain for a 6-month period. The main adjuvants used are amitriptyline (30%), gabapentin (30%), gabapentin with dexamethasone (20%), and dexamethasone alone (20%). The opioids used were tramadol, codeine, and morphine, with 52% of patients receiving morphine as a rescue analgesic. At initial visit, 70% patients had severe pain, 20% had moderate pain, and 10% had mild pain; at the end of study 53.2% patients had no pain, 41.9% patients had mild pain, and only 4.9% patients had moderate pain.

WHO has categorized drugs to be used in the treatment of cancer pain as nonopioid analgesics, adjuvants and opioids. We will consider them individually in Chapters 17–19.

References

1. Moryl N, Coyle N, Foley KM. Managing an acute pain crisis in a patient with advanced cancer: "This is as much of a crisis as a code." *JAMA.* 2008;299:1457–1467.
2. Bottomley DM, Hanks GW. Subcutaneous midazolam infusion in palliative care. *J Pain Symptom Manage.* 1990;5:259–261.
3. Mercadante S, De C-F, Ripamonti C. Propofol in terminal care. *J Pain Symptom Manage.* 1995;10:639–642.
4. Cowan JD, Palmer TW. Practical guide to palliative sedation. *Curr Oncol Rep.* 2002;4:242–249.
5. Fainsinger RL, De Moissac D, Mancini I, et al. Sedation for delirium and other symptoms in terminally ill patients in Edmonton. *J Palliat Care.* 2000;16:5–10.
6. Fainsinger RL, Waller A, Bercovici M, et al. A multicentre international study of sedation for uncontrolled symptoms in terminally ill patients. *J Palliat Med.* 2000;14:257–265.
7. Kohara H, Ueoka H, Takeyama H, et al. Sedation for terminally ill patients with cancer with uncontrollable physical distress. *J Palliat Med.* 2005;8:20–25.
8. Muller-Busch HC, Andres I, Jehser T. Sedation in palliative care—a critical analysis of 7 years experience. *BMC Palliat Care.* 2003;2:2.
9. Mercadante S, Intravaia G, Villari P, et al. Controlled sedation for refractory symptoms in dying patients. *J Pain Symptom Manage.* 2009;37:771–779.
10. Bonica JJ. Treatment of cancer pain: current status and future needs. In: Fields HL, Dubner R, Cervero F, eds. *Advances in pain research and therapy.* New York: Raven Press, 1985:589–616.
11. Foley KM. The management of pain of malignant origin. In: Tyler HR, Dawson DM, eds. *Current neurology.* Boston: Houghton Mifflin, 1979:279–302.
12. Jones WL, Rimer BK, Levy MH, et al. Cancer patients' knowledge, beliefs, and behavior regarding pain control regimens: Implications for education programs. *Patient Educ Couns.* 1984;5:159–164.
13. Taddeini L, Rotschafer JC. Pain syndromes associated with cancer. Achieving effective relief. *Postgrad Med.* 1984;75:101–108.
14. *Cancer Pain Relief.* Geneva, Switzerland. World Health Organization, 1986.
15. Ventafridda V, Tamburini M, Caraceni A, et al. A validation study of the WHO method for cancer pain relief.*Cancer.* 1987;59: 850–856.
16. *Cancer pain relief with a guide to opioid availability*, 2nd ed. Geneva, Switzerland: World Health Organization, 1996.
17. *Cancer pain relief and palliative care.* Geneva, Switzerland: World Health Organization, 1990.
18. Hanks GW, Justins DM. Cancer pain: Management. *Lancet.* 1992;339:1031–1036.
19. Agency for Health Care Policy and Research. *Management of cancer pain. A clinical practice guideline.* 1994;Pub 94–0592
20. Zech DF, Grond S, Lynch J, et al. Validation of World Health Organization Guidelines for cancer pain relief: A 10-year prospective study. *Pain.* 1995;63:65–76.
21. Schug SA, Zech D, Dorr U. Cancer pain management according to WHO analgesic guidelines. *J Pain Symptom Manage.* 1990;5:27–32.
22. Grond S, Zech D, Schug SA, et al. Validation of World Health Organization guidelines for cancer pain relief during the last days and hours of life. *J Pain Symptom Manage.* 1991;6:411–422.
23. Jadad AR, Browman GP. The WHO analgesic ladder for cancer pain management. Stepping up the quality of its evaluation. *JAMA.* 1995;274:1870–1873.
24. Azevedo Sao Leao Ferreira K, Kimura M, et al. The WHO analgesic ladder for cancer pain control, twenty years of use. How much pain relief does one get from using it? *Support Care Cancer.* 2006;14: 1086–1093.
25. Grond S, Radbruch L, Meuser T, et al. Assessment and treatment of neuropathic cancer pain following WHO guidelines. *Pain.* 1999;79:15–20.
26. Zeppetella G, Ribeiro MD. Opioids for the management of breakthrough (episodic) pain in cancer patients. *Cochrane Database Syst Rev.* 2006:CD004311.
27. Mishra S, Bhatnagar S, Gupta D, et al. Management of neuropathic cancer pain following WHO analgesic ladder: a prospective study. *Am J Hosp Palliat Care.* 2008;25:447–451.

CHAPTER 17 ■ NONOPIOID ANALGESICS

The World Health Organization recommended nonopioid analgesic agents and antipyretics as basic drugs for the management of pain, and clinicians should be familiar with the use, efficacy, and adverse effects of these agents. Numerous studies on the pharmacotherapy of cancer pain recommend the use of nonopioid analgesics for management.[1–14] Advantages in using these drugs include their ability to control pain by an independent mechanism from alternative analgesics (eg, in the management of bone pain) or that they may help reduce the dose of opioid required for pain control (opioid-sparing effect).

A wide range of drugs with varying effects and side effects are available. Three groups of drugs are considered nonopioid analgesics: acetylsalicylic acid (ASA), acetaminophen, and nonsteroidal anti-inflammatory drugs (NSAIDs). Although ASA may be considered an NSAID, it merits separate discussion because it is effective, cheap, and widely available.

The basic mechanism of action of all NSAIDs is by inhibition of prostaglandin biosynthesis through effects on the enzyme cyclooxygenase (COX). In addition to peripheral effects, NSAIDs exert a central action at the brain or spinal cord that may influence analgesic effects.[15] The formation of prostaglandins causes inflammation, swelling, pain and fever. Acetaminophen has a different mechanism of action which appears to be a combination of central COX inhibition and a central serotonergic effect.[16] A homogeneous, enzymatically active COX or prostaglandin endoperoxide synthase (PGHS) was first isolated in 1976. This membrane-bound hemoprotein and glycoprotein is found in greatest amounts in the endoplasmic reticulum of prostanoid-forming cells.[17] It exhibits COX activity that both cyclizes arachidonic acid and adds the 15-hydroperoxy group to form PGG_2. The hydroperoxy group of PGG_2 is reduced to the hydroxy group of PGH_2 by a peroxidase that uses a wide variety of compounds to provide the requisite pair of electrons. Both COX and hydroperoxidase activities are contained in the same dimeric protein molecule. NSAIDs inhibit only the COX reaction of PGH synthase. Prostaglandins are important in the regulation of thrombocyte aggregation, inflammatory processes, pain and fever induction, the regulation of blood flow, and many other processes. Structural analysis has shown at least two isoforms of COX, COX-1 and COX-2 (Fig. 17.1). COX-2 is inducible and appears to have both physiologic and pathophysiologic roles (Fig. 17.2).

Epidemiological studies associated a decreased incidence of colorectal cancer with the long-term use of aspirin.[18] Reports also suggested that the use of NSAIDs (in particular sulindac) showed evidence of regression of colorectal adenomas.[19] In subsequent years, the use of other NSAIDs, which inhibit COX enzymes, was linked to reduced cancer risk in multiple tissues including those of the breast, prostate, and lung.[20] Together these studies

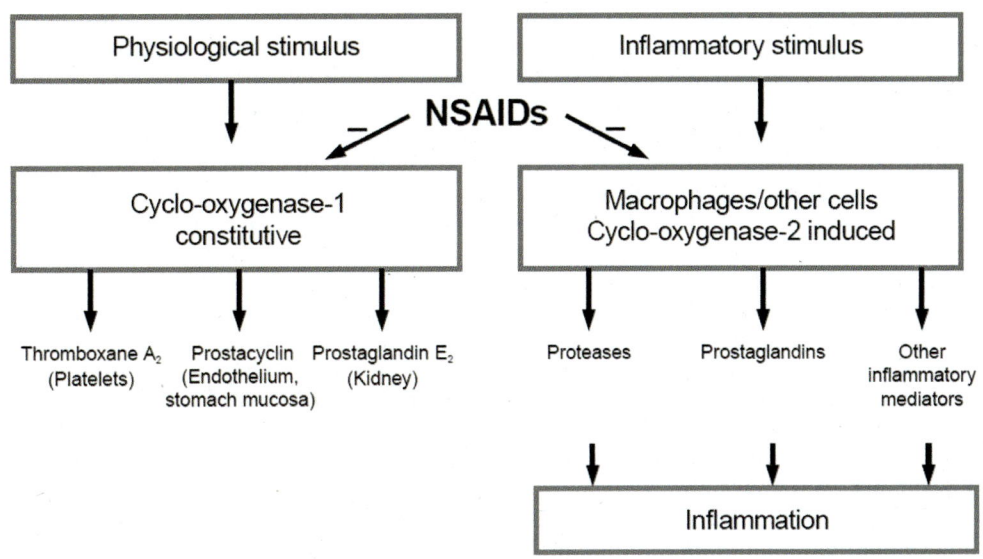

FIGURE 17.1 Regulation of prostaglandin biosynthesis by COX-1 and COX-2. (From Steinmeyer J. Pharmacological basis for the therapy of pain and inflammation with nonsteroidal anti-inflammatory drugs. *Arthritis Res.* 2000;2:379–385. Reprinted with permission of Biomedcentral.)

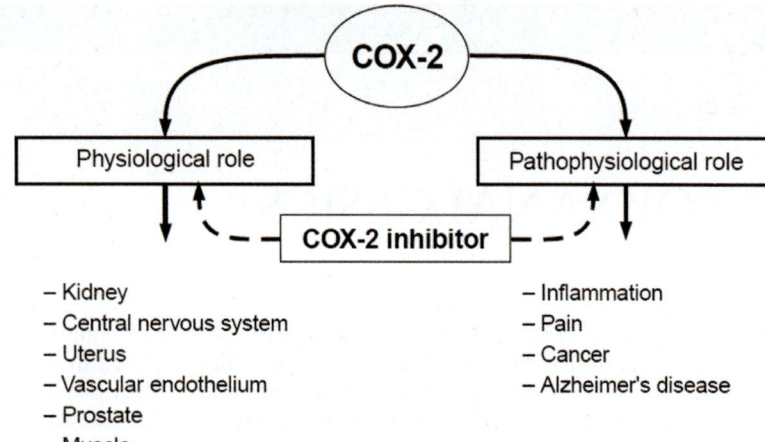

FIGURE 17.2 Physiologic and pathophysiologic functions of COX-2. (Reused with permission from Steinmeyer J. Pharmacological basis for the therapy of pain and inflammation with nonsteroidal anti-inflammatory drugs. *Arthritis Res*. 2000;2(5):379–385. Reprinted with permission of Biomedcentral)

resulted in the identification of a new cancer preventive and/or therapeutic target-COX enzymes, especially COX-2. The overexpression of COX-2, and less consistently, the upstream and downstream enzymes of the prostaglandin synthesis pathway, was demonstrated in multiple cancer types and some preneoplastic lesions.[21] Direct interactions of prostaglandins with their receptors through autocrine or paracrine pathways to enhance cellular survival or stimulate angiogenesis have been proposed as the molecular mechanisms underlying the procarcinogenic functions of COX-2.[21]

THE SALICYLATES

Salicylic or *ortho*-hydroxybenzoic acid belongs to a diverse group of plant phenolics (Fig. 17.3). Several plants of the *Spiraea* genus contain salicylic-like compounds to a significant extent. Salicin is found in the willow, poplar trees, and the black haw plant. Over 160 years ago, the chemical oxidation of salicin resulted in salicylic acid, and the acetylated derivative of this turned into one of the most successful drugs in history, aspirin. Salicylates are compounds with an aromatic ring bearing a hydroxyl group or its functional derivative. Salicylates generally act by virtue of their content of salicylic acid. Substitutions on the carboxyl or hydroxyl groups change the potency or toxicity of salicylate agents. Substitution on the benzene ring has also been accomplished. Diflunisal is a diflurophenyl derivative of salicylic acid. Salicylic acid derivatives include aspirin, sodium salicylate, choline magnesium trisalicylate, salsalate, diflunisal, salicylsalicylic acid, sulphasalazine, and olsalazine. Salicylic acid is so irritating that it can be used only externally; therefore, various derivatives of this acid have been synthesized for systemic use. These comprise two large classes, esters of salicylic acid obtained by substitution in the carboxyl group and salicylate esters of organic acids in which the carboxyl group of salicylic acid is retained and substitution is made in the hydroxyl group. Aspirin is an ester of acetic acid and there are salts of salicylic acid. Salicylate salts such as choline magnesium trisalicylate and salsalate are effective analgesics and produce fewer gastrointestinal (GI) side effects than aspirin. Aspirin selectively acetylates the hydroxyl group of one serine residue (Ser 530) located 70 amino acids from the C terminus of the enzyme.[22] Acetylation leads to irreversible COX inhibition; thus, a new enzyme must be synthesized before more prostanoids are produced.

The two most commonly used preparations of salicylate for systemic effects are sodium salicylate and aspirin. A combination of choline and magnesium salicylate is also available. Mesalamine (5-ASA) is a salicylate used for its local effects in the treatment of inflammatory bowel disease. The drug is not effective orally and is usually administered as a suppository or enema. Sulfasalazine contains mesalamine linked covalently to sulfapyridine. Orally ingested salicylates are absorbed rapidly, partly from the stomach but mostly from the upper small intestine. Appreciable concentrations are found in the plasma in less than 30 minutes; a peak level is reached in about 2 hours and then gradually declines. There is little meaningful difference between the rates of absorption of sodium salicylate, aspirin, and the numerous buffered preparations of salicylates. Rectal absorption of salicylate is usually slower than oral and it is incomplete and unreliable. The plasma half-life for aspirin is approximately 15 minutes; that for salicylate is 2 to 3 hours in low doses and about 12 hours at usual anti-inflammatory doses. Aspirin absorption follows first-order kinetics with an absorption half-life ranging from 5 to 16 minutes. Hydrolysis of aspirin to salicylic acid by nonspecific esterases occurs in the liver and, to a lesser extent, the stomach, so that only 68% of the dose reaches the systemic circulation as aspirin.[23] The serum half-life of salicylic acid is dose-dependent; thus, the larger the dose employed, the longer it will take to reach steady-state. Diflunisal is almost completely absorbed after oral administration, and peak concentrations occur in plasma within 2 to 3 hours. At usual analgesic doses (500 to 750 mg/day) the plasma half-life ranges between 8 and 12 hours.[24]

The antipyretic activity of aspirin probably results from the secondary inhibition of pyrogen-induced release of prostaglandins in the central nervous system (CNS) and possibly from centrally mediated peripheral vasodilation. Aspirin exerts its antiplatelet activity through the inhibition of COX, which is involved in the production of a platelet activator, thromboxane A2 (TXA2), and a platelet inhibitor, prostaglandin I2 (PGI2), also known as prostacyclin.[25] Aspirin acetylates platelet cyclooxygenase and

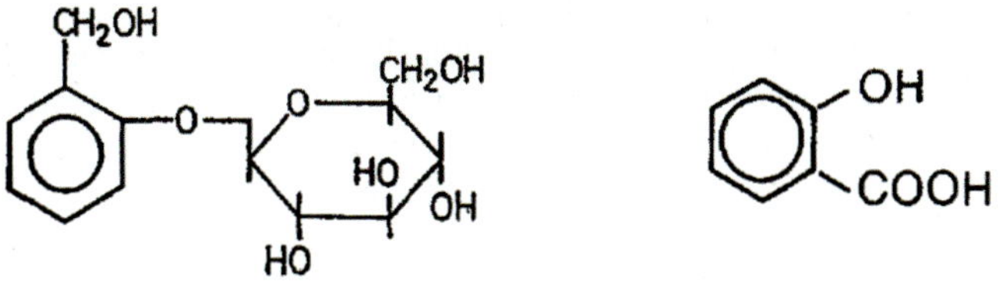

FIGURE 17.3 The molecular structure of salicin and salicylic acid.

prevents the synthesis of thromboxane A_2, a potent vasoconstrictor and inducer of platelet aggregation.

Low doses of aspirin reduce both pain and fever, whereas the anti-inflammatory action of aspirin requires a much higher dose. It is possible that inhibition of COX-1 is the major action of aspirin involved in its analgesic and antipyretic effects, and inhibition of COX-2 is responsible for its anti-inflammatory action.[26] The standard dose of aspirin is 500 to 600 mg every 4 to 6 hours. The administration of more than 4 g/day is likely to lead to toxic effects. A review of aspirin's effect on the renal function of experimental animals following acute and chronic administration[27] revealed that although the findings are inconsistent, chronic administration can cause analgesic-associated nephropathy (AAN).

Nonacetylated salicylates, such as choline magnesium trisalicylate (CMT) and salsalate, have less ulcer-producing potential than aspirin, and at usual clinical doses do not impair platelet aggregation.[28] Kilander and Dotevall[29] compared the effect of aspirin and CMT on gastric and duodenal mucosa by gastroduodenoscopy after 5-day periods of administration in 10 healthy volunteers. Serum salicylate levels were similar in the two groups. All subjects given aspirin developed multiple mucosal lesions, but in only four subjects given CMT were slight mucosal changes noted, suggesting that the risk of developing mucosal lesions is much less during treatment with CMT than with aspirin. Danesh et al.[30] measured parameters of platelet thromboxane biosynthesis 24 hours after ingestion of equivalent salicylate doses (500 mg) of aspirin and CMT. In random order, 10 healthy volunteers received these drugs on 2 separate days, 2 weeks apart. Whereas aspirin significantly prolonged bleeding time and decreased plasma thromboxane generation and serum thromboxane B_2 levels, CMT failed to produce such effects. CMT has no inhibitory effect on platelet thromboxane biosynthesis, and may therefore be considered safer than aspirin for therapeutic use, when inhibition of platelet function can be hazardous. Because of the association with Reye's syndrome, aspirin and other salicylates are contraindicated in children and young adults less than 12 years old with fever associated with viral illness.[31]

The role of salicylates is well established in inflammatory bowel disease (predominantly for ulcerative colitis and to a lesser extent in Crohn disease). Agents used for treatment include 5-aminosalicylic acid (5-ASA) or sulphasalazine (5-ASA in combination with a sulphonamide, sulphapyridine). With the aim of achieving the same efficacy of sulphasalazine but without its major side effects, various preparations of new salicylates (such as mesalazine, olsalazine, and balsalazide) have been formulated to assure targeted release, minor discomfort, and safety in use.[32]

We do not routinely use salicylates for the management of cancer pain, because of our concern about the toxicity associated with these agents, particularly in the immunosuppressed cancer patient, and because of their limited efficacy for pain relief. If this class of medication is deemed useful, we prefer the use of trilisate over the other agents in this group.

ACETAMINOPHEN

Acetaminophen or N-Acetyl-Para-Amino-Phenol (APAP) is one of the most widely used analgesic and antipyretic agents in the world.[33] APAP, indicated for noninflammatory pain and for fever control, is available in a variety of oral preparations and as a suppository. It has potent antipyretic and mild to moderate analgesic actions but very weak anti-inflammatory activity. When administered to humans, it reduces levels of prostaglandin metabolites in urine but does not reduce synthesis of prostaglandins by blood platelets or by the stomach mucosa. Because APAP is a weak inhibitor in vitro of both COX-1 and COX-2, the possibility exists that it also inhibits COX-3,[34] although Hinz et al.[35] stated that APAP has substantial COX-2 inhibition in humans. APAP has been described as a preferential inhibitor of central rather than peripheral cyclooxygenases[36] and is generally considered to be a weak inhibitor of the synthesis of prostaglandins. Others believe the analgesic and antipyretic benefits of APAP are due to its unique ability to selectively block COX products (principally PGE2) in the central and/or peripheral nervous system.[37] The mechanism of the analgesic action also involves the serotonergic system and appears to act predominantly on descending inhibitory pathways.[38] There is a central serotonergic mechanism of action that is not stimulus-dependent although its primary site of action may still be inhibition of prostaglandin synthesis.[39] The use of 5-HT3 antagonists such as tropisetron and granisetron with APAP completely blocked the analgesic effect of APAP in humans.[16] APAP-induced antinociception also involves the cannabinoid system.[40]

APAP is not considered to influence platelet function in vivo. Studies using conventional doses (approximately 1 g) of oral APAP have shown negative results.[41–42] However, Munsterhjelm et al.[43] demonstrated that intravenous APAP (15, 22.5, and 30 mg/kg) inhibited platelet aggregation and TxB_2 release in healthy volunteers in a dose-dependent fashion. No evidence exists for the development of chronic analgesic nephropathy with APAP alone.[44] Epidemiologic studies in healthy individuals have failed to demonstrate a significant correlation between APAP use and chronic renal disease and classic analgesic nephropathy.[45] The only reports on this subject suggest that combination therapy with aspirin[46] or ingestion of toxic doses of APAP[47] may induce nephrotoxicity.

Hepatoxicity is predominantly associated with the use of APAP, and occurs after single, acute, or short-term exposure to larger (>10 g) doses or long-term exposure with lower (<4 g) doses, especially in alcoholics.[48–49] APAP can cause acute liver damage when massive doses are ingested; however, even in overdose situations, the risk of severe liver damage is less than 10% with a mortality rate less than 2%, even before availability of N-acetylcysteine treatment.[50] Benson et al.[51] suggest that APAP can be used safely in patients with liver disease at currently recommended doses and is preferred to aspirin and other NSAIDs because of the absence of inhibitory actions on platelet aggregation or gastrointestinal and renal toxicity.

APAP is metabolized in the liver primarily by glucuronidation and sulfation. With therapeutic doses (≤4 g daily), only 4% is converted by the cytochrome P450 (CYP) system into the reactive toxic intermediate N-acetyl-p-benzoquinoneimine (NAPQI).[52] This toxic metabolite is rendered nontoxic by binding to glutathione. With APAP overdose, CYP enzyme induction, glutathione depletion, or the inhibition of glucuronidation, this reactive metabolite cannot be sufficiently neutralized. Instead, NAPQI reacts with the cysteine group of hepatocellular proteins, which leads to the loss of cell function and cell death. Chronic alcohol use leads to a short-term, two- to threefold increase in hepatic CYP2E1, the major cytochrome responsible for production of the toxic NAPQI metabolite of APAP.[53] Although the minimal amount of APAP needed to produce severe hepatotoxicity in the setting of chronic alcohol use has not been determined, the OTC (Over-The-Counter) Advisory Committee of the FDA recommends that patients who consume three or more alcoholic beverages daily should consult their physicians before use of APAP.[54]

The APAP-alcohol interaction is complex with acute and chronic ethanol having opposite effects. In animals, chronic ethanol causes induction of hepatic microsomal enzymes and increases APAP hepatotoxicity as expected (ethanol primarily induces CYP2E1 and this isoform is important in the oxidative metabolism of APAP).[55-57] However, in man, chronic alcohol ingestion causes only modest (about twofold) and short-lived induction of CYP2E1, and there is no corresponding increase in the toxic metabolic activation of APAP.[58] The APAP-ethanol interaction is not specific for any one isoform of cytochrome P450, and it seems that isoenzymes other than CYP2E1 are primarily responsible for the oxidative metabolism of APAP in man. Acute ethanol inhibits the microsomal oxidation of APAP both in animals and man.[59] This protects against liver damage in animals and there is evidence that it also does so in man.[60] The protective effect disappears when ethanol is eliminated and the relative timing of ethanol and APAP intake is critical.[61-62] Because the minimum safe dose of acetaminophen is not known in the setting of chronic alcohol use, it seems prudent in such situations to avoid acetaminophen altogether, especially during brief periods of abstinence.[63]

Drug interactions with acetaminophen are important in oncology patients. Hylek et al.[64] noted a highly significant dose-response relationship between acetaminophen and coumadin. Patients who reported taking the equivalent of at least 4 regular strength (325-mg) tablets per day for longer than 1 week had a tenfold increased risk of having an INR greater than 6.0 while also taking coumadin. The risk decreased with lower intake of acetaminophen, particularly when taking 6 or fewer 325-mg tablets per week. Parra et al.[65] also noted a clinically significant interaction between coumadin and daily use of acetaminophen but at higher doses of 2 to 4 g per day. Patients with low glutathione stores, such as the elderly, may have an increased risk for drug interaction between coumadin and acetaminophen.[66] In addition, the mechanism of interaction may be due to an effect of acetaminophen or one of its metabolites on factors VII and IX.[67]

Therapeutic dosing of acetaminophen is associated with increased risk of acute liver injury.[68] Use of acetaminophen for 10 days may elevate alanine aminotransferase in moderate alcohol drinkers.[69] Aminotransferase elevations were reported in healthy adults receiving 4 g of acetaminophen daily.[70] Studies on acetaminophen-induced chronic renal failure have produced inconclusive results,[45] although some studies suggest an association between acetaminophen use and adverse chronic renal outcomes.[71-72]

Overall, there are a limited number of studies specifically investigating the role of acetaminophen in cancer pain. In a double-blind, placebo-controlled, cross-over study of 30 cancer patients, Stockler et al.[73] demonstrated that the addition of acetaminophen improved pain and well-being without major side effects in patients on an opioid regimen. Patients received 1 g acetaminophen every 4 hours five times a day for 48 hours. Axelsson et al.[74] recommended the addition of acetaminophen to the use of "strong" opioids for cancer-related pain. Rodriquez et al.[75] reported that combination opioids (codeine or hydrocodone) with acetaminophen was safe and effective in patients with moderate or severe chronic, cancer-related pain although 34% of patients in the codeine/acetaminophen group and 29% in the hydrocodone/acetaminophen group failed to achieve pain relief.

We occasionally use acetaminophen in the management of cancer pain. In general, this drug is well tolerated in the oncology population but its efficacy is limited. It is not unusual for us to use acetaminophen in "pain cocktail" (liquid solution of methadone and other drugs in cherry syrup) for around the clock medication administration. However, opioid and acetaminophen combinations at regular daily dosing intervals may be problematic in reaching potentially toxic levels of acetaminophen and we are careful not to exceed the recommended dosage of approximately 4 g/day.

NONSTEROIDAL ANTI-INFLAMMATORY DRUGS

NSAIDs comprise a group of structurally diverse but similarly acting compounds that are used for relieving signs and symptoms of inflammation, especially in treatment of rheumatic diseases. NSAIDS possess analgesic, anti-inflammatory and antipyretic properties and are widely prescribed for the treatment of pain and inflammation.[76] The main indication for use of NSAIDs is treatment of acute and chronic musculoskeletal pain and common indications for use include chronic polyarthritis, psoriatic arthritis, ankylosing spondylitis, osteoarthritis, gout, inflammatory soft-tissue rheumatism, low back pain, postoperative and post-traumatic inflammation, thrombophlebitis and vasculitis. The discovery of the COX isoforms led to establishing their importance in many nonarthritic or nonpain states where there is an inflammatory component to pathogenesis, including cancer, Alzheimer disease and other neurodegenerative diseases. The applications of NSAIDs and the coxibs in the prevention and treatment of these conditions as well as aspirin and other analogues in the prevention of thromboembolic diseases constitute one of the major therapeutic developments of this century. NSAIDs are recommended for the treatment of mild cancer pain and, in conjunction with opioids, for the treatment of moderate to severe pain.[77] NSAIDs have also been considered effective for certain cancer pain problems, such as bony metastases, although data to support this is limited. NSAIDs may provide additive pain relief when combined with opioids, even over extended periods of time,[78] although most studies investigating the effects of NSAIDs for the treatment of cancer pain are of limited duration.[11] Table 17.1 lists some of the NSAIDs in clinical use.

The maximum efficacy and side effects of each NSAID vary between patients. Similarly, different NSAIDs produce varied effects in the same patient. Three areas of safety concerns are shared by both groups of drugs: gastrointestinal complications (upper gastrointestinal bleeding, perforations or obstruction), cardiovascular safety (mainly myocardial infarction), and renal safety (acute renal failure, hypertension and electrolyte abnormalities). The incidence of renal complications may be increased twofold with NSAIDs or coxibs; there is no evidence for a major difference between the two groups of drugs. Prescribing NSAIDs in non–cancer patients is challenging because clinicians have to consider GI and cardiovascular risks. Current advice suggests that physicians should always prescribe the lowest effective dose for the shortest possible time.[79] The benefits of the combination of NSAID and opioid over opioid monotherapy should be either better pain relief or reduced opioid doses and, consequently, a reduction in the risk of opioid-related side effects. The obvious opioid-related side effects in this situation include constipation, nausea, and sedation, all of which may require additional medications to counter these effects. In order to minimize the risk of gastroduodenal damage in cancer patients taking NSAIDs, drugs such as misoprostol and ranitidine have been advocated.[80] Reviewing the effects of prostaglandin analogues, H2-receptor antagonists (H2RAs), or proton pump inhibitors (PPIs) for the prevention of chronic NSAID-induced upper GI toxicity, Rostom et al.[81] concluded that misoprostol, PPIs, and double dose H2RAs are effective at preventing chronic NSAID related endoscopic gastric and duodenal ulcers. Lower doses of misoprostol were less effective and were still associated with diarrhea. Only misoprostol 800 µg/day has been directly shown to reduce the risk of ulcer complications.

Risk factors for NSAID-induced GI side effects include concomitant use of corticosteroids and/or anticoagulant therapy, history of previous GI side effects, high dosage and long duration of NSAID use, advanced age, and alcoholism. The search for NSAIDs with less GI toxicity led to the introduction of the selective COX-2 inhibitors. A number of established NSAIDs (etodolac, meloxicam, nabumetone) exhibit significant selective COX-2 inhibition.[82–83] Additional potential advantages in the use of COX-2 inhibitors in cancer patients included effects of tumor growth. COX-2 is highly expressed during tumorigenesis and actively contributes to tumor progression,[84] and this effect involves, at least in part, induction of tumor angiogenesis.[85] Several cytokines such as reactive oxygen species (ROS) and mediators of inflammatory pathway such as activation of nuclear factor-κB (NF-κB) and COX-2 leads to an increase in cell proliferation, survival, and inhibition of proapoptotic pathway, ultimately resulting in tumor angiogenesis, invasion and metastasis.[86] Increased

TABLE 17.1

PARTIAL LIST OF NONSTEROIDAL ANTI-INFLAMMATORY DRUGS USED FOR CANCER PAIN

Drug Type	Name/Brand	Typical Starting Dose
Acetaminophen	Tylenol and others	650 mg every 4 hours orally
Aspirin	Multiple	650 mg every 4 hours orally
Ibuprofen	Motrin and others	200–800 mg every 6 hours orally
Choline magnesium trisalicylate	Trilisate	1000–1500 mg 3/d orally
Diclofenac sodium	Voltaren	50–75 mg every 8–12 hours orally
Diflunisal	Dolobid	500 mg every 12 hours orally
Etodolac	Lodine	200–400 mg every 8–12 hours orally
Flurbiprofen	Ansaid	200–300 mg every 4–8 hours orally
Naproxen	Naprosyn	250–750 mg every 12 hours orally
Naproxen sodium	Anaprox	275 mg every 12 hours orally
Oxaprozin	Daypro	600–1200 mg/d orally
Sulindac	Clinoril	150–200 mg every 12 hours orally
Piroxicam	Feldene	10–20 mg/d orally
Nabumetone	Relafen	1000–2000 mg/d orally
Ketoprofen	Orudis	50 mg every 6 hours orally
Ketorolac	Toradol	10 mg every 4–6 hours orally (not to exceed 10 d)

(Modified from Payne R. Limitations of NSAIDs for pain management: Toxicity or lack of efficacy? *J Pain*. 2000;1(3 Suppl):14–18. Copyright 2000, with permission from The American Pain Society.)

COX-2 activity and synthesis of prostaglandins stimulates proliferation, angiogenesis, and invasiveness and inhibits apoptosis.[87] In preclinical models NSAIDs and COX-2 inhibitors possess therapeutic efficacy against established tumors, raising the possibility that COX-2 inhibitors may be used in human cancer treatment.[88] Preliminary human data suggests a potential chemoprevention role in certain cancers (breast, prostate, colon, and lung).[89] Clinical studies are underway to determine the benefit of NSAID use taken as a sole agent or in combination with various chemotherapeutic regimens in reducing cancer risk.[90–96]

NSAID pain relief is typically characterized both by a ceiling dose, beyond which additional increments fail to yield further pain relief or more severe side effects but no further pain relief, and by a lack of demonstrable physical dependence or tolerance. One cannot predict the minimal effective analgesic dose, the ceiling dose, or the toxic dose for the individual patient with cancer pain, and this dose may be higher or lower than the usual dose range recommended for the drug involved. Standard recommended doses for nonopioid drugs derive from studies performed in populations (generally healthy patients with an inflammatory disease) that may have little in common with cancer patients; the latter often have numerous medical problems and use several other drugs increasing the risk of drug–drug interactions).

The successful use of NSAIDs in the cancer patient necessitates a strategy that involves both low initial doses and dose titration with a limited duration of use. With gradual dose escalation, one can usually identify the ceiling dose and reduce the risk of significant toxicity. Because failure with one NSAID does not predict a similar outcome with another, the clinician may need sequential trials of several NSAIDs to identify a drug with a favorable balance between pain relief and side effects.

Topical Nonsteroidal Anti-Inflammatory Drugs

The rationale for topical NSAID delivery is to enable direct application of the drug at the site of pain, as opposed to a transdermal delivery system that uses absorption from the skin into serum to achieve systemic therapeutic levels that will alleviate pain wherever the site. Theoretically, direct application also enhances local drug delivery to affected tissues, minimizes systemic levels to reduce serious adverse events and the risk of drug–drug interactions. NSAIDs have been manufactured in a variety of formulations for topical administration. These include ointment, cream, gel, spray, foam, drops, and patch. Outside of pain relief, there is some interest in the use of topical NSAIDs in other medical disciplines such as ophthalmology as an alternative to corticosteroids[97] and in dermatology for the treatment of actinic keratosis.[98] In the area of pain management, topical NSAIDs are being investigated for postoperative pain management, rheumatologic conditions, acute musculoskeletal pain, and burn injuries. Compared to placebo for the treatment of musculoskeletal pain, topical NSAIDs are significantly better with an NNT of 4.6 (3.8 to 5.9).[99] Possible advantages of topically applied NSAIDs compared to oral administered NSAIDs include less systemic absorption and the potential for fewer side effects.

A topical analgesic drug has three main components: the active drug, the topical excipient chassis, and the penetration enhancer(s). All three components have an effect on the topical drug's properties and resultant clinical profile.[100] The way in which the drug is formulated as a solution, cream, gel, or patch also have significant effects on the clinical profile. For a topical formulation to be effective, it must first penetrate the skin. Only when the drug has entered the lower layers of the skin can it be absorbed by the blood and transported to the site of action, or penetrate deeper into areas where inflammation is occurring. Individual drugs have different degrees of penetration. A balance between lipid and aqueous solubility is needed to optimize penetration, and use of prodrug esters has been suggested as a way of enhancing permeability.[101] Once the drug has reached the site of action, it must be present at a sufficiently high concentration to inhibit COX enzymes and produce pain relief. It is probable that topical NSAIDs exert their action both by local reduction of symptoms arising from periarticular structures, and by systemic delivery to intracapsular structures. Tissue levels of NSAIDs applied topically reach levels high enough to inhibit COX-2.[102] Plasma concentrations achieved by topical delivery are 1% to 10% of those achieved by systemic delivery.[103–104] Drug concentrations in adipose tissue and skeletal muscle after topical administration are the same or higher than those after oral administration, at least with topical diclofenac.[102]

Potential adverse reactions can be considered as cutaneous or systemic reactions. The former tend to be mild, and the more controversial issue is whether systemic reactions are reduced by limiting plasma concentrations. Adverse reactions most commonly involve cutaneous irritation in 2% of patients. The rate of systemic adverse reactions, in particular GI events, is not well defined, but it is clear that reactions such as gastric irritation, asthma and renal impairment, well established complications of oral therapy, can sometimes occur with topical agents. Topical NSAIDs are without the GI adverse events of oral NSAIDs, and should, therefore, be better tolerated. Topical NSAIDs are safer when compared with oral NSAIDs with less risk of gastrointestinal bleeding or renal failure.[105] Differences in tolerability and safety probably reflect considerably lower plasma concentrations with topical NSAIDs.

The topical NSAIDs approved in the United States are a diclofenac epolamine 1.3% patch (Flector Patch), which is applied twice a day for acute pain due to minor sprains, strains, and contusions; and a diclofenac sodium 1% gel (Voltaren Gel Patch), which is applied four times a day to relieve osteoarthritis pain in the hands, knees, or other joints that are amenable to topical treatment. As with oral NSAIDs and coxibs, these topical NSAIDs carry an Food and Drug Administration (FDA)–required "black box" warning of increased cardiovascular risk. We are not aware of any published results on the use of topical NSAIDs in cancer pain, but they may be useful in selected cases.

Use in Cancer Pain

NSAIDs are accepted as an important tool in treating cancer pain and may be combined with opioids for this purpose.[106] Although many NSAIDs are available to treat various painful conditions, it is unclear which agent is most clinically efficacious for relieving cancer-related pain, and if there are clinical differences between these agents that justify their cost differences. Additionally, it is uncertain which opioid and NSAID combinations are the most efficacious for cancer pain or even what may be the additional benefit of combining an NSAID with an opioid in this setting. McNicol et al.[11] assessed and compared the efficacy of various NSAID and NSAID plus opioid combinations in the treatment of cancer pain. They concluded that most studies were of insufficient duration to demonstrate that the long-term use of NSAIDs is safe and effective in patients with cancer. They advised that clinicians should be at least as cautious in using NSAIDs in this population as they would any other population, especially given the probability that a patient with cancer may be on a broad regimen of medications, some of which may increase NSAID-related toxicity. In addition, the selection of a particular NSAID was not conclusively established. The majority of studies demonstrated no difference between different NSAIDs, and of those that did demonstrate a difference, clinical significance was usually marginal.

A significant proportion of chronic cancer pain arises from metastases to bone, and bone cancer pain is one of the most difficult of all persistent pain states to control. Several tumor types including sarcomas and breast, prostate, and lung carcinomas grow in or preferentially metastasize to the skeleton where they proliferate, and induce significant bone remodeling, bone destruction, and cancer pain. Many of these tumors express COX-2.[107] In an animal model of bone cancer pain, Saito et al.[108] examined the effects of oral administration of a COX-1 selective inhibitor, a COX-2 selective inhibitor (celecoxib), and a nonselective COX inhibitor (indomethacin) on bone cancer pain and compared these effects to the effect of orally administered acetaminophen and morphine. Oral administration of acetaminophen, indomethacin, and morphine, but not the selective COX-1 inhibitor or celecoxib, produced an analgesic effect on bone cancer pain. Co-administration of a subanalgesic does of morphine with acetaminophen enhanced the analgesic effect of acetaminophen. Medhurst et al.[109] also failed to demonstrate an analgesic effect from celecoxib in a rat model.

Studies of cancer pain have involved several different NSAIDs. Single- and multiple-dose trials have shown benefit from ibuprofen,[110] naproxen,[111] ketoprofen,[112] and ketorolac.[113] Prolonged subcutaneous infusions of naproxen,[114] diclofenac[115] and ketorolac[116] have also been reported. NSAIDs are widely believed to be especially helpful for the management of malignant bone pain.[117–118] However, specific clinical data about pain-reducing responses to NSAIDs in cancer patients are sparse; many of the assumptions that guide oncologic pain management are based on either clinical impressions or trials in nonmalignant pain.

In 1994, Eisenberg et al.[119] examined the efficacy and safety of NSAIDs in the treatment of cancer-related pain. The authors conducted a meta-analysis of data from 25 randomized controlled trials. The studies provided data on 1545 cancer patients. Although all 25 trials reported analgesic efficacy, only the single-dose studies were comparable for analgesic efficacy analysis. Single doses of placebo produced a 15-36% rate of analgesia, whereas the use of NSAIDs resulted in roughly twice as much pain relief (31% versus 60%). These results support the WHO position that although placebo produces some pain relief in cancer patients, true nonopioid analgesics have a significantly higher analgesic efficacy in patients with cancer pain.[120] The data on comparative efficacy of one NSAID versus another is limited. Four studies compared the single-dose efficacy of aspirin with three other NSAIDs (indoprofen, ketoprofen, and naproxen). The results suggested slightly superior pain relief from NSAIDs compared with aspirin, but were without statistical significance. The dose-response analgesic efficacy of NSAIDs in cancer pain is not yet determined and the results of the meta-analysis are still only suggestive. The dose-response relationship was evaluated by comparing the analgesic efficacy of 600 mg versus 1000 mg of oral aspirin, 100 versus 200 mg of oral indoprofen, and 10 versus 20 mg of intramuscular ketorolac. The two scores used for analgesic efficacy (peak pain intensity difference (PPID) and summed pain intensity difference (SPID)) were approximately 1.3 greater in the high-dose patients than in the low-dose patients, but these differences did not reach statistical significance. The ceiling analgesic effect was tested by comparing pain scores for recommended and supramaximal single doses of three NSAIDs: ketoprofen 100 versus 300 mg and 75 versus 225 mg orally, zomepirac 100 versus 200 orally, and ketorolac 10 and 30 mg versus 90 mg intramuscularly. The recommended and supramaximal doses showed similar efficacy according to all four scores used (PPID, SPID, PPAR (peak pain relief) and TOPAR (total pain relief)), which indicates a ceiling effect. The authors concluded that the meta-analysis precluded testing the hypothesis that NSAIDs are particularly effective for malignant bone pain because of a lack of comparable studies. Well-designed analgesic trials in which bone pain or pain from other specific cancer-related syndromes assessed separately from nonbone pain are required.

In a 2005 Cochrane Database review, McNicol et al.[11] examined the efficacy of NSAIDs or acetaminophen used alone or combined with opioids for cancer pain. Forty-two randomized controlled trials and controlled clinical trials that compared NSAID versus placebo, NSAID versus NSAID, NSAID versus NSAID plus opioid, opioid versus opioid plus NSAID, or NSAID versus opioid involving 3084 patients were reviewed. Studies varied in the agents and dosages used, routes of administration, types of cancer, baseline pain severity, types of pain (nociceptive versus neuropathic), and outcome measures. The length of studies varied. Sixteen of the forty-two study durations were one week or greater. By contrast, eleven studies were single-dose only. None of the studies followed patients for a period of more than 12 weeks. Side effects, although not consistently reported, tended to be minor and occur infrequently. However, many adverse effects such as development of GI ulcer or renal toxicity may not be apparent with short-term dosing. Furthermore, the long-term safety profile of NSAIDs in patients with cancer has not been established in a randomized study. In spite of the limitations of the review, the authors concluded that NSAIDs were more effective in treating cancer pain than placebo, although all of these were single dose studies. There was no evidence to suggest that any one NSAID was superior to another. Comparisons between various NSAID/opioid combinations were inconclusive and there was little clinical difference when combining an NSAID plus an opioid versus either drug alone. The authors were unable to make any conclusions about the long-term safety and efficacy of NSAIDs in cancer patients.

Adverse Effects

Adverse reactions to NSAID therapy are listed in Table 17.2. The ingestion of NSAIDs can produce multiple adverse effects on the kidney[121] and other organ systems.[122] Common side effects of NSAIDs include upper gastrointestinal upset, dizziness, and drowsiness. Multiple doses generally produced more side effects than single doses.

NSAIDs may cause gastric irritation, bleeding, and altered platelet function. Gastric mucosal integrity is maintained by the interplay of three protective networks: prostaglandin synthesis, nitric oxide synthesis and the activity of the enteric nervous system. Patients taking any NSAID require monitoring for gastropathy, renal failure, hepatic dysfunction, and bleeding.[119,123–124] Gastric distress should be ameliorated by the use of a histamine H2 antagonist or sucralfate.[80] Misoprostol is a synthetic analogue of prostaglandin E_1. It inhibits gastric acid production and has cytoprotective effects on the gastroduodenal mucosa. Misoprostol, in a dose of 200 μg taken orally four times a day, is more effective than 150 mg of ranitidine taken orally twice daily in preventing asymptomatic, NSAID-induced gastric ulceration.[125] Side effects include sedation, tremor, abdominal pain, and diarrhea. Mild diarrhea and GI intolerance may occur in 20 to 40% of patients and may limit tolerance to the drug.[126–127]

All NSAIDs should be used cautiously (if at all) in patients with renal insufficiency. Although sulindac may have relatively less effect on the kidney[128] and might seem a safer choice when potent anti-inflammatory effects are desirable in the cancer patient with renal insufficiency, the clinical relevance for this renal-sparing effect is controversial. Nabumetone may require dose adjustment in the elderly, other patients with active rheumatic disease and those with hepatic impairment, but not in patients with mild-to-moderate renal insufficiency.[129]

CARDIOVASCULAR EFFECTS OF NONSTEROIDAL ANTI-INFLAMMATORY DRUGS

In October 2004, rofecoxib was withdrawn from world markets after a randomized placebo-controlled trial found that doses of 25 mg/day increased rates of cardiovascular events (twofold increase in cardiovascular risk) in patients with colorectal polyps.[130] A previous study showed a fivefold increase in thromboembolic cardiovascular events (primarily acute myocardial infarction) among patients treated with 50 mg/day of rofecoxib compared to 1000 mg/day of naproxen.[131] Cardiovascular risks were evident from the start of therapy and continued throughout the study period.[132] A few months later, other selective COX-2 inhibitors, celecoxib[133] and parecoxib with valdecoxib,[134–135] were shown to have similar toxic effects. In 2005, the FDA requested labeling changes from the pharmaceutical manufacturers of NSAIDs that state in a black box warning that patients with cardiovascular disease or risk factors for cardiovascular disease may be at greater risk of cardiovascular outcomes.[136]

Cardiovascular toxicity appears to be a class effect, as studies of other COX-2 inhibitors have reported similar findings.[137] The mechanisms underlying the cardiovascular effects of rofecoxib and other COX-2 inhibitors are not clear, but several possibilities have been proposed. Side effects of rofecoxib include fluid retention and increased blood pressure, both of which may trigger cardiovascular events.[138] Selective COX-2 inhibitors suppress vascular production of prostacyclin (PGI2) without affecting thromboxane A2 synthesis.[139] PGI2 in endothelium inhibits platelet aggregation, causes vasodilation, and prevents the proliferation of vascular smooth muscle cells in vitro. Loss of the antiplatelet and vasodilatory effects of prostacyclin and a relative excess of thromboxane A2 favors vasoconstriction, platelet aggregation, and thrombosis. Depression of PGI2 formation by COX-2 inhibitors can elevate blood pressure, accelerate atherogenesis, and lead to an exaggerated thrombotic response to the rupture of an atherosclerotic plaque.[140]

Celecoxib continues to be widely used, despite meta-analyses of randomized controlled trials showing an increased risk of myocardial infarction.[137,141] Based on the randomized data, celecoxib appears unsafe in doses of 400 mg or more.[137,141] Older nonselective NSAIDs reversibly block both isoforms of COX but vary in their degree of selectivity. Conventional nonaspirin NSAIDs may share the same cardiovascular toxicity to the extent that they are COX-2 selective. McGettigan and Henry[142] did a systematic review and meta-analysis of controlled observational studies to compare the risks of serious cardiovascular events with individual NSAIDs and COX-2 inhibitors. Among older nonselective drugs, diclofenac had the highest risk, with a summary relative risk of 1.40 (95% confidence interval [CI]: 1.16–1.70) and it appears to be harmful at commonly used doses.

TABLE 17.2

SIDE EFFECTS OF NONSTEROIDAL ANTI-INFLAMMATORY DRUGS

System	Symptoms/Signs
Gastrointestinal	Nausea, anorexia, abdominal pain, ulcers, GI hemorrhage, perforation
Cardiovascular	Hypertension, inhibition of platelet activation
Renal	Salt and water retention, edema, deterioration of renal function, hyperkalemia, analgesic nephropathy
Central nervous system	Headache, dizziness, vertigo, confusion, depression
Hypersensitivity	Vasomotor rhinitis, asthma, urticaria, hypotension, shock

(Modified from Mielke CH Jr. Comparative effects of aspirin and acetaminophen on hemostasis. *Arch Intern Med*. 1981;141:305–310.)

Diclofenac is another relatively COX-2–selective drug that has been much less studied than either rofecoxib or celecoxib. It is reported to have a degree of COX-2 selectivity similar to celecoxib.[143] The other drugs had summary relative risks close to 1: naproxen, 0.97 (95% CI: 0.87–1.07); piroxicam, 1.06 (95% CI: 0.70–1.59); and ibuprofen, 1.07 (95% CI: 0.97–1.18). In doses of around 200 mg/day, celecoxib was not associated with an increased risk, but the data did not exclude an increased risk with higher doses. Use of naproxen was not associated with any reduction in risk, as was suggested in a report of a large trial comparing it with rofecoxib.[131] In a study on the effects of COX-3 inhibitors and acute myocardial infarction, Andersohn et al.[144] reported that daily doses of celecoxib less than or equal to 200 mg/day had a multivariate relative risk for acute myocardial infarction of 1.44 (95% CI: 1.12–1.87) and doses exceeding 200 mg/day had a relative risk of 2.46 (95% CI: 1.26–4.81). In reviewing data from 138 randomized trials, Kearney et al.[137] estimated a summary relative risk for COX-2 inhibitors of 1.42 (95% CI: 1.13–1.78). The use of COX-2–selective NSAIDS in patients without major cardiovascular risk factors may also cause harmful effects.[144]

Long-term use of high doses of celecoxib is associated with increased cardiovascular toxicity.[145] Curcumin (diferuloylmethane) is a plant-derived dietary ingredient with potent NF-κB and tumor inhibitory properties. It is the principal curcuminoid of the curry spice turmeric. Curcumin has a surprisingly wide range of beneficial properties, including anti-inflammatory, antioxidant, chemopreventive and chemotherapeutic activity. It is a natural COX-2 inhibitor and when combined with celecoxib synergistically augments (by up to 100%) the growth inhibitory effects of celecoxib this rendering the drug effective at up to tenfold lower doses.[146] At cellular and molecular levels, curcumin has been shown to regulate a number of signaling pathways, including the eicosanoid pathway involving COX and LOX (lipoxygenase).[147] In patients who received 8 g curcumin by mouth daily, it was well tolerated and, despite its limited absorption, had biological activity in some patients with pancreatic cancer.[148] Curcumin exhibits great promise as a therapeutic agent and is currently in human clinical trials for a variety of conditions, including multiple myeloma, pancreatic cancer, myelodysplastic syndromes, colon cancer, psoriasis, and Alzheimer disease. Curcumin synergistically augments the growth inhibition inserted by celecoxib in pancreatic cancer cells expressing COX-2.[149] The synergistic effect was mediated through inhibition of COX-2. Curcumin in combination with celecoxib may enable the use of celecoxib at lower and safer concentrations.

In summary, both selective and nonselective NSAIDs have potential for significant cardiovascular events. There may be differences in the risk for nonselective NSAIDs (in particular doclofenac) because of their different COX-1/COX-2 selectivity. For most patients with conditions who require chronic pain relief, naproxen appears to be the safest NSAID choice from a cardiovascular perspective.[132] For patients at high risk of NSAID-related gastrointestinal tract complications, naproxen plus a proton pump inhibitor is less costly and as effective, and probably safer, than low-dose celecoxib.

Recommendations for Use of Nonsteroidal Anti-Inflammatory Drugs in Cancer Pain

According to the results of the Cochrane review,[11] NSAIDs should not be overlooked as a potential first-line treatment for cancer pain. They may provide additive pain relief for some patients who already are receiving opioids for moderate to severe cancer pain. Caution should be used in interpreting these results. Cancer patients undergoing active treatment of disease are medically very complex with high risk for problems with drug-related toxicities and interactions. Many of these patients are neutropenic and thrombocytopenic and are at risk for bleeding complications (including catastrophic intracranial bleeding) and opportunistic infections. All of the currently available NSAIDs (with the exception of celecoxib for bleeding risk) can potentially cause bleeding or mask the presence of opportunistic infection in immunocompromised patients. The masking of opportunistic infections related to the antipyretic effects of NSAIDs poses particular risk and might even cause lethal complications in patients who are neutropenic, thrombocytopenic, or otherwise immunocompromised.[150] Patients undergoing active radiation therapy or chemotherapy frequently have issues with nausea and vomiting and dehydration. As NSAIDs are relatively contraindicated in situations of relative hypovolemia, NSAIDs should be used with great caution in these patients, if at all. Although it is possible that NSAIDs could be better tolerated than opioids in some situations, there certainly are situations in which the opposite is true. Because cancer pain has a dynamic course, it is necessary to have a repeated assessment to correctly evaluate the possible clinical advantage of NSAIDs, though concomitant and multiple variables may occur to confound the picture.

We recommend limited (less than 2 weeks' exposure) and highly selective use of NSAIDs in the cancer patient with pain. In our experience, most cases of cancer pain, irrespective of source of pain or intensity, can be effectively treated with appropriate opioid use in preference to the use of NSAIDs either alone or in combination with opioids. We are not fearful of using high dose opioids when they are required to manage pain from cancer.

References

1. Colvin L, Fallon M. Challenges in cancer pain management—bone pain. *Eur J Cancer.* 2008;44:1083–1090.
2. Coyle N, Layman-Goldstein M. Pharmacologic management of adult cancer pain. *Oncology (Williston Park).* 2007;21:10–22; discussion 26.
3. Foley KM. Treatment of cancer-related pain. *J Natl Cancer Inst Monogr.* 2004:103–104.
4. Gordin V, Weaver MA, Hahn MB. Acute and chronic pain management in palliative care. *Best Pract Res Clin Obstet Gynaecol.* 2001;15:203–234.
5. Guindon J, Walczak JS, Beaulieu P. Recent advances in the pharmacological management of pain. *Drugs.* 2007;67:2121–2133.
6. Laird B, Colvin L, Fallon M. Management of cancer pain: basic principles and neuropathic cancer pain. *Eur J Cancer.* 2008;44:1078–1082.
7. Lickiss JN. Approaching cancer pain relief. *Eur J Pain.* 2001;5 (Suppl A):5-14.

8. Lucas LK, Lipman AG. Recent advances in pharmacotherapy for cancer pain management. *Cancer Pract.* 2002;10(Suppl 1):S14-20.
9. Maltoni M, Scarpi E, Modonesi C, et al. A validation study of the WHO analgesic ladder: A two-step vs three-step strategy. *Support Care Cancer.* 2005;13:888–894.
10. McDonnell FJ, Sloan JW, Hamann SR. Advances in cancer pain management. *Curr Pain Headache Rep.* 2001;5:265–271.
11. McNicol E, Strassels SA, Goudas L, et al. NSAIDS or paracetamol, alone or combined with opioids, for cancer pain. *Cochrane Database Syst Rev.* 2005:CD005180.
12. Mercadante S. The use of anti-inflammatory drugs in cancer pain. *Cancer Treat Rev.* 2001;27:51–61.
13. Mercadante S, Fulfaro F, Casuccio A. A randomised controlled study on the use of anti-inflammatory drugs in patients with cancer pain on morphine therapy: Effects on dose-escalation and a pharmacoeconomic analysis. *Eur J Cancer.* 2002;38:1358–1363.
14. Swarm R, Anghelescu DL, Benedetti C, et al. Adult cancer pain. *J Natl Compr Canc Netw.* 2007;5:726–751.
15. Malmberg AB, Yaksh TL. Hyperalgesia mediated by spinal glutamate or substance P receptor blocked by spinal cyclooxygenase inhibition. *Science.* 1992;257:1276–1279.
16. Pickering G, Loriot MA, Libert F, et al. Analgesic effect of acetaminophen in humans: first evidence of a central serotonergic mechanism. *Clin Pharmacol Ther.* 2006;79:371–378.
17. Smith WL. Prostaglandin biosynthesis and its compartmentation in vascular smooth muscle and endothelial cells. *Annu Rev Physiol.* 1986;48:251–262.
18. Flossmann E, Rothwell PM. Effect of aspirin on long-term risk of colorectal cancer: consistent evidence from randomised and observational studies. *Lancet.* 2007;369:1603–1613.
19. Giardiello FM, Hamilton SR, Krush AJ, et al. Treatment of colonic and rectal adenomas with sulindac in familial adenomatous polyposis. *N Engl J Med.* 1993;328:1313–1316.
20. Moran EM. Epidemiological and clinical aspects of nonsteroidal anti-inflammatory drugs and cancer risks. *J Environ Pathol Toxicol Oncol.* 2002;21:193–201.
21. Zha S, Yegnasubramanian V, Nelson WG, et al. Cyclooxygenases in cancer: progress and perspective. *Cancer Lett.* 2004;215:1–20.
22. Roth GJ, Majerus PW. The mechanism of the effect of aspirin on human platelets. I. Acetylation of a particulate fraction protein. *J Clin Invest.* 1975;56:624–632.
23. Needs CJ, Brooks PM. Clinical pharmacokinetics of the salicylates. *Clin Pharmacokinet.* 1985;10:164–177.
24. Addison RS, Parker-Scott SL, Eadie MJ, et al. Steady-state dispositions of valproate and diflunisal alone and coadministered to healthy volunteers. *Eur J Clin Pharmacol.* 2000;56:715–721.
25. Yasuda O, Takemura Y, Kawamoto H, et al. Aspirin: Recent developments. *Cell Mol Life Sci.* 2008;65:354–358.
26. Botting R. COX-1 and COX-3 inhibitors. *Thromb Res.* 2003;110:269–272.
27. D'Agati V. Does aspirin cause acute or chronic renal failure in experimental animals and in humans? *Am J Kidney Dis.* 1996;28:S24-9.
28. Stuart JJ, Pisko EJ. Choline magnesium trisalicylate does not impair platelet aggregation. *Pharmatherapeutica.* 1981;2:547–551.
29. Kilander A, Dotevall G. Endoscopic evaluation of the comparative effects of acetylsalicylic acid and choline magnesium trisalicylate on human gastric and duodenal mucosa. *Br J Rheumatol.* 1983;22:36–40.
30. Danesh BJ, McLaren M, Russell RI, et al. Comparison of the effect of aspirin and choline magnesium trisalicylate on thromboxane biosynthesis in human platelets: role of the acetyl moiety. *Haemostasis.* 1989;19:169–173.
31. Glasgow JF. Reye's syndrome: The case for a causal link with aspirin. *Drug Saf.* 2006;29:1111–1121.
32. Campieri M. New steroids and new salicylates in inflammatory bowel disease: A critical appraisal. *Gut.* 2002;50 Suppl 3:III43-6.
33. Peura DA, Lanza FL, Gostout CJ, et al. The American College of Gastroenterology Bleeding Registry: Preliminary findings. *Am J Gastroenterol.* 1997;92:924–928.
34. Botting RM. Mechanism of action of acetaminophen: Is there a cyclooxygenase 3? *Clin Infect Dis.* 2000;31 Suppl 5:S202-10.
35. Hinz B, Cheremina O, Brune K. Acetaminophen (paracetamol) is a selective cyclooxygenase-2 inhibitor in man. *Faseb J.* 2008;22:383–390.
36. Flower RJ, Vane JR. Inhibition of prostaglandin synthetase in brain explains the anti-pyretic activity of paracetamol (4-acetamidophenol). *Nature.* 1972;240:410–411.
37. Warner TD, Mitchell JA. Cyclooxygenases: new forms, new inhibitors, and lessons from the clinic. *Faseb J.* 2004;18:790–804.
38. Pickering G, Esteve V, Loriot MA, et al. Acetaminophen reinforces descending inhibitory pain pathways. *Clin Pharmacol Ther.* 2008;84:47–51.
39. Graham GG, Scott KF. Mechanism of action of paracetamol. *Am J Ther.* 2005;12:46–55.
40. Ottani A, Leone S, Sandrini M, et al. The analgesic activity of paracetamol is prevented by the blockade of cannabinoid CB1 receptors. *Eur J Pharmacol.* 2006;531:280–281.
41. Mielke CH Jr. Comparative effects of aspirin and acetaminophen on hemostasis. *Arch Intern Med.* 1981;141:305–310.
42. Seymour RA, Williams FM, Oxley A, et al. A comparative study of the effects of aspirin and paracetamol (acetaminophen) on platelet aggregation and bleeding time. *Eur J Clin Pharmacol.* 1984;26:567–571.
43. Munsterhjelm E, Munsterhjelm NM, Niemi TT, et al. Dose-dependent inhibition of platelet function by acetaminophen in healthy volunteers. *Anesthesiology.* 2005;103:712–717.
44. Blantz RC. Acetaminophen: Acute and chronic effects on renal function. *Am J Kidney Dis.* 1996;28:S3-6.
45. Barrett BJ. Acetaminophen and adverse chronic renal outcomes: An appraisal of the epidemiologic evidence. *Am J Kidney Dis.* 1996;28:S14-19.
46. Duggin GG. Combination analgesic-induced kidney disease: The Australian experience. *Am J Kidney Dis.* 1996;28:S39-47.
47. Eguia L, Materson BJ. Acetaminophen-related acute renal failure without fulminant liver failure. *Pharmacotherapy.* 1997;17:363–370.
48. Seifert CF, Lucas DS, Vondracek TG, et al. Patterns of acetaminophen use in alcoholic patients. *Pharmacotherapy.* 1993;13:391–395.
49. Whitcomb DC, Block GD. Association of acetaminophen hepatotoxicity with fasting and ethanol use. *JAMA.* 1994;272:1845–50.
50. Prescott LF. Therapeutic misadventure with paracetamol: fact or fiction? *Am J Ther.* 2000;7:99–114.
51. Benson GD, Koff RS, Tolman KG. The therapeutic use of acetaminophen in patients with liver disease. *Am J Ther.* 2005;12:133–141.
52. Rumack BH. Acetaminophen hepatotoxicity: The first 35 years. *J Toxicol Clin Toxicol.* 2002;40:3–20.
53. Riordan SM, Williams R. Alcohol exposure and paracetamol-induced hepatotoxicity. *Addict Biol.* 2002;7:191–206.
54. Novak D, Lewis JH. Drug-induced liver disease. *Curr Opin Gastroenterol.* 2003;19:203–215.
55. Altomare E, Leo MA, Lieber CS. Interaction of acute ethanol administration with acetaminophen metabolism and toxicity in rats fed alcohol chronically. *Alcohol Clin Exp Res.* 1984;8:405–408.
56. Sato C, Matsuda Y, Lieber CS. Increased hepatotoxicity of acetaminophen after chronic ethanol consumption in the rat. *Gastroenterology.* 1981;80:140–148.
57. Walker RM, McElligott TF, Power EM, et al. Increased acetaminophen-induced hepatotoxicity after chronic ethanol consumption in mice. *Toxicology.* 1983;28:193–206.
58. Perrot N, Nalpas B, Yang CS, et al. Modulation of cytochrome P450 isozymes in human liver, by ethanol and drug intake. *Eur J Clin Invest.* 1989;19:549–555.
59. Thummel KE, Slattery JT, Nelson SD, et al. Effect of ethanol on hepatotoxicity of acetaminophen in mice and on reactive metabolite formation by mouse and human liver microsomes. *Toxicol Appl Pharmacol.* 1989;100:391–397.
60. Rumack BH. Acetaminophen overdose in young children. Treatment and effects of alcohol and other additional ingestants in 417 cases. *Am J Dis Child.* 1984;138:428–433.
61. Klotz U, Ammon E. Clinical and toxicological consequences of the inductive potential of ethanol. *Eur J Clin Pharmacol.* 1998;54:7–12.
62. Slattery JT, Nelson SD, Thummel KE. The complex interaction between ethanol and acetaminophen. *Clin Pharmacol Ther.* 1996;60:241–246.
63. Draganov P, Durrence H, Cox C, Reuben A. Alcohol-acetaminophen syndrome. Even moderate social drinkers are at risk. *Postgrad Med.* 2000;107:189–195.
64. Hylek EM, Heiman H, Skates SJ, et al. Acetaminophen and other risk factors for excessive warfarin anticoagulation. *JAMA.* 1998;279:657–662.
65. Parra D, Beckey NP, Stevens GR. The effect of acetaminophen on the international normalized ratio in patients stabilized on warfarin therapy. *Pharmacotherapy.* 2007;27:675–683.

66. Loguercio C, Taranto D, Vitale LM, et al. Effect of liver cirrhosis and age on the glutathione concentration in the plasma, erythrocytes, and gastric mucosa of man. *Free Radic Biol Med*. 1996;20: 483–488.
67. Whyte IM, Buckley NA, Reith DM, et al. Acetaminophen causes an increased International Normalized Ratio by reducing functional factor VII. *Ther Drug Monit*. 2000;22:742–748.
68. Sabate M, Ibanez L, Perez E, et al. Risk of acute liver injury associated with the use of drugs: A multicentre population survey. *Aliment Pharmacol Ther*. 2007;25:1401–1409.
69. Heard K, Green JL, Bailey JE, et al. A randomized trial to determine the change in alanine aminotransferase during 10 days of paracetamol (acetaminophen) administration in subjects who consume moderate amounts of alcohol. *Aliment Pharmacol Ther*. 2007;26: 283–290.
70. Watkins PB, Kaplowitz N, Slattery JT, et al. Aminotransferase elevations in healthy adults receiving 4 grams of acetaminophen daily: A randomized controlled trial. *JAMA*. 2006;296:87–93.
71. Fored CM, Ejerblad E, Lindblad P, et al. Acetaminophen, aspirin, and chronic renal failure. *N Engl J Med*. 2001;345:1801–1808.
72. McLaughlin JK, Lipworth L, Chow WH, et al. Analgesic use and chronic renal failure: A critical review of the epidemiologic literature. *Kidney Int*. 1998;54:679–686.
73. Stockler M, Vardy J, Pillai A, et al. Acetaminophen (paracetamol) improves pain and well-being in people with advanced cancer already receiving a strong opioid regimen: A randomized, double-blind, placebo-controlled cross-over trial. *J Clin Oncol*. 2004;22: 3389–3394.
74. Axelsson B, Stellborn P, Strom G. Analgesic effect of paracetamol on cancer related pain in concurrent strong opioid therapy. A prospective clinical study. *Acta Oncol*. 2008;47:891–895.
75. Rodriguez RF, Castillo JM, Del Pilar Castillo M, et al. Codeine/acetaminophen and hydrocodone/acetaminophen combination tablets for the management of chronic cancer pain in adults: A 23-day, prospective, double-blind, randomized, parallel-group study. *Clin Ther*. 2007;29:581–587.
76. Steinmeyer J. Pharmacological basis for the therapy of pain and inflammation with nonsteroidal anti-inflammatory drugs. *Arthritis Res*. 2000;2:379–385.
77. Grond S, Zech D, Schug SA, et al. The importance of non-opioid analgesics for cancer pain relief according to the guidelines of the World Health Organization. *Int J Clin Pharmacol Res*. 1991; 11:253–260.
78. Zech DF, Grond S, Lynch J, et al. Validation of World Health Organization Guidelines for cancer pain relief: A 10-year prospective study. *Pain*. 1995;63:65–76.
79. Vonkeman HE, van de Laar MA. Nonsteroidal anti-inflammatory drugs: Adverse effects and their prevention. *Semin Arthritis Rheum*. 2008.
80. Valentini M, Cannizzaro R, Poletti M, et al. Nonsteroidal antiinflammatory drugs for cancer pain: comparison between misoprostol and ranitidine in prevention of upper gastrointestinal damage. *J Clin Oncol*. 1995;13:2637–2642.
81. Rostom A, Wells G, Tugwell P, et al. Prevention of chronic NSAID induced upper gastrointestinal toxicity. *Cochrane Database Syst Rev*. 2000:CD002296.
82. Engelhardt G, Bogel R, Schnitzer C, et al. Meloxicam: Influence on arachidonic acid metabolism. Part 1. In vitro findings. *Biochem Pharmacol*. 1996;51:21–28.
83. Meade EA, Smith WL, DeWitt DL. Differential inhibition of prostaglandin endoperoxide synthase (cyclooxygenase) isozymes by aspirin and other non-steroidal anti-inflammatory drugs. *J Biol Chem*. 1993;268:6610–6614.
84. Dubois RN, Abramson SB, Crofford L, et al. Cyclooxygenase in biology and disease. *Faseb J*. 1998;12:1063–1073.
85. Ruegg C, Dormond O. Suppression of tumor angiogenesis by nonsteroidal anti-inflammatory drugs: A new function for old drugs. *ScientificWorldJournal*. 2001;1:808–811.
86. Sarkar FH, Adsule S, Li Y, Padhye S. Back to the future: COX-2 inhibitors for chemoprevention and cancer therapy. *Mini Rev Med Chem*. 2007;7:599–608.
87. de Moraes E, Dar NA, de Moura Gallo CV, et al. Cross-talks between cyclooxygenase-2 and tumor suppressor protein p53: Balancing life and death during inflammatory stress and carcinogenesis. *Int J Cancer*. 2007;121:929–937.
88. Ruegg C, Zaric J, Stupp R. Non steroidal anti-inflammatory drugs and COX-2 inhibitors as anti-cancer therapeutics: hypes, hopes and reality. *Ann Med*. 2003;35:476–487.
89. Harris RE, Beebe-Donk J, Alshafie GA. Cancer chemoprevention by cyclooxygenase 2 (COX-2) blockade: results of case control studies. *Subcell Biochem*. 2007;42:193–212.
90. Agrawal A, Fentiman IS. NSAIDs and breast cancer: A possible prevention and treatment strategy. *Int J Clin Pract*. 2008;62: 444–449.
91. Buchanan FG, Holla V, Katkuri S, et al. Targeting cyclooxygenase-2 and the epidermal growth factor receptor for the prevention and treatment of intestinal cancer. *Cancer Res*. 2007;67: 9380–9388.
92. Xiao H, Yang CS. Combination regimen with statins and NSAIDs: A promising strategy for cancer chemoprevention. *Int J Cancer*. 2008;123:983–990.
93. Xiao H, Zhang Q, Lin Y, et al. Combination of atorvastatin and celecoxib synergistically induces cell cycle arrest and apoptosis in colon cancer cells. *Int J Cancer*. 2008;122:2115–2124.
94. Yip-Schneider MT, Wu H, Njoku V, et al. Effect of celecoxib and the novel anti-cancer agent, dimethylamino-parthenolide, in a developmental model of pancreatic cancer. *Pancreas*. 2008;37: 45–53.
95. Carles J, Font A, Mellado B, et al. Weekly administration of docetaxel in combination with estramustine and celecoxib in patients with advanced hormone-refractory prostate cancer: final results from a phase II study. *Br J Cancer*. 2007;97:1206–1210.
96. Chow LW, Yip AY, Loo WT, et al. Celecoxib anti-aromatase neoadjuvant (CAAN) trial for locally advanced breast cancer. *J Steroid Biochem Mol Biol*. 2008;111:13–17.
97. Schechter BA. Ketorolac tromethamine 0.4% as a treatment for allergic conjuctivitis. *Expert Opin Drug Metab Toxicol*. 2008;4: 507–511.
98. Rivers JK, McLean DI. An open study to assess the efficacy and safety of topical 3% diclofenac in a 2.5% hyaluronic acid gel for the treatment of actinic keratoses. *Arch Dermatol*. 1997;133: 1239–1242.
99. Mason L, Moore RA, Edwards JE, et al. Topical NSAIDs for chronic musculoskeletal pain: systematic review and meta-analysis. *BMC Musculoskelet Disord*. 2004;5:28.
100. Galer BS. All topical NSAIDs not created equal—understanding topical analgesic drug formulations. *Pain*. 2008;139:237–238.
101. Bhandari KH, Newa M, Yoon SI, et al. Evaluation of physicochemical properties, skin permeation and accumulation profiles of ketorolac fatty ester prodrugs. *Biol Pharm Bull*. 2007;30: 2211–2216.
102. Brunner M, Dehghanyar P, Seigfried B, et al. Favourable dermal penetration of diclofenac after administration to the skin using a novel spray gel formulation. *Br J Clin Pharmacol*. 2005;60: 573–577.
103. Radermacher J, Jentsch D, Scholl MA, et al. Diclofenac concentrations in synovial fluid and plasma after cutaneous application in inflammatory and degenerative joint disease. *Br J Clin Pharmacol*. 1991;31:537–541.
104. Taburet AM, Singlas E, Glass RC, et al. Pharmacokinetic comparison of oral and local action transcutaneous flurbiprofen in healthy volunteers. *J Clin Pharm Ther*. 1995;20:101–107.
105. Moore RA, Derry S, McQuay HJ. Topical agents in the treatment of rheumatic pain. *Rheum Dis Clin North Am*. 2008;34:415–432.
106. Jadad AR, Browman GP. The WHO analgesic ladder for cancer pain management. Stepping up the quality of its evaluation. *JAMA*. 1995;274:1870–1873.
107. Sabino MA, Ghilardi JR, Jongen JL, et al. Simultaneous reduction in cancer pain, bone destruction, and tumor growth by selective inhibition of cyclooxygenase-2. *Cancer Res*. 2002;62:7343–7349.
108. Saito O, Aoe T, Yamamoto T. Analgesic effects of nonsteroidal antiinflammatory drugs, acetaminophen, and morphine in a mouse model of bone cancer pain. *J Anesth*. 2005;19:218–224.
109. Medhurst SJ, Walker K, Bowes M, et al. A rat model of bone cancer pain. *Pain*. 2002;96:129–140.
110. Weingart WA, Sorkness CA, Earhart RH. Analgesia with oral narcotics and added ibuprofen in cancer patients. *Clin Pharm*. 1985;4:53–58.
111. Levick S, Jacobs C, Loukas DF, et al. Naproxen sodium in treatment of bone pain due to metastatic cancer. *Pain*. 1988;35: 253–258.
112. Stambaugh J, Drew J. A double-blind parallel evaluation of the efficacy and safety of a single dose of ketoprofen in cancer pain. *J Clin Pharmacol*. 1988;28:S34-9.
113. Yalcin S, Gullu I, Tekuzman G, et al. Ketorolac tromethamine in cancer pain. *Acta Oncol*. 1997;36:231–232.

114. Gottlieb A. Naproxen sodium infusion for exacerbation of cancer pain [letter]. *J Pain Symptom Manage.* 1990;5:73.
115. Hall E. Subcutaneous diclofenac: An effective alternative? [letter]. *Palliat Med.* 1993;7:339–340.
116. Middleton RK, Lyle JA, Berger DL. Ketorolac continuous infusion: A case report and review of the literature. *J Pain Symptom Manage.* 1996;12:190–194.
117. Ashburn MA, Lipman AG. Management of pain in the cancer patient. A*nesth Analg.* 1993;76:402–416.
118. De Jong RH. Drug therapy in cancer pain. *J Med Assoc Ga.* 1991;80:295–300.
119. Eisenberg E, Berkey CS, Carr DB, et al. Efficacy and safety of nonsteroidal antiinflammatory drugs for cancer pain: A meta-analysis. *J Clin Oncol.* 1994;12:2756–2765.
120. *Cancer pain relief with a guide to opioid availability.* 2nd ed. Geneva, Switzerland: World Health Organization, 1996.
121. Nanra RS. Pattern of renal dysfunction in analgesic nephropathy—comparison with glomerulonephritis. *Nephrol Dial Transplant.* 1992;7:384–390.
122. Matzke GR. Nonrenal toxicities of acetaminophen, aspirin, and nonsteroidal anti-inflammatory agents. *Am J Kidney Dis.* 1996;28:S63-70.
123. Doyle D, Hanks DWC, MacDonald N, eds. Monitoring NSAIDS. In: *Oxford textbook of palliative medicine.* Oxford: Oxford University Press, 1993.
124. Hollander D. Gastrointestinal complications of nonsteroidal anti-inflammatory drugs: prophylactic and therapeutic strategies. *Am J Med.* 1994;96:274–281.
125. Raskin JB, White RH, Jaszewski R, et al. Misoprostol and ranitidine in the prevention of NSAID-induced ulcers: A prospective, double-blind, multicenter study. *Am J Gastroenterol.* 1996;91:223–227.
126. Silverstein FE, Graham DY, Senior JR, et al. Misoprostol reduces serious gastrointestinal complications in patients with rheumatoid arthritis receiving nonsteroidal anti-inflammatory drugs. A randomized, double-blind, placebo-controlled trial. *Ann Intern Med.* 1995;123:241–249.
127. Ching CK, Lam SK. A comparison of two prostaglandin analogues (enprostil vs misoprostol) in the treatment of acute duodenal ulcer disease. *J Gastroenterol.* 1995;30:607–614.
128. Swainson CP, Griffiths P. Acute and chronic effects of sulindac on renal function in chronic renal disease. *Clin Pharmacol Ther.* 1985;37:298–300.
129. Davies NM. Clinical pharmacokinetics of nabumetone. The dawn of selective cyclo-oxygenase-2 inhibition? *Clin Pharmacokinet.* 1997;33:404–416.
130. Bresalier RS, Sandler RS, Quan H, et al. Cardiovascular events associated with rofecoxib in a colorectal adenoma chemoprevention trial. *N Engl J Med.* 2005;352:1092–1102.
131. Bombardier C, Laine L, Reicin A, et al. Comparison of upper gastrointestinal toxicity of rofecoxib and naproxen in patients with rheumatoid arthritis. VIGOR Study Group. *N Engl J Med.* 2000;343:1520–1528.
132. Graham DJ. COX-2 inhibitors, other NSAIDs, and cardiovascular risk: The seduction of common sense. *JAMA.* 2006;296:1653–1656.
133. Solomon SD, Pfeffer MA, McMurray JJ, et al. Effect of celecoxib on cardiovascular events and blood pressure in two trials for the prevention of colorectal adenomas. *Circulation.* 2006;114:1028–1035.
134. Nussmeier NA, Whelton AA, Brown MT, et al. Complications of the COX-2 inhibitors parecoxib and valdecoxib after cardiac surgery. *N Engl J Med.* 2005;352:1081–1091.
135. Ott E, Nussmeier NA, Duke PC, Feneck RO, et al. Efficacy and safety of the cyclooxygenase 2 inhibitors parecoxib and valdecoxib in patients undergoing coronary artery bypass surgery. *J Thorac Cardiovasc Surg.* 2003;125:1481–1492.
136. Kuehn BM. FDA panel: Keep COX-2 drugs on market: Black box for COX-2 labels, caution urged for all NSAIDs. *JAMA.* 2005;293:1571–1572.
137. Kearney PM, Baigent C, Godwin J, et al. Do selective cyclo-oxygenase-2 inhibitors and traditional non-steroidal anti-inflammatory drugs increase the risk of atherothrombosis? Meta-analysis of randomised trials. *BMJ.* 2006;332:1302–1308.
138. Zhang J, Ding EL, Song Y. Adverse effects of cyclooxygenase 2 inhibitors on renal and arrhythmia events: meta-analysis of randomized trials. *JAMA.* 2006;296:1619–1632.
139. Grosser T, Fries S, FitzGerald GA. Biological basis for the cardiovascular consequences of COX-2 inhibition: Therapeutic challenges and opportunities. *J Clin Invest.* 2006;116:4–15.
140. Fitzgerald GA. Coxibs and cardiovascular disease. *N Engl J Med.* 2004;351:1709–1711.
141. Caldwell B, Aldington S, Weatherall M, et al. Risk of cardiovascular events and celecoxib: A systematic review and meta-analysis. *J R Soc Med.* 2006;99:132–140.
142. McGettigan P, Henry D. Cardiovascular risk and inhibition of cyclooxygenase: A systematic review of the observational studies of selective and nonselective inhibitors of cyclooxygenase 2. *JAMA.* 2006;296:1633–1644.
143. Patrono C, Patrignani P, Garcia Rodriguez LA. Cyclooxygenase-selective inhibition of prostanoid formation: Transducing biochemical selectivity into clinical read-outs. *J Clin Invest.* 2001;108:7–13.
144. Andersohn F, Suissa S, Garbe E. Use of first- and second-generation cyclooxygenase-2-selective nonsteroidal antiinflammatory drugs and risk of acute myocardial infarction. *Circulation.* 2006;113:1950–1957.
145. Fosbol EL, Gislason GH, Jacobsen S, et al. Risk of myocardial infarction and death associated with the use of nonsteroidal anti-inflammatory drugs (NSAIDs) among healthy individuals: A nationwide cohort study. *Clin Pharmacol Ther.* 2009;85:190–197.
146. Lev-Ari S, Lichtenberg D, Arber N. Compositions for treatment of cancer and inflammation. *Recent Pat Anticancer Drug Discov.* 2008;3:55–62.
147. Rao CV. Regulation of COX and LOX by curcumin. *Adv Exp Med Biol.* 2007;595:213–226.
148. Dhillon N, Aggarwal BB, Newman RA, et al. Phase II trial of curcumin in patients with advanced pancreatic cancer. *Clin Cancer Res.* 2008;14:4491–4499.
149. Lev-Ari S, Zinger H, Kazanov D, et al. Curcumin synergistically potentiates the growth inhibitory and proapoptotic effects of celecoxib in pancreatic adenocarcinoma cells. *Biomed Pharmacother.* 2005;59 Suppl 2:S276-80.
150. Payne R. Limitations of NSAIDs for pain management: Toxicity or lack of efficacy? *J Pain.* 2000;1:14–18.

CHAPTER 18 ■ ADJUVANT DRUGS

There are three main reasons to use adjuvant drugs in cancer patients: to supplement pain relief; to mitigate the adverse effects of analgesic medications (eg, antiemetics and laxatives); and to treat the psychological disturbances such as insomnia, anxiety, depression, and psychosis that so often accompany cancer and its treatment.

ANTIEMETICS

Nausea and vomiting are among the most distressing and feared toxic effects of chemotherapy and radiation therapy.[1] These side effects can result in serious medical problems, increased hospital stay, and impaired quality of life.[2] Chemotherapy-induced nausea and vomiting can be categorized as acute (occurring within 24 hours of therapy), delayed (persisting for 6 to 7 days after therapy), or anticipatory (occurring before chemotherapy administration).[2] Breakthrough and refractory nausea and vomiting describe the symptoms of uncontrolled emesis. Failure of prophylaxis during the first 24 hours after chemotherapy is highly predictive for delayed emesis during the same cycle.[3] Glaus et al.[4] reported that of 247 patients and 38% who received chemotherapy and antiemetics, 13% experienced acute and 38% experienced delayed chemotherapy-induced nausea and vomiting. Of those patients with acute symptoms, 65% had recurrence of symptoms on one or more subsequent days. Thus, a highly effective antiemetic regimen should be employed at the onset of chemotherapy, as opposed to waiting until chemotherapy-induced nausea and vomiting have occurred with initially suboptimal antiemetic treatment. The emetogenicity of cancer chemotherapeutic agents varies significantly and is listed in Table 18.1.

A wide range of treatments are available for emesis prophylaxis. The most frequently used are corticosteroids (methylprednisolone, dexamethasone), 5-HT$_3$ receptor antagonists (ondansetron, granisetron, tropisetron, dolasetron, palonosetron), and neurokinin-1 (NK-1) receptor antagonists (aprepitant).[5] Metoclopramide, lorazepam and other benzodiazepines, and cannabinoids have also been used. Currently, a 5-HT$_3$ receptor antagonist in combination with a corticosteroid and, in certain instances, an NK-1 antagonist are the treatments of choice for prophylaxis against acute emesis following chemotherapy with moderate potential for chemotherapy-induced nausea and vomiting.[6] Various antiemetics and presumed mechanisms of action are listed in Table 18.2.

Even with the emergence of new 5-HT$_3$ receptor and NK-1 antagonists, corticosteroids continue to play an important role in antiemesis for oncology patients. The mechanisms by which corticosteroids are effective as prophylaxis against chemotherapy-induced nausea and

TABLE 18.1

EMETOGENICITY FOR SINGLE-DOSE, INTRAVENOUS CHEMOTHERAPEUTIC AND BIOLOGIC AGENTS

Degree of Emetogenicity (Incidence)	Antineoplastic Agent
High (>90%)	Cisplatin
	Mechlorethamine
	Streptozotocin
	Cyclophosphamide ≥1500 mg/m^2
	Carmustine
	Dacarbazine
Moderate (30–0%)	Oxaliplatin
	Cytarabine >1 g/m^2
	Carboplatin
	Ifosfamide
	Cyclophosphamide <1500 mg/m^2
	Doxorubicin
	Daunorubicin
	Epirubicin
	Idarubicin
	Irinotecan
Low (10–30%)	Paclitaxel
	Docetaxel
	Mitoxantrone
	Topotecan
	Etoposide
	Pemetrexed
	Methotrexate
	Mitomycin C
	Gemcitabine
	Cytarabine ≤100 mg/m^2
	5-Fluorouracil
	Bortezomib
	Cetuximab
	Trastuzumab
Minimal (<10%)	Bleomycin
	Busulfan
	2-Chlorodeoxyadenosine
	Fludarabine
	Vinblastine
	Vincristine
	Vinorelbine
	Bevacizumab

(From Grunberg SM. Antiemetic activity of corticosteroids in patients receiving cancer chemotherapy: dosing, efficacy, and tolerability analysis. *Ann Oncol.* 2007;18:233–240. Reprinted by permission of the European Society for Medical Oncology)

TABLE 18.2

ANTIEMETICS

Agent	Presumed Primary Receptor Site of Action	Dosage/Route	Major Adverse Effects
Metoclopramide	D2 (primarily in GI tract) or 5-HT_3 (only at high doses)	5–20 mg orally or subcutaneously or I.V.	Dystonia, akathisia, esophageal spasm, and colic (in GI obstruction)
Haloperidol	D2 (primarily in CTZ)	0.5–4 mg orally or subcutaneously or I.V. q 6hr	Dystonia and akathisia
Prochlorperazine	D2 (primarily in CTZ)	5–10 mg orally or I.V. q 6h or 25 mg rectally q 6h	Dystonia, akathisia, and sedation
Chlorpromazine	D2 (primarily in CTZ)	10–250 mg orally q 4h, 25–50 mg I.V. or im q 4h, or 50–100 mg rectally q 6h	Dystonia, akathisia, sedation, postural hypotension
Promethazine	H1, muscarinic acetylcholine receptor or D2 (primarily in CTZ)	12.5–25 mg orally or I.V. q 6h or 25 mg rectally q 6h	Dystonia, akathisia, and sedation
Diphenhydramine	H1	25–50 mg orally or I.V. or subcutaneously q 6h	Sedation, dry mouth, urinary retention
Scopolamine	Muscarinic acetylcholine receptor	1.5 mg transdermal patch q 72h	Dry mouth, blurred vision, urinary retention, confusion
Hyoscyamine	Muscarinic acetylcholine receptor	0.125–0.25 mg SL or orally q 4h or 0.25–0.5 mg subcutaneously or I.V. q 4h	Dry mouth, blurred vision, ileus, urinary retention, confusion
Ondansetron	5-HT_3	4–8 mg orally by pill or dissolvable tablet (ODT) or I.V. q 4–8h	Headache, fatigue, constipation
Aprepitant	NK1	40 mg orally qd	

GI, Gastrointestinal; CTZ, chemoreceptor trigger zone. (Modified from Wood GJ, Shega JW, Lynch B, Von Roenn JH. Management of intractable nausea and vomiting in patients at the end of life: "I was feeling nauseous all of the time...nothing was working." *JAMA* 2007;298(10):1196–1207. Copyright 2007 American Medical Association. All rights reserved.)

vomiting are unknown. Antagonism of 5-HT_3 receptors known to be involved in emesis may contribute to the prophylactic effects of corticosteroids in cancer patients.[5] A single intravenous (I.V.) dose of dexamethasone 8 mg given prophylactically before chemotherapy with anthracyclines, carboplatin, or cyclophosphamide completely protected 89.2% of patients against nausea and 61% of patients against vomiting.[7] Moderate-to-severe side effects may occur in patients receiving dexamethasone for prophylaxis against delayed chemotherapy-induced nausea and vomiting and include insomnia (45%), indigestion/epigastric discomfort (27%), agitation (27%), increased appetite (19%), weight gain (16%), and acne (15%) in the week following chemotherapy.[8] Corticosteroids are seldom used as monotherapy for management of emesis and nausea induced by moderately or highly emetogenic chemotherapy.[5]

Management of emesis in oncologic and surgical settings improved with the introduction of 5-HT_3 receptor antagonists. Prophylactic use of these agents is recommended for the prevention of both acute chemotherapy- and radiation-induced nausea and vomiting.[9-10] The 5-HT_3 receptor antagonists widely used in current clinical practice are generally perceived to have comparable efficacy and safety. Although 5-HT_3 receptor antagonists have similar chemical structures, they exhibit differing pharmacologic profiles that result in variations in their pharmacodynamic action. In particular, the elimination half-lives of these compounds differ considerably, with studies in adult cancer patients finding that ondansetron displays the shortest half-life (4 hours), compared with granisetron, for example, which has a mean half-life of 10.6 hours.[11-12] Hydrodolasetron, the active metabolite of dolasetron, has an intermediate elimination half-life of 7.5 hours in cancer patients. The elimination half-life of tropisetron (8 hours) is similar to that of hydrodolasetron; however, this can be increased to as much as 45 h in slow metabolizers of the drug. A further difference in pharmacology between the 5-HT_3-receptor antagonists lies in the nature of their antagonism of 5-HT_3 receptors. Ondansetron displays competitive antagonism at the 5-HT_3 receptor and can be easily displaced by high concentrations of 5-HT_3. Conversely, granisetron and tropisetron exhibit insurmountable, noncompetitive, antagonism of 5-HT_3 receptors.[13] This may have implications for their duration of action with prolonged antiemetic activity beyond that suggested by their plasma half life. Intractable nausea and vomiting antiemetic dosing recommendations are shown in Table 18.3.

The neurokinin-1 (NK1)-receptor antagonists block the action of substance P released in the gut following cytotoxic stimuli. Aprepitant (NK-1 antagonist), when used in combination with a 5-HT_3 receptor antagonist and a corticosteroid, improves control of delayed nausea and vomiting.[14] As Aprepitant is a CYP 3A4 inhibitor and can interfere with dexamethasone metabolism,

TABLE 18.3

INTRACTABLE NAUSEA AND VOMITING: RECOMMENDED DOSES OF ANTIEMETICS

Class	Drug	Route	Recommended dose (once daily)
5-HT$_3$-receptor antagonist	Ondansetron	Oral	24 mg (high), 16 mg (moderate) 8 mg (0.15 mg/kg)*
		I.V.	
	Granisetron	Oral	2 mg
		I.V.	1 mg (0.01 mg/kg)
	Tropisetron	Oral	5 mg
		I.V.	5 mg
	Dolasetron	Oral	100 mg
		I.V.	100 mg (1.8 mg/kg)
	Palonosetron	I.V.	0.25 mg
Steroids	Dexamethasone	Oral or I.V.	12 mg (highly emetogenic, with Aprepitant), 20 mg without Aprepitant; 8 mg (moderately emetogenic); 8 mg (high/moderate) days 2 and 3
NK1-receptor antagonists	Aprepitant	Oral	125 mg on day 1, 80 mg on days 2 and 3

*8 mg twice daily is recommended.
(From Jordan K, Sippel C, Schmoll HJ. Guidelines for antiemetic treatment of chemotherapy-induced nausea and vomiting: past, present, and future recommendations. *Oncologist*. 2007; 12:1143–1150. Copyright 2007 by AlphaMed Press, Inc. Reproduced with permission of AlphaMed Press, Inc.)

the dose of dexamethasone should be reduced when used in combination.[5]

Jordan et al.[15] reviewed the various guidelines for antiemetic treatment of chemotherapy-induced nausea and vomiting. Recommendations were based on guidelines from the Multinational Association of Supportive Care in Cancer, the American Society of Clinical Oncology, and the National Comprehensive Cancer Network. All patients receiving highly emetogenic chemotherapy and selected patients receiving moderately emetogenic chemotherapy should receive an NK-1 antagonist in combination with a 5-HT$_3$ antagonist and/or corticosteroid. Dexamethasone is the preferred agent to use for delayed chemotherapy-induced nausea and vomiting. Patients receiving a low-risk emetogenic regimen should receive a corticosteroid before treatment and no prophylaxis beyond 24 hours for acute nausea and vomiting. For minimally emetogenic chemotherapy, no antiemetic drug should be routinely administered before chemotherapy. We support the use of these guidelines for antiemetic therapy.

Patients undergoing chemotherapy and who are pancytopenic are at risk for significant complications from intractable opioid-induced nausea and vomiting.[16–18] In patients experiencing acute nausea and/or vomiting with opioid use, we recommend the use of I.V. dexamethasone 4 to 8 mg, and/or an orally disintegrating tablet (which may also be given I.V.) ondansetron 8 mg and/or Aprepitant 40 mg for short-term control of symptoms. We do not propose these medications be used long-term for this problem as most opioid-induced vomiting will usually resolve with short-term antiemetic use, opioid dose stabilization, or a change in the type of opioid.

LAXATIVES AND OPIOID-INDUCED BOWEL DYSFUNCTION

Opioid-induced bowel dysfunction (OBD) is a distressing condition that may persist indefinitely in the clinical setting. OBD is characterized by constipation, incomplete evacuation, bloating, and increased gastric reflux. Hard, dry stool, gas distention, incomplete evacuation, and straining are common sequelae. OBD includes inhibition of gastric emptying, peristalsis, and secretions, as well as increased tone of intestinal sphincters.[19] Slowed gastrointestinal (GI) transit, increased fluid absorption, and desiccation of stool can lead to constipation. Opioids induce bowel dysfunction through several effects: block of propulsive peristalsis, inhibition of the secretion of intestinal fluids, and an increase in intestinal fluid absorption.[20–21] Opioids decrease the activity of both excitatory and inhibitory neurons in the myenteric plexus. In addition, they increase smooth muscle tone and inhibit the coordinated peristalsis required for propulsion, leading to disordered, nonpropulsive contractile activity, which contributes to nausea and vomiting as well as constipation.

Constipation is often refractory to stool softeners and laxatives and may limit the ability to deliver effective pain relief by opioid medications. In cancer patients, up to 90% of patients on chronic opioid therapy develop OBD.[22] Three types of receptors for opioid peptides have been identified as having effects on human GI function: δ-, κ-, and μ.[20] Human studies have revealed that μ receptors were more consistently distributed between the myenteric and submucosal plexi, and between the small and large intestines.[23] Because κ-receptors are more abundant in peripheral nerves than in central nerves, stimulation of these receptors may induce fewer central side effects such as euphoria and depression. δ-receptors are found predominantly in the central nervous system (CNS) but are also found in the myenteric and submucosal neurons of the gut, where activation results in inhibition of motility and secretion.[19] Pharmacologic and clinical effects of opioids on different segments of the gastrointestinal tract are shown in Table 18.4.

Several types of pharmacologic agents have been used to treat opioid-induced constipation, including osmotic or lubricant laxatives, stimulant laxatives (oral or rectal), and prokinetics. Fiber bulking agents are organic polymers that retain water in stool. It is important that adequate water be taken concomitantly with fiber. Without sufficient water, fiber may worsen constipation. Many practitioners recommend a combination of a stool softener with a stimulant laxative for patients on chronic opioid therapy. Stool softeners, such as docusate sodium, are detergents that allow better water penetration into stool making it softer and more voluminous. Stimulant laxatives, such as senna and bisacodyl, induce peristalsis via mechanisms that are not well understood. In vitro, applying senna to intestinal mucosa leads to immediate contraction. After optimal titration of these agents, oral osmotics are commonly added to enhance laxation by pulling along water by means of osmotic forces. Osmotics include sugars such as lactulose or sorbitol, magnesium salts such as magnesium citrate, or inert substances such as polyethylene glycol. When these are unsuccessful, rescue oral and rectal interventions are also often needed. Rectal interventions include such agents as bisacodyl suppositories and phosphosoda enemas to soften, lubricate, and mobilize hard, dry distal stool. Often synergism of multiple categories of agents is required for successful laxation.

Opioid antagonists have also been studied in the treatment of OBD. Oral naloxone given in doses between 2 mg to 4 mg three times per day was effective in improving bowel movement frequency, but some patients also experienced reversal of pain relief, and this reversal occurred in spite of using very low doses of naloxone relative to the total dose of opioid taken.[24] In particular, patients using higher doses of opioids appear to be the most vulnerable to the antianalgesic effect of oral naloxone. Naloxone is lipid soluble and easily crosses membranes, but undergoes extensive first-pass metabolism, with only 2% systemic bioavailability.

Peripheral opioid antagonists (alvimopan, methylnaltrexone) may be helpful in this setting. McNicol and Boyce[25] demonstrated that methylnaltrexone and alvimopan were better than placebo in reversing opioid-induced increased gastrointestinal transit time and constipation, and that alvimopan appears to be safe and efficacious in treating postoperative ileus. Methylnaltrexone is a μ-opioid–receptor antagonist with a quaternary amine derivative of naltrexone that prevents substantial entry into most areas of the brain, brain stem, and spinal cord, thereby preserving central analgesic actions of coadministered opioid agonists. Several small brain regions

TABLE 18.4

PHARMACOLOGIC AND CLINICAL EFFECTS OF OPIOIDS ON DIFFERENT SEGMENTS OF GASTROINTESTINAL TRACT

Site	Pharmacologic Effect	Clinical Effect
LOS	Inhibition LOS relaxation	
Gallbladder	Contraction	Biliary pain
	Spasm sphincter of Oddi	Delayed digestion
	Decreased secretion	
Gastroduodenum	Inhibition gastric emptying	Anorexia
	Increase duodenal motility followed by quiescence	Nausea and emesis
	Increased pyloric tone	
	Enhanced gastric acid secretion	
Small bowel	Increase tone/segmentation	Constipation
	Increase transit time	Delayed digestion
	Increase absorption	Hard, dry stool
	Decreased secretion	
Colon	Increase tone, segmentation	Constipation
	Increase transit time	Hard, dry stools
	Increase absorption	Bloating and distension
	Decreased secretion	Spasm, cramps, pain
Anorectum	Decreased rectal sensitivity	Incomplete evacuation
	Increase internal sphincter tone	Straining constipation

LOS, lower esophageal sphincter. (From De Schepper HU, Cremonini F, Park MI, Camilleri M. Opioids and the gut: pharmacology and current clinical experience. *Neurogastroenterol Motil.* 2004;16:383–394. With permission from Wiley-Blackwell.)

known as the circumventricular organs lack a blood–brain barrier,[26] including the vomiting center in the area postrema in the floor of the fourth ventricle. Methylnaltrexone prevents nausea and vomiting in part by gaining access to opioid receptors in the area postrema.[27]

Alvimopan has a greater affinity for the μ-receptor than the κ- or σ-opioid receptors.[28] The polarity of the molecule limits gastrointestinal absorption and CNS penetration. Methylnaltrexone is approved for the treatment of opioid-induced constipation.[29] As a quaternary amine, methylnaltrexone, a μ-opioid-receptor antagonist, has restricted ability to cross the blood–brain barrier. Time to peak effect is approximately 30 minutes after subcutaneous dosing and has an elimination half-life of 8 hours.[30] Portenoy et al.[31] demonstrated that the optimal dose of subcutaneous methylnaltrexone for reversing OBD was ≥5mg. Methylnaltrexone was also approved by the Food and Drug Administration (FDA) in April 2008 for opioid-induced constipation, administered subcutaneously once a day in doses of 8 to 12 mg. Thomas et al.[32] reported on the use of methylnaltrexone in 133 patients (71 placebo, 62 methylnaltrexone) with advanced illness and opioid-induced constipation in a 2-week double-blind, randomized, placebo-controlled study with a 3-month open-label extension. In the methylnaltrexone group, 48% of patients had laxation within 4 hours after the first study dose, compared with 15% in the placebo group, and 52% had laxation without the use of a rescue laxative within 4 hours after two or more of the first four doses, compared with 8% in the placebo group ($P < .001$ for both comparisons). The time to laxation after the first dose was rapid; among patients in the methylnaltrexone group who had a response within 4 hours; half had a response within 30 minutes. The response rate remained consistent throughout the extension trial. The median time to laxation was significantly shorter in the methylnaltrexone group than in the placebo group. Evidence of withdrawal mediated by central nervous system opioid receptors or changes in pain scores was not observed. Abdominal pain and flatulence were the most common adverse events.

Although alvimopan was approved by the FDA in May, 2008, it was only for short-term use (15 doses) in hospitalized patients and was indicated to accelerate the time to upper and lower GI recovery following partial large or small bowel resection surgery with primary anastomosis. In addition, alvimopan should not be used in patients who have received opioids for more than 1 week. This last restriction was included because data presented to the FDA indicated that the 12-mg dose of alvimopan can actually be painful for patients receiving long-term opioid therapy. Dose recommendations for this indication are 12 mg administered 30 minutes to 5 hours before surgery followed by 12 mg bid beginning the day after surgery for a maximum of 7 days or until discharge. Alvimopan is a large polar molecule that does not easily enter the CNS and produces strong peripheral opioid antagonism without affecting central effects such as pain relief. It is available only as an oral preparation. Systemic absorption is approximately 6%.[33] Gonenne et al.[34] demonstrated the effectiveness of alvimopan on codeine-induced constipation in a group of 74 healthy volunteers. Alvimopan 12 mg was given twice daily in the presence and absence of codeine sulfate 30 mg four times/day, or codeine or placebo alone. Codeine delayed gastric, small-bowel, proximal, and overall colonic transit ($P < .05$). Alvimopan reversed codeine's effect on small bowel and colon (ascending colon and overall colonic transit). Alvimopan also accelerated overall colonic transit compared with placebo. Thus, the mean colonic geometric center at 24 hours was 2.33 with placebo/placebo, 3.25 with alvimopan/placebo ($P < .05$), 1.5 with placebo/codeine ($P < .05$), and 2.63 with alvimopan/codeine. The mean geometric colonic center is a research technique used to evaluate colonic transit time. Regions of interest are generated around six segments of the colon to determine the geometric mean of counts in each segment. A weighted numerical value represents the center of the activity as it travels through the colon. A high geometric center implies faster colonic transit times.

In addition to standard recommendations of increasing dietary fiber content and adequate fluid intake, we routinely use a stool softener (docusate) with a bowel stimulant (senna) for opioid-induced constipation. For intractable constipation unresponsive to routine measures, we use subcutaneous methylnaltrexone.

ADJUVANT ANALGESICS

Adjuvant analgesics are medications whose principal indication is not pain relief, but which may provide or enhance pain relief under appropriate circumstances. The common adjunctive analgesics in the setting of cancer pain are corticosteroids, anticonvulsants, and antidepressants. Adjuvant analgesics include general-purpose analgesics, adjuvants used for musculoskeletal pain, and those with specific use for neuropathic, bone, or visceral pain. These drugs play an important role for patients who cannot attain an acceptable balance between pain relief and opioid side effects.

General Purpose Adjuvants

Corticosteroids are the most widely used general-purpose adjuvant analgesics.[35] Steroids are most useful for increased intracranial pressure, acute spinal cord compression, superior vena cava syndrome, metastatic bone pain, neuropathic pain due to infiltration or compression, symptomatic lymphedema, and hepatic capsular distension. Standard doses are dexamethasone 4 to 8 mg/day or prednisone 30 to 60 mg/day or the equivalent in patients with advanced cancer and related symptoms.[36] A very short course of relatively high doses (eg, dexamethasone 100 mg I.V. followed initially by 96 mg per day in divided doses) can help ameliorate an acute episode of severe pain related to a neuropathic lesion (eg, plexopathy or epidural spinal cord compression) or bony metastasis that does not respond adequately to opioids. Once adequate pain relief has been attained, steroid doses should be tapered to the minimum needed to sustain pain relief.

Corticosteroids can also be used to achieve such endpoints as mood elevation, for anti-inflammatory effects, as antiemetics, and as appetite stimulants. The low dose regimen outlined above is appropriate for these purposes. Side effects and toxicity such as myopathy, hyperglycemia, or psychosis may make chronic steroid administration unacceptable for the patient (Table 18.5).

TABLE 18.5
STEROID TOXICITY

Effect	Comments
Adrenal suppression	Commonly seen, varies with dose and duration
Osteoporosis	33% have bone density 2 SD below controls
Psychiatric effects	1.3–18.4%
Infectious complications	Relative risk 1.6 compared to controls
Glucose intolerance	4 times more prevalent than controls
Cutaneous effects	50%–54%
Cushingoid	4 times more prevalent than controls
Hypertension	4–5 times more prevalent than controls
Posterior subcapsular cataracts	9%
Osteonecrosis	1%–2%

(Modified from Campieri M. New steroids and new salicylates in inflammatory bowel disease: A critical appraisal. *Gut.* 2002;50 (Suppl 3):III43–46. With permission from BMJ Publishing Group Ltd.)

Painful cutaneous and mucosal lesions can be managed with topical local anesthetics, such as EMLA cream (eutectic mixture of 2.5% lidocaine and 2.5% prilocaine. EMLA cream should be applied thickly and should be covered with an occlusive dressing. Lidocaine viscous may ameliorate pain associated with oropharyngeal ulceration. A topical lidocaine 5% patch (Lidoderm) may provide pain relief for patients who have failed other topical local anesthetic preparations such as EMLA cream. Besides its pain-relieving abilities, an important characteristic of the topical lidocaine patch is its lack of systemic activity. Studies have shown that Lidoderm results in serum levels approximately one tenth those needed to treat cardiac arrhythmias.[37] Gammaitoni and Davis[38] showed that with the application of four 5% lidocaine patches for 18 hours/day for 3 consecutive days, steady-state plasma concentrations were achieved within 3 days and that maximum plasma concentrations of lidocaine were similar to those reported with 3 lidocaine patches (5%) applied for 12 hours/day for 3 consecutive days. Lidoderm does not appear to cause any systemic side effects or any drug–drug interactions. The lidocaine patch consists of a 10 × 14-cm, nonwoven, polyethylene-backed, and medication-containing adhesive of 5% lidocaine (700 mg/patch) and other inactive ingredients. Patients apply a maximum of three lidocaine patches to intact skin, covering as much of the painful area as possible. The patch is typically left in place for 12 hours but use may also be extended to 24 hours.[38] Unlike other formulations of lidocaine, the lidocaine patch exerts an analgesic effect without causing local anesthesia; the skin underlying its application continues to have normal sensation (ie, no "numbness"). The exact mechanism behind this effect is not known. Theoretically, the formulation may deliver sufficient amounts of lidocaine to block sodium channels on small damaged or dysfunctional pain fibers but insufficient amounts to block sodium channels on large myelinated A-β sensory fibers. The amount of drug absorbed is directly proportional to the skin surface area covered and the duration of patch application. In 1999, the patch was the first agent approved by the FDA for the treatment of PHN. There are also several anecdotal reports of their use in osteoarthritic knee pain and myofascial trigger points. A Cochrane database review reported insufficient evidence to recommend topical lidocaine as a first-line agent in the treatment of postherpetic neuralgia (PHN) with allodynia[39] although Dworkin et al. recommend the agent for first-line treatment.[40] The use of lidocaine patches is very safe with a very low systemic absorption and only local adverse effects (mild skin reactions) have been reported.[41] Up to four patches per day for a maximum of 12 hours may be used to cover the painful area. Titration is not necessary.

We have found that the use of Lidoderm patches is safe and can be effective under certain circumstances in the oncology patient. We routinely use this patch in patients suffering from postherpetic neuralgia. We have also used the Lidoderm patch in chemotherapy-induced peripheral neuropathy, particularly of the lower extremities. In our experience, the results in this situation have been variable. Patients often report difficulty in maintaining patch adhesion in the feet. However, side effects are minimal and there does not appear to be a problem tolerating this medication in the oncology population.

Musculoskeletal Pain Adjuvants

Pain that originates from injury to muscle or connective tissue is not unusual in patients with cancer. Muscle relaxant medications are used primarily to treat spasticity from upper motor neuron syndromes and muscular pain or spasms from peripheral musculoskeletal conditions. Common painful musculoskeletal conditions include fibromyalgia, chronic tension headaches, myofascial pain syndrome, and mechanical low back or neck pain. The efficacy of so-called muscle relaxants and other drugs commonly used for the treatment of musculoskeletal pain has not been evaluated in cancer patients. Various drug categories are considered muscle relaxants such as antihistamines (eg, orphenadrine, Norflex), tricyclic compounds structurally similar to the tricyclic antidepressants (eg, cyclobenzaprine, Flexeril), and others (eg, carisoprodol, Soma, metaxalone, Skelaxin, and methocarbamol, Robaxin). The effects of these drugs are nonspecific and there is no evidence that they relax skeletal muscle in the clinical setting. The most common adverse effect is sedation, which can be additive to other centrally acting drugs, including opioids. The potential for abstinence syndrome, as well as abuse by predisposed patients, suggest caution when discontinuing therapy or when administering these drugs to those patients with a substance abuse history. In particular, we advise particular care when prescribing carisoprodol (Soma) for either short-term or long-term use. This drug is commonly used in the treatment of low back pain. It is a drug of abuse and has been implicated as a cause of impairment in drivers.[42] Clinically, with impairment, patients may display signs similar to those of benzodiazepines with some important differences such as tachycardia, involuntary movements, hand tremor and horizontal gaze nystagmus.[42]

Some studies suggest that patients using carisoprodol for over three months may abuse the medication, especially those individuals with a history of substance abuse.[43] Carisoprodol's active metabolite meprobamate is thought to act through the gamma-aminobutyric acid (GABA) (A)-receptor complex and produces an impairing effect. As the formation of meprobamate from carisoprodol is catalyzed by CYP2C19, patients with impairment of this enzyme system have a lower capacity to metabolize carisoprodol and may therefore have an increased risk of developing concentration dependent side-effects such as drowsiness and hypotension, if treated with ordinary doses of carisoprodol.[44]

Other agents that have been tried for muscle spasms include diazepam, the α_2-adrenergic agonist tizanidine or the GABA (B)-agonist baclofen. Injections of botulinum toxin can be considered for refractory musculoskeletal pain related to muscle spasms. Its duration of action is usually several months.

Tizanidine hydrochloride (Zanaflex) is a centrally-acting α_2-adrenergic receptor agonist used for the treatment of muscle spasticity related to central nervous system diseases.[45-46] Activity at the α_2-receptor results in direct inhibition of excitatory release of amino acids from spinal interneurons and a concomitant inhibition of facilitatory coeruleospinal pathways.[47] Although primarily indicated in the treatment of spasticity, it has been suggested to be helpful in the treatment of chronic neck and lower back pain in patients who have a myofascial component to their pain.[48] However, it should be noted that well controlled studies of the use of tizanidine in the treatment of myofascial pain are lacking. A Cochrane review of skeletal muscle relaxants to treat low back pain (through 2001) showed favorable outcomes for cyclobenzaprine and tizanidine in managing acute but not chronic low back pain.[49] Common side effects of the drug include sedation, dry mouth, asthenia, and dizziness. Tizanidine may produce hypotension in up to 16% of patients.[50] Doses are typically started at 2 to 4 mg and night and titrated slowly. Daily doses should not exceed 36 mg and are administered in divided doses three to four times daily.

Metaxalone (Skelaxin) is an oxazolidone derivative that may be useful for the acute management of peripheral musculoskeletal complaints, but is not effective in treatment of spasticity related to neurological disorders. Typical doses are 800 mg tid or qid. Chou et al.[51] compared the efficacy and safety of a variety of skeletal muscle relaxants for the treatment of spasticity and painful musculoskeletal conditions and concluded that the evidence in favor of metaxalone was fair at best. The benefits of this agent in acute musculoskeletal syndromes may be primarily related to its sedative effects. Of note, Chou et al. also reported that there was very limited or inconsistent data regarding the effectiveness of metaxalone, methocarbamol, chlorzoxazone, baclofen, or dantrolene compared to placebo in patients with musculoskeletal conditions.

In summary, the evidence regarding the clinical use of skeletal muscle relaxants is limited because of poor methodologic design, inadequate assessment methods, and small numbers of patients. Most active comparator trials of patients with spasticity indicated that tizanidine, baclofen, dantrolene, and diazepam improved spasticity equally. There is some evidence to support the use of tizanidine, orphenadrine, carisoprodol, and cyclobenzaprine, but only in the treatment of acute low back pain; the evidence for their long-term use is poor. In general, we rarely prescribe these medications and, if used, they are prescribed only for short-term (less than 1 week) use.

Neuropathic Pain Adjuvants

Patients who suffer from chronic neuropathic pain rarely experience a complete resolution of their symptoms or complete functional restoration with any form of treatment. Neuropathic pain usually has multiple potential etiologies that include non-tumor causes such as central pain from stroke or spinal cord injury, peripheral nerve injury (CRPS Type 2), as well as metabolic causes such as diabetic neuropathy. Clinicians specializing in oncology pain management are likely to encounter diverse sources of neuropathic pain which will also include non-cancer-related issues. The spectrum of problems likely to be encountered includes chemotherapy-induced peripheral neuropathy, postherpetic neuralgia, phantom limb pain, and tumor infiltration of nerves or nerve plexuses. Frequently, treatment strategies for cancer-related neuropathic pain are extrapolated from non-cancer-related neuropathic pain and may not necessarily be efficacious for cancer pain. In the treatment of neuropathic pain that is nonmalignant in origin, most of the randomized controlled trials have been conducted for PHN and painful polyneuropathy whereas there are relatively few trials in other peripheral neuropathic pains (including trigeminal neuralgia), and central pain, and no randomized trials in painful radiculopathies.[41]

Because neuropathic pain represents a complex array of symptoms and heterogeneous group of disorders and medical syndromes, clinicians must be accurate in making a diagnosis of neuropathic pain and not misdiagnosis other conditions that may mimic neuropathic pain such as musculoskeletal pain. Bennett et al.[52] showed that the accuracy in diagnosing neuropathic pain was improved if signs and symptoms such as dysesthesia, tenderness or numbness, evoked pain, evidence of autonomic dysfunction, paroxysmal pain, thermal pain, or allodynia were present. Failure to accurately diagnose neuropathic pain will inevitably lead to less-than-optimal treatment strategies.

The use of adjuvants can contribute substantially to the management of neuropathic pain. The drugs used empirically for this indication include selected antidepressants, anticonvulsants, opioids, tramadol, N-methyl-D-aspartate (NMDA) antagonists, topical lidocaine, cannabinoids, and capsaicin (Table 18.6 and 18.7). Given the great interpatient and intrapatient variability in the response to adjuvants in this setting (including those within the same class), many patients require sequential trials to optimize pain management.

Antiepileptic drugs (AEDs) have been used extensively for the treatment of neuropathic pain but effective pain relief has been achieved in fewer than half of the patients who received this class of drug.[53] Such outcomes may be partially attributable to the large variability in the presentation of each neuropathic pain syndrome and to the lack of a clear understanding of the precise neural mechanisms underlying each clinical symptom. In addition, the

TABLE 18.6

NUMBERS NEEDED TO TREAT (95% CONFIDENCE INTERVAL) WITH VARIOUS ANALGESICS FOR DIFFERENT NEUROPATHIC PAIN STATES

Drug	No. Trials	Central Pain	Peripheral Pain	Painful Polyneuropathy	Postherpetic Neuralgia	Peripheral Nerve Injury	Trigeminal Neuralgia	HIV Neuropathy	Mixed Neuropathic Pain
TCA	16	4.0 (2.6–8.5)	2.3 (2.1–2.7)	2.1 (1.9–2.6)	2.8 (2.2–3.8)	2.5 (1.4–11)	ND	ND	NA
SNRI	2	ND	5.1 (3.9–7.4)	5.1 (3.9–7.4)	ND	NA	ND	ND	ND
Gabapentin/pregabalin	4	MA	4.0 (3.6–5.4)	3.9 (3–4.7)	4.6 (4.3–5.4)	NA	ND	ND	8.0 (5.9–32)
Opioids	6	ND	2.7 (2.1–3.6)	2.6 (1.7–6.0)	2.6 (2.0–3.8)	3.0 (1.5–7.4)	ND	ND	2.1 (1.5–3.3)
Tramadol	1	ND	3.9 (2.7–6.7)	3.5 (2.4–6.4)	4.8 (2.6–27)	ND	ND	NS	ND
NMDA antagonists	5	ND	5.5 (3.4–14)	2.9 (1.8–6.6)	NS	NS	ND	ND	NS
Topical lidocaine	4	ND	4.4 (2.5–17)	ND	NA	ND	ND	NA	4.4 (2.5–17)
Cannabinoids	2	6.0 (3.0–718)	ND	ND	ND	ND	ND	ND	NS
Capsaicin	11	ND	6.7 (4.6–12)	11 (5.5–317)	3.2 (2.2–5.9)	6.5 (3.4–69)	ND	NA	NA

TCA, Tricyclic antidepressant; ND, no studies done; NA, dichotomized data not available; SNRI, serotonin-norepinephrine reuptake inhibitor; NS, relative risk not significant; NMDA, N-methyl-D-aspartate. (Modified from Dworkin RH, O'Connor AB, Backonja M, et al. Pharmacologic management of neuropathic pain: Evidence-based recommendations. *Pain.* 2007;132:237–251.)

relatively high treatment failures with AEDs are associated with the high prevalence of toxicity associated with their use. However, trials indicate that various AEDs, including carbamazepine, oxcarbazepine, valproate, phenytoin, lamotrigine, topiramate, levetiracetam, gabapentin, zonisamide, and tiagabine, are somewhat effective in treating neuropathic pain.[54] However, only gabapentin and pregabalin are currently regarded as first-line treatments in peripheral neuropathic pain.[55] Table 18.8 lists AEDs currently used for neuropathic pain.

Previously, the commonly used AEDs were carbamazepine and valproic acid. Carbamazepine causes enzyme induction, thereby enhancing its own metabolism. Consequently, adverse effects (eg, drowsiness, ataxia) may improve over time. In some oncology patient groups, the use of carbamazepine may prove particularly problematic. Carbamazepine may exacerbate pre-existing chemotherapy-induced suppression of bone marrow. Valproic acid is not very commonly used, because it has a long plasma half-life and is sedative. Because the drug accumulates in the body, it may be necessary to reduce high doses. However, Divalproex sodium (valproic acid and sodium valproate in molar ratio 1:1) in doses of 1000 mg/day has been used successfully in the management of various painful neuropathies (in particular PHN) with a low incidence of side effects.[56] Oxcarbazepine differs from carbamazepine by additional inhibition of several types of voltage-gated calcium channels.[57]

Of concern, AEDs (particularly first generation) are particularly prone to adverse effects associated with drug interactions in cancer patients undergoing chemotherapy.[58] Clinically significant drug interactions have been reported to occur when paclitaxel is administered with doxorubicin, cisplatin, or anticonvulsants (phenytoin, carbamazepine, and phenobarbital).[59] Because paclitaxel undergoes hepatic oxidation via the CYP P450 system, enzyme inducing AEDs decrease paclitaxel levels and thereby reduce the effectiveness of the drug. Protein displacement by drugs of greater affinity for the protein may result in a drug interaction. Use of drugs that are highly bound and undergo elimination by low-extraction hepatic mechanisms may result in reduced total plasma concentrations of the displaced drug and no change in the concentration of unbound drug. Lower concentrations of phenytoin with recurrence of seizures have been observed with the administration of ciplatin,[60] carboplatin,[61] and vinca alkaloids.[62] Phenytoin is a highly protein bound drug that can result in clinically important protein-binding interactions with chemotherapy drugs such as cisplatin and methotrexate.[63] On the contrary, some chemotherapeutic agents (eg, fluoruracil and tamoxifen) can induce higher plasma concentrations of phenytoin.[64-65] AEDs less likely to interact with chemotherapeutic agents include gabapentin, lamotrigine, levetiracetam, and zonisamide.[58] Although some of these newer AEDs are not metabolized by the P450 system, there may be unexpected interactions that do not involve known pathways. However, in comparison to drugs of the first generation (phenobarbital, primidone, phenytoin, carbamazepine, and valproic acid), the potential for interactions and side effects due to enzyme induction or inhibition is reduced by most of the anticonvulsant drugs of the second generation AEDs (gabapentin, lamotrigine, levetiracetam, oxcarbazepine, pregabalin, tiagabine, topiramate, and zonisamide).

The emergence of drugs such as gabapentin, pregabalin, lamotrigine, topiramate, oxcarbazepine, and others have improved the tolerability profile of AEDs. Adverse effects (eg, somnolence, dizziness, ataxia) associated with lamotrigine, however, require a slow titration and,

TABLE 18.7

PREDOMINANT MECHANISM OF ACTION OF DRUGS USED IN TREATMENT OF NEUROPATHIC PAIN

Drug	Predominant mechanism
Amitriptyline	TCA, balanced monoamine reuptake inhibition
Capsaicin (topical)	Depolarizes the nervous membrane via vanilloid receptor type 1, initially stimulates, then blocks, skin nerve fibers
Carbamazepine	Voltage-gated sodium-channel block
Clomipramine	TCA, balanced monoamine reuptake inhibition
Desipramine	TCA, predominantly norepinephrine reuptake inhibition
Dextromethorphan	NMDA-receptor antagonist
Duloxetine	Serotonin-norepinephrine reuptake inhibition
Gabapentin	Binding to the $\alpha_2\delta$ subunit of presynaptic voltage-dependent calcium channels with reduced release of presynaptic transmitters
Imipramine	TCA, balanced monoamine reuptake inhibition
Lidocaine (topical)	Block of peripheral sodium channels and thus of ectopic discharges
Lamotrigine	Presynaptic voltage-gated sodium-channel inhibition and thus reduced release of presynaptic transmitters
Memantine	NMDA-receptor anatagonist
Nortriptyline	Predominantly norepinephrine reuptake inhibition
Oxcarbazepine	Voltage-gated sodium- and calcium-channel block
Oxycodone	μ-opioid receptor agonist
Pregabalin	Binding to the $\alpha_2\delta$ subunit of presynaptic voltage-dependent calcium channels with reduced release of presynaptic transmitters
Tetrahydrocannabinol	Agonist to the CB1 and CB2 subtype of cannabinoid receptors
Topiramate	Voltage-gated sodium-channel block and inhibition of glutamate release by an action on AMPA/kainate receptors
Tramadol	μ-opioid receptor agonist and monoamine reuptake inhibitor
Valproate	Increase of GABA levels in brain and potentiation of GABA-mediated responses
Venlafaxine	Serotonin-norepinephrine reuptake inhibition

TCA, Tricyclic antidepressant; NMDA, N-methyl-D-aspartate; AMPA, a-amino-3-hydroxy-5-methyl-4-isoxazolepropionic acid; GABA, gamma-aminobutyric acid. (From Attal N, Cruccu G, Haanpaa M, et al. EFNS guidelines on pharmacological treatment of neuropathic pain. *Eur J Neurol.* 2006;13:1153–1169. With permission from Wiley-Blackwell.)

although uncommon, the potential for severe rash and Stevens-Johnson syndrome poses some concerns. Gabapentin (Neurontin) has been used for the treatment of neuropathic pain. Gabapentin, a cyclohexane amino acid, is related structurally to GABA, yet is neither GABA-nergic nor a GABA prodrug. The ability of the drug to block voltage-dependent Ca^{2+} channels is the probable reason for its analgesic properties. In animal models, gabapentin reduces glutamate release and reduces the enhanced noxious stimulus-induced spinal release of glutamate.[66] Gabapentin appears to have fewer side effects than the other anticonvulsant agents used for the treatment of neuropathic pain, thus facilitating more aggressive dose titration. Absorption of gabapentin is limited by saturable, active, dose-dependent transport in the gastrointestinal tract.[67]

Pregabalin is associated with analgesic, anxiolytics, and antiepileptic activity.[68–70] Pregabalin selectively binds with high affinity to the $\alpha_2\delta$ subunit of voltage-gated calcium channels, which are widely distributed throughout the central and peripheral nervous systems. This modulates calcium influx in presynaptic nerve terminals to reduce excessive release of several excitatory neurotransmitters. Pregabalin does not block sodium channels, inhibit dopamine, serotonin, or norepinephrine reuptake, or have activity at opioid, serotonin, or dopamine receptors. Binding affinity for the $\alpha_2\delta$ subunit, and potency, is six times more than that of gabapentin.[71] It interacts with the same binding site as gabapentin; the two drugs have similar, but not identical, pharmacologic profiles. Oral pregabalin is absorbed rapidly (peak plasma concentrations occur within 1.5 hours) and exposure is dose proportional. Absorption of pregabalin is not saturable, resulting in a linear pharmacokinetic profile.[72] It has predictable absorption across the GI tract, is neither metabolized nor protein-bound, and has minimal drug-drug interactions.[73] Most of the drug is excreted unchanged in the urine. The mean apparent elimination half-life is 6.3 hours with steady-state concentrations being reached within 24 to 48 hours following administration of multiple doses of pregabalin. Clearance of pregabalin is directly related to creatinine clearance; dosage adjustments are required in patients with impaired renal function.[72] Pregabalin is well tolerated and associated with dose-dependent adverse effects (mostly dizziness and somnolence) that are mild-to-moderate and are usually transient.[74] Recommended doses vary from 150 to 600 mg/day. If pregabalin is to be discontinued, the dose should be gradually tapered over a minimum of 1 week. Table 18.9 compares the clinical and pharmacologic properties of gabapentin and pregabalin.

Oxcarbazepine is an AED with a chemical structure similar to carbamazepine, but with different metabolism. The bioavailability of the oral formulation of oxcarbazepine is high (>95%).[75] It is rapidly absorbed after oral administration, reaching peak concentrations within about 1-3 hours after a single dose. Oxcarbazepine exhibits linear pharmacokinetics and no autoinduction occurs. The elimination half-life is 1 to 5 hours.[76] Oxcarbazepine is better tolerated than carbamazepine and is considered the first-line treatment for trigeminal neuralgia.[77] Oxcarbazepine can provide significant pain relief in several neuropathic pain conditions, including trigeminal neuralgia and painful diabetic neuropathy, and may also be effective in treating neuropathic pain refractory to other AEDs, such as carbamazepine and gabapentin.[78]

TABLE 18.8

ANTIEPILEPTIC DRUGS

Drug	Brand	Mechanism Site of Action	Dose Titration and Range	Remarks
Gabapentin	Neurontin	Ca^{2+} channel	100–4800 mg/day	May stop suddenly; sedation, nausea, ataxia (mostly transient by 2–4 wk)
Pregabalin	Lyrica	Ca^{2+} channel	50 mg tid; ↑ × 7 days to 100 mg tid. Max dose 600 mg/day.	Sedation, ataxia, edema. Cognitive dysfunction.
Carbamazepine	Tegretol	Na^+ channel	400–1800 mg/d. Start low (100 mg bid).	Taper off. Check white blood cell and platelet count. Nausea common. Sedation, ataxia.
Oxcarbazepine	Trileptal	Na^+ channel	600–2400 mg/d. Start low (150 mg bid).	Taper off. Sedation, ataxia, nausea. Hyponatremia.
Lamotrigine	Lamictal	Na^+ channel, ↓glutamate release	25–600 mg/day. Start low 25 mg/day. Follow package insert titration.	Taper off. Skin rash (rarely Stevens-Johnson–dose dependent); sedation, ataxia
Topiramate	Topamax	Mixed Na^+ and Ca^{2+}	15–800 mg/d. Start low (15 mg bid), titrate slowly (weekly).	Taper off. Cognitive dysfunction, weight loss, fatigue.
Levetiracetam	Keppra	Binds to SV2A (Synaptic vesicle protein)	1000–4000 mg/day. Start low (250 mg bid), titrate slowly (weekly).	Somnolence, cognitive dysfunction, mood changes.

Multiple multicenter randomized controlled trials have shown clear efficacy of gabapentin and pregabalin for postherpetic neuralgia and painful diabetic neuropathy.[79] These drugs can be rapidly titrated and are well tolerated. Topiramate, lamotrigine, carbamazepine, and oxcarbazepine are alternatives for the treatment of painful diabetic neuropathy, but should be titrated slowly. Caraceni et al.[80] reported on the analgesic effect of gabapentin in 121 patients with neuropathic pain with cancer, partially controlled with opioids. Gabapentin was titrated from 600 mg/day to 1800 mg/day in addition to stable opioid dose. There was a significant difference of average pain intensity between gabapentin (pain score, 4.6) and placebo group (pain score, 5.4; $P = .0250$). Xiao et al.[81] tested gabapentin as a potential analgesic for paclitaxel- and vincristine-evoked pain in an animal model. Paclitaxel- and vincristine-evoked mechano-allodynia and mechano-hyperalgesia were significantly reduced by gabapentin, but only with repeated dosing. Paclitaxel-evoked painful peripheral neuropathy was associated with an increased expression of the $\alpha(2)\delta-1$ subunit in the spinal dorsal horn, but not in the dorsal root ganglia, suggesting that gabapentin's mechanisms of action for this type of neuropathy may include normalization of the nerve injury-evoked increase in calcium channel $\alpha_2\delta$ subunit expression. Dunteman[82] reported on the use of oral

TABLE 18.9

COMPARISON OF GABAPENTIN AND PREGABALIN

Structure	Gabapentin	Pregabalin
Bioavailability	27%–60%	90%
T_{max} (hours)	2–3	1
Plasma protein binding	<3%	0
Potency	+	++++++
$T_{1/2}$ (hours)	5–7	5.5–6.7
Metabolism	None	None
Elimination	Renal (100% unchanged)	Renal (92%–99% unchanged)
Dosing	tid	bid/tid
Average neuropathic pain dose	1800–3600 mg/day	150–600 mg/day
Time to effective dose	9 days	1 day

(From Gajraj NM. Pregabalin: Its pharmacology and use in pain management. *Anesth Analg*. 2007; 105:1805–1815.)

levetiracetam titrated over days to two weeks in seven patients with neoplasms involving neural structures (four invading the brachial plexus, and three the lumbosacral plexus). The maximum levetiracetam dose ranged from 500 mg to 1500 mg BID. All patients experienced improved pain control after the addition of levetiracetam; opioid use decreased by at least an estimated 70%, without drug-related adverse events. Like gabapentin and pregabalin, levetiracetam lacks any significant drug–drug interactions.

Tsavaris et al.[83] reported on the use of gabapentin monotherapy for the treatment of chemotherapy-induced neuropathy in 75 patients who received a fixed low dose of gabapentin (800 mg/day). Gabapentin produced a complete response in 25.3%, a partial response in 44%, a minor response in 25.3%, and no response in 5.3%. Approximately 25% of patients receiving gabapentin experienced mild somnolence, but none discontinued the drug for this reason. This study has limitations as there was no blinding of active drug and no placebo arm. In addition, restrictions in the use of gabapentin dose may not reveal additional responders to gabapentin at higher doses.

In our practice, we do not use first generation AEDs in the management of neuropathic pain, except for carbamazepine for the management of trigeminal neuralgia. Our preference is for second generation AEDs; we typically use gabapentin, pregabalin, and oxcarbazepine. Our experience is that these drugs are generally well tolerated in oncology patients. We do not routinely prescribe high doses of gabapentin (doses exceeding 3600 mg/day).

Tricyclic antidepressants (TCAs) have been used to treat neuropathic pain, depression, and sleep disorders. TCAs have long been the drugs of first choice in the treatment of neuropathic pain. Max et al. reported that the character of the pain complaint did not predict response to antidepressants.[84] Amitriptyline and imipramine are both widely available. Alternative TCAs, available in most countries, may be more suitable for some patients. Nortriptyline has less sedating properties than amitriptyline; desipramine is relatively non-sedative and has minimal anticholinergic effects. Starting doses depend on the patient's age, weight, previous use of such drugs, and concurrent medications. A dose as low as 10 mg may be appropriate for some patients, but most can begin with 25 to 50 mg. The dose should be increased to 30 to 50 mg as rapidly as tolerated (usually in terms of sedation, postural hypotension, and dry mouth). After that, increase the dose weekly to a maximum of 150 mg/day until the pain is relieved or adverse effects preclude further escalation. Pain reduction, independent of changes in mood,[85] occurs in many patients after a few days on doses of 50 to 100 mg.[86-87] In a Cochrane Database review, Saarto and Wiffen[88] reported on the use of TCAs for neuropathic pain. TCAs are effective for neuropathic pain, with a number needed to treat (NNT) of 3.6 (95% confidence interval [CI]: 3–4.5) and relative ratio (RR) of 2.1 (95% CI: 1.8–2.5) for the achievement of at least moderate pain relief. There is limited evidence for the effectiveness of the newer selective serotonin reuptake inhibitors (SSRIs). Venlafaxine has an NNT of 3.1 (95% CI: 2.2–5.1) and RR of 2.2 (95% CI: 1.5–3.1). The number needed to harm (NNH) for major adverse effects defined as an event leading to withdrawal from a study was 28 (95% CI: 17.6–68.9) for amitriptyline and 16.2 (95% C: 8–436) for venlafaxine. The NNH for minor adverse effects was 6 (95% CI: 4.2–10.7) for amitriptyline and 9.6 (95% CI: 3.5–13) for venlafaxine.

The analgesic effects of the antidepressants are related to multiple mechanisms. These drugs may increase neurotransmitter availability in endogenous monoamine-mediated pain-modulating pathways that use 5-HT or norepinephrine. They may also interact with endogenous opioid systems.[89] TCAs are classified as tertiary amines (amitriptyline, imipramine, doxepin, clomipramine) and secondary amines (nortriptyline, desipramine). In general, the secondary amines are better tolerated. TCAs can cause a variety of side effects ranging from mild and inconvenient to life threatening. Adverse effects include somnolence, mental clouding, and anticholinergic effects, such as dry mouth, blurred vision, or constipation. More serious anticholinergic problems include precipitation of acute-angle closure glaucoma, tachycardia, severe constipation, or urinary retention. The most common serious cardiovascular complication of most TCAs is orthostatic hypotension. TCAs are essentially free of any other serious adverse effects in patients without cardiovascular disease but in patients with preexisting bundle-branch disease, there is a risk of heart block.[90]

Although antidepressants are helpful in the treatment of painful polyneuropathies, there is relatively little information on their efficacy in cancer pain patients. Berger et al.[91] using claims data from a large U.S. insurance company noted that the use of AEDS and TCAs is relatively low in cancer patients with painful neuropathies and limited to those who also receive other analgesic and adjuvant medications. Of 956 patients, 14% received TCAs and 17% received AEDs. Gabapentin was the most widely used AED (92%) and amitriptyline the most widely used TCA (79%). Those who received AEDs or TCAs were more likely to have diabetes and spinal pain. Kautio et al.[92] studied the effect of amitriptyline in the treatment of chemotherapy-induced neuropathy in 44 patients. Patients were treated with low-dose amitriptyline for 8 weeks (starting dose of 10 mg/day, then dose titration of 10 mg/week up to 50 mg/day, followed by a stable dose for more than 4 weeks). Although amitriptyline was well tolerated, it failed to improve sensory neuropathic symptoms.

Antidepressants that inhibit synaptic uptake of 5-HT_3, norepinephrine, or other monamines are potentially analgesic. Selective 5-HT_3 and norepinephrine reuptake inhibitors (SSNRIs) are potentially analgesic, with less evidence supporting the analgesic efficacy of the SSRIs. Duloxetine is approved by the FDA for the treatment of painful diabetic peripheral neuropathy and fibromyalgia. The optimal dose of duloxetine for the treatment of these conditions is 60 mg/day.[93] The most common adverse effects are nausea, somnolence, dizziness, and fatigue.

In order to provide clear guidelines for the drug treatment of nonmalignant neuropathic pain, a task force of the European Federation of Neurological Societies (EFNS) reported on treatments for painful polyneuropathies (predominantly painful diabetic neuropathy), PHN, trigeminal neuralgia, and central pain (spinal cord injury, poststroke pain, and multiple sclerosis (Table 18.10).[41] For painful peripheral neuropathy (with the exception of HIV-associated polyneuropathy), the medications with

TABLE 18.10

EUROPEAN FEDERATION OF NEUROLOGICAL SOCIETIES CLASSIFICATION OF EVIDENCE FOR DRUG TREATMENTS IN PAINFUL POLYNEUROPATHY (PPN), POST HERPETIC NEURALGIA (PHN), TRIGEMINAL NEURALGIA (TN), AND CENTRAL PAIN

Pain Condition	First-Line Recommendations	Second/Third-Line Recommendations
Painful polyneuropathy	Gabapentin	Lamotrigine
	Pregabalin	Opioids
	TCAs	SNRIs
		Tramadol
Postherpetic neuralgia	Gabapentin	Capsaicin
	Pregabalin	Opioids
	Lidocaine, topical (in patients with small area of pain-allodynia)	Tramadol
		Valproate
	TCAs	
Trigeminal neuralgia	Oxcarbazepine	Surgery
	Carbamazepine	
Central pain	Amitriptyline	Cannabinoids
	Gabapentin	Lamotrigine
	Pregabalin	Opioids

TCA, Tricyclic antidepressant; SNRI, serotonin-norepinephrine reuptake inhibitor.

established efficacy are TCA, duloxetine, venlafaxine, gabapentin, pregabalin, opioids, and tramadol. The balanced TCAs (amitriptyline and imipramine) at adequate doses seem to have the highest efficacy. A TCA or gabapentin/pregabalin was recommended as first choice. Serotonin-norepinephrine reuptake inhibitors (SNRIs), duloxetine, and venlafaxine were considered second choice because of moderate efficacy, but were safer and had fewer contraindications than TCAs and should be preferred to TCA, particularly in patients with cardiovascular risk factors. The optimal dosage of duloxetine is 60 mg/day: 120 mg/day are no better than 60 mg; 20 mg/day are ineffective. High doses of venlafaxine (150 to 225 mg/day) are effective, although lower doses (75 mg/day) are weakly or not at all effective. Immediate-release venlafaxine is associated with adverse CNS and somatic symptoms such as agitation, diarrhea, increased liver enzymes, hypertension, and hyponatremia; the extended release formulation seems to be far more tolerable, the main side-effects being GI disturbances. Opioids are considered second or third line therapy. Effective doses range 10 to 120 mg/day for oxycodone and 15 to 300 mg/day for morphine. Treatments with lack of proven efficacy include capsaicin, mexiletine, oxcarbazepine, SSRI, topiramate, memantine, mianserin, and topical clonidine. Carbamazepine was considered to have little utility for this condition and there are safety concerns for its ongoing use. For trigeminal neuralgia, carbamazepine (200 to 1200 mg/day) and oxcarbazepine (600 to 1800 mg/day) are recommended as first line. Baclofen or lamotrigine may be added in patients refractory to carbamazepine or oxcarbazepine, particularly if the patient cannot undergo or refuses surgery. Several less studied neuropathic conditions, such as phantom limb pain, postsurgical neuropathic pain, and Guillain–Barré syndrome, appear to be similarly responsive to most current drugs used in other neuropathic conditions (eg, TCAs, gabapentin, opioids), but results are based on limited numbers.

We do not aggressively pursue the option of prescribing TCAs for tumor-related neuropathic pain. We do use TCAs commonly for the treatment of chemotherapy-induced neuropathy but our experiences in this area have been variable and the results are not predictable. Patients with PHN often report pain relief with TCAs and we routinely use TCAs for this condition. With the above exceptions, we have found that these medications are often poorly tolerated in the oncology patient, particularly at higher dosages.

Bone Pain Adjuvants

Bone-seeking radiopharmaceuticals are used to deliver medium- to high-energy β-particle radiation to skeletal sites involved with tumor. This can result in more effective antitumor activity while sparing normal tissues the damaging effects of radiation. Radiopharmaceuticals are bone precursors that will be concentrated by metastatic lesions producing a significant osteoblastic response in bone. The use of radiopharmaceuticals is discussed in the section "Focused Management Strategies for Painful Bone Metastases" in Chapter 23.

Bisphosphonates are frequently used in the treatment of metastatic bone disease and the hypercalcemia related to malignancy. This class of drugs currently represents the standard care for the prevention and treatment of skeletal-related complications from metastatic bone disease. The aims of bisphosphonates for metastatic bone disease are to prevent skeletal-related events, reduce bone pain, and improve quality of life. Bisphosphonates are taken up by bone at sites of active bone metabolism. They inhibit osteoclast maturation and function and ultimately cause osteoclast apoptosis. Although initially developed to treat predominantly osteolytic bone metastases (eg, multiple myeloma and breast cancer), bisphosphonates are increasingly used to treat osteoblastic lesions such as those in prostate cancer. The five most often used bisphosphonates in metastatic bone disease are oral clodronate and ibandronate, and intravenous pamidronate, zoledronate, and ibandronate. Among these all but one, clodronate, are nitrogen-containing bisphosphonates. Although the primary intent of bisphosphonate use is considered to be the reduction of overall skeletal events, clinical trials have established that these agents have an analgesic effect on patients with metastatic bone pain from a variety of tumors. The results vary considerably, and comparison of bisphosphonates across studies is difficult because of differences in patient populations and the methods for assessing bone pain and analgesic use.[94]

Some I.V. bisphosphonates have been associated with occasional renal toxicity in the clinical setting. Preclinical studies have also shown that there may be considerable differences among bisphosphonate renal safety profiles.[95] There appear to be variations in the risk for histopathologic damage and the ability to cause cumulative toxicity during intermittent dosing. Reasons for the differences among bisphosphonates are not fully understood; however, research shows that they may be influenced by pharmacokinetic properties such as renal tissue half-life or protein binding and intracellular potency.[95] All of the bisphosphonates may induce renal damage, probably by proximal tubular degeneration and single-cell necrosis. Bisphosphonate therapy has also been associated with osteonecrosis of the mandibular and maxillary bone[96]; this has been particularly associated with zoledronate.[97] With this complication, pain and oral discomfort are often the first symptom. The most common clinical finding was an area of ulcerated mucosa and exposed devitalized bone. The exposed bone had a yellow-white discoloration and the surrounding soft-tissue areas were often inflamed due to secondary mucosal infection and painful. Management of this complication includes cessation of bisphosphonate therapy for more than 6 months, long-term antibiotics, hyperbaric oxygen administration in some cases, and various surgical restorative procedures.[97]

The physiologic role of calcitonin is the preservation of osseal integrity through reduced osteoclast activity. As such, the role of calcitonin in the management of tumor pain relates to bone metastases. Because of its antiresorptive effects (by inhibiting osteoclasts and analgesic activity), it has been hypothesized that calcitonin has a likely benefit for bone pain. Calcitonin is a hormone produced in the thyroid glands of some animals. It has a hypocalcemic action that is due primarily to the inhibition of osteoclastic bone resorption, and secondarily by action on the kidneys that results in increased urinary excretion of calcium and phosphorus. Naturally occurring porcine calcitonin, synthetic salmon calcitonin (salcatonin), and synthetic human calcitonin are in clinical use. Salcatonin is the most potent, and is used to control bone pain from malignant neoplasms. The use of calcitonin for the relief of metastatic bone pain is not very common, and little information is available about its use in this context. The most frequent routes of administration are subcutaneous and intranasal. The current analgesic dose of the intranasal route is 200 UI/day, and the optimal dose of subcutaneous route is not well defined

Repeated doses of calcitonin reduced bone pain in one trial,[98] but not in another.[99] Reports indicate that neuraxial (epidural and intrathecal) administration can reduce metastatic cancer pain,[100] but this mode of administration requires further evaluation in controlled randomized clinical trials. Martinez-Zapata et al.[101] concluded that limited evidence currently available does not support the use of calcitonin to control pain from bone metastases. We do not use calcitonin for bone pain on a regular basis.

Bone metastases arise, in general, from blood-borne spread of a primary tumor site. Consequentially, even patients with localized bone pain usually have occult sites of metastasis, and many patients develop new pain at new sites. Hemibody irradiation has attracted some interest in this setting. A large randomized trial using hemibody irradiation demonstrated reduced requirements for further bone radiation therapy when patients receive the treatment at the time of presentation of local bone pain.[102] However, the role of such prophylactic therapy in clinical practice remains uncertain at this time. Scarantino et al.[103] evaluated the effect of fractionated hemibody irradiation in the treatment of osseous metastases. The maximum tolerated dose of fractionated (2.50 Gy) HBI was 17.5 Gy and the major dose limiting toxicity was hematological (thromboleukopenia).

Visceral Pain Adjuvants

Although they are commonly prescribed, there is little evidence for the efficacy of adjuvant agents for the management of bladder spasm, tenesmoid pain, and colicky intestinal pain. A trial of nonsteroidal anti-inflammatory drugs (NSAIDs) may help patients with painful bladder spasms.[104] Although there is no well-established pharmacotherapy for painful rectal spasms, diltiazem can help in the management of proctalgia fugax.[105] The treatment of pain caused by inoperable bowel obstruction has been described above. Octreotide may relieve bowel obstructive symptoms by decreasing gastric secretions. Two classes of antisecretory drugs are used to reduce GI secretions: anticholinergics (eg, scopolamine), and somatostatin analogues (Octreotide). The two drugs have different mechanisms of action. The anticholinergic activity of scopolamine decreases tone and peristalsis in smooth muscle by competitive inhibition of muscarinic receptors at the smooth muscle level and by impairment of ganglionic neural transmission in the bowel wall.[106] Octreotide modulates GI function by reducing gastric acid secretion, slowing intestinal motility, decreasing bile flow, increasing mucous production, and reducing splanchnic blood flow.[107-108] Ripamonti et al.[109] compared the effectiveness of octreotide and scopolamine in 17 patients with inoperable bowel obstruction. Patients received either octreotide 0.3 mg/day or scopolamine 60 mg/day for 3 days by continuous subcutaneous infusion. Both drugs equally reduced colicky abdominal pain. Octreotide significantly reduced the amount of secretions drained by nasogastric tube and allowed earlier removal of the drainage tube compared to scopolamine. The authors considered octreotide as the first-choice antisecretory drug when a rapid reduction in GI secretions was necessary. Corticosteroids may have a role in reducing peritumoral inflammatory edema and improving intestinal transit. In a systematic review on the medical treatment of inoperative malignant bowel obstruction, Mercadante et al.[110] considered octreotide superior to hyoscine butylbromide and data supporting the use of corticosteroids was less convincing.

There are no satisfactory medications for the treatment of visceral pain. Pharmacologic advances in this area have been slow but are currently an active area of research. Our preference is to use opioids preferentially for visceral pain, even though the use of opioids for this problem is complicated by opioid-induced bowel dysfunction. We do not have experience with the use of corticosteroids and octreotide for visceral pain.

PSYCHOTROPIC DRUGS

A psychotropic drug may be defined as any drug capable of affecting the mind, emotions, or behavior. Drugs that are used for medicinal purposes include the antidepressants, psychostimulants, neuroleptics, anticonvulsants, and anxiolytics. Many patients with advanced cancer benefit from a psychotropic drug for the management of physical and psychosocial symptoms.[111] Some patients use psychotropics for pain relief (eg, tricyclic antidepressants for nerve injury pain), whereas others need an antiemetic (eg, haloperidol for opioid-induced nausea). Still others require an anxiolytic such as clonazepam or alprazolam. Some require a night sedative and others an antidepressant for identifiable depression. The concurrent use of two centrally acting drugs (eg, opioid with psychotropic drug or two psychotropic drugs together) is more likely to produce sedation in ill and malnourished cancer patients than in others. Indications for the use of neuroleptics in cancer patients include acute confusional states (delirium), nausea and vomiting, and pain. For pain, data from the 1960s has supported the use of methotrimeprazine in various pain syndromes, especially for patients who are anxious or agitated.[112] Other phenothiazines such as chlorpromazine and prochlorperazine are useful antiemetics but probably have limited use as analgesics. Fluphenazine in combination with TCAs may be useful for neuropathic pain.[113] Neuroleptic use is limited by the occurrence of adverse events, in particular, acute dystonic reactions, tremor and rigidity, akathisia, and tardive dyskinesia. Furthermore, neuroleptics are inhibitors of the CYP2D6 isoenzyme and may therefore interfere with the metabolism of other drugs.

Anxiolytics such as alprazolam and clonazepam have been suggested to be useful as adjuvant analgesics.[114-115] Reddy and Patt reported insufficient evidence to support the contention that the benzodiazepines have meaningful analgesic properties in most clinical circumstances.[116] Treatment with the benzodiazepines may reduce complaints of pain, but this seems to be an indirect effect related to their psychotropic properties, such as alleviation of anxiety and, in selected cases, depression. Further, long-term use of alprazolam is not without issues and this drug should be used with caution for nonpsychiatric indications.[117] Benzodiazepines are used widely in medical practice, especially as anxiolytics/hypnotics and as anticonvulsants. These agents can be poorly tolerated, eg, because of residual daytime sedation, anterograde amnesia, delirium, paradoxical agitation, or drug interactions.[118] Although generally not considered as analgesics, benzodiazepines may inhibit some of the ectopic activity in peripheral nerves following nerve injury and this has led to the use of benzodiazepines in the management of neuropathic pain.[116] Clonazepam has been used successfully in the treatment of selected neuropathic conditions such as phantom limb pain[119] and tic douloureux.[120] For phantom limb pain, Bartusch[119] reported on the use of clonazepam 0.5 mg tid in 2 patients over an extended period of time without major side effects. Hugel et al.[115] reported on the successful use of clonazepam in doses up to 2 mg/day in 10 opioid-tolerant patients with neuropathic cancer pain. Clonazepam was started at 0.5 mg/day, increased to 1 mg/day if pain was not adequately controlled, and further increased to 2 mg/day dependent on response or the occurrence of side effects. Five patients were excluded because of clonazepam-induced side effects at 1 mg/day or because regular opioid doses were increased during clonazepam titration.

Although we commonly use psychotropic drugs for the treatment of psychological symptoms such as anxiety disorders, we do not use them as primary analgesic therapy.

CANNABINOIDS

Cannabinoids, the active components of *Cannabis sativa*, act by mimicking endogenous substances (endocannabinoids) that activate specific cell surface receptors. The endocannabinoid system is a complex signaling system of cannabinoid receptors (cannabinoid receptors CB1 and CB2), endogenous ligands and enzymes responsible for their biosynthesis and inactivation. The system is involved in a broad range of functions and in a growing number of pathologic conditions. Studies of the endogenous cannabinoids (endocannabinoids) have demonstrated that they are present in most tissues and that in some pain states, such as neuropathic pain, levels of endocannabinoids are elevated at key sites involved in pain processing.[121] There is increasing evidence that endocannabinoids are able to inhibit cancer cell growth in culture as well as in animal models.[122]

The isolation of the main constituent, Δ9-tetrahydrocannabinol (THC), and the discovery of the endocannabinoid system, resulted in studies on the pharmacologic activity of cannabinoids. Cannabinoids exert various palliative effects in cancer patients. In addition, cannabinoids inhibit the growth of different types of tumor cells, including glioma cells,[123] possibly pancreatic cancer,[124] and reduce the inflammatory response in acute pancreatitis.[125] Two oral formulations of cannabinoids, dronabinol (Marinol) and nabilone (Cesamet) are approved by the FDA for use in chemotherapy-induced nausea and vomiting refractory to conventional antiemetic therapy. Cannabinoids stimulate appetite and food intake and may have a role in the management of cancer-induced cachexia.[126]

Sativex, a cannabis-derived oromucosal spray containing equal proportions of THC (partial CB1 receptor agonist) and cannabidiol (CBD, a noneuphoriant, anti-inflammatory analgesic with CB1 receptor antagonist and endocannabinoid modulating effects) was approved in Canada in 2005 for treatment of central neuropathic pain in multiple sclerosis, and in 2007 for intractable cancer pain.[127] The effectiveness of nabilone (Cesamet) therapy was assessed in managing pain and symptoms experienced by 47 advanced-cancer patients.[128] Patients taking nabilone showed a borderline improvement in appetite and had a lower rate of starting NSAIDs, tricyclic antidepressants, gabapentin, dexamethasone, metoclopramide, and ondansetron and a greater tendency to discontinue these drugs. Abrams et al. demonstrated that inhaled cannabis was well tolerated and effectively relieved chronic neuropathic pain from HIV-associated sensory neuropathy.[129] In some states, medical use of marijuana is allowed for certain conditions including HIV, cancer, multiple sclerosis, and epilepsy. However, the U.S. Supreme Court ruled that the federal government has the power to arrest and prosecute patients and their suppliers even if the marijuana is permitted under state law because of its authority under the federal Controlled Substances Act to regulate interstate commerce in illegal drugs.[130] In practical terms, it is not yet clear what effect the Court's decision will have on patients. One of the main challenges for the medical use of cannabinoids appears to be the development of safe and effective methods of use that lead to therapeutic effects but avoid adverse psychoactive effects.

We occasionally prescribe THC for oncology patients for appetite stimulation and nausea control. Our experience is that this drug has variable efficacy and does not appear to have significant pain-relieving effects.

KETAMINE

Ketamine is an anesthetic with dissociative, analgesic and psychedelic properties; its mechanism of action in pain management is primarily as a noncompetitive NMDA receptor antagonist. Ketamine has a complex mechanism of action that is further complicated by stereoselectivity; however, antagonism of glutamate NDMA receptors is thought to underlie its analgesic, dissociative, and neuroprotective effects.[131] Ionotropic glutamate receptors of the NMDA subtype are highly expressed in the CNS and are involved in excitatory synaptic transmission and synaptic plasticity. NMDA receptors are present in several regions of the CNS, especially the dorsal horn, and the limbic system. The receptors respond to L-aspartate and L-glutamate and are involved in numerous processes, such as cerebral plasticity, learning and memory, brain damage after ischemia, and pain, especially in the development and maintenance of chronic painful states. The NMDA receptor requires binding at both glycine (NR1 subunit) and glutamate (NR2 subunit) binding sites for ion channel activation.[132] Ketamine inhibits the NMDA receptor by two distinct mechanisms which involve blocking the open channel and thereby reduces channel mean open time, and by decreasing the frequency of channel opening by an allosteric mechanism.[133] NMDA receptor antagonists have therapeutic potential in numerous CNS disorders ranging from acute neurodegeneration (eg, stroke and trauma), chronic neurodegeneration (eg, Parkinson disease, Alzheimer disease, Huntington disease, amyotrophic lateral sclerosis [ALS]) to symptomatic treatment (eg, epilepsy, Parkinson disease, drug dependence, depression, anxiety, and chronic pain).[134]

Ketamine is metabolized in the liver to an active metabolite, norketamine. The potency of norketamine is approximately one-third that of ketamine. Ketamine metabolites are excreted renally with an elimination half-life of 2 to 3 hours in adults.[135] The oral and rectal bioavailability is only 16%.[136] After oral administration, peak effects are attained in 15 to 30 min. This is considerably slower than intravenous administration (peak effect 1 to 5 min) and is caused by incomplete GI absorption and first-pass metabolism. Peak plasma levels of ketamine are considerably lower after oral administration than after parenteral administration. Grant et al.[136] measured the pharmacokinetic and analgesic effects of intramuscular (I.M.) and oral ketamine in a dose of 0.5 mg/kg in six healthy volunteers. Although peak levels of oral ketamine were approximately one quarter that of I.M. ketamine, equal degrees of pain relief and periods of analgesia were observed in a tourniquet ischemia test model. Following oral administration of ketamine, norketamine levels are three times higher than I.V. administration which may account for a significant role in the analgesic effects of oral ketamine.

Ketamine has been used as an adjuvant to opioids in the treatment of refractory cancer pain, particularly in low or subanesthetic doses.[137-138] Lossignol et al.[138] reported on the use of ultra-low dose ketamine in 12 cancer patients with refractory cancer pain despite high opioid doses. All patients had visceral, somatic, and/or neuropathic pain at different sites. An intravenous test dose of 5 mg of ketamine was given (which was repeated if initially unsuccessful). After a successful test dose, patients received a continuous infusion of ketamine (1.5 mg/kg/day) mixed with half the last morphine dose. This mixture was continued until death and adjusted accordingly. The prolonged use of ketamine allowed a reduction in the total daily dose of morphine required (range: 200 to 1200 mg) by 50% and allowed eight patients to go home with a portable pump with morphine and ketamine during a relatively long period of time (range: 7 to 350 days, median: 58 days). Side effects were moderate (dizziness) and were limited to the test phase. Although the number of patients was small, there was a tendency to a plateau in the doses required despite rapid tumor progression.

Subanesthetic test doses of ketamine were reported by Mercadante et al.[139] in a randomized, double-blind, crossover, double-dose study. A slow bolus of subhypnotic doses of ketamine (0.25 mg/kg or 0.50 mg/kg) was given to ten cancer patients whose pain was unrelieved by morphine. Ketamine, but not saline solution, significantly reduced the pain intensity in almost all the patients at both doses. This effect was more relevant in patients treated with higher doses. Hallucinations occurred in 4 patients, and an unpleasant sensation ("empty head") was also reported by two patients.

The primary role of ketamine in such low doses is as an *antihyperalgesic, antiallodynic,* or *tolerance-protective* agent.[140] It appears to have a role in the treatment of opioid-resistant or "pathologic" pain (central sensitization with hyperalgesia or allodynia, opioid-induced hyperalgesia, neuropathic pain) rather than as an analgesic in its own right. Low-dose ketamine also has "preventive analgesia" properties.

Ketamine is prescribed with opioids for the treatment of cancer pain in a variety of different countries. Treatment with low-dose ketamine is relatively inexpensive. Bell et al.[141] systemically reviewed the literature to determine the effectiveness of ketamine in relieving cancer pain. The majority of studies were case reports, open-label audits, or open-label, uncontrolled trials. A total of 32 such reports were identified. Ketamine was used to treat refractory cancer pain, often described as neuropathic. Twenty-eight reports described improvement of pain relief with ketamine. In the majority of cases, ketamine improved opioid-mediated pain relief. The most common opioid was morphine, but in some cases ketamine was given as an adjuvant to fentanyl, hydromorphone, or diamorphine, or combinations of these opioids. Ketamine also was used as the sole analgesic. Adverse effects were related to higher doses of ketamine. The most commonly reported adverse effects were sedation and hallucination. The route of ketamine administration included oral, intramuscular bolus, subcutaneous bolus and infusion, intravenous bolus and infusion, epidural bolus, and intrathecal infusion. Ketamine doses ranged from 1 mg/kg/day subcutaneous infusion to 600 mg/day intravenously and 67.2 mg/day intrathecally. Treatment duration ranged from 4 hours to 1 year. However, the authors concluded that the evidence base for ketamine as an adjuvant to opioids for cancer pain is weak. The available literature allows for only a cautious conclusion that there is promise in the potential efficacy of ketamine as an adjuvant to opioids for cancer pain. Neuraxial administration of ketamine is discussed further in Chapter 22

We do not prescribe oral ketamine in our practice. However, we have found intravenous ketamine by continuous infusion in limited dose (less than 10 mg/hour) beneficial for the management of postoperative pain, particularly in the opioid tolerant population.

MEMANTINE

Many NMDA receptor antagonists produce highly undesirable side effects at doses within their putative therapeutic range. This has unfortunately led to the conclusion that the use of NMDA receptor antagonism is not a valid therapeutic approach. Memantine is an orally active NMDA receptor antagonist. It is an uncompetitive NMDA receptor antagonist at therapeutic concentrations achieved in the treatment of dementia and is essentially devoid of such side effects at doses within the therapeutic range.[142] This has been attributed to memantine's moderate potency and associated rapid, strongly voltage-dependent blocking kinetics. Memantine preferentially blocks excessive NMDA receptor activity without disrupting normal activity. Memantine does this through its action as an uncompetitive, low-affinity, open-channel blocker; it enters the receptor-associated ion channel preferentially when it is excessively open, and, most importantly, its off-rate is relatively fast so that it does not substantially accumulate in the channel to interfere with normal synaptic transmission.[143] Potentially important differences between memantine and ketamine include effects on gating of blocked channels and binding of memantine to two sites on NMDA receptors. Because modulation of NMDA receptor activity can increase or decrease excitability of neuronal circuits, subtle differences in the mechanisms of action of NMDA receptor antagonists can strongly impact on their clinical effects.[144] Because memantine is noncompetitive and is a relatively low-moderate affinity NMDA antagonist, this may be due to the strong voltage dependency and rapid unblocking kinetics of memantine, resulting in memantine blocking the pathologic, but not the physiologic, activation of NMDA receptors.[134]

Memantine is well absorbed after oral administration and has linear pharmacokinetics over the therapeutic dose range. It is excreted predominantly in the urine, unchanged, and has a terminal elimination half-life of about 60 to 80 hours. Starting doses are 5 mg once daily with a target dose of 20 mg/day. Memantine differs from many other NMDA receptor channel blockers in that it is well tolerated and does not cause psychotomimetic effects at therapeutic doses.[145]

Memantine may have efficacy in the management of neuropathic pain.[146] Relatively high doses of memantine selectively block thermal hyperalgesia and mechanical allodynia in some models of chronic and neuropathic pain without obvious effects on motor reflexes.[134] In an animal neuropathic pain model, memantine directly blocked spinothalamic cells and significantly reduced responses in these cells to cutaneous stimulation.[147] There is limited information in humans on the use of memantine for pain management. Memantine appears to be effective in some case reports of phantom limb pain[148] and CRPS pain.[149] However, 2 randomized controlled trials for the relief of phantom limb pain failed to demonstrate a significant clinical benefit from the use of 30 mg/day of memantine.[150-151] There also appears to be limited responses to pain associated with diabetic neuropathy and PHN.[152] Regarding cancer-related pain, there is also very limited information. Grande et al.[137] reported on the successful use of memantine 20 mg/day in a patient with severe spinal pain secondary to tumor. The patient's pain was well controlled with memantine and other medications until his demise 3 months later.

Memantine is a promising agent for the management of cancer pain. We have limited experience using this drug and are particularly interested in its efficacy for chemotherapy-induced peripheral neuropathy. This drug appears to be well tolerated in the oncology population in doses less than 30 mg/day.

References

1. Sun CC, Bodurka DC, Weaver CB, et al. Rankings and symptom assessments of side effects from chemotherapy: Insights from experienced patients with ovarian cancer. *Support Care Cancer*. 2005; 13:219–227.
2. Schnell FM. Chemotherapy-induced nausea and vomiting: The importance of acute antiemetic control. *Oncologist*. 2003;8:187–198.
3. Sharma R, Tobin P, Clarke SJ. Management of chemotherapy-induced nausea, vomiting, oral mucositis, and diarrhoea. *Lancet Oncol*. 2005;6:93–102.

4. Glaus A, Knipping C, Morant R, et al. Chemotherapy-induced nausea and vomiting in routine practice: A European perspective. *Support Care Cancer*. 2004;12:708–715.
5. Grunberg SM. Antiemetic activity of corticosteroids in patients receiving cancer chemotherapy: dosing, efficacy, and tolerability analysis. *Ann Oncol*. 2007;18:233–240.
6. Herrstedt J, Koeller JM, Roila F, et al. Acute emesis: Moderately emetogenic chemotherapy. *Support Care Cancer*. 2005;13:97–103.
7. Italian Group for Random Emitic Research. Randomized, double-blind, dose-finding study of dexamethasone in preventing acute emesis induced by anthracyclines, carboplatin, or cyclophosphamide. *J Clin Oncol*. 2004;22:725–729.
8. Vardy J, Chiew KS, Galica J, et al. Side effects associated with the use of dexamethasone for prophylaxis of delayed emesis after moderately emetogenic chemotherapy. *Br J Cancer*. 2006;94:1011–1015.
9. Gralla RJ, Osoba D, Kris MG, et al. Recommendations for the use of antiemetics: Evidence-based, clinical practice guidelines. American Society of Clinical Oncology. *J Clin Oncol*. 1999;17:2971–2994.
10. Kris MG, Hesketh PJ, Herrstedt J, et al. Consensus proposals for the prevention of acute and delayed vomiting and nausea following high-emetic-risk chemotherapy. *Support Care Cancer*. 2005;13:85–96.
11. Carmichael J, Cantwell BM, Edwards CM, et al. A pharmacokinetic study of granisetron (BRL 43694A), a selective 5-HT3 receptor antagonist: Correlation with anti-emetic response. *Cancer Chemother Pharmacol*. 1989;24:45–49.
12. Roila F, Del Favero A. Ondansetron clinical pharmacokinetics. *Clin Pharmacokinet*. 1995;29:95–109.
13. Newberry NR, Watkins CJ, Sprosen TS, et al. BRL 46470 potently antagonizes neural responses activated by 5-HT3 receptors. *Neuropharmacology*. 1993;32:729–735.
14. Schwartzberg LS. Chemotherapy-induced nausea and vomiting: which antiemetic for which therapy? *Oncology (Williston Park)*. 2007;21:946–953.
15. Jordan K, Sippel C, Schmoll HJ. Guidelines for antiemetic treatment of chemotherapy-induced nausea and vomiting: past, present, and future recommendations. *Oncologist*. 2007;12:1143–1150.
16. Bellm LA, Epstein JB, Rose-Ped A, et al. Patient reports of complications of bone marrow transplantation. *Support Care Cancer*. 2000;8:33–39.
17. Fishman ML, Thirlwell MP, Daly DS. Mallory-Weiss tear. A complication of cancer chemotherapy. *Cancer*. 1983;52:2031–2032.
18. Palmer K. Acute upper gastrointestinal haemorrhage. *Br Med Bull*. 2007;83:307–324.
19. Kurz A, Sessler DI. Opioid-induced bowel dysfunction: Pathophysiology and potential new therapies. *Drugs*. 2003;63:649–671.
20. De Schepper HU, Cremonini F, Park MI, Camilleri M. Opioids and the gut: Pharmacology and current clinical experience. *Neurogastroenterol Motil*. 2004;16:383–394.
21. Wood JD, Galligan JJ. Function of opioids in the enteric nervous system. *Neurogastroenterol Motil*. 2004;16 Suppl 2:17–28.
22. Sykes NP. The relationship between opioid use and laxative use in terminally ill cancer patients. *Palliat Med*. 1998;12:375–382.
23. Sternini C, Patierno S, Selmer IS, Kirchgessner A. The opioid system in the gastrointestinal tract. *Neurogastroenterol Motil*. 2004;16 Suppl 2:3–16.
24. Liu M, Wittbrodt E. Low-dose oral naloxone reverses opioid-induced constipation and analgesia. *J Pain Symptom Manage*. 2002;23:48–53.
25. McNicol ED, Boyce D, Schumann R, Carr DB. Mu-opioid antagonists for opioid-induced bowel dysfunction. *Cochrane Database Syst Rev*. 2008:CD006332.
26. Saper CB, Breder CD. The neurologic basis of fever. *N Engl J Med*. 1994;330:1880–1886.
27. Yuan CS. Methylnaltrexone mechanisms of action and effects on opioid bowel dysfunction and other opioid adverse effects. *Ann Pharmacother*. 2007;41:984–993.
28. Neary P, Delaney CP. Alvimopan. *Expert Opin Investig Drugs*. 2005;14:479–488.
29. Lang L. The Food and Drug Administration approves methylnaltrexone bromide for opioid-induced constipation. *Gastroenterology*. 2008;135:6.
30. Yuan CS, Foss JF, O'Connor M, et al. Effects of enteric-coated methylnaltrexone in preventing opioid-induced delay in oral-cecal transit time. *Clin Pharmacol Ther*. 2000;67:398–404.
31. Portenoy RK, Thomas J, Moehl Boatwright ML, et al. Subcutaneous methylnaltrexone for the treatment of opioid-induced constipation in patients with advanced illness: A double-blind, randomized, parallel group, dose-ranging study. *J Pain Symptom Manage*. 2008;35:458–468.
32. Thomas J, Karver S, Cooney GA, et al. Methylnaltrexone for opioid-induced constipation in advanced illness. *N Engl J Med*. 2008;358:2332–2343.
33. Foss JF, Fisher DM, Schmith VD. Pharmacokinetics of alvimopan and its metabolite in healthy volunteers and patients in postoperative ileus trials. *Clin Pharmacol Ther*. 2008;83:770–776.
34. Gonenne J, Camilleri M, Ferber I, et al. Effect of alvimopan and codeine on gastrointestinal transit: A randomized controlled study. *Clin Gastroenterol Hepatol*. 2005;3:784–791.
35. Watanabe S, Bruera E. Corticosteroids as adjuvant analgesics. *J Pain Symptom Manage*. 1994;9:442–445.
36. Twycross R. The risks and benefits of corticosteroids in advanced cancer. *Drug Saf*. 1994;11:163–178.
37. Rowbotham MC, Davies PS, Verkempinck C, Galer BS. Lidocaine patch: Double-blind controlled study of a new treatment method for postherpetic neuralgia. *Pain*. 1996;65:39–44.
38. Gammaitoni AR, Alvarez NA, Galer BS. Pharmacokinetics and safety of continuously applied lidocaine patches 5%. *Am J Health Syst Pharm*. 2002;59:2215–2220.
39. Khaliq W, Alam S, Puri N. Topical lidocaine for the treatment of postherpetic neuralgia. *Cochrane Database Syst Rev*. 2007:CD004846.
40. Dworkin RH, O'Connor AB, Backonja M, et al. Pharmacologic management of neuropathic pain: Evidence-based recommendations. *Pain*. 2007;132:237–251.
41. Attal N, Cruccu G, Haanpaa M, et al. EFNS guidelines on pharmacological treatment of neuropathic pain. *Eur J Neurol*. 2006;13:1153–1169.
42. Bramness JG, Skurtveit S, Morland J. Impairment due to intake of carisoprodol. *Drug Alcohol Depend*. 2004;74:311–318.
43. Reeves RR, Carter OS, Pinkofsky HB, et al. Carisoprodol (soma): Abuse potential and physician unawareness. *J Addict Dis*. 1999;18:51–56.
44. Dalen P, Alvan G, Wakelkamp M, Olsen H. Formation of meprobamate from carisoprodol is catalysed by CYP2C19. *Pharmacogenetics*. 1996;6:387–394.
45. Nance PW, Bugaresti J, Shellenberger K, et al. Efficacy and safety of tizanidine in the treatment of spasticity in patients with spinal cord injury. North American Tizanidine Study Group. *Neurology*. 1994;44:S44-51.
46. Smith C, Birnbaum G, Carter JL, et al. Tizanidine treatment of spasticity caused by multiple sclerosis: results of a double-blind, placebo-controlled trial. US Tizanidine Study Group. *Neurology*. 1994;44:S34-42.
47. Coward DM. Tizanidine: Neuropharmacology and mechanism of action. *Neurology*. 1994;44.
48. Malanga G, Reiter RD, Garay E. Update on tizanidine for muscle spasticity and emerging indications. *Expert Opin Pharmacother*. 2008;9:2209–2215.
49. Van Tulder MW, Touray T, Furlan AD, et al. Muscle relaxants for non-specific low back pain. *Cochrane Database Syst Rev*. 2003:CD004252.
50. Nance PW, Sheremata WA, Lynch SG, et al. Relationship of the antispasticity effect of tizanidine to plasma concentration in patients with multiple sclerosis. *Arch Neurol*. 1997;54:731–736.
51. Chou R, Peterson K, Helfand M. Comparative efficacy and safety of skeletal muscle relaxants for spasticity and musculoskeletal conditions: A systematic review. *J Pain Symptom Manage*. 2004;28:140–175.
52. Bennett MI, Smith BH, Torrance N, Lee AJ. Can pain can be more or less neuropathic? Comparison of symptom assessment tools with ratings of certainty by clinicians. *Pain*. 2006;122:289–294.
53. Sindrup SH, Jensen TS. Efficacy of pharmacological treatments of neuropathic pain: An update and effect related to mechanism of drug action. *Pain*. 1999;83:389–400.
54. Johannessen Landmark C. Antiepileptic drugs in non-epilepsy disorders: Relations between mechanisms of action and clinical efficacy. *CNS Drugs*. 2008;22:27–47.
55. Finnerup NB, Otto M, McQuay HJ, et al. Algorithm for neuropathic pain treatment: An evidence based proposal. *Pain*. 2005;118:289–305.
56. Kochar DK, Garg P, Bumb RA, et al. Divalproex sodium in the management of post-herpetic neuralgia: A randomized double-blind placebo-controlled study. *QJM*. 2005;98:29–34.

57. Schmidt D, Elger CE. What is the evidence that oxcarbazepine and carbamazepine are distinctly different antiepileptic drugs? *Epilepsy Behav.* 2004;5:627–635.
58. Yap KY, Chui WK, Chan A. Drug interactions between chemotherapeutic regimens and antiepileptics. *Clin Ther.* 2008;30:1385–1407.
59. Baker AF, Dorr RT. Drug interactions with the taxanes: Clinical implications. *Cancer Treat Rev.* 2001;27:221–233.
60. Neef C, de Voogd-van der Straaten I. An interaction between cytostatic and anticonvulsant drugs. *Clin Pharmacol Ther.* 1988;43:372–375.
61. Dofferhoff AS, Berendsen HH, vd Naalt J, et al. Decreased phenytoin level after carboplatin treatment. *Am J Med.* 1990;89:247–248.
62. Sylvester RK, Lewis FB, Caldwell KC, et al. Impaired phenytoin bioavailability secondary to cisplatinum, vinblastine, and bleomycin. *Ther Drug Monit.* 1984;6:302–305.
63. Relling MV, Pui CH, Sandlund JT, et al. Adverse effect of anticonvulsants on efficacy of chemotherapy for acute lymphoblastic leukaemia. *Lancet.* 2000;356:285–290.
64. Gilbar PJ, Brodribb TR. Phenytoin and fluorouracil interaction. *Ann Pharmacother.* 2001;35:1367–1370.
65. Rabinowicz AL, Hinton DR, Dyck P, Couldwell WT. High-dose tamoxifen in treatment of brain tumors: Interaction with antiepileptic drugs. *Epilepsia.* 1995;36:513–515.
66. Coderre TJ, Kumar N, Lefebvre CD, Yu JS. Evidence that gabapentin reduces neuropathic pain by inhibiting the spinal release of glutamate. *J Neurochem.* 2005;94:1131–1139.
67. Stewart BH, Kugler AR, Thompson PR, Bockbrader HN. A saturable transport mechanism in the intestinal absorption of gabapentin is the underlying cause of the lack of proportionality between increasing dose and drug levels in plasma. *Pharm Res.* 1993;10:276–281.
68. Belliotti TR, Capiris T, Ekhato IV, et al. Structure-activity relationships of pregabalin and analogues that target the alpha(2)-delta protein. *J Med Chem.* 2005;48:2294–2307.
69. Lauria-Horner BA, Pohl RB. Pregabalin: A new anxiolytic. *Expert Opin Investig Drugs.* 2003;12:663–672.
70. Taylor CP, Angelotti T, Fauman E. Pharmacology and mechanism of action of pregabalin: The calcium channel alpha2-delta (alpha2-delta) subunit as a target for antiepileptic drug discovery. *Epilepsy Res.* 2007;73:137–150.
71. Jones DL, Sorkin LS. Systemic gabapentin and S(+)-3-isobutyl-gamma-aminobutyric acid block secondary hyperalgesia. *Brain Res.* 1998;810:93–99.
72. Randinitis EJ, Posvar EL, Alvey CW, et al. Pharmacokinetics of pregabalin in subjects with various degrees of renal function. *J Clin Pharmacol.* 2003;43:277–283.
73. Stacey BR, Swift JN. Pregabalin for neuropathic pain based on recent clinical trials. *Curr Pain Headache Rep.* 2006;10:179–184.
74. Gajraj NM. Pregabalin: Its pharmacology and use in pain management. *Anesth Analg.* 2007;105:1805–1815.
75. Flesch G. Overview of the clinical pharmacokinetics of oxcarbazepine. *Clin Drug Investig.* 2004;24:185–203.
76. May TW, Korn-Merker E, Rambeck B. Clinical pharmacokinetics of oxcarbazepine. *Clin Pharmacokinet.* 2003;42:1023–1042.
77. Cruccu G, Gronseth G, Alksne J, et al. AAN-EFNS guidelines on trigeminal neuralgia management. *Eur J Neurol.* 2008;15:1013–1028.
78. Carrazana E, Mikoshiba I. Rationale and evidence for the use of oxcarbazepine in neuropathic pain. *J Pain Symptom Manage.* 2003;25:S31-5.
79. Eisenberg E, River Y, Shifrin A, Krivoy N. Antiepileptic drugs in the treatment of neuropathic pain. *Drugs.* 2007;67:1265–1289.
80. Caraceni A, Zecca E, Bonezzi C, et al. Gabapentin for neuropathic cancer pain: A randomized controlled trial from the Gabapentin Cancer Pain Study Group. *J Clin Oncol.* 2004;22:2909–2917.
81. Xiao W, Boroujerdi A, Bennett GJ, Luo ZD. Chemotherapy-evoked painful peripheral neuropathy: Analgesic effects of gabapentin and effects on expression of the alpha-2-delta type-1 calcium channel subunit. *Neuroscience.* 2007;144:714–720.
82. Dunteman ED. Levetiracetam as an adjunctive analgesic in neoplastic plexopathies: case series and commentary. *J Pain Palliat Care Pharmacother.* 2005;19:35–43.
83. Tsavaris N, Kopterides P, Kosmas C, et al. Gabapentin monotherapy for the treatment of chemotherapy-induced neuropathic pain: A pilot study. *Pain Med.* 2008;9:1209–1216.
84. Max MB, Lynch SA, Muir J, et al. Effects of desipramine, amitriptyline, and fluoxetine on pain in diabetic neuropathy. *N Engl J Med.* 1992;326:1250–1256.
85. McQuay HJ, Tramer M, Nye BA, et al. A systematic review of antidepressants in neuropathic pain. *Pain.* 1996;68:217–227.
86. McQuay HJ, Carroll D, Glynn CJ. Low dose amitriptyline in the treatment of chronic pain. *Anaesthesia.* 1992;47:646–652.
87. Sindrup SH, Gram LF, Brosen K, et al. The selective serotonin reuptake inhibitor paroxetine is effective in the treatment of diabetic neuropathy symptoms. *Pain.* 1990;42:135–144.
88. Saarto T, Wiffen PJ. Antidepressants for neuropathic pain. *Cochrane Database Syst Rev.* 2007:CD005454.
89. Gray AM, Spencer PS, Sewell RD. The involvement of the opioidergic system in the antinociceptive mechanism of action of antidepressant compounds. *Br J Pharmacol.* 1998;124:669–674.
90. Glassman AH. Cardiovascular effects of tricyclic antidepressants. *Annu Rev Med.* 1984;35:503–511.
91. Berger A, Dukes E, Mercadante S, Oster G. Use of antiepileptics and tricyclic antidepressants in cancer patients with neuropathic pain. *Eur J Cancer Care (Engl).* 2006;15:138–145.
92. Kautio AL, Haanpaa M, Saarto T, Kalso E. Amitriptyline in the treatment of chemotherapy-induced neuropathic symptoms. *J Pain Symptom Manage.* 2008;35:31–39.
93. Goldstein DJ, Lu Y, Detke MJ, et al. Duloxetine vs. placebo in patients with painful diabetic neuropathy. *Pain.* 2005;116:109–118.
94. Gralow J, Tripathy D. Managing metastatic bone pain: The role of bisphosphonates. *J Pain Symptom Manage.* 2007;33:462–472.
95. Body JJ. Bisphosphonates in metastatic bone disease: Renal safety matters. *Oncologist.* 2005;10(Suppl 1):1-2.
96. Migliorati CA, Schubert MM, Peterson DE, Seneda LM. Bisphosphonate-associated osteonecrosis of mandibular and maxillary bone: An emerging oral complication of supportive cancer therapy. *Cancer.* 2005;104:83–93.
97. Magopoulos C, Karakinaris G, Telioudis Z, et al. Osteonecrosis of the jaws due to bisphosphonate use. A review of 60 cases and treatment proposals. *Am J Otolaryngol.* 2007;28:158–163.
98. Hindley AC, Hill EB, Leyland MJ, Wiles AE. A double-blind controlled trial of salmon calcitonin in pain due to malignancy. *Cancer Chemother Pharmacol.* 1982;9:71–74.
99. Blomqvist C, Elomaa I, Porkka L, et al. Evaluation of salmon calcitonin treatment in bone metastases from breast cancer—a controlled trial. *Bone.* 1988;9:45–51.
100. Blanchard J, Menk E, Ramamurthy S, Hoffman J. Subarachnoid and epidural calcitonin in patients with pain due to metastatic cancer. *J Pain Symptom Manage.* 1990;5:42–45.
101. Martinez-Zapata MJ, Roque M, Alonso-Coello P, et al. Calcitonin for metastatic bone pain. *Cochrane Database Syst Rev.* 2006;3:CD003223.
102. Poulter CA, Cosmatos D, Rubin P, et al. A report of RTOG 8206: A phase III study of whether the addition of single dose hemibody irradiation to standard fractionated local field irradiation is more effective than local field irradiation alone in the treatment of symptomatic osseous metastases. *Int J Radiat Oncol Biol Phys.* 1992;23:207–214.
103. Scarantino CW, Caplan R, Rotman M, et al. A phase I/II study to evaluate the effect of fractionated hemibody irradiation in the treatment of osseous metastases—RTOG 88-22. *Int J Radiat Oncol Biol Phys.* 1996;36:37–48.
104. Cardozo LD, Stanton SL. A comparison between bromocriptine and indomethacin in the treatment of detrusor instability. *J Urol.* 1980;123:399–401.
105. Castell DO. Calcium-channel blocking agents for gastrointestinal disorders. *Am J Cardiol.* 1985;55:210B-213B.
106. Gomez A, Martos F, Bellido I, et al. Muscarinic receptor subtypes in human and rat colon smooth muscle. *Biochem Pharmacol.* 1992;43:2413–2419.
107. Mercadante S, Spoldi E, Caraceni A, et al. Octreotide in relieving gastrointestinal symptoms due to bowel obstruction. *Palliat Med.* 1993;7:295–299.
108. Pandha HS, Waxman J. Octreotide in malignant intestinal obstruction. *Anticancer Drugs.* 1996;7 Suppl 1:5–10.
109. Ripamonti C, Mercadante S, Groff L, et al. Role of octreotide, scopolamine butylbromide, and hydration in symptom control of patients with inoperable bowel obstruction and nasogastric tubes: A prospective randomized trial. *J Pain Symptom Manage.* 2000;19:23–34.
110. Mercadante S, Casuccio A, Mangione S. Medical treatment for inoperable malignant bowel obstruction: A qualitative systematic review. *J Pain Symptom Manage.* 2007;33:217–223.

111. Bruera E, Neumann CM. The uses of psychotropics in symptom management in advanced cancer. *Psychooncology*. 1998;7:346–358.
112. Beaver WT, Wallenstein SL, Houde RW, Rogers A. A comparison of the analgesic effects of methotrimeprazine and morphine in patients with cancer. *Clin Pharmacol Ther*. 1966;7:436–466.
113. Gomez-Perez FJ, Rull JA, Dies H, et al. Nortriptyline and fluphenazine in the symptomatic treatment of diabetic neuropathy. A double-blind cross-over study. *Pain*. 1985;23:395–400.
114. Fernandez F, Adams F, Holmes VF. Analgesic effect of alprazolam in patients with chronic, organic pain of malignant origin. *J Clin Psychopharmacol*. 1987;7:167–169.
115. Hugel H, Ellershaw JE, Dickman A. Clonazepam as an adjuvant analgesic in patients with cancer-related neuropathic pain. *J Pain Symptom Manage*. 2003;26:1073–1074.
116. Reddy S, Patt RB. The benzodiazepines as adjuvant analgesics. *J Pain Symptom Manage*. 1994;9:510–514.
117. Juergens S. Alprazolam and diazepam: Addiction potential. *J Subst Abuse Treat*. 1991;8:43–51.
118. Buclin T, Mazzocato C, Berney A, et al. Psychopharmacology in supportive care of cancer: A review for the clinician. IV. Other psychotropic agents. *Support Care Cancer*. 2001;9:213–222.
119. Bartusch SL, Sanders BJ, D'Alessio JG, et al. Clonazepam for the treatment of lancinating phantom limb pain. *Clin J Pain*. 1996;12:59–62.
120. Court JE, Kase CS. Treatment of tic douloureux with a newanticonvulsant (clonazepam). *J Neurol Neurosurg Psychiatry*. 1976;39:297–299.
121. Jhaveri MD, Richardson D, Chapman V. Endocannabinoid metabolism and uptake: novel targets for neuropathic and inflammatory pain. *Br J Pharmacol*. 2007;152:624–632.
122. Bifulco M, Laezza C, Gazzerro P, et al. Endocannabinoids as emerging suppressors of angiogenesis and tumor invasion (review). *Oncol Rep*. 2007;17:813–816.
123. Aguado T, Carracedo A, Julien B, et al. Cannabinoids induce glioma stem-like cell differentiation and inhibit gliomagenesis. *J Biol Chem*. 2007;282:6854–6862.
124. Michalski CW, Oti FE, Erkan M, et al. Cannabinoids in pancreatic cancer: correlation with survival and pain. *Int J Cancer*. 2008;122:742–750.
125. Michalski CW, Laukert T, Sauliunaite D, et al. Cannabinoids ameliorate pain and reduce disease pathology in cerulein-induced acute pancreatitis. *Gastroenterology*. 2007;132:1968–1978.
126. Osei-Hyiaman D. Endocannabinoid system in cancer cachexia. *Curr Opin Clin Nutr Metab Care*. 2007;10:443–448.
127. Russo EB. Cannabinoids in the management of difficult to treat pain. *Ther Clin Risk Manag*. 2008;4:245–259.
128. Maida V, Ennis M, Irani S, et al. Adjunctive nabilone in cancer pain and symptom management: A prospective observational study using propensity scoring. *J Support Oncol*. 2008;6:119–124.
129. Abrams DI, Jay CA, Shade SB, et al. Cannabis in painful HIV-associated sensory neuropathy: A randomized placebo-controlled trial. *Neurology*. 2007;68:515–521.
130. Okie S. Medical marijuana and the Supreme Court. *N Engl J Med*. 2005;353:648–651.
131. Ho CM, Su CK. Ketamine attenuates sympathetic activity through mechanisms not mediated by N-methyl-D-aspartate receptors in the isolated spinal cord of neonatal rats. *Anesth Analg*. 2006;102:806–810.
132. Kew JN, Kemp JA. Ionotropic and metabotropic glutamate receptor structure and pharmacology. *Psychopharmacology (Berl)*. 2005;179:4–29.
133. Orser BA, Pennefather PS, MacDonald JF. Multiple mechanisms of ketamine blockade of N-methyl-D-aspartate receptors. *Anesthesiology*. 1997;86:903–917.
134. Parsons CG, Danysz W, Quack G. Memantine is a clinically well tolerated N-methyl-D-aspartate (NMDA) receptor antagonist—a review of preclinical data. *Neuropharmacology*. 1999;38:735–767.
135. Clements JA, Nimmo WS. Pharmacokinetics and analgesic effect of ketamine in man. *Br J Anaesth*. 1981;53:27–30.
136. Grant IS, Nimmo WS, Clements JA. Pharmacokinetics and analgesic effects of I.M. and oral ketamine. *Br J Anaesth*. 1981;53:805–810.
137. Grande LA, O'Donnell BR, Fitzgibbon DR, et al. Ultra-low dose ketamine and memantine treatment for pain in an opioid-tolerant oncology patient. *Anesth Analg*. 2008;107:1380–1383.
138. Lossignol DA, Obiols-Portis M, Body JJ. Successful use of ketamine for intractable cancer pain. *Support Care Cancer*. 2005;13:188–193.
139. Mercadante S, Arcuri E, Tirelli W, et al. Analgesic effect of intravenous ketamine in cancer patients on morphine therapy: A randomized, controlled, double-blind, crossover, double-dose study. *J Pain Symptom Manage*. 2000;20:246–252.
140. Visser E, Schug SA. The role of ketamine in pain management. *Biomed Pharmacother*. 2006;60:341–348.
141. Bell RF, Eccleston C, Kalso E. Ketamine as adjuvant to opioids for cancer pain. A qualitative systematic review. *J Pain Symptom Manage*. 2003;26:867–875.
142. Rogawski MA, Wenk GL. The neuropharmacological basis for the use of memantine in the treatment of Alzheimer's disease. *CNS Drug Rev*. 2003;9:275–308.
143. Lipton SA. Failures and successes of NMDA receptor antagonists: molecular basis for the use of open-channel blockers like memantine in the treatment of acute and chronic neurologic insults. *NeuroRx*. 2004;1:101–110.
144. Johnson JW, Kotermanski SE. Mechanism of action of memantine. *Curr Opin Pharmacol*. 2006;6:61–67.
145. Parsons CG, Gilling K. Memantine as an example of a fast, voltage-dependent, open channel n-methyl-d-aspartate receptor blocker. *Methods Mol Biol*. 2007;403:15–36.
146. Buvanendran A, Kroin JS. Early use of memantine for neuropathic pain. *Anesth Analg*. 2008;107:1093–1094.
147. Carlton SM, Rees H, Tsuruoka M, et al. Memantine attenuates responses of spinothalamic tract cells to cutaneous stimulation in neuropathic monkeys. *Eur J Pain*. 1998;2:229–238.
148. Hackworth RJ, Tokarz KA, Fowler IM, et al. Profound pain reduction after induction of memantine treatment in two patients with severe phantom limb pain. *Anesth Analg*. 2008;107:1377–1379.
149. Sinis N, Birbaumer N, Gustin S, et al. Memantine treatment of complex regional pain syndrome: A preliminary report of six cases. *Clin J Pain*. 2007;23:237–243.
150. Maier C, Dertwinkel R, Mansourian N, et al. Efficacy of the NMDA-receptor antagonist memantine in patients with chronic phantom limb pain—results of a randomized double-blinded, placebo-controlled trial. *Pain*. 2003;103:277–283.
151. Wiech K, Kiefer RT, Topfner S, et al. A placebo-controlled randomized crossover trial of the N-methyl-D-aspartic acid receptor antagonist, memantine, in patients with chronic phantom limb pain. *Anesth Analg*. 2004;98:408–413, table of contents.
152. Sang CN, Booher S, Gilron I, et al. Dextromethorphan and memantine in painful diabetic neuropathy and postherpetic neuralgia: Efficacy and dose-response trials. *Anesthesiology*. 2002;96:1053–1061.

CHAPTER 19 ■ OPIOID ANALGESICS

Cancer pain is often undertreated even in developed countries with abundant resources and easy access to oral, parenteral, and transdermal opioids.[1] However, problems in developing nations are more complex, and these medications are often not readily available to the majority of patients in Latin and South America, Eastern Europe, Asia, and Africa.[2] Furthermore, the ratio of cost of opioids to income is higher in developing countries.[3] In spite of the efforts by the World Health Organization (WHO) and others to make oral opioids available, too little progress has been made in relieving cancer pain in developing countries. Unfortunately, developing countries account for 75% of the world's population and bear more than half the global cancer burden.

Drug therapy is the cornerstone in the treatment of pain in the cancer patient. Opioids are the essential category of drug for use in most cancer patients with pain.[4] In some situations, particularly with rapid opioid escalation due to either worsening pain or the development of opioid tolerance, the addition of a second opioid may have merit.[5] Furthermore, because patients have significant and unpredictable variations in response to opioids (both in terms of pain relief and side effects), use of these medications must be largely governed by trial and error. As such, the clinician caring for cancer patients must be familiar with all the available drugs in this category. It is not sufficient to be familiar with one or two opioids. Rather, comprehensive care of the cancer patient with pain requires detailed knowledge of the pharmacology (both pharmacokinetics and pharmacodynamics) of a wide array of currently available opioids. Modifications in formulation have resulted in prolongation of activity over standard or IR formulations. These modifications have resulted in the availability of sustained-release (SR), controlled-release (CR), and extended-release (ER) products. These products include morphine (SR, ER, CR), oxycodone (CR), oxymorphone (ER), and fentanyl (transdermal). Traditionally, opioids are best administered orally. However, other modes of opioid drug delivery such as by implantable osmotic pump,[6] by inhalation,[7] by iontophoresis,[8] or transmucosally[9] are either under investigation or in clinical use.

For millennia, opium derived from secretions of *Papaver somniferum* seedpods have been utilized for analgesic purposes. Opium contains two chemical classes of alkaloids, phenantrenes and benzyl-isoquinolines. One of the phenantrene alkaloids, thebaine, present in 0.2% to 0.8% of the opium derived from *Papaver somniferum* and in 90% of that extracted from morphine-free *Papaver bracteatum*, is extremely toxic and lacks analgesic properties. Morphine, an opium alkaloid, was isolated in 1803 by Serturner and was later found to be primarily responsible for the analgesic properties of opium. The word "opioid" is a generic term for naturally occurring, semisynthetic, and synthetic drugs that combine with opioid receptors to produce physiological effects and which are stereospecifically antagonized by naloxone. For clinical purposes, opioids can be classified according to their receptor interactions (agonist, partial agonist, and agonist-antagonist). Pure (full) μ-agonists (most of the currently used opioids such as morphine, hydromorphone, oxycodone, hydrocodone) are conventionally used for moderate- to severe-intensity pain.[10] Partial agonists, such as buprenorphine, are avidly bound to the μ-receptor such that reversal of effects with standard clinical doses of naloxone may be difficult.[11] Agonist-antagonist opioids, such as pentazocine, butorphanol, and nalbuphine appear to exert their agonist analgesic effect through κ-receptors with an antagonist effect at μ-receptors.[12]

Insights into receptor biology, pharmacogenetics, and pharmacological antagonism help refine the use of established opioids and may result in the development of more selective drugs with improved clinical profiles. Opioids act on different receptors or receptor subtypes, and individual receptor profiles may influence the degree of pain relief attainable and the occurrence of opioid-related adverse events.[13] There are at least three major types of opioid receptors identified on the basis of pharmacological response, in vitro radioligand binding affinities, and in vivo localization of labeled drug in tissue homogenates or sections. These receptors are μ (MOR), κ (KOR), and δ (DOR). Identification of receptors allowed opioids to be grouped according to similarities in the activation of their receptor types. These receptors have been identified on cell bodies in the dorsal root ganglion (DRG) and on central terminals of primary afferent neurons within the dorsal horn of the spinal cord.[14] In the early 1990s, the opioid receptors were cloned.[15] Although the receptor most commonly associated with pain relief is the μ-receptor, specific δ- and κ-agonists can also mediate antinociception at spinal and supraspinal sites. MOR is the primary target mediating analgesic, euphoric, and reinforcing effects of morphine.[16] DOR agonists are associated with pain relief and euphoria, whereas KOR agonists produce pain relief, miosis, sedation, and dysphoria.

Individual variations to pain perception may in part be accounted for by variation in levels of μ-opioid receptor expression and responses to different opioids.[17] In addition, variable patient responses to different opioids may be influenced by genetic variation and subtle differences in mechanism of action and potency.[18] Basic science research is beginning to identify the allelic variants that underlie such antinociceptive variability using a multiplicity of animal models, and genetic approaches are being exploited to accelerate this process.[19] Other factors that may explain interpatient variability in opioid responsiveness include polymorphisms in the μ-receptor regulatory region,[20] pharmacokinetic differences due to cytochrome P450 monooxygenase heterogeneity, and use of concomitant medications that may predispose to pharmacokinetic and pharmacodynamic drug interactions.

Opioids are small peptides primarily involved in nociception and immune responses;[21] they act through specific receptors (μ, δ, and κ) expressed in nervous and immune systems, which are also targets of substances of abuse. Opioid and chemokine systems can reciprocally influence each other's function at different levels; for example, μ-opioid ligands regulate expression and function of chemokine receptors in immune cells via heterologous desensitization.[22-23]

Opioid receptors belong to the G protein–coupled receptor (GPCR) family and they signal via a second messenger (cyclic AMP) or an ion channel (K^+). GPCRs regulate the function of ion channels, which play an essential role in the function of neurons by mediating and regulating of selective ion concentrations across the cell membrane.[24] GPCRs are widely distributed in the nervous system, and mediate key physiological processes including cognition, mood, appetite, pain, and synaptic transmission.[25] mRNA for all the opioid receptors have been demonstrated in the dorsal root ganglion and small-diameter primary afferent neurons. MOR, DOR, and KOR are members of the GPCR superfamily. A fourth major opioid receptor has been cloned—nociceptin/orphanin FQ receptor or opioid receptor-like 1 (ORL1).[26] Its function is not clear. Opioids have different affinities to the μ opioid receptor and potency is sometimes classified as low (eg, codeine) or high (eg, fentanyl). μ-opioid receptors are found in the periphery (following inflammation), at pre- and postsynaptic sites in the spinal cord dorsal horn, and in the brain stem, thalamus, and cortex, in what constitutes the ascending pain transmission system. In addition, μ-opioid receptors are found in the midbrain periaqueductal gray, the nucleus raphe magnus, and the rostral ventral medulla, where they comprise a descending inhibitory system that modulates spinal cord pain transmission. At a cellular level, opioids decrease calcium ion entry, resulting in a decrease in presynaptic neurotransmitter release (eg, substance P release from primary afferents in the spinal cord dorsal horn). They also enhance potassium ion efflux, resulting in the hyperpolarization of postsynaptic neurons and a decrease in synaptic transmission. A third mode of opioid action is the inhibition of GABAergic transmission in a local circuit (eg, in the brain stem, where gamma-aminobutyric acid (GABA) acts to inhibit a pain-inhibitory neuron). This disinhibitory action of the opioid has the net effect of exciting a descending inhibitory circuit.

The administration of opioids results in a variety of effects including pain relief, miosis, bradycardia, sedation, hypothermia, insensitivity to various stimuli, and depression of flexor reflexes. Opioids can modulate endocrine processes[27-28] and can also affect the immune response.[29] Although gender differences in opioid response have been reported in humans, with some studies reporting greater sensitivity in women[30-32] and others reporting greater sensitivity in men,[33-35] others have reported no differences.[36-37] Craft[38] suggests that animal studies demonstrate gender differences in a variety of behavioral effects of opioids. This author suggests that μ-agonists are more potent and in some cases more efficacious in male than in female rats and that women were more sensitive than men to the reinforcing and locomotor stimulant effects of opioids. Furthermore, there also appears to be gender differences in opioid-related side effects such as respiratory depression, nausea, urinary retention, and altered immune function, as well as the rate at which opioid tolerance and dependence develop. Craft suggests that estradiol may be an important modulator of opioid effects and may be the primary mechanism by which adult women differ from adult men in opioid sensitivity. The anatomic and physiologic characteristics of the periaqueductal gray and its descending projections to the rostral ventromedial medulla may account for gender difference in morphine potency.[39]

The expression of opioid receptors on cells of the immune system was first implicated by the ability of opioids to alter immune function.[40] Since then, pharmacologic, molecular, and, more recently, immunologic evidence for the expression of opioid receptors on immune cells have been reported.[41-43] The regulation of cytokine, chemokine, and cytokine receptor expression may also be a critical component of the immunomodulatory activity of the opioids.[44] Increased expression of chemokines is associated with a wide range of inflammatory diseases and pathologies. MOR activation by opioids results in altered transcriptional and protein regulation of several cytokines, chemokines, and chemokine receptors. By contrast with MOR, KOR activation exhibits a broad inhibitory influence on cytokine, chemokine, and chemokine receptor expression.[44] Cytokines represent some of the principal mediators of immune function by mediating and regulating the innate and adaptive immunity and stimulating the growth and the differentiation of cells in the immune system. Proinflammatory cytokines can enhance neuronal excitability and perpetuate neuropathic pain. In addition, proinflammatory cytokines can suppress the ability of opioids to control pain and contribute to opioid tolerance and dependence/withdrawal.[45] Acute and long-term administration of exogenous opioids is known to have inhibitory effects on antibody and cellular immune responses, natural killer (NK) cell activity, cytokine expression, and phagocytic activity.[46] Opioid receptor signaling has been implicated in the regulation of cell proliferation and cell death in various cells expressing opioid receptors.[47] The observed tumor-suppressive effects of morphine suggest the intriguing possibility that morphine might be useful as an adjunct in cancer therapy not only to reduce cancer pain but also tumor growth.[48] Other opioids also appear to induce apoptosis. Methadone induced cell death not only in anticancer drug-sensitive and apoptosis-sensitive leukemia cells but also in doxorubicin-resistant, multidrug-resistant, and apoptosis-resistant leukemia cells.[49] Several important pathways that control cell proliferation, survival, and apoptosis have been reported to be associated with the nonanalgesic effects of opioids, which may be mediated through both opioid receptor signaling and other non-opioid receptor molecular entity-mediated signaling.[50] Opioid-induced general suppression of the immune system might jeopardize other potentially favorable outcomes. Although data are very limited in this area, one animal study suggests that chronic morphine treatment

TABLE 19.1

OPIOID CLASSIFICATION OF ACTIVE METABOLITES BASED ON CLINICAL RELEVANCE

No known or minimal metabolite activity	Active metabolite clinically not important	Active metabolite clinically important
Alfentanil	Buprenorphine	Codeine
Butorphanol	Hydromophone	Dextropropoxyphene[a]
Fentanyl	Nalbuphine	Dihydrocodeine
Levorphanol	Nalorphine	Diacetylmorphine
Methadone	Oxymorphone	Hydrocodone
Pentazocine		Morphine
Remifentanil		Oxycodone
Sufentanil		Meperidine[b]
		Tramadol

[a]Cardiotoxic.
[b]Neurotoxic.
(Modified from Coller JK, Christrup LL, Somogyi AA. Role of active metabolites in the use of opioids. *Eur J Clin Pharmacol.* 2009;65(2):121–139.)

may have resulted in accelerated tumor growth probably as a consequence of general immunosuppression.[51] At this time, it is unknown whether the administration of opioids and the association with immunosuppression has clinical implications in cancer patients.

Opioid alkaloids are extensively metabolized, mainly in the liver, and predominantly excreted by the kidneys. All opioids are eliminated by hepatic metabolism, principally oxidation (catalyzed by CYP450) and conjugation (catalyzed by transferases such as UDP-glucuronyl transferase). In many cases the primary metabolites formed are then further metabolized via secondary pathways (phase I—functionalization followed by phase II—conjugation). Opioids, which are alkyl ethers at the 3-phenolic hydroxyl group, such as codeine, hydrocodone, and oxycodone, are subject to O-dealkylation; this reaction is catalyzed by CYP2D6 and is therefore subject to considerable genetic polymorphism. Many opioids are subject to N-demethylation into nor-derivatives, including morphine, codeine, dihydrocodeine, oxycodone, and tramadol. Many analgesic and psychoactive drugs are metabolized by one of three P450 enzymes. The major cytochrome in humans is 3A4, which is involved in 50% of all microsomal drug metabolism and is responsible for the metabolism of methadone, fentanyl, and certain selective selective serotonin-reuptake inhibitors (SSRIs). Opioid N-demethylation is also catalyzed mainly but not exclusively by CYP3A4. Glucuronidation reactions take place on free hydroxyl groups on opioids (eg, morphine, oxymorphone, nalbuphine). Overall, glucuronidation of opioids is mainly mediated by the UDP glucuronosyltransferase UGT2B7. About 90% of a morphine dose is converted into metabolites; principally the glucuronide conjugates morphine-3-glucuronide (M3G, 50%) and morphine-6-glucuronide (M6G, 10%).[52–53] M3G does not bind to opioid receptors and is not an agonist.[54] M6G has analgesic efficacy and has a superior side effect profile compared with morphine. Several opioids have metabolites with activity comparable to or even greater than the parent drug, with the best example being the conversion to morphine from codeine (Table 19.1). This has clinical relevance, especially in the elderly and those with renal dysfunction, because many of the active metabolites are more renally eliminated than the parent opioid (eg, morphine and M6G).[55] In other situations, the metabolites are analgesically inactive but have evidence of toxicity (eg, normeperidine and neurotoxicity, nordextropropxyphene, and cardiotoxicity). Liver dysfunction may not only reduce the blood/plasma clearance of drugs eliminated by hepatic metabolism or biliary excretion; it can also affect plasma protein binding, which in turn could influence the processes of distribution and elimination.[56] The hepatic metabolism of morphine, meperidine, pentazocine, and alfentanil is significantly reduced in patients with cirrhosis, leading to changes in drug disposition that should be considered in dosage regimens.[57]

Unexpected degree and duration of effect of morphine metabolites can occur in patients with severely impaired renal function given morphine or derivatives in whom there is accumulation of metabolites.[58] The elimination half-life of M3G varied between 14.5 and 118.8 hours (mean 49.6 hours) in renal failure patients, which was distinctly different from the 2.4 to 6.7 hours (mean 4.0 hours) found in patients with normal kidney function.[59] Hydromorphone is metabolized principally by conjugation with glucuronic acid to form hydromorphone-3-glucuronide (H3G). After repeated doses, the steady-state plasma concentrations of both H3G and M3G exceed the respective plasma concentrations of the parent opioids to a similarly large extent (20- to 50-fold) in both adults and children.[60–62] Due to the polar nature of the glucuronide conjugates, these metabolites can accumulate relative to the parent opioid in patients with renal impairment such that plasma concentration ratios of 100:1 have been reported.[62–63] M3G has been shown to evoke a range of neuroexcitatory behaviors including altered body posture, myoclonic jerks, and seizures[64–66] in a dose-dependent manner.[67] M3G is considered the likely reason for neuroexcitatory behaviors (myoclonus, allodynia, and seizures) observed in some patients receiving high doses of chronically administered systemic morphine for the treatment of cancer pain.[68] There are also reports of myoclonus in cancer patients dosed chronically with hydromorphone with speculation that H3G may be the causative agent.[69] In an experimental model, Wright et al.[70] demonstrated that H3G produced dose-dependent behavioral excitation similar to M3G and that H3G was approximately 2.5-fold more potent than M3G. The authors suggested that if H3G crosses the blood–brain barrier with equivalent efficiency to M3G, then the myoclonus, allodynia, and seizures observed in some patients dosed chronically with large systemic doses of hydromorphone were almost certainly caused by the accumulation of sufficient H3G in the central nervous system (CNS) to evoke behavioral excitation.

SELECTION OF OPIOID THERAPY

The effective clinical use of opioid drugs requires familiarity with drug selection, routes of administration, dosage guidelines, and potential adverse effects. Several factors must be considered if opioids are to be used effectively. These include:

- The patient's previous opioid exposure and preferences
- Severity and nature of disease
- Age of patient
- Extent of cancer, particularly hepatic and renal involvement altering normal opioid pharmacokinetics (Table 19.2).
- Concurrent disease
- Available formulations

The specific pathogenic mechanism that underlies a patient's cancer pain should not be a factor in deciding which opioid to use, because the mechanism of pain does not reliably predict the response to opioid therapy.[71] This particularly applies to situations in which neuropathic mechanisms dominate the pain complaint. Opioids should be used as first-line therapy in such situations, particularly if the pain is considered moderate to severe in intensity.

Short-acting agents (eg, morphine IR, hydrocodone IR, hydromorphone IR, oxycodone IR, oxymorphone IR, transmucosal fentanyl) may be favored initially because they are easier to titrate than long-acting agents (eg, morphine controlled release [CR], oxycodone CR, oxymorphone extended release [ER], and transdermal fentanyl [TTS]). Short-acting opioids are characterized by a rapid rise and fall in serum opioid levels, whereas serum levels of long-acting opioids increase slowly to therapeutic levels, remain there for an extended period, and then slowly decline.[72] In general, the clinical circumstance dictates the choice of a short- or long-acting opioid. For example, the treatment of acute or postoperative pain usually requires frequent titration, and short-acting opioids, with duration of action of 2 to 4 hours, are preferred. Conversely, the treatment of cancer pain or chronic, moderate to severe nonmalignant pain usually can be treated with a long-acting oral agent, with a duration of action of 12 to 24 hours, with less need for titration. In patients being treated with long-acting agents, short-acting opioids are usually provided as rescue medication for breakthrough pain. Because of the substantial interpatient variability in opioid responsiveness, clinicians who prescribe opioids for the treatment of cancer pain should be familiar with at least three different opioids appropriate for the management of moderate to severe pain.[73]

The opioids used most commonly in the treatment of cancer pain are listed in Table 19.3. During the past decade, several long-acting oral opioid formulations have been developed for once- or twice-daily administration, and a transdermal fentanyl patch is also available for administration every 72 hours. Long-acting formulations of opioids are recommended to provide around-the-clock pain relief. With appropriately prescribed long-acting opioids, patients do not typically experience a significant disruption in cognitive functioning but instead may experience moderate improvement of some aspects of cognitive functioning, as a consequence of pain relief and concomitant improvement of well-being and mood.[74] In addition, patients are often able to improve sleep patterns, have increased control over their own pain management, become more independent of caregivers, and experience improved compliance with treatment strategies.[75] Although most of the commonly used CR oral opioid formulations (eg, oxycodone CR, morphine CR) are recommended by the manufacturer to be given every 12 hours, many patients with chronic, moderate to severe pain need to use these agents more frequently than every 12 hours to achieve adequate, sustained pain relief.[76]

Opioids should be administered by the most comfortable and convenient route that meets the specific needs of the individual patient. The regimen for opioid medications should generally provide around-the-clock analgesia with provision for rescue doses for the management of exacerbations of the pain not covered by the regular dosage. At all times, uncontrolled pain should be addressed by gradual increase in the opioid dose until either pain control is achieved or intolerable and unmanageable adverse effects supervene. The management of pain with opioid analgesics demands frequent patient assessment and a readiness to reevaluate the therapeutic plan in the setting of either inadequate relief or adverse effects.

There is no single optimal or maximal dose of an opioid analgesic drug. In general, for progressive, tumor-related pain, the appropriate dose of an opioid is one that relieves a patient's pain throughout the dosing interval without causing unmanageable or intolerable adverse events.[77] The initial dose may be based on the severity of pain and known response to previous analgesic therapy, if any.[78] Aggressive upward titration to a stable dose (ie, one

TABLE 19.2

EFFECTS OF RENAL FAILURE ON OPIOID PHARMACOKINETICS

Opioid	Effect
Dihydrocodeine	Decreased clearance
Dextropropoxyphene	Increased norpropoxyphene (toxic metabolite)
Morphine	Increased morphine-6-glucuronide (active metabolite)
Meperidine	Increased normeperidine (toxic metabolite)

TABLE 19.3

ORAL AND TRANSDERMAL OPIOIDS USED IN THE PRIMARY TREATMENT OF CANCER PAIN

Opioid	Initial Dose and Frequency	Pharmacokinetics	Most Common Adverse Events	Comments
Hydrocodone IR	5–10 mg q4–6h	T_{max} = 1.3 hours; $T_{1/2}$ = 3.8 hours	Light-headedness, dizziness, sedation, nausea	Dosage ceiling related to combination with aspirin or acetaminophen. Available in United States in combination only.
Meperidine IR	50–150 mg q3–4h	Duration of action shorter than morphine. T_{max} = 1–2 hours $T_{1/2}$ = 3–5 hours (normal renal/hepatic function); 7–11 hours (hepatic dysfunction)	Light-headedness, dizziness, sedation, nausea	Not recommended for routine use.
Morphine IR	5–30 mg q4h	T_{max} = 1.2 hours $T_{1/2}$ = 2–4 hours	Constipation, light-headedness, dizziness	Useful for initial dose titration and for breakthrough pain
Morphine ER	Based on dose of morphine IR; administered q12h	T_{max} MS Contin = 2.3 hours T_{max} Kadian = 9.5 hours T_{max} Avinza = 6.3 hours $T_{1/2}$ = 2–4 hours	Constipation, light-headedness, dizziness	Available in different preparations (Ms Contin, Oramorph, Kadian, Avinza)
Oxycodone IR	5–10 mg q4h	T_{max} = 1.5 hours $T_{1/2}$ = 3.2 hours	Drowsiness, light-headedness, nausea	Useful for initial dose titration and for breakthrough pain; if compounded with aspirin or acetaminophen, may impose a dosage ceiling
Oxycodone CR	Based on dose of oxycodone IR or previous opioid; administered q12h	T_{max} = 3.2 hours $T_{1/2}$ = 4.5 hours	Constipation, nausea, somnolence	Immediate release component (approx. 30% of total dose); equianalgesic dose ratio to oxymorphone ER is 2:1
Oxymorphone IR	5-10 mg q4-6h	T_{max} = 0.5 hours $T_{1/2}$ = 7.3-9.4 hours	Nausea, dizziness	Useful for initial dose titration and for breakthrough pain
Oxymorphone ER	Based on dose of oxymorphone IR or previous opioid; administered q12h	T_{max} = 3.5 hours; $T_{1/2}$ = 7.3–9.4 hours	Nausea, dizziness	Dose and dose interval should be adjusted according to patient needs; little need for rescue medication in clinical trials
Transdermal fentanyl	One patch applied to skin q72h	T_{max} = 27–38 hours $T_{1/2\,(apparent)}$ = 7 hours	Nausea, vomiting	Useful for patients with gastrointestinal dysfunction; poor adhesion to skin may limit use in some patients
Methadone	5 mg bid	T_{max} = 2.5–4 hours $T_{1/2}$ = 18–36 hours	Nausea, vomiting	Prolonged QTc; difficult titration for uncontrolled pain; risk of drug accumulation. Does not require renal pathways for elimination.

that provides adequate pain relief throughout the dosing interval) is predicated on continuing assessment of the effectiveness of therapy. Patients rarely benefit from combinations of opioids given in suboptimal doses; ideally clinicians should prescribe a single opioid analgesic and titrate to a stable dose.[78] However, it is important to recognize that there is significant interpatient variability with regard to responsiveness to different opioid drugs, and patients who respond poorly to one opioid may respond favorably to another.[79] In situations in which pain is not related to the tumor or its progression, unlimited opioid dose escalation may be inappropriate and the concepts of pain management need to shift from those of cancer pain to chronic pain not caused by cancer.[80]

An ongoing opioid regimen should include provisions for rescue doses for the treatment of breakthrough pain.

The rationale for providing rescue medication instead of increasing the dose of the around-the-clock opioid is to prevent overmedication and associated adverse events. Often, there is a narrow therapeutic window between an opioid dosage sufficient to achieve pain relief and one that is associated with unacceptable adverse events.[81] For patients treated with a long-acting opioid, an IR or short-acting opioid formulation (often the same drug) may be used as the rescue medication. We recommend that the rescue drug be started at a dose equivalent to approximately 10% of the 24-hour baseline dose and titrated upward to achieve adequate pain relief.[82] The dosing frequency of the rescue drug depends on the time to peak effect and the route of administration; in general, we administer oral rescue doses as frequently as every 2 hours if needed, but typically tend to start at every 3 to 4 hours as needed.[83] If breakthrough pain occurs frequently, we advocate increasing the dose or shorten the dosing interval of around-the-clock opioid or increase the dose of the rescue opioid. A key principle in treating breakthrough pain is to optimize the background pain control by appropriately adjusting the around-the-clock opioid regimen.

Hanks et al.[78] reported on the recommendations of the European Association for Palliative Care (EAPC) on the use of morphine and alternative opioids in cancer pain. These recommendations provide practical strategies for dealing with difficult situations. The opioid of first choice for moderate to severe cancer pain is morphine. The optimal route of administration of morphine is by mouth. Ideally, two types of formulation are required: normal-release (for dose titration) and modified-release (for maintenance treatment). The simplest method of dose titration is with a dose of normal-release morphine given every 4 hours with the same dose for breakthrough pain. This "rescue" dose may be given as often as required (up to hourly) and the total daily dose of morphine should be reviewed daily. The regular dose can then be adjusted to take into account the total amount of rescue morphine. If pain returns consistently before the next regular dose is due, the regular dose should be increased. In general, normal-release morphine does not need to be given more often than every 4 hours and modified-release (MR) morphine more often than 12 or 24 hours (according to the intended duration of the formulation). Patients stabilized on regular oral morphine require continued access to a rescue dose to treat "breakthrough" pain. Several countries do not have a normal-release formulation of morphine, though such a formulation is necessary for optimal pain management. A different strategy is needed if treatment is started with MR morphine. Changes to the regular dose should not be made more frequently than every 48 hours, which means that the dose titration phase will likely be prolonged. For patients receiving normal-release morphine every 4 hours, a double dose at bedtime is a simple and effective way of avoiding being woken by pain. Several MR formulations are available. There is no evidence that the 12-hourly formulations (tablets, or capsules) are substantially different in their duration of effect and relative analgesic potency. The same is true for the 24-hour formulations though there is less evidence to evaluate. If patients are unable to take morphine orally, the preferred alternative route is subcutaneous. There is generally no indication for giving morphine intramuscularly for chronic cancer pain because subcutaneous administration is simpler and less painful. The average relative potency ratio of oral morphine to subcutaneous morphine is between 1:2 and 1:3 (ie, 20 to 30 mg of morphine by mouth is equianalgesic to 10 mg by subcutaneous injection). In patients requiring continuous parenteral morphine, the preferred method of administration is by subcutaneous infusion. Intravenous infusion of morphine may be preferred in patients who already have an indwelling intravenous line; with generalized edema; who develop erythema, soreness, or sterile abscesses with subcutaneous administration; with coagulation disorders; or with poor peripheral circulation. The average relative potency ratio of oral to intravenous morphine is between 1:2 and 1:3.

The buccal, sublingual, and nebulized routes of administration of morphine are not recommended, because there is no evidence of clinical advantage over the conventional routes. Oral transmucosal fentanyl citrate (OTFC) is an effective treatment for "breakthrough pain" in patients stabilized on regular oral morphine or an alternative step 3 opioid. Successful pain management with opioids requires that adequate analgesia be achieved without excessive adverse effects. By these criteria the application of the WHO and the EAPC guidelines (using morphine as the preferred step 3 opioid) permit effective control of chronic cancer pain in the majority of patients. In a small minority of patients adequate relief without excessive adverse effects may depend on the use of alternative opioids, spinal administration of analgesics, or nondrug methods of pain control. A small proportion of patients develop intolerable adverse effects with oral morphine (in conjunction with a nonopioid and adjuvant analgesic as appropriate) before achieving adequate pain relief. In such patients a change to an alternative opioid or a change in the route of administration should be considered. Hydromorphone or oxycodone, if available in both normal release and MR formulations for oral administration, are effective alternatives to oral morphine. Methadone is an effective alternative but may be more complicated to use compared with other opioids because of pronounced interindividual differences in its plasma half-life, relative analgesic potency, and duration of action. Its use by nonspecialist practitioners is not recommended. Transdermal fentanyl is an effective alternative to oral morphine but is best reserved for patients whose opioid requirements are stable. It may have particular advantages for such patients if they are unable to take oral morphine, as an alternative to subcutaneous infusion. Spinal (epidural or intrathecal) administration of opioid analgesics in combination with local anesthetics or clonidine should be considered in patients who derive inadequate analgesia or suffer intolerable adverse effects despite the optimal use of systemic opioids and nonopioids.

MORPHINE

Oral morphine was first recommended in England in the 1950s for the treatment of cancer pain. This was often in the form of a "Brompton Cocktail," which contained cocaine and alcohol in addition to morphine or diamorphine. Although many compounds produce morphine-like pain relief and other effects, morphine is the standard opioid against which all new analgesics are measured. Morphine, usually as the sulfate or hydrochloride salt, is available in four oral formulations—an elixir or solution, an IR tablet, a number of different preparations of MR tablets or capsules, and MR suspensions. Chronic subcutaneous infusions of morphine are used in cancer patients; however, significant intra- and interpatient variability in morphine, M6G, and M3G concentrations have been reported with chronic infusions.[84] The reasons for this variability and its clinical implications are unknown. Subcutaneous administration of morphine results in less interpatient variability than oral morphine and smoother and more stable plasma concentrations.[85] Oral absorption of IR morphine (tablets and solution) is almost complete. Peak plasma concentrations are 5 to 10 times lower than those obtained following parenteral administration.[53,86–87] Peak plasma concentrations usually occur within the first hour after oral administration of morphine in solution[88] and slightly later with IR tablets.[87] Both short-acting formulations have a rapid effect, and pain relief lasts for approximately 4 hours. By contrast, CR morphine tablets produce delayed peak plasma concentrations after 2 to 4 hours,[89–90] the peak is attenuated, and analgesia usually lasts for 12 hours.[91] Following oral administration, there is rapid and extensive first-pass metabolism. The average bioavailability is 30% to 40%, but is quite variable (19% to 47%).[53,92–93] Although short-acting opioids are appropriate for immediate pain relief and dosage titration, long-acting opioids, generally indicated for once-daily (q24 hours) or twice-daily (q12 hours) dosing, are recommended for around-the-clock control in patients with moderate to severe chronic pain. Absolute bioavailability following administration of CR morphine is similar to other oral solutions and no dosage adjustment is required when converting between IR and CR formulations.[86] The elimination half-life of CR morphine is similar to that of IR formulations. CR agents are specially formulated to control the rate of dissolution of opioid from the dosage form, enabling a slow release of the analgesic, followed by an increase to therapeutic level, plateau, and ultimate decline in concentration. This ER delivery system maintains blood levels of opioid within the therapeutic window with minimal fluctuation.

Sublingual and buccal administration of morphine appear to be equally efficacious as oral morphine and these routes may be suitable for patients who cannot take oral medications. However, these routes do not appear to offer any advantages in terms of speed of onset of the drug or more extensive absorption compared to other IR preparations. Rectal administration is often not a viable alternative because of the necessary frequency of administration of IR formulations and the lack of patient acceptance. The rectal route of administration shows similar plasma concentrations and bioavailability compared to the oral route.[94] Elderly patients (>60 years of age) have reduced distribution volumes, which may result in higher peak plasma concentrations and reduced clearance of morphine.[95–96] Patients with impaired renal function have increased sensitivity to morphine and may experience severe and prolonged respiratory depression when treated with morphine.[97–98] Long-term treatment with escalating doses of morphine does not appear to change the pharmacokinetics of morphine or its metabolites, suggesting that escalating doses can be administered to cancer patients with disease progression or opioid tolerance.[99]

In a Cochrane review, Wiffen and McQuay[100] reported that oral morphine is an effective analgesic in patients who suffer pain associated with cancer and remains the gold standard for moderate to severe pain. Morphine has a wide therapeutic range, is effective by different routes of administration, is available in most countries, and is relatively inexpensive. Furthermore, WHO recommends that oral morphine is part of the essential drug list. In this review it was not possible to demonstrate the superiority of one modified-release product over another, either by brand or by length of time release. Some preparations had the practical advantage of a formulation as microcapsules for those who cannot readily swallow tablets.

The standard for long-acting opioids is generally considered to be controlled-release morphine. In the United States, five preparations of controlled- or slow-release morphine are now available. These agents exist in either tablet or capsule form. Most tablet formulations adsorb morphine onto a hydrophilic polymer that is embedded in a hydrophobic matrix. Upon ingestion, gastrointestinal (GI) fluid dissolves the tablet surface and hydrates the hydrophilic polymer to produce a gel layer through which morphine is released at a rate determined by the type of hydrophilic polymer, hydrophobic matrix, or their ratio. MS Contin and Oramorph SR are produced in a resin matrix that dissolves and releases morphine over approximately a 12-hour period. The controlled-release form of morphine incorporates two different classes of macromolecules which provide gradual, measured release of morphine by dissolution and diffusion. One of these macromolecules is a cellulose polymer of variable branching and molecular weights. Slow release of morphine is related to binding of water as the polymer passes through the GI tract largely unchanged. The other macromolecule consists of aliphatic alcohols. Inclusion of both macromolecules results in both hydrophilic and hydrophobic molecular effects. This system regulates morphine release rate proportional to the hydrophilic and hydrophobic components. On aqueous contact, the drug-containing cellulose matrix becomes hydrated and relatively porous but otherwise remaining intact. Water absorption allows the drug to diffuse smoothly and evenly. Morphine release rate is determined by the size of the pores and by the barrier created by the aliphatic alcohol. The rate of release is not significantly altered by pH.

The efficacy and safety of MS Contin and Oramorph SR for patients with cancer pain has been confirmed by multiple studies. In a study comparing the pharmacokinetic profiles of MS Contin and Oramorph SR by administering a single 60-mg dose to 18 healthy volunteers, significant differences between the drugs for maximum plasma concentration ($P < .001$), area under the plasma concentration curve from zero to 12 hours ($P < .01$), and apparent elimination half-life ($P < .001$) were observed, indicating that the two morphine preparations were not bioequivalent.[101] Patients should be instructed not to chew on or crush these preparations as this may result in a potentially toxic dose of morphine. Although the product insert for both MS Contin and Oramorph SR recommends using these drugs every 12 hours, we have found that it is frequently necessary to prescribe them every 8 hours, particularly when higher doses (doses >200 mg/day) are required.

A form of CR morphine, Kadian, is available in clear capsules containing small polymer-coated pellets of drug and is recommended for once a day use. An individual capsule contains multiple pellets (eg, a 100-mg capsule contains on average 300 pellets). Each of the pellets contains a morphine sulfate-containing core that essentially functions as a separate drug reservoir. Kadian is available as 10, 20, 30, 50, 60, 80, 100, and 200 mg capsules. Following multiple doses of 100 mg capsules every 24 hours, the T_{max} was approximately 10.3 hours. On a fixed dosing regimen to patients with chronic pain from malignancy, steady state is achieved in about 2 days. The nature of the core, the nature of the polymer coat, and the thickness of the coat collectively control the release of morphine from each pellet. The outer gelatin capsule rapidly dissolves in the stomach. The polymer coating has three components: an insoluble layer consisting of ethylcellulose, which has an enteric component (methacrylic acid copolymer, which is insoluble and relatively hydrophobic at pH 1.2); a water-soluble component (polyethylene glycol which is soluble and hydrophilic at pH 1.2); and a plasticizer (diethyl phthalate). As the core coating is partially soluble at an acidic pH, some release of morphine will occur in the stomach. As pH increases in the intestine, the remaining coating dissolves and significant drug absorption occurs in both the small and large intestines.

The pharmacokinetic profile of Kadian offers some advantages over MS Contin and Oramorph SR.[102] MS Contin has a short time to C_{max} with significant fluctuations in plasma concentrations at steady-state.[103] Although Kadian and MS Contin administered every 12 hours have similar total plasma morphine concentrations (as measured by area under the curve), Kadian exhibited a significantly higher C_{min}, less fluctuation in plasma morphine concentration throughout the dosing interval, a longer T_{max}, and a greater time that the plasma morphine concentration was ≥75% of C_{max}.[103] Another advantage of Kadian is its use by sprinkling (ie, breaking the capsule and sprinkling the pellets onto an easily ingested substance such as apple sauce or Guinness) which does not affect the time-release mechanism. Patients with swallowing difficulties may find Kadian a more suitable formulation as it can also be administered through a gastrostomy tube.

Avinza utilizes a combination of immediate- and extended-release beads. Upon ingestion, 10% of the beads release morphine immediately while the residual beads gradually release their morphine content over the next 24 hours. The fumaric acid component of the extended-release system of Avinza limits the daily dose to a maximum of 1600 mg because of the potential for renal toxicity from high doses of fumaric acid. Avinza is a once-daily, extended-release oral morphine preparation. The controlled-release formulation utilizes SODAS (Spheroidal Oral Drug Absorption System) technology. This multiparticulate product is designed to provide a rapid onset of action together with a sustained therapeutic effect over 24 hours. Avinza is available in 30-, 60-, 90-, and 120-mg capsules. The capsule can be opened and the entire bead content sprinkled on a small amount of applesauce or put down a feeding tube. The beads should not be chewed or crushed. Within the GI tract, due to the permeability of the ammoniomethacrylate copolymers of the beads, fluid enters the beads and solubilizes the drug. This is mediated by fumaric acid, which acts as an osmotic agent and a local pH modifier. The resultant solution then diffuses out in a predetermined manner which prolongs the in vivo dissolution and absorption phases. It has a pharmacokinetic profile that exhibits less peak-to-trough fluctuation (%FI) in plasma concentration while providing analgesia statistically identical to that produced by MS Contin (CR morphine sulfate), OxyContin (oxycodone HCl controlled-release) and six doses of oral morphine sulfate administered every 4 hours. Compared to twice-daily controlled-release morphine, Avinza had a 19% lower maximum concentration (C_{max}), a 66% higher minimum concentration (C_{min}), and a 44% lower peak-to-trough fluctuation over the 24-hour period. In addition, Avinza maintained concentrations above 50% and 75% of the C_{max} longer than controlled-release morphine.[104] In 2005, the Food and Drug Administration (FDA) issued a black box warning regarding alcohol use with Avinza suggesting that alcohol may cause dose-dumping.

Although some clinicians advocate the use of CR morphine when initiating morphine therapy in cancer patients, others suggest the best approach is to start treatment with an immediate-release preparation because dosage can be modified every 4 hours according to patients' needs.[78] Once the effective dosage is determined, it can be converted to a longer-acting preparation with the use of a short-acting opioid for breakthrough pain. De Conno et al.[105] reported on the use of immediate-release morphine (5 or 10 mg initial doses) given every 4 hours with a double dose given at bedtime and uptitrated according to response resulted in adequate pain control in 75% of 159 cancer patients during the first 5 days of treatment. Overall, 50% and 75% of patients achieved pain control within 8 and 24 hours after starting immediate-release morphine, respectively. The most commonly reported adverse events were somnolence (24%), constipation (22%), vomiting (13%), nausea (10%), and confusion (7%). The use of a double dose of IR morphine at bedtime instead of single doses repeated every 4 hours throughout the night has been recommended by EAPC.[78] However, Dale et al.[106] failed to find a significant difference between the two regimens, in terms of pain control.

The intracellular protein β-arrestin$_2$ appears to be an important regulator of MOR desensitization. In β-arrestin$_2$ knockout mice, morphine analgesia was increased and prolonged.[107] Genetic variation in β-arrestin$_2$ is associated with the need to switch from morphine to an alternative opioid, although variation in genes involved in MOR signaling may influence the clinical response to morphine in cancer patients.[108] Catechol-o-methyltransferase (COMT) inactivates dopamine, epinephrine, and norepinephrine in the nervous system. A common functional polymorphism (Val158Met) leads to a three- to fourfold variation in the COMT enzyme activity. The Val158Met polymorphism affects pain perception, and subjects with the Met/Met genotype have the most pronounced response to experimental pain. Genetic variation in the COMT gene may contribute to variability in the efficacy of morphine in cancer pain treatment.[109]

When we select morphine as the opioid of choice for the treatment of tumor pain, we usually use a long-acting preparation for baseline pain control. Our preference is to use Avinza because of its exceptional duration of action. We commonly use a short-acting, immediate release opioid for the control of breakthrough pain; in most instances, this will be morphine sulfate, immediate release. Our standard dose for breakthrough medication is up to 10% of the 24-hour long-acting dose. Breakthrough medication dose intervals are based on the known duration of action of the drug (typically every 3 to 4 hours). The long-acting medication dose is first adjusted to control the background pain. Once this is satisfactorily controlled, breakthrough medication is adjusted proportionally.

OXYCODONE

Oxycodone is a semisynthetic opioid that is a derivative of the opium alkaloid thebaine. It has been in use for over 80 years, mainly as the hydrochloride or terephthalate salt. Oxycodone has a lipid solubility similar to morphine.[110] Oxycodone is a MOR-specific ligand with clear agonist properties. The μ-opioid receptor binding affinity of oxycodone is less than that of morphine or methadone.[111] Oxycodone has been suggested to be a κ-opioid receptor agonist.[112] This is not likely, as animal studies have shown that oxycodone and oxymorphone analgesia are fully antagonized by the μ-opioid receptor antagonist naloxone, whereas there was no antagonistic effect of the κ-opioid receptor antagonist norbinaltorphimine.[113]

Oxymorphone, the active metabolite of oxycodone that accounts for approximately 11% of the oxycodone metabolized, has a significantly higher MOR affinity.[114] Kalso et al. suggested that the analgesic effect of oxycodone was due to the presence of pharmacologically active metabolites in circulation.[115] Oxymorphone, although possessing analgesic activity, is present in the plasma only in low concentrations. The role of metabolites in the analgesic effects of oxycodone was investigated in healthy volunteers.[114] The central opioid effects of oxycodone could be explained by the pharmacokinetic-pharmacodynamic of the parent drug alone. Although the potent active metabolite noroxymorphone was present at relatively high concentrations in the circulation, it did not appear to penetrate the blood brain barrier to a significant extent. Furthermore, other metabolites either demonstrated low potency or were present in circulation at very low levels. The main known metabolic pathways of oxycodone are through O-demethylation to oxymorphone and via N-demethylation to noroxycodone. Noroxycodone is a considerably weaker analgesic than oxycodone and does not appear to contribute to the analgesic effect of oxycodone.

The conversion of oxycodone to oxymorphone, as well as the conversion of noroxycodone to noroxymorphone is catalyzed by CYP2D6. The contribution of oxymorphone to the analgesic effect is controversial. Recently, Zwisler et al.[116] suggested that oxycodone analgesia was dependent on both oxycodone and oxymorphone. In a human experimental model, differences in pain detection and tolerance thresholds were demonstrated between CYP2D6 poor metabolizers and extensive metabolizers with oxycodone administration. For single sural nerve stimulation, there was a less pronounced increase in thresholds on oxycodone in pain detection (9% vs. 20%, $P = .02$, a difference of 11%; 95% confidence interval [CI]: 2%–20%) and pain tolerance thresholds (15% vs. 26%, $P = .037$, a difference of 10%; CI: 1%–20%) for poor metabolizers compared with extensive metabolizers. In the cold pressor test, there was less reduction in pain AUC on oxycodone for poor metabolizers compared with extensive metabolizers (14% vs. 26%, $P = .012$, a difference of 12%; CI: 3%–22%).

Oxycodone and its metabolites are excreted primarily via the kidney and elimination is impaired by renal failure. Patients with renal dysfunction (creatinine clearance <60 mL/min) show peak plasma oxycodone and noroxycodone concentrations 50% and 20% higher, respectively, and AUC values for oxycodone, noroxycodone, and oxymorphone 60%, 50%, and 40% higher than normal subjects, respectively.[117] Oxycodone is well absorbed, when orally administered. Approximately 60% of an oral dose (range: 50% to 87%) is bioavailable. With the controlled-release oxycodone tablets, 38% of the available dose is rapidly absorbed with a mean half-life of 37 minutes, providing a fast onset of pain relief, within 1 hour.[118] Pharmacologic effects of oxycodone include anxiolysis, euphoria, feelings of relaxation, respiratory depression, constipation, miosis, and cough suppression, as well as pain relief. Common side effects associated with oxycodone (OxyContin or oxycodone IR) are constipation (23%), nausea (23%), somnolence (23%), dizziness (13%), pruritus (13%), vomiting (12%), dry mouth (6%), and sweating (5%).

After oral administration, oxycodone is rapidly absorbed to produce an initial peak plasma oxycodone in about 2 hours.[115,119] Once peak plasma concentrations are reached, oxycodone concentrations decline, rapidly, with an apparent terminal half-life ranging from 3.0 to 5.7 hours.[119–120] The rapid absorption and quick elimination after oral administration of oxycodone (bioavailability of oxycodone is >60%), mandates frequent dosing to maintain plasma concentrations within the therapeutic analgesic range. The elimination half-life of CR oxycodone is 4.5 hours compared to 3.2 hours for IR oxycodone. Given the shortness of its half-life of elimination, steady-state of plasma concentrations is achieved within 24 to 36 hours of initiation of dosing with oxycodone CR. The higher oral-intravenous ratio of oxycodone (0.7) compared with that of morphine (0.31) reflects the greater oral bioavailability of oxycodone compared to morphine.[121]

Oxycodone was first introduced in the United States in fixed combination with acetaminophen, acetylsalicylic acid, or with nonsteroidal anti-inflammatory drugs (NSAIDs). It is now also available as a single agent in CR and IR formulations. CR oxycodone exhibits a biphasic absorption pattern with two apparent absorption half-times of 0.6 and 6.9 hours. Thirty-eight percent of the available dose is rapidly absorbed, with a mean half-life of 37 minutes, providing onset of analgesia within 1 hour.[118] The relative oral bioavailability of OxyContin to IR oral dosage forms is 100%. OxyContin administered per rectum produces an area under the curve (AUC) 39% greater and a C_{max} 9% higher than tablets administered by mouth, suggesting an increased risk of adverse events with rectal administration.

In the treatment of cancer-related pain, the oral requirement for oxycodone is less than morphine, but oxycodone is less potent intravenously.[115,121] According to Beaver et al.,[122–123] twice the amount of oxycodone in milligrams is required orally than intramuscularly for equianalgesia; intramuscular oxycodone is two thirds as potent as intramuscular morphine. IR oxycodone is well-tolerated in steady-state pharmacodynamic studies.[120–121,124] Kalso and Vainio[121] utilized oxycodone hydrochloride and morphine in a double-blind crossover study of 20 patients who were experiencing severe cancer pain. No major differences in the side effects between the two opioids were observed, although morphine led to more nausea than oxycodone and hallucinations occurred only during morphine treatment. Maddocks et al.[125] stated that morphine-induced delirium in cancer patients was ameliorated when they were changed to oxycodone.

OxyContin, a CR preparation of oxycodone, is now available in strengths of 10, 15, 20, 30, 40, 60, and 80 mg. Mandema et al.[118] showed that the pharmacokinetics of the CR dosage form permitted 12-hourly dosing. Oxycontin absorption is characterized by a rapid initial component ($t_{1/2}$abs = 37 min) accounting for 38% of the available dose and a slower component ($t_{1/2}$abs = 6.2 hours) accounting for 62% of the available dose.

Steady-state pharmacodynamic profiles of Oxycontin and MS Contin were compared in 27 patients with chronic cancer pain in a double-blind, randomized, crossover design.[126] When oxycodone was given initially, the total opioid consumption ratio of oxycodone to morphine was 2:3; when given after morphine, it was 3:4. Patients reported similar adverse experiences but significantly more vomiting occurred with morphine, and constipation was more common with oxycodone. The two opioids provided comparable pain relief in this study. Reid et al.[127] evaluated the efficacy and tolerability of oxycodone in cancer-related pain in a systematic review of randomized controlled trials. The authors found no clinically important differences between the analgesic efficacy and the adverse effect profile of oxycodone compared with morphine. In essence, the efficacy and tolerability of oxycodone was similar to morphine, supporting its use as an opioid for cancer-related pain.

We use oxycodone routinely in the management of pain in the cancer patient. It is usually well tolerated and easy to titrate. The availability of a wide variety of dosing formats (in both tablet and liquid) facilitates the use of this medication. However, we are concerned about the relatively large immediate dose available in the CR formulation (30%) and its euphoric effects. This may be problematic in patients who are at risk to abuse opioid medications.

OXYMORPHONE

Oxymorphone is a semisynthetic μ-opioid agonist that has been available in parenteral form since 1959. It is a pyridine-ring unsubstituted pyridomorphinan. Structurally, oxymorphone is more closely related to hydromorphone. It is available as a hydrochloride salt. It has a greater analgesic potency than morphine. It is available as parenteral injection, suppository and oral formulations (Table 19.4).

TABLE 19.4

FORMULATIONS OF OXYMORPHONE

Route	Formulation	Dose/concentration
Oral	Immediate-release tablet	5 mg, 10 mg
Oral	Extended-release tablet	5 mg, 7.5 mg, 10 mg, 15 mg, 20 mg, 30 mg, and 40 mg
Parenteral	Ampoules	1 mg/mL
Rectal	Suppository	5 mg

The antinociceptive effects of oxymorphone are mediated predominantly through μ- and δ-receptors.[128] The oral bioavailability of oxymorphone is approximately 10%. The half-life is influenced by the route of administration. The recommended dosing has been every 6 hours, which is longer than most IR opioids. Steady-state conditions are achieved after 3 to 4 days. Oxymorphone is subject to hepatic first-pass effects and is renally excreted. Oxymorphone undergoes extensive hepatic metabolism via conjugation with glucuronic acid to create oxymorphone 3-glucuronide, and the keto group is reduced to form 6-OH-oxymorphone. Hale et al.[129] found a 2:1 dose ratio for oxycodone (CR) relative with oxymorphone (ER). Oxymorphone IR reaches T_{max} at 0.5 hrs after single doses (5, 10, or 20 mg) with a terminal elimination half-life of approximately 7.3 to 9.4 hours in healthy volunteers.[130] Ingestion of food along with oxymorphone increases the C_{max} by 38% to 50% and it may be advisable to take the drug on an empty stomach. Oxymorphone ER is a tablet formulation that utilizes the proprietary TIMERx technology (Penwest Pharm) which allows 12-hour dosing. This CR technology inserts the opioid into an agglomerated hydrophilic matrix which releases the drug (as water penetrates the matrix) to sustain plasma levels during the 12-hour dosing interval. The elimination half-life of oxymorphone ER is similar to the half-life of oxymorphone IR. Steady-state conditions were achieved after 3 days of 12-hour dosing and T_{max} occurred at 1.5 to 3.5 hours.[130] Consumption of alcohol with oxymorphone ER may increase release of oxymorphone by 31%. The absolute oral bioavailability is approximately 10% suggesting that patients may be switched from parenteral to oral oxymorphone by giving 10 times the parenteral doses in divided doses. Oxymorphone should be considered a more potent opioid than morphine with no reported CYP450 system interactions[131] and an otherwise similar profile to that of other available opioids. As with other opioids, renal and hepatic impairment require monitoring and dose adjustment.

Sloan et al.[132] compared oxymorphone ER and oxycodone CR in patients (N = 86) with moderate to severe cancer pain. Patients were first stabilized for 3 days or longer on morphine CR or oxycodone CR. Those who attained stable pain relief for at least 3 days (three or fewer rescue doses of opioid per day) entered the first 7-day treatment period (period 1) at the stabilized dose of the titrated medication with no dosage adjustments. All patients who were treated for 7 days at their stabilized dose of either morphine CR or oxycodone CR were then crossed over to oxymorphone ER at an estimated equianalgesic dosage and treated for an additional 7 days (period 2). During periods 1 and 2, the oral IR formulation of the study medication was available as rescue medication. Each dose of rescue medication was approximately 10% of the total daily dose of scheduled medication. Similar daily pain intensity scores during the last 2 days of the initial treatment phase (morphine CR or oxycodone CR) compared with those during the last 2 days of the oxymorphone ER treatment phase indicate that equivalent analgesia was achieved after patients had been rotated to oxymorphone ER. This also suggests that the long-acting formulation can maintain drug levels in a stable fashion. Patients taking oxymorphone ER needed less breakthrough medication than patients taking morphine CR. The tolerability/safety profiles (eg, nausea, drowsiness, and somnolence) were similar between the two drugs. There were no significant differences in daily pain intensity scores between oxymorphone ER and either morphine or oxycodone. Gabrail et al.[133] noted that 47 adult patients with cancer who were taking oxycodone CR were readily converted to oxymorphone ER and required half the milligram dose to stabilize their pain. Within 72 hours, most patients achieved a stable dose that provided adequate relief with similar opioid adverse events.

We have found oxymorphone to be a useful drug in the oncology population. The drug is generally well tolerated in our patient population. It has a similar pharmacokinetic profile to other CR opioids such as MS Contin and OxyContin, but it does not have the immediate-release component associated with latter.

HYDROMORPHONE

Hydromorphone (Dilaudid) is a short-half-life opioid that is versatile because of its many routes of administration. Hydromorphone is a semisynthetic opioid agonist and is a hydrogenated ketone analogue of morphine. It was synthesized in Germany in 1921 and introduced into clinical medicine in 1926. It is commercially available in most countries as the hydrochloride salt. Absorption of oral hydromorphone is mainly from the upper small intestine. Onset of action is within 30 minutes and the duration of action is approximately 4 hours. Bioavailability is low owing to extensive presystemic liver elimination. The mean proportion of the oral dose absorbed is 62 ± 33%, but variability is wide.[134] Low oral bioavailability and interindividual variation determine the oral–parenteral relative milligram potency ratio, which is 5:1 with repeated administration.[134-135] Hydromorphone is metabolized in the liver and undergoes conjugation to H3G. Hydromorphone also undergoes reduction to dihydromorphine and dihydroisomorphine. H3G can produce dose-dependent behavioral excitation if it crosses the blood brain barrier.[70] In renal failure the mean ratio of H3G to hydromorphone may increase to 100:1, perhaps producing neuropsychological effects including cognitive impairment.[63,136]

The short elimination half-life of hydromorphone requires at least q4hr administration of the drug to maintain adequate plasma levels. Equianalgesic dose equivalence of hydromorphone to morphine is approximately 1:5. Quigley[137] concluded that hydromorphone was a potent analgesic, as predicted for a μ-opioid receptor agonist and its efficacy was dose related. The adverse effect profile of hydromorphone was also predictable and similar to other μ-opioid agonists. Hydromorphone has no clinical superiority over other opioid analgesics. An ER form called Palladone was available for a short time in the United States before being voluntarily withdrawn from the market when an FDA advisory released in July 2005 warned of a high overdose potential if taken with alcohol ("dose dumping").

Oral hydromorphone use in our patient population is limited because of the current unavailability of a long-acting oral preparation. We do use it in the management of breakthrough pain.

METHADONE

Methadone is a synthetic opioid and is a phenylheptylamine structure. It is a potent μ- and δ-opioid receptor agonist. In animal studies, it also has antagonist activity at N-methyl-D-aspartic acid (NMDA) receptors, resulting in some interest in the use of this drug for various neuropathic pain syndromes.[138]

Methadone is an attractive alternative opioid for the management of cancer pain because of its analgesic efficacy, good oral bioavailability, and lack of known neuroactive metabolites. Unfortunately, the substitution of methadone for another opioid is not simple. Clinically, methadone has large interindividual pharmacokinetic variability, a potential for delayed toxicity and a widely varying dose ratio when switching from different opioids. Methadone is available as the lipophilic hydrochloride powder that can be used for the preparation of oral, rectal, and parenteral solutions and is available commercially in a variety of preparations. It is commonly available as a racemic mixture of two isomers, levorotatory (L) methadone and dextrorotatory (D) methadone, although pure L-methadone is available in some countries. Clinical effects of the racemic mixture are pain relief, meiosis, respiratory depression, antidiuresis and suppression of the abstinence syndrome in opioid addicts. L-methadone is the much more potent isomer in man and is believed to be almost entirely responsible for the analgesic properties.

Methadone is well absorbed by all routes. Oral administration is followed by rapid gastrointestinal absorption with measurable plasma levels at 30 minutes. Methadone is rapidly absorbed from the stomach, with little absorption occurring beyond the pylorus.[139] The peak plasma levels after an oral dose occur at four hours and begin to decline 24 hours after dosing. The analgesic effect of an oral dose begins within 30 to 60 minutes and generally lasts for 4 to 6 hours.[140] Oral bioavailability is high, generally more than 85%. The recommended dose to be given parenterally is between 50% and 80% of the oral dose.[141] Significant interindividual variation in half-life has been observed in practice, with an average half-life of approximately 24 hours but a range of 13 to 100 hours[141–142] (Table 19.5). This has significant clinical implications with such variability at steady state dosing and often results in the accumulation of methadone in tissues with

TABLE 19.5

KEY PHARMACOKINETIC PARAMETERS FOR METHADONE

Parameter	Value	Range
Bioavailability	70% to 80%	36% to 100%
Tmax	2.5 to 4 hours	1 to 5 hours
Vdβ	4.0 L/kg	1.9 to 8.0 L/kg
Protein Binding	87%	81%–97%
Half-life	20 to 35 hours	5 to 130 hours

(With permission from Liu M, Wittbrodt E. Low-dose oral naloxone reverses opioid-induced constipation and analgesia. *J Pain Symptom Manage.* 2002;23:48–53.)

chronic administration. This can lead to significant toxicity. Methadone is metabolized almost exclusively by the liver by type I CYP450 group of enzymes. Elimination of methadone is mediated by hepatic oxidative biotransformation, renal N-demethylation, and urinary and fecal clearance. Methadone is predominantly excreted in the feces. It does not accumulate in renal failure and does not appreciably filter during hemodialysis. Chronic administration results in increased metabolite to methadone ratios, suggesting that autoinduction of hepatic microsomal enzymes does occur. Renal impairment is not thought to impair clearance.[143]

Methadone has several advantages, including excellent oral and rectal absorption (oral bioavailability varies from 41% to 99%), no known active metabolites, high potency, high lipid solubility, low cost, and longer administration intervals. It may also offer enhanced pain relief due to incomplete cross-tolerance with other μ-opioid receptor agonist drugs.[144–147]

The potency of methadone is much greater than previously recognized, especially with repeated-dose administration.[146–149] Standard equianalgesic tables underestimate methadone versus hydromorphone potency.[150] This mandates a highly individualized and cautious approach when rotating patients with cancer pain from any other opioid to methadone. At the initiation of treatment, repeated doses of methadone at fixed intervals may lead to its accumulation and overdose effects. This has raised concerns about its use in cancer pain, particularly in situations that require rapid dose escalation.[151]

There are large interindividual variations in methadone pharmacokinetics with rapid and extensive distribution phases ($t_{1/2}\alpha$ = 2 to 3 hours; $t_{1/2}\beta$ = 15 to 60 hours). Considerably longer elimination half-lives, even extending to 120 hours, have been reported.[152] Relatively high daily doses of methadone (40 to 50 mg/day) have been used in patients with chronic renal disease.[143]

Concomitant administration of CYP3A4 inducers will increase methadone metabolism, potentially causing a reduction in methadone plasma concentrations. This may result in the need for larger doses of methadone during the period of interaction. In addition, doses of methadone may need to be reduced when a CYP3A4 inducer is discontinued. Known inducers of CYP3A4 include rifampin, rifabutin, carbamazepine, phenytoin, phenobarbital, and abacavir. The commonly used dietary supplement for depression, St. John's wort, has also been shown to lower the plasma concentrations of methadone.[153] Many methadone-related deaths may be caused by drug interactions rather than administration of methadone alone.[154] Drugs that potentially interact with methadone include inhibitors of CYP3A4 and CYP2D6. Drugs that inhibit CYP3A4 include fluconazole, fluvoxamine, fluoxetine, paroxetine, HIV-1 protease inhibitors, and likely erythromycin and ketoconazole. In addition to CYP3A4 inhibitors affecting methadone's clearance, methadone itself acts as a CYP3A4 inhibitor and therefore has the potential to interact with other CYP3A4 substrates.[155]

Unexpected deaths have been associated with the use of methadone.[156–157] The presumed mechanism of death in these cases was once thought to be respiratory depression from overdose. However, evidence now suggests that methadone administration is associated with prolongation of QTc interval and cases of torsades de pointes (TdP) ventricular arrhythmia.[158–160] Torsades de pointes is most often caused by drugs that block the rapidly activating component of the delayed rectifier potassium current (Ikr) channels in cardiac myocytes. The human ether-a-go-go related gene (HERG) encodes for a major subunit of the Ikr channel.[161] In vitro studies have revealed that methadone can block the cardiac HERG potassium channel.[158–162] In addition, methadone has negative chronotropic properties[163] and it has been observed that drug-induced TdP is often triggered during periods of bradycardia.[164] Women have a slightly longer QTc interval than men; a prolonged QTc interval may be defined as >450 ms for men and >470 ms for women. Although there is disagreement over the exact risk QTc prolongation confers, measurements over 500 ms significantly increase the risk for torsades de pointes.[165] Additionally, increases in the QTc interval > 40 over baseline also increase this risk.[165–166] Pearson and Woosley[167] reported on adverse events associated with methadone to the FDA MedWatch program from 1969 to 2002 and noted the occurrence of torsades de pointes and QT prolongation to be 0.78% and 0.29%, respectively. The mean dose of methadone was 410 ± 349 mg/day, range 29 to 1680 mg/day. Female gender, interacting medications, hypokalemia, hypomagnesemia, and structural heart disease were identified as potential risk factors. Most adverse events required hospitalization or resulted in prolonged hospitalization; 8% were fatal. Krantz et al.[168] provided cardiac safety consensus recommendations for physicians prescribing methadone (Table 19.6). Electrocardiograph (ECG) screening may be performed on an individual basis in patients receiving methadone with multiple risk factors for QTc prolongation, including a family history of long QTc syndrome or early sudden cardiac death or electrolyte depletion, and on initiation of therapy with a CYP450 inhibitor or other QTc interval-prolonging drug, including cocaine. Moreover, urgent evaluation that includes ECG screening is warranted for patients receiving methadone with unexplained syncope or generalized seizures; if marked QTc interval prolongation is present, torsade de pointes should be suspected and methadone discontinued.

Methadone is actively used as a potent analgesic for cancer pain, with the advantages of a long half-life, lack of known active metabolites, high lipid solubility, good oral

TABLE 19.6

CARDIAC SAFETY RECOMMENDATIONS FOR METHADONE USE

Recommendation 1 (Disclosure)	Clinicians should inform patients of arrhythmia risk when they prescribe methadone.
Recommendation 2 (Clinical History)	Clinicians should ask patients about any history of structural heart disease, arrhythmia, and syncope.
Recommendation 3 (Screening)	Obtain a pretreatment electrocardiogram for all patients to measure the QTc interval and then a follow-up electrocardiogram within 30 days and annually. Additional electrocardiography is recommended if the methadone dosage exceeds 100 mg/day or if patients have unexplained syncope or seizures.
Recommendation 4 (Risk Stratification)	If the QTc interval is greater than 450 ms but less than 500 ms, discuss potential risks and benefits with patients and monitor them more frequently. If the QTc interval exceeds 500 ms, consider discontinuing or reducing the methadone dose, eliminating contributing factors, such as drugs that promote hypokalemia, or using an alternative therapy.
Recommendation 5 (Drug Interactions)	Clinicians should be aware of interactions between methadone and other drugs that possess QT interval-prolonging properties or slow the elimination of methadone.

(Used with permission from Krantz MJ, Martin J, Stimmel B, Mehta D, Haigney MC. QTc interval screening in methadone treatment. *Ann Intern Med Online*. 2009;150(6):387–395. Copyright 2009. Reprinted with permission of American College of Physicians-Journals.)

and rectal bioavailability, low cost, and theoretical benefit over other opioids in the setting of neuropathic pain. Bruera et al.[169] compared the effectiveness and side effects of methadone and morphine as first-line treatment with opioids for cancer pain. During a 4-week period, patients were randomly assigned to receive methadone (7.5 mg orally every 12 hours and 5 mg every 4 hours as needed) or morphine (15 mg sustained release every 12 hours and 5 mg every 4 hours as needed). A total of 103 patients were randomly assigned to treatment (49 in the methadone group and 54 in the morphine group). The groups had similar baseline scores for pain, sedation, nausea, confusion, and constipation. Patients receiving methadone had more opioid-related drop-outs (11 of 49; 22%) than those receiving morphine (three of 54; 6%; $P = .019$). The opioid escalation index at days 14 and 28 was similar between the two groups. More than three fourths of patients in each group reported a 20% or more reduction in pain intensity by day 8. The proportion of patients with a 20% or more improvement in pain at 4 weeks in the methadone group was 0.49 (95% CI: 0.34–0.64) and was similar in the morphine group (0.56; 95% CI: 0.41–0.70). The rates of patient-reported global benefit were nearly identical to the pain response rates and did not differ between the treatment groups. The authors concluded that methadone did not produce superior analgesic efficiency or overall tolerability at 4 weeks compared with morphine as a first-line strong opioid for the treatment of cancer pain. In a Cochrane review, Nicholson[170] concluded that methadone was no more effective than morphine for cancer-related nerve related pain and that methadone had a similar side effect profile, but these side effects may be more apparent with repeated dosing.

As with other potent opioids, caution must be exercised in elderly patients, in patients with encephalopathy or a major organ failure, in those who are difficult to monitor, and in patients who are noncompliant with treatment regimens. In addition, caution is suggested in situations where rapid control of severe pain is required. Substantial interindividual variation in the relationship between changes in plasma concentration and pain relief can occur in patients with chronic pain receiving methadone.[171] Information about interpatient variation in pain perception has led to the concept of individualization of methadone dosing in the management of cancer pain.

We commonly prescribe methadone for the treatment of cancer pain. We use this medication in either a "pain cocktail" or tablet format. We are very cautious in converting to or from this drug with other opioids. We typically do not prescribe this drug to patients who have been noncompliant with opioid instructions. Compared to other opioids commonly used in the management of cancer pain, we believe that methadone is a unique drug that should be used cautiously, particularly by the inexperienced prescriber. The possibility of a life-threatening cardiac arrhythmia with this drug as well as the possibility of drug accumulation in a relatively short time period is particularly concerning. We recommend obtaining an ECG (for QTc measurement) before starting this drug and at yearly intervals thereafter if methadone treatment is continued. We believe that methadone is a useful and probably unique drug in the management of cancer pain. Its role is well established but it clearly has hazards that remain to be accurately defined.

LEVORPHANOL

Although structurally related to morphine, levorphanol has high affinity for a number of receptor subtypes, including both κ1 and κ3.[172] Levorphanol infusions resulted in tolerance to both morphine and levorphanol, whereas morphine infusions selectively produced tolerance to morphine, suggesting that the unidirectional tolerance of morphine may occur because of the selectivity of morphine for μ receptors compared to levorphanol's ability to interact more potently with other receptor subtypes.[173] Levorphanol (levo-3-hydroxy-N-methyl morphinan) should be considered an agonist to μ1-, κ3-, and δ-opioid receptors.[174–175] In addition, it also appears to have NMDA receptor antagonist effects[176] and also a monoamine reuptake inhibitor.[177] Leorphanol is the levoenantiomer of dextromethorphan. Levorphanol has a long half-life (12 to 16 hours), and is available in both oral and parenteral formulations. It is not well absorbed sublingually from the buccal mucosa.[178] Levorphanol is metabolized in the liver to produce a 3-glucuronide metabolite and is renally excreted.[179] Drug concentrations peak 30 minutes after parenteral injection and 1 hour after oral dose.[179] The duration of pain relief ranges from 6 to 15 hours. With repeated dosing, the half-life can be as long as 30 hours.[179] The initial oral dose should be 2 mg and can be repeated every 6 hours. The parenteral dose is approximately one half the oral dose. With repeated dosing, drug accumulation and accidental overdose may occur. Strategies for use of levorphanol are similar to those suggested for methadone. Levorphanol may be considered 4 to 8 times as potent as morphine, but a sliding scale for conversion from morphine to levorphanol has been suggested.[180] To convert oral morphine equivalent doses <100 mg, use a conversion ratio of 12:1; from 100 to 299 mg, a ratio of 15:1; from 300 to 599 mg, a ratio of 20:1; and from 600 to 799 mg, a ratio of 25:1.

We have rarely used this drug for cancer pain. It is often not available in our local pharmacies. We do not see unique advantages to this drug over methadone.

FENTANYL

Fentanyl is a synthetic μ agonist derivative of phenylpiperidine and is a chemical congener of the reversed ester of meperidine. It has a short duration of action: 30 to 60 minutes after a single intravenous bolus of 100 μg, mainly due to its large volume of distribution and redistribution and uptake into fatty tissues. It is characterized by high potency and lipophilicity and is 75 to 100 times more potent than morphine on a molar basis. Transdermal, transmucosal/buccal, and parenteral formulations are available. At steady-state conditions after parenteral administration, half-life is primarily determined by redistribution which results in a short duration of effect. The combination of high potency, low molecular weight, and high lipid solubility makes fentanyl an ideal medication for transdermal administration.[181]

Transdermal Fentanyl

Fentanyl patches have been in use since the early 1990s. The original patch (which is described as a reservoir patch) consists of a backing layer to protect the patch from the environment, a liquid drug reservoir, a membrane which controls the rate of drug transfer, and an adhesive layer to secure the patch to the skin surface. The drug reservoir contains fentanyl (2.5 mg/10 cm^2 of system size) and ethanol (alcohol) [0.1 ml/10 cm^2 system size] gelled with hydroxyethyl cellulose. The surface area of the patch determines the amount of fentanyl released. However, a significant amount of fentanyl remains in a transdermal system after 3 days of continuous use. Adequate policies for patch disposal have not been established.[182] Abuse of reservoir fentanyl patches is not restricted to transdermal application and there are reports of I.V. injection of patch contents[183-184] as well as oral / transmucosal administration,[185-187] rectal insertion,[188] and inhalation.[189] New transdermal-fentanyl systems that have an adhesive matrix but no drug reservoir or rate-controlling membrane are available. D-TRANS Matrix delivery system has fentanyl dissolved in a polyacrylate adhesive to form a drug-in-adhesive layer, which in conjunction with the stratum corneum provides the rate-controlling element. The matrix adheres directly to the skin without adhesive edges or layers. This system compared with established reservoir and matrix fentanyl patches appears to be equivalent in terms of efficacy[190] and bioequivalence[191] in the management of severe cancer-related pain. A generic drug-in-adhesive fentanyl patch was approved for use by the FDA in October 2008. However, some of these patches contain metal in a layer of the patch and the FDA has issued a warning about the risk of a burn if the patch is worn during a magnetic resonance imaging (MRI) scan.

Reservoir transdermal therapeutic system fentanyl (TTS-fentanyl) patches are designed to release drug for up to 3 days at a controlled rate influenced more by the system than the skin. The patches are manufactured such that the amount of drug released is proportionate to the surface area of the patch. In bioavailability studies, 92% of the fentanyl dose delivered from the TTS into the skin reaches the systemic circulation as unchanged fentanyl.[192] After skin penetration, fentanyl is taken up by the cutaneous microcirculation and from there into the general circulation. Appearance of fentanyl in the systemic circulation is influenced not only by skin permeability but also by local blood flow.

After the initial transdermal fentanyl patch application, there is a significant delay before steady-state blood levels are achieved, resulting in prolonged time to adequate pain relief. This lag period can vary from 1 hour to over 30 hours (mean value, 13 hours). After application of the first TTS, the skin absorbs fentanyl, and a fentanyl depot concentrates in the upper skin layers. Thereafter, fentanyl becomes available to the systemic circulation, and it takes several hours latency until clinical fentanyl effects can be observed. The plateau of plasma fentanyl concentration is achieved during the second 12-hour period of the first patch.[193] Half-life values after patch removal vary between 13 and 25 hours.[194-195] After removal, a depot of fentanyl (about 10% of the dose) remains in the stratum corneum, and absorption continues maintaining plasma levels.[196] Solassol et al.[193] investigated the intra- and inter-individual pharmacokinetic variability of fentanyl with TTS delivery in 29 cancer patients. Large patient-to-patient variations in pharmacokinetic parameters occurred, although intraindividual variability was limited. Significant variations in the fraction of fentanyl absorbed from the patch occurred (18% to 100%) with a mean estimated bioavailability of 78%. In a study of 108 cancer patients using TTS-fentanyl, large interindividual variability in the amount of remaining fentanyl in the patches occurred.[197] For 58.1% of patches, absorption was 60% to 84%; for 33.2% of them, it was lower; and for 8.8%, it was higher than this range. The intraindividual variability ranged from 2.8% to 75.1%. The bioavailability of fentanyl was statistically different according to patient age. Patients more than 75 years of age absorbed 50% of the fentanyl during the selected 72-hour period, whereas patients less than 65 years of age absorbed 66%. Moreover, there is a significant difference in the percentage of absorbed fentanyl according to the type of cancer. Absorption was higher in patients with breast or digestive cancer than in those with lung cancer.

Fentanyl release from the reservoir is relatively constant. Drug release is driven by the concentration gradient existing between the saturated solution of drug in the reservoir and the lower concentration in the skin as regulated by the copolymer release membrane and diffusion through layers of the skin. The patch is labeled with a nominal flux which is the average amount of drug delivered in a patient with average skin thickness. Thus, patch application should not occur in regions of thickened skin such as areas of increased callosities.

After sequential 48- or 72-hour applications, patients reach and maintain steady state serum concentrations that are determined by individual variation in skin permeability and body clearance of fentanyl. A number of studies demonstrate that constant serum levels are maintained with the second transdermal system and that fluctuations of serum levels are small after the first 72 hours.[192,195] Application of external heat to a patch increases the rate of fentanyl uptake in the systemic circulation because of increased cutaneous blood flow. It is important to advise patients to avoid exposing the application site to direct external heat sources, such as heating pads, heat lamps, or hot tubs, which may result in serious overdose.[198]

In the treatment of cancer pain, TTS-fentanyl can provide continuous administration of a potent opioid in the absence of needles and expensive drug-infusion pumps. The management of cancer pain with TTS-fentanyl has been the subject of many studies.[199–207] Pharmacokinetic studies indicate a relative steady state 15 to 20 hrs after application of the patch, suggesting the possibility of early titration with TTS-fentanyl at 24 hours intervals.[208–209] The long-term efficiency of TTS-fentanyl was evaluated in 51 cancer patients, most of whom had bone metastases by Donner et al.[200] Patients used TTS-fentanyl for an average of 158 days (range: 15 to 855 days) at a final dose of 233.3 μg/hours (range: 25 to 700 μg/hours). Dose increases were predominantly related to disease progression and not drug tolerance. Insufficient pain relief resulted in discontinuation of fentanyl in 16% of patients. Most patients changed patches every 3 days, but 24% of patients required more frequent changing (varying from 48 to 60 hours). Overall, pain relief was assessed as good throughout the study. Constipation and the need for laxatives occurred less frequently than with previously administered oral morphine.

Payne et al.[205] compared 504 advanced cancer patients who received either TTS-fentanyl or sustained-release oral forms of morphine. The mean dose of fentanyl was 84.4 μg/hours (range: 25 to 400 μg/hours), and the mean dose of morphine per 24 hours was 195 mg (range: 15 to 3000 mg). Although patients who received TTS-fentanyl were more satisfied, pain intensity rating and sleep adequacy were not different. Side effects were less with fentanyl. However, because assessment of side effects was global in nature, the investigators could not distinguish between the frequency or impact of individual, particular side effects. Gourlay reported that open comparative studies against sustained-release formulations of morphine (Ms Contin, Oramorph SR) suggested essentially equivalent effects for pain relief, measures of quality of life, and physical functioning, and adverse effects, except for a lower frequency of constipation or use of laxatives with transdermal fentanyl.[196]

The most common formulation-unique side effects are caused by the adhesive used to attach the systems to the skin, and include erythema, itching, and occasional pustule formation (>1%) with an overall frequency of cutaneous side effects of approximately 10%.[196] It is our opinion that the TTS-fentanyl system is a first-line treatment modality for moderate to severe cancer pain. When appropriately used and titrated, pain control is satisfactory with high levels of patient satisfaction. When compliance with oral medications is a problem, transdermal fentanyl has particular advantages. In addition, TTS is useful for patients who cannot take medications by mouth. We do use this drug delivery system frequently in the treatment of pain from cancer.

Iontophoretic Transdermal Fentanyl

Iontophoresis is a method of transdermal administration of drug in which electrically charged components are propelled through the skin by an external electric field. Delivery requires the creation of an external electrical current from positive and negative terminals in which the intra- and extracellular ions that are present in the dermis complete an electrical loop. The basic principle consists of the placement of two oppositely charged electrodes on the skin. The drug which has to be in ionic form is brought under the active electrode bearing the same charge as the drug. As the ions carry current through the skin barrier, the circuit is completed whereby the charged molecules are repelled from the active electrode into the skin from where they reach the systemic circulation. Because iontophoresis may enable transdermal administration with a rapid achievement of steady state and the ability to regulate drug delivery, this may be of potential benefit for both acute pain and breakthrough pain. Iontophoresis has been approved by the FDA to deliver lidocaine and fentanyl. The IONSY is a self-contained preprogrammed fentanyl iontophoretic transdermal system (ITS) that adheres to the patient's skin and delivers fentanyl from a gel reservoir by iontophoresis. It has been approved by the FDA for use in the treatment of acute postoperative pain in hospitalized patients. The system delivers 40 μg fentanyl per on-demand dose and can deliver up to 6 doses per hour for a total of 80 doses per system. Each dose is delivered over a 10-minute period, during which the system is unresponsive to additional medication requests. The pharmacokinetics of fentanyl ITS vary considerably compared with intravenous fentanyl during the first 10 hours of dosing, which is largely due to differences in absorption.[210] The initial fentanyl dose received iontophoretically is actually 16 μg, with the full 40-μg dose being achieved as a function of time after 10 hours of continued therapy. At this time, the system is primarily indicated for the treatment of inpatient postoperative pain.[8] There are no published trials of the system for cancer-related pain. The device appears somewhat limited for this indication because of the availability of only a one-dose system.

Oral Transmucosal Fentanyl

The FDA has approved the use of transmucosal fentanyl for the management of procedure-associated pain and for the management of breakthrough pain in opioid-tolerant cancer patients. The main clinical application for this preparation is for breakthrough and incident pain in the cancer patient.[211] Oral transmucosal fentanyl citrate (OTFC) units consist of a lozenge with a handle. The original product was manufactured by dissolving fentanyl in a sucrose solution. It is now manufactured in a sugar-free formulation. The lozenge is available with 200, 400, 800, 1200, and 1600 μg per lozenge. The unit dissolves in saliva: some of the fentanyl diffuses across the oral mucosa, and the remainder is swallowed; partial absorption occurs in the stomach and intestine. Patients must be taught to apply the lozenge to the buccal mucosa or under the tongue, smearing avoids first-pass metabolism in the liver whereas swallowing does not. The lozenge is designed to be consumed within 15 minutes. Onset of effect is rapid (5 to 15 min), peak analgesic effect occurs in approximately 25 minutes, and the duration of effect is usually about 120 minutes. One quarter of the available dose is transmucosally absorbed in 15 minutes; an additional one quarter is absorbed through the gastric mucosa during 90 minutes.[212] Unique advantages of OFTC include rapid onset of pain relief, absence of the need to ingest medication by swallowing, relative ease of titration, and simplicity of use. In addition, if office titration of OTFC is used, immediate effect of the drug may be observed and breakthrough dose quickly established. Patients may also be directly observed using this drug, compliance assessed and dose modifications implemented. It is important to realize that the dose of OTFC required to control breakthrough pain is not predicted by the around-the-clock opioid dose.[213] Consequently, each patient should be titrated to a dose that is effective for control of breakthrough pain.

Farrar et al.[214] studied OTFC for breakthrough pain in a double-blind, randomized trial of 130 cancer patients. Patients were started on 200 μg OFTC and titrated to an effective dose for breakthrough pain up to the maximum available dose (1600 μg) over a 2-week period. If patients achieved satisfactory pain relief with OTFC, they moved to a double-blind phase, which was designed as a 10-period crossover. In the 80 patients who completed the study, patients receiving placebo required significantly more additional rescue medication than those treated with active drug (34% vs. 15%). OTFC resulted in significantly larger changes in pain intensity and better pain relief than placebo at all time points (two-tailed $P < 0.0001$). The most frequent opioid-related adverse events reported as possibly related to OTFC were dizziness (17%), nausea (14%), somnolence (8%), constipation (5%), asthenia (5%), confusion (4%), vomiting (3%), and pruritus (3%). OTFC was compared with MSIR for management of breakthrough pain in 134 cancer patients receiving a fixed scheduled opioid regimen in a double-blind, double-dummy, randomized, multiple crossover study.[215] OTFC was more effective than MSIR in treating breakthrough pain in terms of pain intensity, pain relief, and global performance of medication scores. In a Cochrane review, Zeppetella concluded that OTFC was an effective treatment in the management of breakthrough pain.[216]

Buccal Fentanyl

The fentanyl buccal tablet (FBT) incorporates a novel drug delivery platform, OraVescent technology, which employs an effervescence-type reaction to enhance fentanyl absorption through the buccal mucosa and facilitate rapid systemic exposure to the analgesic. Sublingual FBT placement is a viable alternative to buccal placement in patients who may require an alternate administration site.[217] Transient pH changes accompany the effervescence reaction, and increase both the rate of tablet dissolution (at a lower pH) and membrane permeation (at a higher pH) of fentanyl.[218] Darwish et al.[219] compared the relative bioavailability of FBT versus OFTC in a healthy volunteer study and reported a higher C_{max} with a more rapid onset for FBT. In cancer patients with and without oral mucositis, FBT 200 μg had a median T_{max} of 25.0 min (range; 15 to 45 min) in patients with mucositis and 22.5 min (range: 10 to 121 min) in patients without mucositis.[220] Approximately 30% smaller dose of FBT achieved systemic exposures comparable to OTFC.[9]

A single dose of FBT 100 to 800 μg provided clinically significant improvements in pain intensity from 15 to 60 minutes after the dose.[221]

Portenoy et al.[222] in a randomized placebo-controlled study of FBT in patients with cancer pain found that mean measures of the analgesic effect of buccal fentanyl separated from placebo as early as 15 minutes after administration and the extent of separation increased up to and including the 60-minute time point. A clinically significant reduction in pain intensity occurred by 15 minutes in 13% of episodes treated with fentanyl; by 30 minutes, this level of response was observed in 48% of episodes. Pain intensity decreased from a mean of 6.9 at baseline to 4.6 at 30 minutes. Slatkin et al.[223] demonstrated FBT was effective for the management of BTP in opioid-tolerant patients with chronic cancer pain and that the drug had a rapid onset (<10 minutes) of pain relief. Currently, FBT and OTFC are approved by the FDA only for the management of breakthrough pain in cancer patients.

Fentanyl is a well tolerated and effective drug in cancer patients. In our patient population, the patch is a very convenient and effective formulation for relief of chronic pain. However, rapidly progressive tumor-associated pain requiring frequent dose escalation of opioid (24- to 48-hour changes) is problematic. Furthermore, some patients have complained about patch adhesiveness (particularly in patients who are physically very active or who are febrile). Patients with extreme wasting disorders (such as may occur with advanced cancer) may also find drug absorption by this route inadequate. FBT and OFTC preparations are excellent for the management of breakthrough cancer pain and are our drug of choice for this indication.

BUPRENORPHINE

Buprenorphine is a potent, semisynthetic opioid analgesic derived from thebaine. The drug displays the characteristics of an agonist at the μ receptors and antagonist at the κ receptors. Although buprenorphine has shown some pharmacologic effects on δ and κ opioid receptors, the action on the μ receptors appears to be responsible for most of the analgesic effects associated with this compound. Clinically, buprenorphine is a potent opioid at low doses but has a relatively diminished potency at higher doses that is characteristic of a partial opioid agonist.[224] Buprenorphine may precipitate a withdrawal syndrome in those who are opioid tolerant. Buprenorphine slowly dissociates from the μ receptor compared to other opioids, although it only partially or poorly activates the receptor. By contrast with morphine and fentanyl, buprenorphine uniquely upregulates μ receptors.[225] Oral absorption of buprenorphine is only 14% and is due to metabolism by CYP3A4 in the gastrointestinal tract and first-pass hepatic clearance.

Outside of the United States, a transdermal delivery system (TDS) is available.[226] This buprenorphine matrix patch is available in three doses, which release 35, 52.5, and 70 μg/hour, respectively; these rates correspond to daily doses of 0.8, 1.2, and 1.6 mg buprenorphine or approximately 60, 90, and 120 milligrams per day equivalent of oral morphine. A multicenter, open-labeled, uncontrolled, prospective, observational clinical practice study involving 1,223 patients with moderate to severe chronic pain demonstrated that transdermal buprenorphine was effective in alleviating cancer and noncancer pain and was overall well tolerated.[227] These patients also experienced a significant improvement ($P < .001$) in quality of life scores and reported very good to good pain relief ($P < .001$).

Buprenorphine was first marketed in the United States in 1985 as a Schedule V opioid analgesic. Until recently, the only available buprenorphine product in the United States has been a low-dose (0.3 mg/ml) injectable formulation under the brand name, Buprenex. Buprenorphine is intended for the treatment of pain (Buprenex) and opioid addiction (Suboxone and Subutex). We have not used buprenorphine for cancer pain management. The use of Suboxone for drug addiction is discussed in Chapter 20, "Management of the Patient Misusing Medications."

HYDROCODONE

Hydrocodone is a semisynthetic opioid derived from codeine and thebaine and is a Schedule III drug. It is metabolized by CYP P450 2D6 and transformed into another μ agonist, hydromorphone.[228] The usefulness of hydrocodone is limited by its preparation in fixed combinations with nonopioid analgesics (aspirin, acetaminophen, and ibuprofen). Combination hydrocodone has different trademark names, such as Vicodin, Norco, Lortab, Lorcet, and Zydone (containing acetaminophen), Lortab ASA (containing aspirin), and Vicoprofen (containing ibuprofen) with varying strengths of hydrocodone (2.5, 5.0, 7.5, and 10 mg). The strength of the nonopioid component differs in these preparations; it is important not to exceed toxic doses when prescribing these medications for breakthrough pain, particularly when using acetaminophen combinations. Pure hydrocodone tablets or capsules are not available in the United States.

The FDA has approved hydrocodone for use as an antitussive and as an analgesic. Homsi et al.[229] reported that median hydrocodone doses associated with the best response for the treatment of cough in advanced cancer was 10 mg/day (range: 5 to 30 mg/day) and associated side effects (dry mouth, nausea, and drowsiness) were tolerable and mild. Hydrocodone is the most frequently prescribed opioid in the United States with an estimated 130 million prescriptions in 2006, up from approximately 88 million in 2000.[230] The prevalence of hydrocodone use is reported to be 3% among 8th-grade students, 7% in 10th-grade students, and 10% in 12th-grade students.[231] Using data from the 2005 U.S. National Survey on Drug Use and Health on nonprescribed use of pain relievers among adolescents in the United States, Wu et al.[232] noted that approximately one in 10 adolescents aged 12 to 17 years reported nonprescribed use of pain relievers in their lifetime (9.3% in men and 10.3% in women) and the mean age of first nonprescribed use was 13.3 years. Among all nonprescribed users, 52% reported having used hydrocodone products (Vicodin, Lortab, Lorcet, Lorcet Plus, and hydrocodone), 50% had used propoxyphene (Darvocet or Darvon) or codeine (Tylenol with codeine), and 24% had used oxycodone products (OxyContin, Percocet, Percodan, and Tylox).

Rodriquez et al.[233] compared the analgesic efficacy and tolerability of hydrocodone/acetaminophen and tramadol in 118 patients with chronic cancer pain. Hydrocodone/acetaminophen was effective in relieving pain in 56.5% of the patients at the starting dose of 25 mg/2500 mg/day. An additional 14.5% of the patients responded to a double dose, and the remaining 29% of patients did not experience any pain relief from hydrocodone administration. One dose of tramadol at 200 mg/day produced pain relief in 62% of the patients and alleviated pain in another 11% of patients at a dose of 400 mg/day, and the remaining 27% of patients did not experience pain relief from tramadol. There was no difference in terms of analgesic efficacy between the two treatments, although Tramadol produced milder side effects compared to hydrocodone.

We rarely use hydrocodone preparations in the management of cancer pain. This is primarily because of the limitations in dosage imposed by the nonopioid combination and the current lack of a long-acting preparation.

CODEINE/DIHYDROCODEINE

Codeine has been used medicinally since the 1800s as an analgesic and antitussive agent. It is intended mainly for the management of mild to moderate intensity pain, and is prescribed usually in combination with aspirin or acetaminophen. Codeine is a prodrug which acts on μ-opioid receptors via its metabolite morphine, which is formed almost exclusively by the genetically polymorphic enzyme CYP2D6. The plasma half-life and duration of action of codeine are usually in the range of 2 to 4 hours, although there is some variability. Codeine use is limited by the increasing incidence of side effects at doses above 1.5 mg per kg of body weight.[234–235] Codeine is metabolized by CYP2D6 to morphine.[236] Patients with a deficiency of CYP2D6 enzymes or those taking inhibitors of CYP2D6, such as quinidine, cimetidine, or fluoxetine, may not be able to convert codeine into morphine and therefore may get little or no analgesic effect from codeine.[237–239] The presence of polymorphisms in CYP2D6 defines poor versus extensive metabolizers. Extensive metabolizers convert 6% to 9% of administered codeine to morphine, compared with only a trace in poor metabolizers.[240] Consequently, an analgesic response to codeine occurs in extensive metabolizers only, even though both groups are responsive to the effects of morphine itself. Poor metabolizers may experience the side effects, but not the analgesic effects of codeine.[241] Like other opioids, codeine causes a delay of gastric emptying and induces spastic constipation. Mikus et al.[242] demonstrated a delay in orocecal transit time after codeine use in extensive metabolizers of codeine versus poor metabolizers, suggesting that the effect of codeine on GI motility is predominantly mediated by its morphine metabolite.

Dihydrocodeine is an equianalgesic codeine analogue, and is metabolized to dihydromorphine, dihydrocodeine-6-O-, dihydromorphine-3-O- and dihydromorphine-6-O-glucuronide, and nordihydrocodeine. Dihydrocodeine has active metabolites (dihydromorphine and dihydromorphine-6-glucuronide).[243] Dihydromorphine and its 6-O-glucuronide may provide a relevant contribution to the pharmacologic effects of dihydrocodeine.[244] The O-demethylation of dihydrocodeine to dihydromorphine is mediated by CYP2D6, resulting in different metabolic profiles in extensive and poor metabolizers. In the United States, it is available only in combination with acetaminophen or aspirin. Brands available include DHC Plus (16 and 32 mg), Panlor SS (32 mg), ZerLor (32 mg), Panlor DC (16 mg), and Synalgos DC (16 mg). Duration of effect is approximately 6 hours. When taken in higher than normal initial therapeutic doses, dihydrocodeine tends to produce euphoria. For postoperative pain management, a single 30 mg dose of dihydrocodeine was not sufficient to provide adequate pain relief. Statistical superiority of ibuprofen 400 mg over dihydrocodeine (30 mg or 60 mg) was also shown.[245]

We rarely use codeine or dihydrocodeine for cancer pain management. We are concerned about the inability to predict poor metabolizers (and subsequent lack of efficacy) of these drugs.

PROPOXYPHENE (DEXTROPROPOXYPHENE)

Propoxyphene is a synthetic weak opioid introduced into the United States in 1957. Dextropropoxyphene has a similar chemical structure to methadone but it is a weak opioid analgesic with an number needed to treat (NNT) of 7.7.[246] Its affinity for the μ-receptor is less than 10% compared with morphine.[55] Propoxyphene is indicated for the treatment of mild to moderate pain. For postoperative pain management, the combination of dextropropoxyphene 65 mg with acetaminophen 650 mg shows similar efficacy to tramadol 100 mg for single-dose studies but with a lower incidence of adverse effects. Ibuprofen 400 mg has a lower (better) NNT than both dextropropoxyphene 65 mg plus acetaminophen 650 mg and tramadol 100 mg.[246] Dextroproxyphene is most frequently prescribed in combination with acetaminophen or aspirin and is available as the HCl salt napsylate salt. Medications include Darvon, the original propoxyphene hydrochloride product, and Darvocet-N 100, containing propoxyphene napsylate and acetaminophen. Some authors recommend avoiding use of the drug in the elderly because of its complex pharmacokinetics and pharmacodynamics.[247] The elimination half-life of the parent compound is 6 to 12 hrs and 30 to 36 hours for norpropoxyphene.[247] Time to peak effect is 2 to 2.5 hours with onset of analgesic activity in 30 to 60 minutes. Oral bioavailability is 30% to 70%.

The major metabolite of propoxyphene is nordextropropoxyphene, a nonopioid that is renally excreted; however, accumulation of this metabolite may precipitate CNS depression, cardiac depression, and respiratory depression.[97] Nordextropropoxyphene is cardiotoxic and increases the PR interval in animal studies.[248] Norpropoxyphene accumulates in cardiac tissue and may cause cardiac toxicity.[98] Ulens et al.[249] demonstrated that proxyphene and norpropoxyphene showed affinity for HERG cardiac K^+ channels at concentrations similar to those reported in propoxyphene-induced fatalities and that the drug-HERG interaction accounts, at least in part, for the cardiotoxic effects of propoxyphene and norpropoxyphene. Regulators in the United Kingdom in 2005 began a gradual withdrawal of the propoxyphene-and-acetaminophen combination coproxamol from the market, although certain patients are still allowed access to the medication.

We do not use propoxyphene nor do we advocate its use for cancer pain management.

TRAMADOL

Tramadol is a codeine analogue that possesses opioid agonist features and activates the spinal pain inhibitory system. It acts centrally and has a low affinity for μ-opioid receptors (approximately tenfold less than that of codeine and 6000-fold less than that of morphine).[250] Thus, affinity for opioid receptors alone is not sufficient to account for the analgesic action of tramadol. A further mode of tramadol action has been identified as the inhibition of the reuptake of monoamines, such as norepinephrine and serotonin released from nerve endings. Although μ-opioid receptors and monoamine transporters are thought to be the sites of tramadol activity, additional sites probably exist. Several studies have shown that some GPCRs and ligand-gated ion channels are also targets for tramadol.[250] The Gs- and Gi-coupled receptors might also be targets for tramadol.

The second mode of analgesic action of tramadol is its influence on the descending pain inhibitory system. The effects are mainly on two pathways. The first originates from the periaqueductal gray matter in the midbrain and has synapses in the nucleus raphe magnus, from which fibers project to the spinal cord. Serotonin (5HT) is a synaptic transmitter in this pathway. The second main pathway originates from the locus coeruleus in the pons, and also projects to the spinal cord. Norepinephrine is utilized in this pathway, which inhibits nociceptive transmission in the spinal cord via an α-adrenergic mechanism. The periaqueductal gray, the raphe magnus in the medulla oblongata, and the dorsal horns in the spinal cord possess significant amounts of endogenous opioid peptides and opioid receptors. Activation of the descending pain inhibitory system is connected by stimulating interneurones, which inhibit transmission of nociceptive impulses in the synapses in the dorsal horn of the spinal cord by the action of endogenous opioids. The mechanism of the analgesic action of tramadol comprises activation of both descending serotoninergic and noradrenergic pathways.[251]

Tramadol is available in IR and ER preparations. After a single dose of IR, it is rapidly absorbed and reaches C_{max} in approximately 2 hours. The mean bioavailability after a single oral dose is 68% but increases to about 90% to 100% after multiple doses, possibly because of saturation of the liver first-pass effect.[252] The elimination half-life is approximately 5 hours. Tramadol is metabolized by the highly polymorphic enzyme cytochrome P450 (CYP) 2D6. Patients with different CYP2D6 genotypes may respond differently to tramadol in terms of pain relief and adverse events.[253]

The most frequent adverse effects associated with tramadol include dizziness, nausea, constipation, somnolence, and flushing. Respiratory depression does not appear to be a problem with long-term use of tramadol, but some experimental data with the use of high doses of intravenous tramadol (4 mg/kg) in cats resulted in respiratory depression that was reversed with naloxone.[254] In clinical practice, respiratory depression has been observed during cancer pain treatment with tramadol in patients with renal impairment.[255] This was associated with the accumulation of the active metabolite (M1), which has a longer elimination half-life than the parent compound, and mainly acts on μ opioid receptors. Tramadol has been reported to induce dizziness, dry mouth, nausea, constipation, and somnolence with significantly more dropouts compared with placebo.[256-257] There is an increased risk of seizures in patients with a history of epilepsy or receiving drugs which may reduce the seizure threshold. Serotonin syndrome may occur if tramadol is used as an add-on treatment to other serotoninergic medications (particularly SSRIs; serotonin syndrome is discussed further in "Serotonin Syndrome" below). Tramadol should be initiated at low dosages, particularly in the elderly patient (50 mg once daily) and then titrated as tolerated. The effective dosages appear to be in the range of 200 to 400 mg/day.

The analgesic efficacy of tramadol and morphine was compared in 20 cancer patients.[258] Morphine was found to be four times as potent as tramadol. Side effects such as nausea and constipation were less with tramadol, but pain control was less satisfactory. Leppert and Luczak[252] reviewed the role of tramadol in cancer pain management. Tramadol appeared to have a role in reducing opioid requirements when combined with other opioids.[259]

For the treatment of neuropathic pain, there is some interest in the use of tramadol. Tramadol (mean dosage 275 mg/day, up to 400 mg/day) was shown moderately effective only on some measures of spontaneous pain intensity in PHN, with an NNT = 4.8 (CI: 2.6–26.9);[260] in this study, only patients with pain lasting for less than 1 year were included, thus, several patients tended to recover spontaneously during the trial, which accounts for the high rate of placebo response. For patients with painful peripheral neuropathy (diabetic neuropathy being the most common example), tramadol in doses of 200–400 mg/day provided effective relief with an NNT = 3.4 (CI: 2.3–6.4).[257,261]

We believe that patients with cancer pain who are most likely to benefit from tramadol are those with mild-to-moderate pain that has not been relieved by acetaminophen, who cannot tolerate NSAIDs, and who wish to avoid taking, stabilize, or reduce their opioid dose. The role of tramadol in the management of neuropathic pain secondary to cancer or its treatment is unclear at this time. We do use this medication under these circumstances, particularly for the treatment of chemotherapy-induced neuropathy, although we have had limited success. Tramadol is not a primary cancer pain drug in our practice.

PARENTERAL ADMINISTRATION OF OPIOIDS

Intravenous Opioid Therapy

Parenteral routes should be considered for patients who require rapid onset of analgesia, and for highly tolerant patients who require doses that cannot otherwise be conveniently administered.[262] Intravenous opioids allow for rapid control of pain. Ideally, patients with severe, uncontrolled pain who require intravenous therapy should start treatment in a monitored in-patient setting. High doses of intravenous opioids via patient-controlled analgesia (PCA) or by continuous infusion offer a means of rapidly controlling increasing severe pain. Because of high interindividual variation in opioid requirements, one must ascertain previous opioid exposure and consider the patient's tolerance. Flexibility for individual titration and the PCA modality are important considerations for patients requiring intravenous opioid therapy. Once patients begin opioid therapy for tumor pain control, doses should be titrated according to patient comfort or the appearance of intolerable side effects. For severe pain, we employ a minimum lockout interval of 6 minutes. However, for patients with inadequate pain control and minimal opioid-related side effects, we increase incremental doses by 50% every 4 hours. We also order additional nurse-administered loading doses to achieve pain control. When the pain is under control, it is possible to continue therapy safely at home with the aid of a home infusion service.[263–265]

Enting et al.[266] prospectively evaluated 100 patients with unrelieved cancer pain on conventional oral or systemic opioid therapy who were switched to parenteral opioids. Opioids used for parenteral therapy included morphine, fentanyl, and sufentanil. The main objectives were to evaluate the analgesic efficacy and side effects of parenteral opioids selected for uncontrolled cancer pain or intolerable side effects and to estimate the proportion of patients requiring further treatment options, including opioid rotation, spinal analgesia, or a sedation procedure. Patients were evaluated on the second day and again when a clinical decision was made to continue or change parenteral opioid treatment after a median of 6 days. Patients predominantly had lung carcinoma (19%), breast carcinoma (19%), head and neck carcinoma (15%), or colorectal carcinoma (11%). Ninety-eight patients (98%) had progressive disease. The median duration of survival was 45 days (range: 6 to 1152 days). Forty-two patients (42%) had nociceptive pain, and 58 patients (58%) had neuropathic pain. The most prevalent sites of pain were the lower back, pelvis, or lower extremities (29%). In 19 patients, multiple pain sites were present. Mean pain intensity at rest decreased significantly from 6.3 to 4.4 at 48 hours and to 3.4 at the end of treatment. Mean pain intensity during movement decreased significantly from 8.4 to 5.7 at 48 hours and to 4.6 at the end of treatment. Clinically important pain control at rest was seen in 52% of patients at 48 hours, in 71% of patients at the end of treatment; and clinically important pain control during movement was seen in 43% of patients at 48 hours and in 61% of patients at the end of treatment. The proportion of patients with mild pain increased significantly both at rest and during movement. Side effects were present in 78% of patients, and they resolved completely in 32% of patients. The median intravenous morphine equivalent dose increased from 80 mg per day to 135 mg per day at 48 hours and to 201 mg per day at the end of treatment. Results were not different for opioid rotation or for change of route only, nor did the start of antitumor treatment influence the results. In 34% of patients, it was decided to rotate to a second-line parenteral opioid or to start either spinal analgesia or a sedation procedure after a median of 6 days. During follow-up, 18% of patients who were discharged with parenteral opioids (and 6% of all patients) needed a further change of treatment. This study reflects our clinical experience.

Intravenous therapy can employ any of several opioids: morphine, hydromorphone, fentanyl, sufentanil, and methadone. The use of opioids (such as methadone) with properties of NMDA receptor antagonism may improve pain control by attenuating the development of tolerance to morphine.[267] This degree of incomplete cross-tolerance is probably unique to methadone[148] and may stem from isomers of methadone interacting with the NMDA receptor to reverse tolerance, and thereby reduce dose requirements.[268]

Postoperative pain studies comparing opioid-related side effects failed to show a difference between morphine and hydromorphone[269] and morphine, meperidine, and fentanyl.[270] Coda et al.[271] found differences in efficacy and side effects for morphine, hydromorphone, and sufentanil in bone marrow transplantation patients with severe oral mucositis pain. The pain relief achieved in all three opioid groups was nearly equivalent, whereas measures of side effects, especially for the combination of sedation, sleep, and mood disturbances were statistically lower in the morphine group than in hydromorphone or sufentanil groups. Daily opioid consumption patterns showed continual dose escalation during the first week of therapy for all three opioids, coincident with worsening mucositis. Morphine consumption reached a plateau by day 5, whereas hydromorphone and sufentanil consumption continued to rise until days 7 and 9, respectively. Sufentanil dose requirement increased by approximately tenfold compared to morphine and hydromorphone, whose requirements increased only fivefold, suggesting the possibility of development of acute pharmacologic tolerance in some patients with this phenylpiperidine opioid.

Knowledge of intravenous opioid pharmacokinetics and pharmacodynamics informs opioid selection for the management of severe cancer pain. Coda et al.[272] defined the intravenous dose-effect characteristics of hydromorphone. Bolus doses of 10, 20, and 40 μg/kg of hydromorphone in human subject volunteers produced log linear dose-dependent analgesia. Onset of analgesia after an intravenous bolus was rapid, within 5 minutes, and the maximum analgesic effect was seen between 10 and 20 minutes after maximum plasma concentrations with analgesia lasting approximately 2 hours after a bolus injection. Hydromorphone was approximately three to five times as potent as morphine on a milligram basis.[272-273] Peak CNS effects of methadone coincide with peak plasma concentrations, thus corresponding well to the observed early onset of action of 3 to 5 minutes after intravenous administration.[171]

Morphine, on the other hand, has a slower onset of action, probably related to its relatively poorer lipid solubility. Hug et al. administered an I.V. bolus of morphine to dogs and showed that the peak concentration in CSF did not occur for approximately 15 to 30 minutes.[274] Fentanyl, a highly lipophilic opioid, has a rapid analgesic onset and time to peak effect (less than 6 minutes).[275] Intermittent boluses of opioids (such as fentanyl) with rapid onset and early peak effect offer advantages for patients whose predominant pain stems from activity or weight-bearing and occurs intermittently. Patients with constant, severe, intractable cancer pain and large opioid requirements may benefit from the use of intravenous methadone by PCA and continuous infusion. This approach offers some advantages over the more hydrophobic drugs such morphine and hydromorphone. The more rapid peak analgesic effect and longer elimination half-life of methadone foster earlier intense analgesia with prolonged analgesic effect, particularly after patients reach steady state plasma levels with repeat administration.

Systemic opioid therapy has limitations: most commonly, drowsiness and sedation are dose limiting. In such situations, we recommend alternate therapies (eg, neuraxial analgesia). Less frequently, CNS side effects of high-dose opioids will occur. These include hyperexcitability, myoclonus, confusion, and hyperalgesia.[276] Myoclonus, the most common problem for patients receiving high-dose opioid infusion therapy, initially is localized, but it can spread and eventually progress to grand mal seizures. These effects can occur with opioids administered via different routes (oral, parenteral, and neuraxial). The cause of opioid-induced myoclonus is still unknown. Some speculate that the active metabolite of morphine, M3G, may be responsible for the hyperalgesia and myoclonus seen with high-dose morphine therapy.[277] Intravenous hydromorphone in doses >60 mg/day has resulted in hyperalgesia and myoclonus. Doses of I.V. morphine >60 mg/hour have resulted in similar problems. Although treatments including phenobarbital loading and clonazepam have occasionally proved helpful,[278] definitive treatment for myoclonus usually involves either dose reduction and/or a change in opioid.[279] Switching to intravenous methadone therapy may also prove helpful. If these strategies fail, one should consider alternative pain management techniques.[280]

Subcutaneous Opioid Therapy

Continuous subcutaneous infusion of opioids is both an efficacious and safe method to control the chronic pain of the home-bound and hospitalized patient.[265,281–283] Hypothetically, absorption of opioid from the subcutaneous compartment into the systemic circulation should be slow, but it is not, even for morphine.[284] Moulin et al.[285] reported equianalgesic responses in a comparison of I.V. versus subcutaneous infusions of hydromorphone. Breakthrough pain control was equal in both groups and only occasionally did patients experience undue dermal irritation or recurrent infection. Various opioids are suitable for subcutaneous infusion: morphine, hydromorphone, methadone, fentanyl, and sufentanil.

Hydromorphone's solubility, its high bioavailability by continuous subcutaneous infusion (78%),[285] and the availability of a high-concentration preparation (10 mg/mL), make it a good choice for subcutaneous infusion. Parenteral hydromorphone is six times as soluble in aqueous solutions as morphine and five times as potent, allowing for smaller injection or infusion volumes in patients who require parenteral opioids.[286]

Continuous subcutaneous infusions offer a safe, simple, effective alternative to intravenous infusion when patients cannot take medications orally. Moulin et al.[285] compared the safety and efficacy of subcutaneous versus intravenous infusion of hydromorphone in cancer patients. Pain intensity, pain relief, mood, and sedation did not differ between the two techniques. The mean bioavailability of hydromorphone from subcutaneous infusion was 78% of that with intravenous infusion. Simplicity, technical advantages, and cost-effectiveness are clear advantages of continuous subcutaneous opioid infusion into the chest wall or trunk. Paix et al.[287] described the successful substitution of subcutaneous fentanyl and sufentanil for morphine, noting the effective substitution of sufentanil for fentanyl when the patient needs higher doses of a lipophilic opioid. Nelson et al.[288] compared continuous intravenous and subcutaneous morphine for chronic cancer pain and concluded that both routes were equianalgesic for most patients when administered as a continuous infusion. Stuart-Harris et al.[289] studied the pharmacokinetics of morphine after subcutaneous bolus injection and subcutaneous infusion. Although bioequivalence was demonstrated between the subcutaneous bolus and I.V. routes of morphine administration, the bioavailability of morphine after subcutaneous infusion was significantly lower than after I.V. administration. C_{max} (nmol/L) of morphine after I.V. injection was 283 ±74 and did not differ significantly from subcutaneous bolus (262 ±49) but did differ from subcutaneous infusion (46 ±8). T_{max} (h) was 0.08 (0.08 to 0.08) for I.V. versus 0.25 (0.17 to 0.25) for subcutaneous bolus and 4.0 (3.5 to 5.0) for subcutaneous infusion. T_{max} values for I.V. differed significantly for both subcutaneous bolus injection and infusion.

Most patients will require a weekly change of the site of subcutaneous infusion.[282] Our usual initial concentrations of morphine and hydromorphone are 5 mg/mL and 1 mg/mL, respectively, calculated according to the hourly infusion rate. Ideally, the subcutaneous rate should not exceed 2 mL/hours although some have established considerably higher rates (rates of 20 to 80 mL/hours by adding hyaluronidase to the infusion to promote hypodermoclysis)[290]. One might expect a longer time to peak plasma levels after bolus injection with subcutaneous use than with intravenous use and consequently the subcutaneous route requires a longer lockout interval (10 to 15 minutes compared to 6 to 8 minute for the intravenous). PCA doses may equal 25% to 50% of the hourly infusion rate every 10 to 15 minutes as needed. Subcutaneous administration of opioids may prove impractical in patients with generalized edema who develop erythema, soreness, or sterile abscesses with subcutaneous administration, in patients with coagulation disorders, and in patients with very poor peripheral circulation.

We have found that I.V. administration of opioids is superior to the subcutaneous route mainly because of the rapid onset of a bolus dose administered by patient-controlled modalities. Many of our patients have established long-term intravenous access for cancer treatment and this may be used to conveniently administer opioids. We do not routinely use subcutaneous infusions for the management of pain from cancer.

OPIOIDS NOT RECOMMENDED FOR ROUTINE USE IN CANCER PAIN CONTROL

Several opioids are not recommended for the control of moderate to severe cancer pain (Table 19.7), and we never prescribe them for patients with pain due to cancer. These are meperidine, pentazocine, butorphanol, dezocine, nalbuphine, and dextropropoxyphene. Meperidine has a short half-life and its metabolite, normeperidine, is toxic.[291] Normeperidine can produce CNS hyperexcitability, presenting as nervousness to tremors, twitches, multifocal myoclonus, and grand mal seizures. Although excreted by the kidneys, the accumulation of normeperidine may lead to toxicity even with normal renal function. Meperidine also has a potential lethal interaction with monoamine oxidase inhibitors.[292]

Mixed agonist-antagonists such as pentazocine, butorphanol, dezocine, and nalbuphine present other problems. Although these agonist-antagonists are often classified as a κ-receptor agonist and a μ-receptor antagonist, they are more accurately described as a partial agonist at both κ and μ receptors. These agents have a low maximal effi-

TABLE 19.7

OPIOIDS NOT RECOMMENDED FOR CANCER PAIN MANAGEMENT

Drug	Reason
Meperidine	Normeperidine accumulation (increased seizure risk
Pentazocine	Reversal of μ-receptor activity; ceiling effect, may induce fibrous myopathy
Butorphanol	Reversal of μ-receptor activity; ceiling effect; dysphoria
Dezocine	Reversal of μ-receptor activity; ceiling effect
Nalbuphine	Reversal of μ-receptor activity; ceiling effect
Dextropropoxyphene	Nordextropropoxyphene accumulation

cacy and have the potential to reverse μ-receptor analgesia, and even precipitate a physical-withdrawal syndrome when taken by patients already receiving full agonists such as morphine.[12] In addition, agonist-antagonist opioids have a ceiling effect.[12,293]

Propoxyphene 65 mg of hydrochloride, equivalent to 100 mg of napsylate salt, is a poor choice for routine use because of its long half-life and the risk of accumulation of nordextropropoxyphene, a toxic metabolite.[97] It is also considered a weak opioid with a NNT of 7.7. Dextropropoxyphene is renally excreted and accumulation may cause CNS, respiratory, and myocardial depression.[97] Acute toxicity may cause seizures.

LONG-TERM USE OF OPIOIDS

Although cancer prevalence is increasing, new and effective treatments for cancer mean that most patients are living well past 5 years after their diagnosis date, and many are returning to the workforce. The National Cancer Institute (NCI) reported that the survival rate at 5 years has made an extraordinary improvement over the last 20 years.[294] Colon cancer survival has increased by 65% and breast cancer shows 89% improvement. Prostate cancer shows the most improvement of all cancers, with a 100% increase in 5-year survival. As patients live longer with cancer, concern is growing about both the health-related quality of life of those diagnosed with cancer and the quality of care they receive. Cancer care progresses through different stages, including diagnosis, treatment, survivorship, and sometimes end-of-life care. Among the most common symptoms of cancer and treatments for cancer are pain, depression, and fatigue.[295] These symptoms may persist or appear, even after treatment for the cancer ends.

Our strategies for the long-term use of opioids generally follow standard guidelines for chronic pain[296] and require a complete review of the patient's history, both for pain complaints and other issues such as concurrent medical problems, psychosocial status, medication history, cancer case history, and appropriate recent diagnostic testing. A directed physical examination should also be performed. A pain diagnosis and differential diagnosis should be made and key factors influencing the pain complaint should be outlined. Once a diagnosis is made, the prescribing clinician should ask three key questions:

1. Is this patient's pain complaint responsive to opioids?
2. Are opioids indicated for this particular patient?
3. What dose of opioid am I prepared to titrate to?

In general, most tumor-related pain processes (nociceptive and neuropathic) will be opioid responsive and, as such, the decision to use opioids in tumor-related pain will be relatively straightforward. However, in patients whose pain complaint is non–tumor-related and chronic (eg, myofascial in origin), opioids may not be considered the primary treatment modality but may have a limited role in rehabilitation of the pain process. With regards to dose titration, most clinicians do not appear to have problems in prescribing appropriate doses to patents with tumor-related pain processes but may exercise more caution for chronic nonmalignant processes in the cancer patient with pain. Once a determination is made that opioids have a role in pain management, steps in cancer pain management will usually include an individualized use of opioids appropriate for the pain complaint, anticipation and management of opioid-related adverse events, and possible consideration of opioid rotation.[77] It is important to realize that each patient is unique with regard to response to analgesic pharmacotherapy. This, in turn, has led to an increase in the number of opioid agents and formulations available. Various professional societies and governmental and regulatory agencies have developed standards and guidelines for long-term opioid prescription.[10,297–300] These guidelines usually include recommendations for careful, comprehensive assessment of the pain complaint and close monitoring of the response to opioid therapy (Table 19.8). Patients should be educated about their pain complaint and the factors contributing to that complaint. Patients should be told of the reasons for their pain. If the reasons for the patient's pain are unclear, additional testing may be necessary. It is the treating clinician's responsibility to provide a diagnosis to the patient. If the clinician cannot establish a diagnosis, the patient should be informed of this. Monitoring of opioid dose and use is the responsibility of the prescriber. Each prescriber should formulate a plan for ongoing assessment of the patient's compliance with drug prescriptions and related treatment plans. Informed consent implies a process through which a patient arrives at a decision regarding a future course of treatment after obtaining information from the practitioner. Informed consent for the suggested treatment plan should be obtained from the patient and any risks (including long-term opioid-related issues) should be outlined. Appropriate consultation should be sought for problems outside the scope of practice of the treating clinician. This may include help with the treatment of refractory depression or help with drug addiction. Medical records should be meticulously maintained. Additional records from other clinicians involved in the treatment of the patient should be obtained and documented. Ideally, there should only be one prescriber for pain medications, and, where possible, one pharmacy where these drugs are obtained.

Reluctance to prescribe opioids may occur because of physician concerns of regulatory scrutiny as well as the potential for patient dependence, misuse, and abuse.

TABLE 19.8

STANDARDS FOR LONG-TERM OPIOID PRESCRIPTION

Comprehensive patient evaluation
Diagnosis and differential diagnosis for pain complaint and factors contributing to pain complaint
Patient education
Informed consent and written treatment plan
Monitoring
Consultation
Accurate medical record keeping
Compliance with controlled substance laws and regulations

Given the ramifications of improper opioid use, it is important that the physician and patient reach an understanding regarding the specific circumstance for which opioids are prescribed. An opioid contract or agreement has been recommended by some pain specialists and primary care physicians as a key component in outlining instructions and expectations for appropriate opioid use and patients' rights and responsibilities.[301–304] Some professional societies, such as the American Academy of Pain Medicine, have published prototype opioid contracts. These contracts usually contain formal and explicit written agreements between physicians and patients. Although published individual contracts differ, content characteristics typically include terms of treatment, patient responsibilities, emergency issues, and legal considerations. There is some controversy about the value of opioid contracts in certain patient populations, the nature of the information included, and their ability to accomplish positive outcomes. Some authors argue that the challenge in deciding about implementing opioid contracts in clinical practice relates to the multiplicity of potential objectives they might serve, to a lack of empirical evidence regarding their effectiveness, and to ethical concerns over their implementation.[302]

Some authors also recommend the use of routine urine toxicology testing in the management of patients on chronic opioid therapy.[305] It is believed that urine testing is a practical, inexpensive, and valuable tool in general medical practice for patient guidance, treatment planning, and dosage determination in opioid-treated chronic pain patients.[306] In addition, random urine toxicology screens among patients prescribed opioids for pain reveal a high incidence of abnormal findings.[307] Abnormal findings include the absence of a prescribed opioid, the presence of an additional nonprescribed controlled substance, and the detection of an illicit substance.

The proper role of opioid contracts in the management of patients with chronic pain to whom the long-term administration of opioids is contemplated or employed is not currently well defined. In general, we do not endorse the routine use of an opioid contract or agreement in cancer pain. We believe that the use of these written contracts adds stigma to a form of therapy which is already fraught with misunderstanding and prejudice. High-quality patient care requires ongoing open communication between patients and clinicians and a clear understanding of the goals and requirements of treatment. Although a formal written contract may accomplish these goals, this may not be desirable or necessarily appropriate for all patients. Many patients whom we encounter have fears and concerns surrounding opioid use and we believe the introduction of a formal contract early in our encounter with these patients may jeopardize our relationship with the patient and result in additional misunderstanding in the role of opioid in their care. Clinicians should determine on a case-by-case basis how to optimally provide documentation to treat a patient with long-term opioids; this may or may not involve an opioid contract. Finally, we do not advocate routine urine toxicology screening in patients receiving long-term opioid therapy. However, certain aberrant drug behaviors may be predictive of substance abuse disorders in patients receiving opioids for chronic pain.[308] Such behaviors include oversedation, feeling intoxicated, early refills, and increasing dosage without approval; these may be useful as screening issues in predicting patients at greatest risk for a current substance use disorder. Strong predictors for opioid misuse by chronic pain patients include a personal history of illicit drug and alcohol abuse but no one procedure or set of predictor variables is sufficient to identify patients at risk.[309] We do not hesitate to order urine toxicology when we believe this test to be warranted by the patient's behavior. However, we always explain to the patient what we will do with the results when we discuss ordering this test. In ordering a urine toxicology, we always ask for gas chromatography, mass spectrometry analysis to be included with the test.

OPIOID-RELATED SIDE EFFECTS

The side effects or toxicities associated with opioids can significantly distress the patient and impair normal functioning. Effective opioid intervention requires careful dose titration targeted at an optimal pain relief to side effect ratio. Table 19.9 lists the major side effects and indicates the frequency with which they occur. Most patients will report more than one side effect, although a few will report only constipation.

The distress imposed by one or more side effects typically determines the upper limit or the rate of dose titration. Patients with similar pain problems differ markedly in side effect burden even when they receive similar dosages of a single opioid drug. For a given patient, a specific drug may cause a heavy side effect burden, whereas an alternative drug delivered at equianalgesic concentrations may produce a mild side effect burden. For this reason, adept prescribers often ask about a patient's previous experiences with opioid drugs in an attempt to avoid trial-and-error drug selection.

Because marked interindividual differences exist among patients, the best predictor of patient response to an opioid is the patient's past experience with that drug.

TABLE 19.9

OPIOID-RELATED SIDE EFFECTS

Side Effect	Frequency with Oral Long-Acting Opioids	Does Symptom Diminish with Tolerance?
Constipation	Very common	No
Sedation	Common	Yes
Nausea	Common	Yes
Cognitive impairment	Occasional	Yes
Pruritus	Occasional	Yes
Dysphoria	Occasional	Yes
Hypnogogic imagery	Rare	Yes
Myoclonus	Rare with oral route	No
Respiratory depression	Very rare	Yes

Although the side effect burden depends in part on the idiosyncratic fit between the patient and the drug administered, it depends primarily on dose magnitude and the rate of dose increase. With increments in drug dosage or rapid rates of titration, the probability of a particular side effect occurring typically increases and the severity of any existing side effect increases as well.

The severity of the side effect burden also depends on the duration of drug use. Fortunately, patients develop tolerance to most side effects more rapidly than to pain relief.[310] Consequently, the longer a patient uses an opioid, the fewer the side effects and the less severe persisting side effects become.

Assessment and treatment of side effects are basic aspects of opioid therapy. When side effects are strong and poorly controlled, patients are likely to report poor pain relief as well. Patients tend to take opioids on an "as-needed" rather than an "around-the-clock" basis. Often, they will use the drug only when the pain becomes unbearable. Moreover, intermittent drug use prevents patients from developing tolerance to side effects, so bothersome side effects never abate. Side effects are also a significant source of discomfort and suffering in their own right. The extremely nauseated patient feels miserable, tends to avoid comforting social interactions, and cannot engage in productive activity. The cognitively impaired patient cannot cope effectively with the simple mental demands of everyday life and becomes increasingly dependent on others. In these and other ways, untreated side effects compromise the quality of life in patients using opioids for pain relief.

Opioid-related side effects occur because of opioid receptor pharmacodynamics and/or the production of toxic metabolites. Activation of μ2-receptors appears to cause certain side effects, such as sedation and respiratory depression, but other side effects are linked to other receptor types or subtypes.[311] Evidence exists that κ-receptor agonism contributes to dysphoria as well as to pain relief.[293] σ-receptor agonism produces purely negative effects: dysphoria, depersonalization, and psychotomimetic experiences such as hypnogogic imagery.[312] The σ-receptor is a naloxone-inaccessible opioid receptor, so standard opioid receptor antagonism does not relieve these side effects. However, this receptor has a high affinity for haloperidol, and this may antagonize negative side effects.[313]

Some side effects result from the toxic metabolites associated with a particular drug. The side effects associated with the accumulation of normeperidine and norpropoxyphene are well recognized.[97,291] The role of M3G, a metabolite of morphine, is less clear because it does not bind to opioid receptors and yet it seems to exert antagonist effects.[277,314] Some authors speculate that the antagonist effects of M3G are responsible for some of morphine's side effects, including myoclonus.[277]

Prevention or Minimizing Opioid-Related Side Effects

Optimal use of opioids requires minimizing or preventing the side effects ascribed to this class of drugs. For patients with constant pain, rapidly shifting to a long-acting preparation as soon as dose titration with a short-acting drug is accomplished may help attenuate side effects. If side effects are significant, the clinician should allow time for tolerance to develop, which usually takes 3 to 7 days. Protecting the patient from severe side effects during this period is appropriate and will not prevent tolerance development. For example, a patient with nausea could benefit from a one-week course of antiemetic medication at the outset of opioid therapy.

If side effects do not diminish satisfactorily over time, there are two alternatives: changing the opioid or introducing supplementary medications that control the side effects. Changing from one opioid to another may enhance pain relief and reduce opioid-related side effects, particularly if incomplete cross tolerance to opioid effect is experienced.[142,148,279,315–316] Changing the route of administration for a particular drug, such as morphine, may eliminate certain difficult side effects in some patients.[317] It is possible to alleviate many of the most difficult side effects pharmacologically when necessary. For example, administering methylphenidate can help protect the cognitive functioning of patients using high doses of opioids.[318–319] Table 19.10 lists common side effects and their treatments.

In cancer patients, certain pathophysiologic conditions commonly contribute to side effect problems or may even masquerade as side effects. Renal insufficiency in patients using morphine can lead to accumulation of M6G, which in turn can exacerbate side effects. Nausea is a frequent opioid toxicity, but it has other potential causes which must be considered: gastric irritation, constipation or other changes in gut motility, chemotherapy, or hypercalcemia induced by bone metastases. Similarly, sedation and confusion may accompany opioid use, but other potential causes in the cancer patient such as raised intracranial pressure, metabolic disturbances (eg, hypercalcemia), sepsis, or concomitant drug use merit consideration. We have found that opioid-induced changes in mental status are less probable when the patient has been on a stable opioid dose without recent significant dose escalation.

TABLE 19.10

PHARMACOLOGIC TREATMENTS FOR OPIOID-RELATED SIDE EFFECTS

Side Effect	Treatment
Constipation	Stool softener, laxative, opioid rotation
Sedation	Methylphenidate, modafinil
Pruritus	Diphenhydramine, hydroxyzine
Nausea	Prochlorperazine, haloperidol, metoclopramide, ondansetron, antihistamine
Dysphoria	Haloperidol, opioid rotation
Hypnogogic imagery	Haloperidol
Cognitive impairment	Methylphenidate, modafinil, opioid rotation
Respiratory depression	Naloxone
Myoclonus	Clonazepam, dose reduction, opioid rotation

OPIOID EFFECTS ON COGNITION, MOTOR SKILLS, AND DRIVING ABILITY

A major concern that has arisen as long-term opioid therapy becomes an accepted standard for patients with chronic, moderate-to-severe pain is the effect of long-term opioid use on cognition and motor skills[320] such as driving.[321] Results have been inconsistent regarding decrements in cognitive performance. Patients with chronic pain who have been using opioids for more than 3 days exhibit relatively few differences when cognitive performance is compared with performance before taking opioids or with that of a comparable patient population not taking opioids.[322] The majority of research has revealed that the greatest potential impairment in cognitive function from opioids occurs during the first several days of use. During longer periods, impairment has been demonstrated primarily in studies that have compared patients with significant pain with healthy volunteers. The negative effects of opioids on cognition may be balanced by enhanced cognitive function with the relief of pain.[322] Questions still remain concerning the mechanisms responsible for opioid-induced cognitive impairment, interpatient variability with regard to opioid-related cognitive impairment, and the identification of predictors for cognitive impairment in patients receiving long-term opioid therapy. Each of these areas deserves further study.

The effects of opioid use, specifically on driving ability, has become a contentious issue, predictably because a growing number of patients are taking opioids and driving, and also because insurers may seek to assign liability in cases of motor vehicle accidents involving drivers who use opioids. When given in single doses to healthy volunteers, opioids impair reaction time, muscle coordination, attention, and short-term memory sufficiently to affect driving and other skilled activities.[323] A pilot study examined the effects of medically prescribed, chronic, stable opioid use on the driving abilities of 16 patients with persistent, nonmalignant pain; chronic opioid use did not significantly impair the perception, cognition, coordination, and behavior measured in off-road tests that have been regarded as requisite for on-road driving.[324] Vainio et al.[323] examined the effects of continuous morphine medication on the driving ability of cancer patients. They conducted psychological and neurological tests, originally designed for professional motor vehicle drivers, in two groups of cancer patients who were similar apart from their experience of pain. Twenty-four patients received continuous morphine (mean 209-mg oral morphine daily) for cancer pain; and 25 were pain free without regular analgesics. Though the results were a little worse in the patients taking morphine, there were no significant differences between the groups in intelligence, vigilance, concentration, fluency of motor reactions, or division of attention. Of the neural function tests, reaction times (auditory, visual, associative), thermal discrimination, and body sway with eyes open were similar in the two groups; only balancing ability with closed eyes was worse in the morphine group. These results indicate that, in cancer patients receiving long-term morphine treatment with stable doses, morphine has only a slight and selective effect on functions related to driving.

Galski et al. published a structured, evidence-based review on the issue of opioids and driving.[324] Forty-eight reports were identified that studied the following areas: psychomotor ability; cognitive function; effect of opioid dosing on psychomotor ability; motor vehicle driving violations and motor vehicle accidents; and driving impairment as measured in driving simulators and off- and on-road driving. There was moderate, generally consistent evidence for no impairment of psychomotor abilities of opioid-maintained patients, strong, consistent evidence in multiple studies for no impairment of psychomotor abilities immediately after being given doses of opioids, and consistent evidence for no impairment as measured in driving simulators. Overall, the majority of studies in the evidence-based review appeared to indicate that patients who use opioids are not impaired by the opioids with regard to driving ability. Byas-Smith et al. reported that many patients with chronic pain, even if treated with potent analgesics such as morphine and hydromorphone at equivalent average daily morphine doses of 118 mg, showed comparable driving ability as normal subjects.[325]

Clearly, opioids may affect cognitive function and impair driving ability in patients who are opioid-naive or in patients who are not on stable opioid regimens. Whether some degree of "cognitive tolerance" develops with chronic opioid use is unknown. Other unresolved questions include the effects of different types of opioids, dose effects, and interactions with other medications on driving ability. These are areas for further investigation, preferably with well-designed, well-controlled studies. At our institution, patient guidelines are provided regarding opioid medications and driving but we do not interdict driving for those on stable doses without impairments (Appendix E).

The effects of morphine on alertness and cognition in patients with advanced cancer were studied by Clemons et al.[326] Twenty-nine subjects were recruited into three groups: healthy volunteers (16 subjects without cancer and not on opioids), inpatients and outpatients with advanced cancer not taking any opioids (6 subjects), and inpatients and outpatients with advanced cancer on a stable and regular dose of oral morphine (7 subjects). Subjects were tested with a battery of tests designed to test the global effects of alertness on cognitive function on either five or six occasions. The New Adult Reading Test, Reaction Time and Stroop Color-Word Tests failed to show any difference between the two cancer groups, although they did show a difference between the healthy controls and the cancer patients, suggesting that the tests were sensitive to the effects of cancer but not to the effects of morphine. The Stroop Color-Word Test is a complex measure of cognitive function and the difference between healthy volunteers and cancer/no morphine patients suggests that advanced cancer itself may be impairing performance. The authors noted that the cancer/morphine patients subjectively felt less "generally well," less "alert," less "active," more "depressed," had poorer "concentration," and were more "anxious" than either of the other groups.

Opioids can cause or exacerbate confusion and these effects may range from mild impairment in concentration to frank delirium with disorientation, disorganized thinking, perceptual distortions, and hallucinations. Hallucinations are the product of σ-receptor activation and can occur in the context of intact cognitive function.[327] Obviously, when this problem occurs it is important to consider other causes of altered mental status. When a confusional state is due to opioids, it generally follows a recent increase in dose and will usually resolve with tolerance or as the dose is reduced. Rapid discontinuation of the opioid will result in severe pain, withdrawal symptoms, and possible exacerbation of confusion; this should be avoided. Dysphoria is probably more common than euphoria following opioid administration in patients with cancer.

Modafinil is an FDA-approved medication with wakefulness-promoting properties. Preclinical studies of modafinil suggest a complex profile of neurochemical and behavioral effects, distinct from those of amphetamine. Cognitive dysfunction may be a particularly important emerging treatment target for modafinil. Modafinil (at well-tolerated doses) improves function in several cognitive domains, including working memory and episodic memory, and other processes dependent on prefrontal cortex and cognitive control.[328] It appears to be well-tolerated, with a low rate of adverse events and a low liability to abuse. Modafinil may also have a role in the management of opioid-induced sedation.[329] Typical doses of modafinil start at 100 mg taken orally in the morning.

TOLERANCE AND HYPERALGESIA

Side effects of opioids after initial administration include sedation, nausea, vomiting, respiratory depression, miosis, constipation, and euphoria/dysphoria. Studies have shown that tolerance to sedation, nausea, and respiratory depression can occur rapidly, whereas tolerance to constipation and miosis is minimal. Tolerance to the sedative and cognitive effects of opioids can occur rapidly. Usually sedation and cognitive impairment occur at the start of treatment or after a dose increase. With prolongation of use, most opioid-related side effects diminish. On the other hand, continued use of opioids may cause tolerance and physical dependence. A notable feature of physical dependence is the hyperalgesic response during opioid withdrawal.[330–331] Hyperalgesia can also occur in the absence of opioid withdrawal.[332–333] Using quantitative sensory testing as a means for detection, Chen et al.[334] demonstrated decreased heat pain threshold and exacerbated temporal summation in opioid tolerant chronic pain patients. Patients in this study must have had a stable pain condition for at least 3 months and also have been on opioid therapy (taking at least 30 mg daily equivalent dose of morphine) for at least 3 months.

Opioid tolerance refers to the diminished opioid analgesic effect during opioid therapy. Opioid tolerance is a phenomenon in which repeated exposure to an opioid results in decreased therapeutic effect of the drug or need for a higher dose to maintain the same effect. Prolonged use of opioids is known to result in antinociceptive tolerance, in which higher doses of the opioid are required to elicit the same amount of pain relief or antinociception.[335–336] In practice, physical dependence and tolerance do not prevent the effective use of these drugs and the evidence for the development of tolerance to the analgesic effects of opioids with chronic administration has been mixed. Exposure to opioids can result in a need to increase the dose over time to maintain a desired analgesic effect. Typically, this has been attributed to the development of tolerance. However, dose escalation can also be expected as a result of opioid-induced hyperalgesia. Mechanistically, tolerance reflects a desensitization of antinociceptive pathways to opioids, whereas hyperalgesia involves a sensitization of pronociceptive pathways. Morphine tolerance may be attributed to enhancement of glutamatergic neurotransmission, in particular to increased function of the NMDA receptor. In an electrophysiologically defined subpopulation of dorsal horn neurons, Zhao and Joo demonstrated enhanced NMDA receptor function after chronic morphine exposure which was shown to be mechanistically dependent on morphine concentration and sensitive to both NMDA and μ-opioid receptor antagonism.[337] Administration of very high doses of certain opioids can produce allodynia and possibly hyperalgesia on rare clinical occasions. The allodynic/hyperalgesic state is not reversed by opioid antagonists and can become aggravated when the dose of the causative opioid agonist is further escalated.[338] As soon as a high-dose, opioid-induced allodynic/hyperalgesic state is suspected, dose reduction of the causative agent and/or substitution of the causative agent with an opioid agonist less likely to cause such symptoms are appropriate next steps aiming at attenuating or eliminating these symptoms.

Many of the studies of opioid tolerance were in cancer patients with severe pain and showed that they maintained a stable opioid dose (for weeks to years) even with different routes of administration.[339–340] Patients with stable disease often remain on a stable dose for weeks or months.[341] Collin et al.[342] demonstrated a relationship between tumor progression and escalation of opioid doses over time such that the development of opioid tolerance as a result of chronic opioid use was unlikely in cancer patients with pain. Although it is generally agreed that tolerance to the analgesic properties of opioids occurs in patients with malignant pain, dose escalation is thought to be mostly a result of disease progression rather than the development of pharmacodynamic tolerance.

Unexpected hyperalgesia and allodynia associated with opioid administration can be seen with both acute and chronic administration of opioids or with opioid withdrawal. Opioid-induced hyperalgesia (OIH) may be defined as a paradoxical state of nociceptive sensitization caused by exposure to opioids.[343] Clinically, OIH may manifest as apparent opioid tolerance, worsening pain despite increasing opioid doses, and abnormal or unusual pain symptoms. The paradoxical phenomenon of OIH can be related to the altered balance between pronociceptive and antinociceptive (ie, endogenous inhibitory modulation) processes.[344] Findings from clinical and preclinical studies suggest that opioid exposure can paradoxically induce hyperalgesic states and patients may become more sensitive to pain. This situation is thought to result from neuroplastic changes in the CNS and peripheral nervous system leading to sensitization of pronociceptive pathways. Clinically relevant concentrations of remifentanil induce rapid, persistent increases in NMDA responses that mirror the development of remifentanil-induced

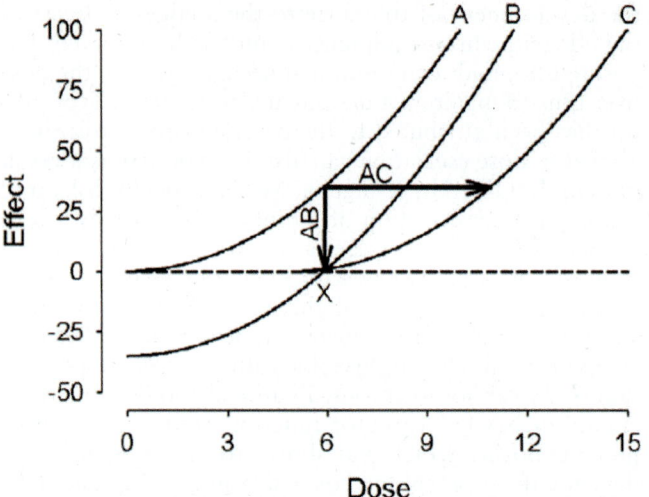

FIGURE 19.1 Alterations in opioid dose versus analgesic relationship with chronic opioid administration. Curve A represents the relationship in opioid-naive patients. Curve B shows patients developing OIH. Curve C shows opioid tolerance. Arrow AB and AC indicate the shift of the opioid dose-versus-analgesic effect relationship with the occurrence of OIH and tolerance. Both tolerance and OIH result in a decreased effectiveness of a given drug dose (X). OIH, Opioid-induced hyperalgesia. (Reused with permission from Carroll IR, Angst MS, Clark JD. Management of perioperative pain in patients chronically consuming opioids. Reg Anesth Pain Med. 2004;29:576–591.)

hyperalgesia and tolerance.[345] Of interest, modulation of microglia activation by suppression of TNF-α, IL-1β, and IL-6 may be potentially useful for the treatment of neuropathic pain and for the prevention of tolerance to morphine.[346]

OIH should be distinguished from tolerance, although clinically, these conditions can be difficult to separate Fig. 19.1). In tolerance, desensitization of opioid antinociceptive pathways over time can be reversed by increasing the opioid dose. In patients with OIH, dose increases will paradoxically aggravate the problem and worsen the underlying pain complaint.[343] Proposed mechanisms for OIH include sensitization of primary afferent neurons, enhanced production and release of excitatory neurotransmitters and diminished reuptake of neurotransmitters, sensitization of second order neurons to excitatory neurotransmitters, and neuroplastic changes in the rostral ventromedial medulla that may increase descending facilitation via "on-cells" leading to up-regulation of spinal dynorphin and enhanced primary afferent neurotransmitter release and pain.[343] Management of OIH includes reduction of opioid dose, opioid rotation, or the use of adjuvant therapies, where appropriate.

In humans, much of the evidence for OIH is based on studies on intraoperative infusions of short-acting opioids.[347] Opioids such as morphine have been reported to induce hyperalgesia in humans and animals.[335] In preclinical studies, sustained opioid exposure across multiple days has been shown to reduce sensory thresholds, resulting in hypersensitivity to tactile stimulation (ie, allodynia) and to noxious thermal stimulation (ie, hyperalgesia).[348] Opioid-induced hyperalgesia has mostly been observed in cancer patients who receive very high and escalating opioid doses.[338] Morphine has been implicated in virtually all reported cases. Recognition of this phenomenon can be difficult in a clinical setting of cancer pain where multiple factors can confound the picture. In a mixed cancer pain and non–cancer pain population, Reznikov et al.[349] found no differences in threshold pain for punctuate, pressure, and heat as well as the intensity of suprathreshold heat pain in opioid-compared to nonopioid-treated patients. In chronic back pain, Fillingim et al.[350] failed to show a difference between patients taking opioids and nonopioids with regard to back pain severity and to experimental ischemic pain tolerance.

Opioid-induced hyperalgesia should be recognized as a syndrome of neuroexcitatory effects which includes hyperalgesia, allodynia, myoclonus, and seizures, in a setting where patients are administered large doses of systemic morphine or its structural analogues. The predominant symptom of opioid-induced hyperalgesia is severe allodynia (touch-evoked pain) and is often accompanied by myoclonus. Putting a blanket on or gently turning a bed-ridden patient can evoke excruciating pain. Further dose escalation will exacerbate pain complaints or symptoms. Management strategies for hyperalgesia usually require a reduction in opioid dosage. There are case reports of cancer patients with high dose opioid-induced hyperalgesia whose pain resolved after reduction in dose.[351–352] In general, however, there is a lack of controlled clinical studies and proven approaches to differentiate and manage pharmacologic tolerance and OIH.

SEROTONIN SYNDROME

Serotonin syndrome is a potentially life-threatening adverse drug reaction caused by excessive serotonergic agonism in central and peripheral nervous system serotonergic receptors. The syndrome is most commonly reported with exposure to more than one serotonergic agent. It arises when pharmacologic agents increase serotonin neurotransmission at postsynaptic $5HT_{1A}$ and $5HT_{2A}$ receptors through increased serotonin synthesis, decreased serotonin metabolism, increased serotonin release, inhibition of serotonin reuptake, or direct agonism of the serotonin receptors. Symptoms are characterized by a triad of neuroexcitatory features, which include neuromuscular hyperactivity (tremor, clonus, myoclonus, hyperreflexia and, in advanced stages, pyramidal rigidity); autonomic hyperactivity (diaphoresis, fever, tachycardia, and tachypnea); and altered mental status (agitation, excitement, and, in advanced stages, confusion).[353] Clinical diagnostic criteria remain poorly defined and unvalidated, and there are no diagnostic studies to confirm the diagnosis.

Toxicity becomes obvious when the second serotonergic agent is added. The onset of frank toxicity is usually rapid and the patient's status can rapidly deteriorate after the first or second dose of the second serotonergic drug. The serotonin toxic patient is often initially alert, even hypervigilant, with tremor and hyperreflexia. Ankle clonus and myoclonus may be elicited. Neuromuscular signs are initially greater in the lower limbs, and become more generalized as toxicity increases. Patients may exhibit pronounced tremors. Autonomic features may develop

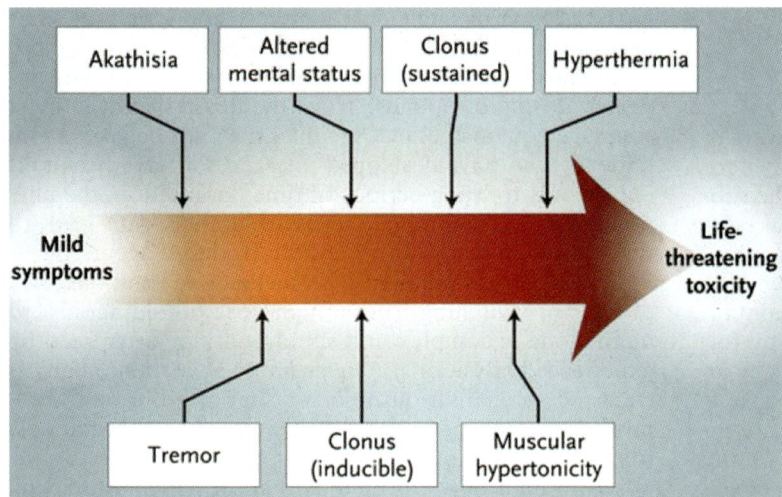

FIGURE 19.2 Serotonin syndrome: spectrum of clinical findings. Manifestations of the serotonin syndrome range from mild to life-threatening. The *vertical arrows* suggest the approximate point at which clinical findings initially appear in the spectrum of the disease, but all findings may not be consistently present in a single patient with the serotonin syndrome. Severe signs may mask other clinical findings. For example, muscular hypertonicity can overwhelm tremor and hyperreflexia. (Reused with permission from Boyer E and Shannon M. The serotonin syndrome. *N Engl J Med.* 2005;352(11):1112–1120. Copyright 2005 Massachusetts Medical Society. All rights reserved.)

with fever, sweating, mydriasis, tachycardia, and tachypnea. The features of serotonin syndrome are illustrated in Fig. 19.2.

The etiology is often the result of therapeutic drug use, intentional overdosing of serotonergic agents, or complex interactions between drugs that directly or indirectly modulate the serotonin system. Different classes of drugs exhibit distinct degrees to which they can elevate serotonin. Severe forms of the syndrome usually result from overdose, but can be induced by monotherapy. The most severe cases usually arise from interactions involving SSRIs, monoamine oxidase inhibitors (MAOIs), serotonin precursors, and other substances with serotonergic actions, including some drugs of abuse (eg, lysergic acid diethylamide [LSD] and 3,4-methylenedioxymethamphetamine [MDMA; Ecstasy]).[354] The syndrome occurs in approximately 14% to 16% of persons who overdose on SSRIs.[355] Antibiotics such as Linezolid can be associated with serotonin syndrome.[356] Analgesics such as meperidine, dextromethorphan, and tramadol have also been implicated.[357-358] Animal studies indicate that tramadol, meperidine, and dextromethorphan exhibit monoamine reuptake inhibitory effects[359] and increase 5HT levels by this effect. Fentanyl has also been implicated as a causative agent of serotonin syndrome as a result of interactions with citalopram[360] and paroxetine.[361] Oxycodone (in an interaction with fluvoxamine) has also been reported as a cause.[354] The phenylpiperidine series opioids, meperidine, tramadol, methadone and fentanyl (and congeners), and dextromethorphan and propoxyphene, are all weak serotonin re-uptake inhibitors.[177] Drugs and drug interactions associated with serotonin syndrome are listed in Table 19.11.

Diagnosis and withholding the offending agents is important. Management strategies include the provision of supportive care, the control of agitation, administration of $5HT_{2A}$ antagonists, and the control of autonomic instability. Rapid changes in the patient's clinical status will usually require monitoring in intensive care. Severe, late-stage serotonin toxicity may impair ventilation and require ventilatory support. If medication treatment is necessary, cyproheptadine and chlorpromazine may be useful. Oral doses of 12 to 32 mg of cyproheptadine in 24 hours may be required.[362] Initial doses are 12 mg and then 2 mg every 2 hours if symptoms continue.[363]

Serotonin syndrome has been reported in cancer patients, as they are frequent recipients of prescriptions for many of the drugs that are known to precipitate this syndrome.[364-368] Clinicians must be aware of the possibility of drug interactions that can lead to serotonin syndrome and take prompt action when early signs and symptoms are manifested by their patients.

TABLE 19.11

DRUGS AND DRUG INTERACTIONS ASSOCIATED WITH SEROTONIN SYNDROME

Class	Drug(s)
SSRIs	Sertaline, fluoxetine, fluvoxamine, paroxetine, and citalopram
Antidepressants	Trazodone, nefazodone, buspirone, clomipramine, and venlafaxime
MAOIs	Phenelzine, moclobemide, clorgiline, and isocarboxazid
Anticonvulsants	Valproate
Analgesics	Meperidine, fentanyl, tramadol, pentazocine
Antiemetics	Ondansetron, granisetron, metoclopramide
Antimigraine	Sumatriptan
Bariatric	Sibutramine
Antibiotics	Linezolide, ritonavir
OTC cough remedies	Dextromethorphan
Drugs of abuse	LSD
Dietary supplements/ herbal products	St. John's wort, ginseng, tryptophan
Other	lithium

SSRIs, selective serotonin-reuptake inhibitors; MAOIs, monoamine oxidase inhibitors; OTC, over the counter; LSD, lysergic acid diethylamide. (Reused with permission from Boyer E and Shannon M. The serotonin syndrome. *N Engl J Med.* 2005;352(11):1112–1120. Copyright 2005 Massachusetts Medical Society. All rights reserved.)

OPIOID ROTATION IN CANCER PAIN

Opioid rotation was first described in 1993.[369] It refers to the practice of converting from one opioid to another for a variety of clinical reasons and has recently been the subject of a number of reviews.[370–374] Ashby[375] has also coined the term "opioid substitution" for this practice and suggests the term "opioid rotation" be reserved for "the sequential use of different available opioids to maintain pain control which is thought to be compromised by tolerance to a particular opioid." Opioid rotation may be an important option when the opioid analgesic response is inadequate and/or if opioid-related adverse events are intolerable or unmanageable.[376–377] Reasons for initiating opioid rotation are listed in Table 19.12. In cancer patients the most common reasons for opioid rotation are intolerable side effects such as cognitive failure, hallucinations, myoclonus, nausea, and uncontrollable pain.[315,375]

In all cases of opioid rotation, patients must be followed up closely to assess the adequacy of pain relief and the effect on opioid-related adverse events. As with any opioid regimen, subsequent dose adjustments will probably be necessary. Use of opioid rotation requires familiarity with a range of opioids and with the use of equianalgesic dose tables (Table 19.13). However, it is also important to consider that the evidence to support dose ratios in standard equianalgesic tables refers largely to the context of single-dose administration; that does not necessarily reflect the clinical realities of chronic opioid administration in the treatment of cancer pain with repeated dosing of opioids. Thus, the doses shown in most standard equianalgesic dose tables may not be accurate in patients who have developed tolerance or have been taking opioids for long periods of time. In addition, the phenomenon of incomplete cross-tolerance can lead to unexpected potency in the newly introduced agent.[79]

Special care is required with methadone rotations. The process of switching from a high-dose opioid agonist to methadone is complex and should only be attempted by experienced physicians.[378] Even among experienced physicians, occasional serious toxicity can occur during the administration of methadone.[379] Contrary to expectations, toxicity occurs more frequently in patients previously exposed to high doses of opioids than in patients receiving low doses. Manfredi et al.[146] described the conversion of four patients receiving high continuous infusions of either morphine or hydromorphone to methadone. All four patients had excellent pain relief without significant side effects at a dose that, according to the conversion charts, was approximately 3% of the calculated equianalgesic dose of hydromorphone. When converting from continuous I.V. hydromorphone to continuous I.V. methadone, use much lower doses than those suggested by the opioid conversion charts as starting doses. We reported on the conversion of a patient receiving approximately 2,000 mg/day of morphine intravenously by PCA

TABLE 19.12

REASONS FOR UNDERTAKING OPIOID ROTATIONS

1. Reduced ability to control pain due to:
   a. Worsening of existing pain or underlying disease process
   b. Pharmacodynamic factors:
      Development of opioid analgesic tolerance
   c. Pharmacokinetic factors:
      Drug absorption (inability to swallow oral medications, poor vascular status, edema limiting transdermal delivery)
      Interaction with other drugs
      Changes in protein binding
      Biotransformation and metabolism (accumulation of metabolites)
      Reduced clearance—renal failure

2. Development of intolerable side effects/opioid toxicity:
   a. Gastrointestinal (ie, constipation, nausea, vomiting)
   b. Central nervous system (ie, sedation, somnolence, dysphoria, hallucinations, myoclonus)
   c. Cardiovascular (ie, orthostatic hypotension due to histamine release)

3. Practical concerns:
   a. Dose required to produce analgesia exceeds maximum daily dose (patients taking combination products, eg, acetaminophen)
   b. Cost of drugs
   c. Drug availability
   d. Need for large volumes of drug to be delivered
   e. Changes in route of administration

(From Souter KJ, Fitzgibbon D. Equianalgesic dose guidelines for long-term opioid use—theoretical and practical considerations. *Semin Anesth Periop Med Pain.* 2004;23:271–280. With permission from Elsevier.)

TABLE 19.13

STEADY STATE EQUIANALGESIC OPIOID CONVERSIONS

Rotation[a]	Parenteral	Oral	Comments
Morphine to oxycodone	1:0.7	2:1	Bidirectional difference
Oxycodone to morphine (parenteral oxycodone not available in United States)	0.7:1	1:1.5	
Morphine to hydromorphone	5:1	5:1	Bidirectional difference
Hydromorphone to morphine	1:3.5	1:3.5	
Morphine to methadone	1:1 (initially)	<100 mg[b] 3:1 101 to 300mg 5:1 301 to 600mg 10:1 601 to 800mg 12:1 801 to 1000mg 15:1 >1000 mg 20:1	Equianalgesic dose ratio depends on dose and is similar for all non-methadone opioids.[b]
Hydromorphone to methadone	1:1 (initially then consider 5:1 or scale similar to MS)	1:1 (for low dose[c])	Recommend conversion to morphine equivalent and then use similar scale
Hydromorphone to fentanyl	20:1	Convert to IV	TM Fentanyl—titrate 200 μg if opioid naive, 400 μg if not
Morphine to fentanyl (mg)	100:1 (initially)	Oral to transdermal 100:1 (safe start) 70:1 (likely necessary)	IV fentanyl to TTS TTS dose approx 30% to 60%
Morphine to meperidine	1:10	1:10	No difference between routes
Morphine to butorphanol	1:0.2	15 mg morphine = 1 spray (1mg)	Nasal bioavailability = I.V. route
Morphine to nalbuphine	1:1	NA	

[a]If pain is *poorly* controlled, execute full conversion. If pain is *well* controlled, execute conservative conversion.
[b]Previous daily dose of morphine
[c]Exercise caution when converting to methadone. Frail or elderly patients, or those on high doses of morphine equivalent, may require in-hospital conversion. Begin with a loading dose and titrate to pain score and side effects over the next few days. The predicted maintenance dose is calculated from the conversion ratios noted above. The original opioid is then discontinued and on the first 2 days, an optional loading dose of 25% to 50% extra is used, allowing for saturation of body tissues. Begin with a q6h dosing interval and graduate to 8- to 12-hour intervals over several days. Ensure the provision of sufficient short-acting opioids for breakthrough pain during the transition period.
I.V., Intravenous; NA, not applicable. (Reused with permission from Souter KJ, Fitzgibbon D. Equianalgesic dose guidelines for long-term opioid use—theoretical and practical considerations. *Semin Anesth Periop Med Pain.* 2004;23:271–280.)

and continuous infusion to methadone by the same treatment modalities.[147] Although the patient required 1,800 mg of methadone on the first day of conversion, the total daily dose decreased to one tenth of the initial dose on day 3 once the patient reached steady state plasma levels. Bruera et al. provided some guidelines for the conversion of patients from high dose oral opioids to oral methadone.[148] They recommended decreasing the previous opioid dose by one third during the first 24 hours and replacing it with methadone using an equianalgesic dose ratio. One mg of oral methadone is equal to 10 mg of oral morphine (ie, a patient receiving 1000 mg of oral morphine per day will switch to 660 mg of oral morphine per day plus 33 mg of oral methadone during the first day). Administer methadone every 8 hours by the oral route. During the second day, if pain control is adequate, the patient requires a further one third decrease in the dose of the previous opioid. The dose of the methadone should only increase if the patient experiences moderate to severe pain. Manage transient episodes of pain with intermittent rescue doses of short-acting opioids. During day 3, discontinue the final third of the previous opioid and maintain the patient on regular methadone every 8 hours, plus approximately 10% of the daily methadone dose as an extra dose orally for breakthrough pain. Assess pain and methadone requirements frequently until a stable methadone dose is reached. Until the equianalgesic dose ratio of parenteral and oral opioids to methadone is clearly established, patients receiving high doses of oral/parenteral opioids who require conversion to methadone should undergo this conversion only under close supervision and preferably in an in-patient environment. In general, the safe use of methadone to control cancer pain requires meticulous follow-up care and anticipatory downward dose titration.

OPIOIDS AND GENOMICS

Advances in biotechnology have led to improved understanding of the human genome. Our understanding of opioid-induced pain relief is quickly expanding because of the development of genomic and proteomic research. Since genetics and other pharmacokinetic/pharmacodynamic causes may affect opioids differently, a patient not responding to one opioid should not be labeled *opioid resistant,* because another opioid may work. Genetic causes for intervariability of the clinical response to opioids have been known for several years. In humans, pain genetics is difficult to investigate as the various experimental pain stimuli are different from the myriad of clinical pain responses, and the genes involved are only now being elucidated. Moreover, to assign a major genetic component to clinical pain problems remains difficult, whereas in experimental pain the elucidation of genetic factors can be more readily identified, as precise quantitation of the experimental noxious stimulus can be controlled.

Molecular pain genetics is a relatively new and rapidly expanding research field that advances conventional pain research into the modern era. Developments in molecular technology have now made it possible to assess the contribution of genes in pain treatment and control.[380] Molecular pain research addresses physiologic and pathological pain at the cellular, subcellular, and molecular levels. These studies integrate pain research with molecular biology, genomics, proteomics, modern electrophysiology, and neurobiology. Advances in molecular biology have made it possible to rapidly obtain the amino acid sequence of neuropeptide precursors—either by cloning and sequencing the cDNA that encodes the precursor, or by reconstructing the arrangement of exons and introns in a neuropeptide-coding gene through genomic approaches. The databases generated from these molecular approaches have been used to design probes to identify the cells that express the gene, or to ascertain the rate of expression of the gene, and even to predict the post-translational modifications that can generate functional neuropeptides from a biologically inert precursor.[381] Parallel studies on the receptors and molecules that bind such neuropeptides, as well as how the signaling cascades are affected before and after noxious stimulation, have also been ongoing over the last decade.

Bioinformatics and genomics are closely related disciplines that hold great promises for the advancement of research and development in complex biomedical systems, as well as public health, drug design, comparative genomics, and personalized medicine. Genomics is the study of all of the nucleotide sequences, including structural genes, regulatory sequences, and coding/noncoding DNA segments, in the chromosomes of an organism. Functional genomics can be defined as the search for the physiologic role of a gene when only its primary sequence is known.

Proteomics is the study of the function of all (or a large percentage of) expressed proteins. Proteomics describes the science and methodology of the investigation of the proteome, which quantitatively describes the composition of proteins in a cell, a tissue, or an organism. Proteomics is complementary to genomic approaches, which investigate DNA and RNA. Unlike genomics, proteomics provides information about protein isoforms, post-translational protein modifications such as glycosylations and phosphorylations, protein–protein interactions, and protein stability and degradation.[382] Whereas genomic DNA are relatively constant, the transcriptome (RNA) and proteome (proteins) differ strongly from cell to cell and are constantly modulated through biochemical interactions with the genome and the environment. Proteomic studies have generated numerous datasets of potential diagnostic, prognostic, and therapeutic significance in human cancer.[383] Shui et al.[384] undertook a proteomic analysis of spinal protein expression in rats exposed to repeated intrathecal injection of morphine primarily to investigate the neuroadaptive changes in the spinal cord that are thought to underlie molecular mechanisms in the development of morphine tolerance and dependence. They found eight proteins that were significantly up-regulated or down-regulated in the spinal cord after morphine tolerance development, including proteins involved in targeting and trafficking of glutamate receptors and opioid receptors, proteins involved in oxidative stress, and cytoskeletal proteins. The authors believed that the identified proteins may serve as potential molecular targets for prevention of the development of morphine tolerance and physical dependence.

Improved information on the human genome has resulted in a better understanding into the subtle elements underlying variable drug effects which may be a cause of patient morbidity. Efforts have also been made to begin ascribing a function to each of the 30,000 or so genes that constitute the human genome. Even before all of the functions are known, it may then be possible to identify subtle abnormalities in DNA sequences. The simplest type of variation or polymorphism derives from a single base mutation in DNA that substitutes one nucleotide for another (single-nucleotide polymorphism [SNP]). The effect of any particular SNP, ie, the resulting phenotype, will depend on the impact of the resulting substitution of the encrypted amino acid on the respective protein. Having detected a SNP, it is possible using gene-association studies to link the abnormal gene with either a disease process or with an abnormal response to a drug. Genetics are not the only possible cause for interindividual variability, and the "classic" causes for variability, such as organ function, comedication or underlying disease, have to be taken into consideration before assigning an unexpected drug response to a genetic cause.

As with any biological system, the mechanisms underlying pain signal transduction, transmission, and spinal and central processing are subject to variations between individuals owing to their genetic codes. Different phenotypes are potentially produced when genes undergo variations (or mutations) from the normal (or "wild-type") form. These gene variations are called polymorphisms; although significant genotype differences can be attributed to a SNP and each gene is usually subject to more than one SNP, whether a specific SNP is responsible for an associated phenotype is more complicated to determine. This is because some genetic variants do not result in an alteration of a phenotype (even if they do give a specific "fingerprint" adequate for forensic analysis). For example, it has been calculated that for neuropathic pain, there are at least 20 candidate genes whose SNPs could influence points on the pain pathways.[385] These include SNPs of genes which encode cytokines, kinins, ion channels, and the opioid receptors. Genetic factors regulating pharmacokinetics (metabolizing enzymes, transporters) and pharmacodynamics (receptors and signal transduction elements) contribute to variability in drug responses. Even when a particular SNP is found associated with disease, it is important to note that the presence of a SNP does not imply causation, but rather that the variant may be in close proximity to a region of DNA involved with the clinical effect. Whereas some SNPs have been shown to be related to disease, others are not.

Genetic predisposition, including (but not limited to) variants in specific genes, can influence the experience, sensation, and behavioral response of pain. These may include factors that influence the synthesis of receptors and neurotransmitters and catabolic enzymes. The catechol-O-methyltransferase (COMT) enzyme metabolizes dopamine, epinephrine, and norepinephrine, and is a key modulator of dopaminergic and adrenergic neurotransmission. The involvement of catecholamines in pain modulation is known from clinical[386] and experimental[387] studies. A common functional polymorphism (Val158Met) leads to a three- to fourfold variation in the COMT enzyme activity. The Val158Met polymorphism affects pain perception, and subjects with the Met/Met genotype have the most pronounced response to experimental pain.[388] Rakvag et al.[109] studied the influence of the COMT Val158Met polymorphism on the efficacy of morphine in a cohort of 207 patients suffering from cancer pain. Patients with the Val/Val genotype (N = 44) needed more morphine (155 ±160 mg/day) compared with the Val/Met (117± 100 mg/day; N = 96) and the Met/Met genotype (95 ±99 mg/day; N = 67) groups (P = .025). This difference is not explained by other factors such as duration of morphine treatment, performance status, time since diagnosis, perceived pain intensity, adverse symptoms, or time until death. These results suggest that genetic variation in the COMT gene may contribute to variability in the efficacy of morphine in cancer pain treatment. The findings also suggest that genetic variability in genes relevant to nonopioid systems can influence the clinical efficacy of opioids.

Clinical variations in responses to drugs may be caused by the effect of genetic variation on both receptors (pharmacodynamics) and on factors that determine drug concentrations (pharmacokinetics). As stated above, in humans, the important opioid receptors for pain are of three varieties: the μ (MOR), κ (KOR), and δ-opioid receptor (DOR).[389] A fourth opioid-like receptor, the orphanin or ORL-1 receptor, has been identified, but its role in pain mechanisms is still poorly understood. MOR is a preferred target of morphine, and it appears to play a crucial role in mediating major clinical effects of morphine, including pain relief, tolerance, and dependence.[390] Opioid receptors are each encoded by specific genes, which share 60% to 70% of identical DNA code between MOR, KOR, and DOR.[391] The remaining 30% to 40% variations in genetic coding lead to the functional differences between receptor types. The receptor which has been most closely studied is the MOR, which has been found to have over 20 SNPs, ten of which are known to lead to amino acid changes in the resulting receptor protein. Some of these occur rarely and not all have been shown to have functional significance in humans or animals. The most common SNP is a substitution, at the gene's 118 position, of adenine by guanine; this SNP is thus referred to as 118A > G or A118G. One or both of the base pairs is substituted (ie, causing AG or GG genotypes) in 20% to 30% of the population and the homozygous GG genotype has been found to occur in about 10% to 12% of whites.[392] Gender differences have also been reported in relation to another nonopioid gene, which encodes the melanocortin-1 receptor (MC-1R).[32] In addition to influencing skin and hair color phenotypes, this gene influences pain experience and response to opioids. At least six common SNPs exist for the MC-1R gene, the three most common of them occurring in about 11% of whites.[393] Some SNPs result in red hair and fair skin; in these individuals, there is an abnormally higher response to the KOR-binding opioids phenazocine and oxycodone.[32]

Ross et al.[108] studied the clinical response to morphine and the genetic variation in four candidate genes (MOR, βarrestin$_2$, stat6, and UGT2B7) in 162 cancer patients who had responded to morphine (117 controls) versus those who switched to alternate opioids who had failed to achieve adequate pain relief with morphine (39 switchers). UGT2B7 (uridine diphosphate-glucuronysltransferase 2B7) metabolizes morphine and it is unclear if polymorphisms in UGT2B7 influence clinical responses to morphine. Animal studies support the physiologic role of βarrestin$_2$ in MOR desensitization.[107] As such, it can regulate the number of functional receptors expressed on the cell surface at a given time. Functional studies have highlighted the role of stat6 (known to be highly polymorphic), which causes an increase in MOR gene expression.[394] The authors reported that genetic variation in the βarrestin$_2$ gene was associated with the need to switch from morphine to an alternative opioid; switchers were more likely to carry the T allele at position 8622. Polymorphisms in the MOR gene were not significantly different in switchers compared with controls.

MOR, encoded by the gene OPRM1, has been the focus of numerous genetic studies because this receptor is the primary site of action for many endogenous opioid peptides, including β-endorphin and enkephalin, as well as being the major target of opioid analgesics.[19] About 100 variants in the MOR gene OPRM1 have been identified,[395] with more than 20 producing amino acid changes and having polymorphic frequencies of more than 1%.[392] The most commonly identified SNP is A118G (allele frequency 2% to 48% ethnicity dependent), resulting in an amino-acid exchange at position 40 from asparagine to aspartate, leading to the loss of a putative N-glycosylation site in the extracellular receptor region. Mutations of OPRM1 are primary candidates for genetic influences on opioid effects. Genetic differences in perception or processing of pain account for an important part of the variability of clinical opioid effects. Sequence variability in the gene encoding human OPRM1 may create a receptor with altered expression, structure, or function, and as a consequence may increase or decrease an individual's susceptibility to substance dependence.[396] In addition, the pharmacokinetics and pharmacodynamics of morphine are under the influence of several polymorphic genes. Campa et al.[397] studied the effect of two genes, ABCB1/MDR1 (a major determinant of morphine bioavailability), and OPRM1 (which encodes for MOR) on gene polymorphisms for morphine pain relief. One hundred forty-five cancer patients undergoing morphine therapy were genotyped for the SNP C3435T of ABCB1/MDR1 and for the A80G SNP of OPRM1. Pain relief variability was significantly ($P<0.0001$) associated with both polymorphisms. Combining the extreme genotypes of both genes, the association between patient polymorphism and pain relief improved ($P < .00001$), allowing the detection of three groups: strong responders, responders, and nonresponders, with sensitivity close to 100% and specificity more than 70%. Reyes-Gibby et al.[398] explored the joint effects of OPRM1 and COMT genes in predicting morphine dose for cancer pain relief. The joint effects of genes can be expected to enhance, suppress, or have no effect on the phenotypic outcome of interest. The authors used genotype and clinical data from a pharmacokinetic study of morphine in 207 inpatients treated with stable morphine dose for at least 3 days. There was significant variation in morphine dose requirement by genotype groups: Carriers of COMT Val/Val and Val/Met genotype required (63% and 23%, respectively), higher morphine dose compared to carriers of Met/Met genotype ($P = .02$). Carriers of OPRM1 GG genotype required 93% higher morphine dose compared to carriers of AA genotypes ($P = .012$). For joint effects, the authors found that carriers of the OPRM1 AA and COMT Met/Met genotype required the lowest morphine dose to achieve pain relief (87 mg/day) and those with neither Met/Met nor AA genotype needed the highest morphine dose (147 mg/day). The significant joint effects for the Met/Met and AA genotypes ($P < .012$) persisted, even after controlling for demographic and clinical variables in the multivariable analyses. These findings provide empirical support for the importance of joint effects of the OPRM1 and COMT gene in the clinical efficacy of morphine. Furthermore, because pain is prevalent not just in cancer patients but in other diseases, the COMT and OPRM1 genotypes may be relevant information to consider when implementing pain therapy.

Prediction of therapeutic efficacy of opioids in individuals based on information on variability in opioid pharmacology may help establish improved personalized pain management with opioids. For this reason, exploring genetic factors that affect opioid pharmacology has significant import. The analgesic action of opioids is dependent on metabolic enzymes, transporters, and molecules involved in the opioid signal transduction pathways. There are numerous enzymes which metabolize lipid-soluble opioids into more water-soluble metabolites to facilitate elimination. Genetic polymorphisms in CYP genes also would cause interindividual variations in the plasma levels of opioids and their efficacies. CYP2D6 catalyzes the biotransformation of codeine, tramadol, dihydrocodeine, oxycodone, hydrocodone, dextropropoxyphene, and partly that of methadone. Mutations of the CYP2D6 gene include SNPs, nucleotide insertions, and deletions up to the deletion of the whole gene.[399] CYP2D6 alleles are differently distributed in Chinese or Japanese and in African Americans compared with whites. Codeine pain relief is closely related to the pharmacogenetics of CYP2D6.[239] Since O-demethylation of codeine into morphine is impaired in poor metabolizers of debrisoquine/sparteine, codeine is devoid of analgesic effects in these poor metabolizers as well as in situations when CYP2D6 is pharmacologically inhibited. This is known to be the case in 10% of white men.[400]

Pharmacologic data generated from genetically modified murine models add to the development of genotyping technologies and resultant new human sequencing projects have lead to an accumulation of information about genomic polymorphisms associated with the function of these molecules and opioid sensitivity are rapidly increasing.[401] We believe that the care of the patient with pain due to cancer will take on new meanings as the fields of genomics and proteomics expands. New diagnostic tests will lead to targeted opioid therapy with higher efficacy and fewer side effects.

References

1. Deandrea S, Montanari M, Moja L, et al. Prevalence of undertreatment in cancer pain. A review of published literature. *Ann Oncol.* 2008;19:1985–1991.
2. Joranson DE, Ryan KM. Ensuring opioid availability: methods and resources. *J Pain Symptom Manage.* 2007;33:527–532.
3. De Lima L, Sweeney C, Palmer JL, et al. Potent analgesics are more expensive for patients in developing countries: A comparative study. *J Pain Palliat Care Pharmacother.* 2004;18:59–70.
4. Maltoni M, Scarpi E, Modonesi C, et al. A validation study of the WHO analgesic ladder: A two-step vs three-step strategy. *Support Care Cancer.* 2005;13:888–894.
5. Mercadante S, Villari P, Ferrera P, et al. Addition of a second opioid may improve opioid response in cancer pain: Preliminary data. *Support Care Cancer.* 2004;12:762–766.
6. Fisher DM, Kellett N, Lenhardt R. Pharmacokinetics of an implanted osmotic pump delivering sufentanil for the treatment of chronic pain. *Anesthesiology.* 2003;99:929–937.
7. Ward ME, Woodhouse A, Mather LE, et al. Morphine pharmacokinetics after pulmonary administration from a novel aerosol delivery system. *Clin Pharmacol Ther.* 1997;62:596–609.
8. Viscusi ER. Patient-controlled drug delivery for acute postoperative pain management: A review of current and emerging technologies. *Reg Anesth Pain Med.* 2008;33:146–158.
9. Darwish M, Kirby M, Robertson P Jr, et al. Absolute and relative bioavailability of fentanyl buccal tablet and oral transmucosal fentanyl citrate. *J Clin Pharmacol.* 2007;47:343–350.
10. *Cancer pain relief with a guide to opioid availability*, 2nd ed. Geneva, Switzerland: World Health Organization, 1996.
11. Van Dorp E, Yassen A, Sarton E, et al. Naloxone reversal of buprenorphine-induced respiratory depression. *Anesthesiology.* 2006;105:51–57.
12. Hoskin PJ, Hanks GW. Opioid agonist-antagonist drugs in acute and chronic pain states. *Drugs.* 1991;41:326–344.
13. Ripamonti C, Dickerson ED. Strategies for the treatment of cancer pain in the new millennium. *Drugs.* 2001;61:955–977.
14. Stein C, Schafer M, Hassan AH. Peripheral opioid receptors. *Ann Med.* 1995;27:219–221.
15. Kieffer BL. Recent advances in molecular recognition and signal transduction of active peptides: receptors for opioid peptides. *Cell Mol Neurobiol.* 1995;15:615–635.
16. Matthes HW, Maldonado R, Simonin F, et al. Loss of morphine-induced analgesia, reward effect and withdrawal symptoms in mice lacking the mu-opioid-receptor gene. *Nature.* 1996;383:819–823.
17. Uhl GR, Sora I, Wang Z. The mu opiate receptor as a candidate gene for pain: Polymorphisms, variations in expression, nociception, and opiate responses. *Proc Natl Acad Sci U S A.* 1999;96:7752–7755.
18. Klepstad P, Dale O, Skorpen F, et al. Genetic variability and clinical efficacy of morphine. *Acta Anaesthesiol Scand.* 2005;49:902–908.
19. Flores CM, Mogil JS. The pharmacogenetics of analgesia: Toward a genetically-based approach to pain management. *Pharmacogenomics.* 2001;2:177–194.
20. Chevlen E. Opioids: A review. *Curr Pain Headache Rep.* 2003;7:15–23.
21. McCarthy L, Wetzel M, Sliker JK, et al. Opioids, opioid receptors, and the immune response. *Drug Alcohol Depend.* 2001;62:111–123.
22. Chen C, Li J, Bot G, Szabo I, et al. Heterodimerization and cross-desensitization between the mu-opioid receptor and the chemokine CCR5 receptor. *Eur J Pharmacol.* 2004;483:175–186.
23. Grimm MC, Ben-Baruch A, Taub DD, et al. Opiates transdeactivate chemokine receptors: Delta and mu opiate receptor-mediated heterologous desensitization. *J Exp Med.* 1998;188:317–325.
24. Pan HL, Wu ZZ, Zhou HY, et al. Modulation of pain transmission by G-protein-coupled receptors. *Pharmacol Ther.* 2008;117:141–161.

25. Lim WK. GPCR drug discovery: novel ligands for CNS receptors. *Recent Pat CNS Drug Discov.* 2007;2:107–112.
26. Mollereau C, Parmentier M, Mailleux P, et al. ORL1, a novel member of the opioid receptor family. Cloning, functional expression and localization. *FEBS Lett.* 1994;341:33–38.
27. Maggi R, Pimpinelli F, Martini L, et al. Inhibition of luteinizing hormone-releasing hormone secretion by delta-opioid agonists in GT1-1 neuronal cells. *Endocrinology.* 1995;136:5177–5181.
28. Schafer MK, Martin R. Opioid peptides in the pituitary: A hormone, a paracrine modulator and a peptide in search of a function. *Biol Chem Hoppe Seyler.* 1994;375:737–740.
29. Roy S, Loh HH. Effects of opioids on the immune system. *Neurochem Res.* 1996;21:1375–1386.
30. Gear RW, Gordon NC, Heller PH, et al. Gender difference in analgesic response to the kappa-opioid pentazocine. *Neurosci Lett.* 1996;205:207–209.
31. Gear RW, Miaskowski C, Gordon NC, et al. Kappa-opioids produce significantly greater analgesia in women than in men. *Nat Med.* 1996;2:1248–1250.
32. Mogil JS, Wilson SG, Chesler EJ, et al. The melanocortin-1 receptor gene mediates female-specific mechanisms of analgesia in mice and humans. *Proc Natl Acad Sci U S A.* 2003;100:4867–4872.
33. Cepeda MS, Carr DB. Women experience more pain and require more morphine than men to achieve a similar degree of analgesia. *Anesth Analg.* 2003;97:1464–1468.
34. Larijani GE, Goldberg ME, Gratz I, et al. Analgesic and hemodynamic effects of a single 7.5-mg intravenous dose of morphine in patients with moderate-to-severe postoperative pain. *Pharmacotherapy.* 2004;24:1675–1680.
35. Zacny JP, Beckman NJ. The effects of a cold-water stimulus on butorphanol effects in males and females. *Pharmacol Biochem Behav.* 2004;78:653–659.
36. Fillingim RB, Ness TJ, Glover TL, et al. Experimental pain models reveal no sex differences in pentazocine analgesia in humans. *Anesthesiology.* 2004;100:1263–1270.
37. Olofsen E, Romberg R, Bijl H, et al. Alfentanil and placebo analgesia: no sex differences detected in models of experimental pain. *Anesthesiology.* 2005;103:130–139.
38. Craft RM. Sex differences in analgesic, reinforcing, discriminative, and motoric effects of opioids. *Exp Clin Psychopharmacol.* 2008;16:376–385.
39. Loyd DR, Murphy AZ. The role of the periaqueductal gray in the modulation of pain in males and females: Are the anatomy and physiology really that different? *Neural Plast.* 2009;2009:462879.
40. Wybran J, Appelboom T, Famaey JP, et al. Suggestive evidence for receptors for morphine and methionine-enkephalin on normal human blood T lymphocytes. *J Immunol.* 1979;123:1068–1070.
41. Bidlack JM, Khimich M, Parkhill AL, et al. Opioid receptors and signaling on cells from the immune system. *J Neuroimmune Pharmacol.* 2006;1:260–269.
42. Bidlack JM, Saripalli LD, Lawrence DM: kappa-Opioid binding sites on a murine lymphoma cell line. *Eur J Pharmacol.* 1992;227:257–265.
43. Carr DJ, DeCosta BR, Kim CH, et al. Opioid receptors on cells of the immune system: Evidence for delta- and kappa-classes. *J Endocrinol.* 1989;122:161–168.
44. Finley MJ, Happel CM, Kaminsky DE, et al. Opioid and nociceptin receptors regulate cytokine and cytokine receptor expression. *Cell Immunol.* 2008;252:146–154.
45. Watkins LR, Hutchinson MR, Milligan ED, et al. "Listening" and "talking" to neurons: Implications of immune activation for pain control and increasing the efficacy of opioids. *Brain Res Rev.* 2007;56:148–169.
46. Vallejo R, de Leon-Casasola O, Benyamin R. Opioid therapy and immunosuppression: A review. *Am J Ther.* 2004;11:354–365.
47. Tegeder I, Geisslinger G. Opioids as modulators of cell death and survival—unraveling mechanisms and revealing new indications. *Pharmacol Rev.* 2004;56:351–369.
48. Gupta K, Kshirsagar S, Chang L, et al. Morphine stimulates angiogenesis by activating proangiogenic and survival-promoting signaling and promotes breast tumor growth. *Cancer Res.* 2002;62:4491–4498.
49. Friesen C, Roscher M, Alt A, et al. Methadone, commonly used as maintenance medication for outpatient treatment of opioid dependence, kills leukemia cells and overcomes chemoresistance. *Cancer Res.* 2008;68:6059–6064.
50. Chen YL, Law PY, Loh HH. The other side of the opioid story: modulation of cell growth and survival signaling. *Curr Med Chem.* 2008;15:772–778.
51. Ishikawa M, Tanno K, Kamo A, et al. Enhancement of tumor growth by morphine and its possible mechanism in mice. *Biol Pharm Bull.* 1993;16:762–766.
52. Lotsch J, Stockmann A, Kobal G, et al. Pharmacokinetics of morphine and its glucuronides after intravenous infusion of morphine and morphine-6-glucuronide in healthy volunteers. *Clin Pharmacol Ther.* 1996;60:316–325.
53. Osborne R, Joel S, Trew D, et al. Morphine and metabolite behavior after different routes of morphine administration: Demonstration of the importance of the active metabolite morphine-6-glucuronide. *Clin Pharmacol Ther.* 1990;47:12–19.
54. Mignat C, Wille U, Ziegler A. Affinity profiles of morphine, codeine, dihydrocodeine and their glucuronides at opioid receptor subtypes. *Life Sci.* 1995;56:793–799.
55. Coller JK, Christrup LL, Somogyi AA. Role of active metabolites in the use of opioids. *Eur J Clin Pharmacol.* 2009;65:121–139.
56. Verbeeck RK. Pharmacokinetics and dosage adjustment in patients with hepatic dysfunction. *Eur J Clin Pharmacol.* 2008;64:1147–1161.
57. Tegeder I, Lotsch J, Geisslinger G. Pharmacokinetics of opioids in liver disease. *Clin Pharmacokinet.* 1999;37:17–40.
58. Faura CC, Collins SL, Moore RA, et al. Systematic review of factors affecting the ratios of morphine and its major metabolites. *Pain.* 1998;74:43–53.
59. Sawe J, Odar-Cederlof I. Kinetics of morphine in patients with renal failure. *Eur J Clin Pharmacol.* 1987;32:377–382.
60. Babul N, Darke AC, Hain R. Hydromorphone and metabolite pharmacokinetics in children. *J Pain Symptom Manage.* 1995;10:335–337.
61. Hagen N, Thirlwell MP, Dhaliwal HS, et al. Steady-state pharmacokinetics of hydromorphone and hydromorphone-3-glucuronide in cancer patients after immediate and controlled-release hydromorphone. *J Clin Pharmacol.* 1995;35:37–44.
62. Milne RW, Nation RL, Somogyi AA. The disposition of morphine and its 3- and 6-glucuronide metabolites in humans and animals, and the importance of the metabolites to the pharmacological effects of morphine. *Drug Metab Rev.* 1996;28:345–472.
63. Babul N, Darke AC, Hagen N. Hydromorphone metabolite accumulation in renal failure. *J Pain Symptom Manage.* 1995;10:184–186.
64. Gong QL, Hedner T, Hedner J, et al. Antinociceptive and ventilatory effects of the morphine metabolites: morphine-6-glucuronide and morphine-3-glucuronide. *Eur J Pharmacol.* 1991;193:47–56.
65. Labella FS, Pinsky C, Havlicek V. Morphine derivatives with diminished opiate receptor potency show enhanced central excitatory activity. *Brain Res.* 1979;174:263–271.
66. Yaksh TL, Harty GJ, Onofrio BM. High dose of spinal morphine produce a nonopiate receptor-mediated hyperesthesia: Clinical and theoretic implications. *Anesthesiology.* 1986;64:590–597.
67. Bartlett SE, Cramond T, Smith MT. The excitatory effects of morphine-3-glucuronide are attenuated by LY274614, a competitive NMDA receptor antagonist, and by midazolam, an agonist at the benzodiazepine site on the GABAA receptor complex. *Life Sci.* 1994;54:687–694.
68. Smith MT. Neuroexcitatory effects of morphine and hydromorphone: Evidence implicating the 3-glucuronide metabolites. *Clin Exp Pharmacol Physiol.* 2000;27:524–528.
69. Babul N, Darke AC. Putative role of hydromorphone metabolites in myoclonus. *Pain.* 1992;51:260–261.
70. Wright AW, Mather LE, Smith MT. Hydromorphone-3-glucuronide: A more potent neuro-excitant than its structural analogue, morphine-3-glucuronide. *Life Sci.* 2001;69:409–420.
71. Cherny NI. Opioid analgesics: Comparative features and prescribing guidelines. *Drugs.* 1996;51. 713–37.
72. McCarberg BH, Barkin RL. Long-acting opioids for chronic pain: Pharmacotherapeutic opportunities to enhance compliance, quality of life, and analgesia. *Am J Ther.* 2001;8:181–186.
73. Cherny NJ, Chang V, Frager G, et al. Opioid pharmacotherapy in the management of cancer pain: A survey of strategies used by pain physicians for the selection of analgesic drugs and routes of administration. *Cancer.* 1995;76:1283–1293.
74. Tassain V, Attal N, Fletcher D, et al. Long term effects of oral sustained release morphine on neuropsychological performance in patients with chronic noncancer pain. *Pain.* 2003;104:389–400.

75. Ferrell B, Wisdom C, Wenzl C, et al. Effects of controlled-released morphine on quality of life for cancer pain. *Oncol Nurs Forum.* 1989;16:521–526.
76. Marcus DA, Glick RM. Sustained-release oxycodone dosing survey of chronic pain patients. *Clin J Pain.* 2004;20:363–366.
77. Levy MH. Pharmacologic treatment of cancer pain. *N Engl J Med.* 1996;335:1124–1132.
78. Hanks GW, Conno F, Cherny N, et al. Morphine and alternative opioids in cancer pain: The EAPC recommendations. *Br J Cancer.* 2001;84:587–593.
79. Galer BS, Coyle N, Pasternak GW, et al. Individual variability in the response to different opioids: report of five cases. *Pain.* 1992;49:87–91.
80. Fitzgibbon DR, Galer BS. The efficacy of opioids in cancer pain syndromes. *Pain.* 1994;58:429–431.
81. Coluzzi PH. Oral patient-controlled analgesia. *Semin Oncol.* 1997;24:S16–35–42.
82. Pappagallo M, Dickerson ED, Hulka S. Palliative care and hospice opioid dosing guidelines with breakthrough pain (BP) doses. *Am J Hosp Palliat Care.* 2000;17:407–413.
83. Cherny N, Ripamonti C, Pereira J, et al. Strategies to manage the adverse effects of oral morphine: An evidence-based report. *J Clin Oncol.* 2001;19:2542–2554.
84. Vermeire A, Remon JP, Rosseel MT, et al. Variability of morphine disposition during long-term subcutaneous infusion in terminally ill cancer patients. *Eur J Clin Pharmacol.* 1998;53:325–330.
85. Mikkelsen Lynch P, Butler J, et al. A pharmacokinetic and tolerability evaluation of two continuous subcutaneous infusion systems compared to an oral controlled-release morphine. *J Pain Symptom Manage.* 2000;19:348–356.
86. Hoskin PJ, Hanks GW, Aherne GW, et al. The bioavailability and pharmacokinetics of morphine after intravenous, oral and buccal administration in healthy volunteers. *Br J Clin Pharmacol.* 1989;27:499–505.
87. Sawe J, Dahlstrom B, Rane A. Steady-state kinetics and analgesic effect of oral morphine in cancer patients. *Eur J Clin Pharmacol.* 1983;24:537–542.
88. Sawe J. High-dose morphine and methadone in cancer patients. Clinical pharmacokinetic considerations of oral treatment. *Clin Pharmacokinet.* 1986;11:87–106.
89. Savarese JJ, Goldenheim PD, Thomas GB, et al. Steady-state pharmacokinetics of controlled release oral morphine sulphate in healthy subjects. *Clin Pharmacokinet.* 1986;11:505–510.
90. Poulain P, Hoskin PJ, Hanks GW, et al. Relative bioavailability of controlled release morphine tablets (MST continus) in cancer patients. *Br J Anaesth.* 1988;61:569–574.
91. Hanks GW. Controlled-release morphine (MST Contin) in advanced cancer. The European experience. *Cancer.* 1989;63:2378–2382.
92. Brunk SF, Delle M. Morphine metabolism in man. *Clin Pharmacol Ther.* 1974;16:51–57.
93. Sawe J, Dahlstrom B, Paalzow L, et al. Morphine kinetics in cancer patients. *Clin Pharmacol Ther.* 1981;30:629–635.
94. Westerling D, Lindahl S, Andersson KE, et al. Absorption and bioavailability of rectally administered morphine in women. *Eur J Clin Pharmacol.* 1982;23:59–64.
95. Baillie SP, Bateman DN, Coates PE, et al. Age and the pharmacokinetics of morphine. *Age Ageing.* 1989;18:258–262.
96. Owen JA, Sitar DS, Berger L, et al. Age-related morphine kinetics. *Clin Pharmacol Ther.* 1983;34:364–368.
97. Davies G, Kingswood C, Street M. Pharmacokinetics of opioids in renal dysfunction. *Clin Pharmacokinet.* 1996;31:410–422.
98. Chan GL, Matzke GR. Effects of renal insufficiency on the pharmacokinetics and pharmacodynamics of opioid analgesics. *Drug Intell Clin Pharm.* 1987;21:773–783.
99. Sawe J, Svensson JO, Rane A. Morphine metabolism in cancer patients on increasing oral doses—no evidence for autoinduction or dose-dependence. *Br J Clin Pharmacol.* 1983;16:85–93.
100. Wiffen PJ, McQuay HJ. Oral morphine for cancer pain. *Cochrane Database Syst Rev.* 2007:CD003868.
101. Hunt TL, Kaiko RF. Comparison of the pharmacokinetic profiles of two oral controlled-release morphine formulations in healthy young adults. *Clin Ther.* 1991;13:482–488.
102. Broomhead A, Kerr R, Tester W, et al. Comparison of a once-a-day sustained-release morphine formulation with standard oral morphine treatment for cancer pain. *J Pain Symptom Manage.* 1997;14:63–73.
103. Gourlay GK, Cherry DA, Onley MM, et al. Pharmacokinetics and pharmacodynamics of twenty-four-hourly Kapanol compared to twelve-hourly MS Contin in the treatment of severe cancer pain. *Pain.* 1997;69:295–302.
104. Portenoy RK, Sciberras A, Eliot L, et al. Steady-state pharmacokinetic comparison of a new, extended-release, once-daily morphine formulation, Avinza, and a twice-daily controlled-release morphine formulation in patients with chronic moderate-to-severe pain. *J Pain Symptom Manage.* 2002;23:292–300.
105. De Conno F, Ripamonti C, Fagnoni E, et al. The MERITO Study: A multicentre trial of the analgesic effect and tolerability of normal-release oral morphine during 'titration phase' in patients with cancer pain. *Palliat Med.* 2008;22:214–221.
106. Dale O, Piribauer M, Kaasa S, et al. A double-blind, randomized, crossover comparison between single-dose and double-dose immediate-release oral morphine at bedtime in cancer patients. *J Pain Symptom Manage.* 2009;37:68–76.
107. Bohn LM, Lefkowitz RJ, Gainetdinov RR, et al. Enhanced morphine analgesia in mice lacking beta-arrestin 2. *Science.* 1999;286:2495–2498.
108. Ross JR, Rutter D, Welsh K, et al. Clinical response to morphine in cancer patients and genetic variation in candidate genes. *Pharmacogenomics J.* 2005;5:324–336.
109. Rakvag TT, Klepstad P, Baar C, et al. The Val158Met polymorphism of the human catechol-O-methyltransferase (COMT) gene may influence morphine requirements in cancer pain patients. *Pain.* 2005;116:73–78.
110. Poyhia R, Seppala T. Liposolubility and protein binding of oxycodone in vitro. *Pharmacol Toxicol.* 1994;74:23–27.
111. Chen ZR, Irvine RJ, Somogyi AA, et al. Mu receptor binding of some commonly used opioids and their metabolites. *Life Sci.* 1991;48:2165–2171.
112. Ross FB, Smith MT. The intrinsic antinociceptive effects of oxycodone appear to be kappa-opioid receptor mediated. *Pain.* 1997;73:151–157.
113. Lemberg KK, Kontinen VK, Siiskonen AO, et al. Antinociception by spinal and systemic oxycodone: why does the route make a difference? In vitro and in vivo studies in rats. *Anesthesiology.* 2006;105:801–812.
114. Lalovic B, Kharasch E, Hoffer C, et al. Pharmacokinetics and pharmacodynamics of oral oxycodone in healthy human subjects: role of circulating active metabolites. *Clin Pharmacol Ther.* 2006;79:461–479.
115. Kalso E, Vainio A, Mattila MJ, et al. Morphine and oxycodone in the management of cancer pain: Plasma levels determined by chemical and radioreceptor assays. *Pharmacol Toxicol.* 1990;67:322–328.
116. Zwisler ST, Enggaard TP, Noehr-Jensen L, et al. The hypoalgesic effect of oxycodone in human experimental pain models in relation to the CYP2D6 oxidation polymorphism. *Basic Clin Pharmacol Toxicol.* 2009;104:335–344.
117. Kalso E. Oxycodone. *J Pain Symptom Manage.* 2005;29:S47-56.
118. Mandema JW, Kaiko RF, Oshlack B, et al. Characterization and validation of a pharmacokinetic model for controlled-release oxycodone. *Br J Clin Pharmacol.* 1996;42:747–756.
119. Leow KP, Smith MT, Watt JA, et al. Comparative oxycodone pharmacokinetics in humans after intravenous, oral, and rectal administration. *Ther Drug Monit.* 1992;14:479–484.
120. Leow KP, Smith MT, Williams B, et al. Single-dose and steady-state pharmacokinetics and pharmacodynamics of oxycodone in patients with cancer. *Clin Pharmacol Ther.* 1992;52:487–495.
121. Kalso E, Vainio A. Morphine and oxycodone hydrochloride in the management of cancer pain. *Clin Pharmacol Ther.* 1990;47:639–646.
122. Beaver WT, Wallenstein SL, Rogers A, et al. Analgesic studies of codeine and oxycodone in patients with cancer. II. Comparisons of intramuscular oxycodone with intramuscular morphine and codeine. *J Pharmacol Exp Ther.* 1978;207:101–108.
123. Beaver WT, Wallenstein SL, Rogers A, et al. Analgesic studies of codeine and oxycodone in patients with cancer. I. Comparisons of oral with intramuscular codeine and of oral with intramuscular oxycodone. *J Pharmacol Exp Ther.* 1978;207:92–100.
124. Glare PA, Walsh TD. Dose-ranging study of oxycodone for chronic pain in advanced cancer. *J Clin Oncol.* 1993;11:973–978.
125. Maddocks I, Somogyi A, Abbott F, et al. Attenuation of morphine-induced delirium in palliative care by substitution with infusion of oxycodone. *J Pain Symptom Manage.* 1996;12:182–189.

126. Heiskanen T, Kalso E. Controlled-release oxycodone and morphine in cancer related pain. *Pain.* 1997;73:37–45.
127. Reid CM, Martin RM, Sterne JA, et al. Oxycodone for cancer-related pain: meta-analysis of randomized controlled trials. *Arch Intern Med.* 2006;166:837–843.
128. Ananthan S, Khare NK, Saini SK, et al. Identification of opioid ligands possessing mixed micro agonist/delta antagonist activity among pyridomorphinans derived from naloxone, oxymorphone, and hydromorphone [correction of hydropmorphone]. *J Med Chem.* 2004;47:1400–1412.
129. Hale ME, Dvergsten C, Gimbel J. Efficacy and safety of oxymorphone extended release in chronic low back pain: results of a randomized, double-blind, placebo- and active-controlled phase III study. *J Pain.* 2005;6:21–28.
130. Adams MP, Ahdieh H. Single- and multiple-dose pharmacokinetic and dose-proportionality study of oxymorphone immediate-release tablets. *Drugs R D.* 2005;6:91–99.
131. Adams M, Pieniaszek HJ Jr, Gammaitoni AR, et al. Oxymorphone extended release does not affect CYP2C9 or CYP3A4 metabolic pathways. *J Clin Pharmacol.* 2005;45:337–345.
132. Sloan P, Slatkin N, Ahdieh H. Effectiveness and safety of oral extended-release oxymorphone for the treatment of cancer pain: A pilot study. *Support Care Cancer.* 2005;13:57–65.
133. Gabrail NY, Dvergsten C, Ahdieh H. Establishing the dosage equivalency of oxymorphone extended release and oxycodone controlled release in patients with cancer pain: A randomized controlled study. *Curr Med Res Opin.* 2004;20:911–918.
134. Vallner JJ, Stewart JT, Kotzan JA, et al. Pharmacokinetics and bioavailability of hydromorphone following intravenous and oral administration to human subjects. *J Clin Pharmacol.* 1981;21:152–156.
135. Ritschel WA, Parab PV, Denson DD, et al. Absolute bioavailability of hydromorphone after peroral and rectal administration in humans: saliva/plasma ratio and clinical effects. *J Clin Pharmacol.* 1987;27:647–653.
136. Fainsinger R, Schoeller T, Boiskin M, et al. Palliative care round: Cognitive failure and coma after renal failure in a patient receiving captopril and hydromorphone. *J Palliat Care.* 1993;9:53–55.
137. Quigley C. Hydromorphone for acute and chronic pain. *Cochrane Database Syst Rev.* 2002:CD003447.
138. Fischer BD, Carrigan KA, Dykstra LA. Effects of N-methyl-D-aspartate receptor antagonists on acute morphine-induced and l-methadone-induced antinociception in mice. *J Pain.* 2005;6:425–433.
139. Toombs JD, Kral LA. Methadone treatment for pain states. *Am Fam Physician.* 2005;71:1353–1358.
140. Ayonrinde OT, Bridge DT. The rediscovery of methadone for cancer pain management. *Med J Aust.* 2000;173:536–540.
141. Davis MP, Walsh D. Methadone for relief of cancer pain: A review of pharmacokinetics, pharmacodynamics, drug interactions and protocols of administration. *Support Care Cancer.* 2001;9:73–83.
142. Ripamonti C, Zecca E, Bruera E. An update on the clinical use of methadone for cancer pain. *Pain.* 1997;70:109–115.
143. Kreek MJ, Schecter AJ, Gutjahr CL, et al. Methadone use in patients with chronic renal disease. *Drug Alcohol Depend.* 1980;5:197–205.
144. Leng G, Finnegan MJ. Successful use of methadone in nociceptive cancer pain unresponsive to morphine. *Palliat Med.* 1994;8:153–155.
145. Crews JC, Sweeney NJ, Denson DD. Clinical efficacy of methadone in patients refractory to other mu-opioid receptor agonist analgesics for management of terminal cancer pain. Case presentations and discussion of incomplete cross-tolerance among opioid agonist analgesics. *Cancer.* 1993;72:2266–2272.
146. Manfredi PL, Borsook D, Chandler SW, et al. Intravenous methadone for cancer pain unrelieved by morphine and hydromorphone: Clinical observations. *Pain.* 1997;70:99–101.
147. Fitzgibbon DR, Ready LB. Intravenous high-dose methadone administered by patient controlled analgesia and continuous infusion for the treatment of cancer pain refractory to high-dose morphine. *Pain.* 1997;73:259–261.
148. Bruera E, Pereira J, Watanabe S, et al. Opioid rotation in patients with cancer pain. A retrospective comparison of dose ratios between methadone, hydromorphone, and morphine. *Cancer.* 1996;78:852–857.
149. Lawlor PG, Turner KS, Hanson J, et al. Dose ratio between morphine and methadone in patients with cancer pain: A retrospective study. *Cancer.* 1998;82:1167–1173.
150. Ripamonti C, DeConno F, Groff L, et al. Equianalgesic dose/ratio between methadone and other opioid agonists in cancer pain: Comparison of two clinical experiences. *Ann Oncol.* 1998;9:79–83.
151. Fainsinger R, Schoeller T, Bruera E. Methadone in the management of cancer pain: A review. *Pain.* 1993;52:137–147.
152. Plummer JL, Gourlay GK, Cherry DA, et al. Estimation of methadone clearance: Application in the management of cancer pain. *Pain.* 1988;33:313–322.
153. Izzo AA. Drug interactions with St. John's Wort (Hypericum perforatum): A review of the clinical evidence. *Int J Clin Pharmacol Ther.* 2004;42:139–148.
154. Corkery JM, Schifano F, Ghodse AH, et al. The effects of methadone and its role in fatalities. *Hum Psychopharmacol.* 2004;19:565–576.
155. Boulton DW, Arnaud P, DeVane CL. A single dose of methadone inhibits cytochrome P-4503A activity in healthy volunteers as assessed by the urinary cortisol ratio. *Br J Clin Pharmacol.* 2001;51:350–354.
156. Ballesteros MF, Budnitz DS, Sanford CP, et al. Increase in deaths due to methadone in North Carolina. *JAMA.* 2003;290:40.
157. Hickman M, Madden P, Henry J, et al. Trends in drug overdose deaths in England and Wales 1993-98: methadone does not kill more people than heroin. *Addiction.* 2003;98:419–425.
158. Kornick CA, Kilborn MJ, Santiago-Palma J, et al. QTc interval prolongation associated with intravenous methadone. *Pain.* 2003;105:499–506.
159. Krantz MJ, Lewkowiez L, Hays H, et al. Torsade de pointes associated with very-high-dose methadone. *Ann Intern Med.* 2002;137:501–504.
160. Walker PW, Klein D, Kasza L. High dose methadone and ventricular arrhythmias: A report of three cases. *Pain.* 2003;103:321–324.
161. Sanguinetti MC, Jiang C, Curran ME, et al. A mechanistic link between an inherited and an acquired cardiac arrhythmia: HERG encodes the IKr potassium channel. *Cell.* 1995;81:299–307.
162. Katchman AN, McGroary KA, Kilborn MJ, et al. Influence of opioid agonists on cardiac human ether-a-go-go-related gene K(+) currents. *J Pharmacol Exp Ther.* 2002;303:688–694.
163. Rendig SV, Amsterdam EA, Henderson GL, et al. Comparative cardiac contractile actions of six narcotic analgesics: morphine, meperidine, pentazocine, fentanyl, methadone and l-alpha-acetylmethadol (LAAM). *J Pharmacol Exp Ther.* 1980;215:259–265.
164. Wesley RC Jr, Turnquest P. Torsades de pointe after intravenous adenosine in the presence of prolonged QT syndrome. *Am Heart J.* 1992;123:794–796.
165. Bednar MM, Harrigan EP, Anziano RJ, et al. The QT interval. *Prog Cardiovasc Dis.* 2001;43:1–45.
166. Roden DM. Drug-induced prolongation of the QT interval. *N Engl J Med.* 2004;350:1013–1022.
167. Pearson EC, Woosley RL. QT prolongation and torsades de pointes among methadone users: reports to the FDA spontaneous reporting system. *Pharmacoepidemiol Drug Saf.* 2005;14: 747–753.
168. Krantz MJ, Martin J, Stimmel B, et al. QTc Interval Screening in Methadone Treatment. *Ann Intern Med.* 2009;120:387–395.
169. Bruera E, Palmer JL, Bosnjak S, et al. Methadone versus morphine as a first-line strong opioid for cancer pain: A randomized, double-blind study. *J Clin Oncol.* 2004;22:185–192.
170. Nicholson AB. Methadone for cancer pain. *Cochrane Database Syst Rev.* 2007:CD003971.
171. Inturrisi CE, Colburn WA, Kaiko RF, et al. Pharmacokinetics and pharmacodynamics of methadone in patients with chronic pain. *Clin Pharmacol Ther.* 1987;41:392–401.
172. Tive L, Ginsberg K, Pick CG, et al. Kappa 3 receptors and levorphanol-induced analgesia. *Neuropharmacology.* 1992;31:851–856.
173. Moulin DE, Ling GS, Pasternak GW. Unidirectional analgesic cross-tolerance between morphine and levorphanol in the rat. *Pain.* 1988;33:P 233-9.
174. Wang Y, Li JG, Huang P, et al. Differential effects of agonists on adenylyl cyclase superactivation mediated by the kappa opioid receptors: Adenylyl cyclase superactivation is independent of agonist-induced phosphorylation, desensitization, internalization, and down-regulation. *J Pharmacol Exp Ther.* 2003;307:1127–1134.
175. Zhang A, Xiong W, Bidlack JM, et al. 10-Ketomorphinan and 3-substituted-3-desoxymorphinan analogues as mixed kappa and micro opioid ligands: synthesis and biological evaluation of their binding affinity at opioid receptors. *J Med Chem.* 2004;47:165–174.

176. Stringer M, Makin MK, Miles J, et al. D-morphine, but not l-morphine, has low micromolar affinity for the non-competitive N-methyl-D-aspartate site in rat forebrain. Possible clinical implications for the management of neuropathic pain. *Neurosci Lett.* 2000;295:21–24.
177. Codd EE, Shank RP, Schupsky JJ, et al. Serotonin and norepinephrine uptake inhibiting activity of centrally acting analgesics: structural determinants and role in antinociception. *J Pharmacol Exp Ther.* 1995;274:1263–1270.
178. Weinberg DS, Inturrisi CE, Reidenberg B, et al. Sublingual absorption of selected opioid analgesics. *Clin Pharmacol Ther.* 1988;44:335–342.
179. Dixon R, Crews T, Inturrisi C, et al. Levorphanol: Pharmacokinetics and steady-state plasma concentrations in patients with pain. *Res Commun Chem Pathol Pharmacol.* 1983;41:3–17.
180. McNulty JP. Can levorphanol be used like methadone for intractable refractory pain? *J Palliat Med.* 2007;10:293–296.
181. Jeal W, Benfield P. Transdermal fentanyl. A review of its pharmacological properties and therapeutic efficacy in pain control. *Drugs.* 1997;53:109–138.
182. Marquardt KA, Tharratt RS, Musallam NA. Fentanyl remaining in a transdermal system following three days of continuous use. *Ann Pharmacother.* 1995;29:969–971.
183. Lilleng PK, Mehlum LI, Bachs L, et al. Deaths after intravenous misuse of transdermal fentanyl. *J Forensic Sci.* 2004;49:1364–1366.
184. Tharp AM, Winecker RE, Winston DC. Fatal intravenous fentanyl abuse: four cases involving extraction of fentanyl from transdermal patches. *Am J Forensic Med Pathol.* 2004;25:178–181.
185. Kramer C, Tawney M. A fatal overdose of transdermally administered fentanyl. *J Am Osteopath Assoc.* 1998;98:385–386.
186. Liappas IA, Dimopoulos NP, Mellos E, et al. Oral transmucosal abuse of transdermal fentanyl. *J Psychopharmacol.* 2004;18: 277–280.
187. Woodall KL, Martin TL, McLellan BA. Oral abuse of fentanyl patches (Duragesic): seven case reports. *J Forensic Sci.* 2008;53:222–225.
188. Coon TP, Miller M, Kaylor D, et al. Rectal insertion of fentanyl patches: A new route of toxicity. *Ann Emerg Med.* 2005;46:473.
189. Marquardt KA, Tharratt RS. Inhalation abuse of fentanyl patch. *J Toxicol Clin Toxicol.* 1994;32:75–78.
190. Hair PI, Keating GM, McKeage K. Transdermal matrix fentanyl membrane patch (matrifen): In severe cancer-related chronic pain. *Drugs.* 2008;68:2001–2009.
191. Marier JF, Lor M, Morin J, et al. Comparative bioequivalence study between a novel matrix transdermal delivery system of fentanyl and a commercially available reservoir formulation. *Br J Clin Pharmacol.* 2007;63:121–124.
192. Varvel JR, Shafer SL, Hwang SS, et al. Absorption characteristics of transdermally administered fentanyl. *Anesthesiology.* 1989;70:928–934.
193. Solassol I, Bressolle F, Caumette L, et al. Inter- and intraindividual variabilities in pharmacokinetics of fentanyl after repeated 72-hour transdermal applications in cancer pain patients. *Ther Drug Monit.* 2005;27:491–498.
194. Muijsers RB, Wagstaff AJ. Transdermal fentanyl: An updated review of its pharmacological properties and therapeutic efficacy in chronic cancer pain control. *Drugs.* 2001;61:2289–2307.
195. Portenoy RK, Southam MA, Gupta SK, et al. Transdermal fentanyl for cancer pain. Repeated dose pharmacokinetics. *Anesthesiology.* 1993;78:36–43.
196. Gourlay GK. Treatment of cancer pain with transdermal fentanyl. *Lancet Oncol.* 2001;2:165–172.
197. Solassol I, Caumette L, Bressolle F, et al. Inter- and intra-individual variability in transdermal fentanyl absorption in cancer pain patients. *Oncol Rep.* 2005;14:1029–1036.
198. Frolich MA, Giannotti A, Modell JH. Opioid overdose in a patient using a fentanyl patch during treatment with a warming blanket. *Anesth Analg.* 2001;93:647–648.
199. Donner B, Zenz M, Tryba M, et al. Direct conversion from oral morphine to transdermal fentanyl: A multicenter study in patients with cancer pain. *Pain.* 1996;64:527–534.
200. Donner B, Zenz M, Strumpf M, et al. Long-term treatment of cancer pain with transdermal fentanyl. *J Pain Symptom Manage.* 1998;15:168–175.
201. Grond S, Zech D, Lehmann KA, et al. Transdermal fentanyl in the long-term treatment of cancer pain: A prospective study of 50 patients with advanced cancer of the gastrointestinal tract or the head and neck region. *Pain.* 1997;69:191–198.
202. Korte W, de Stoutz N, Morant R. Day-to-day titration to initiate transdermal fentanyl in patients with cancer pain: short- and long-term experiences in a prospective study of 39 patients. *J Pain Symptom Manage.* 1996;11:139–146.
203. Payne R. Transdermal fentanyl: suggested recommendations for clinical use. *J Pain Symptom Manage.* 1992;7:S40-4.
204. Payne R, Chandler S, Einhaus M. Guidelines for the clinical use of transdermal fentanyl. *Anticancer Drugs.* 1995;6 Suppl 3:50–53.
205. Payne R, Mathias SD, Pasta DJ, et al. Quality of life and cancer pain: satisfaction and side effects with transdermal fentanyl versus oral morphine. *J Clin Oncol.* 1998;16:1588–1593.
206. Zech DF, Grond SU, Lynch J, et al. Transdermal fentanyl and initial dose-finding with patient-controlled analgesia in cancer pain. A pilot study with 20 terminally ill cancer patients. *Pain.* 1992;50:293–301.
207. Zech DF, Lehmann KA. Transdermal fentanyl in combination with initial intravenous dose titration by patient-controlled analgesia. *Anticancer Drugs.* 1995;6(Suppl 3):44-9.
208. Gourlay GK, Mather LE. Pharmacokinetics and Pharmacodynamics. In: Lehmann KA, Zech D, eds. Transdermal Fentanyl. Berlin: Springer-Verlag, 1991:119–140.
209. Sandler AN, Baxter AD, Katz J, et al. A double-blind, placebo-controlled trial of transdermal fentanyl after abdominal hysterectomy. Analgesic, respiratory, and pharmacokinetic effects. *Anesthesiology.* 1994;81:1169–1180.
210. Sathyan G, Jaskowiak J, Evashenk M, et al. Characterisation of the pharmacokinetics of the fentanyl HCl patient-controlled transdermal system (PCTS): Effect of current magnitude and multiple-day dosing and comparison with IV fentanyl administration. *Clin Pharmacokinet.* 2005;44(Suppl 1):7-15.
211. Fine PG, Marcus M, De Boer, AJ, et al. An open label study of oral transmucosal fentanyl citrate (OTFC) for the treatment of breakthrough cancer pain. *Pain.* 1991;45:149–153.
212. Streisand JB, Varvel JR, Stanski DR, et al. Absorption and bioavailability of oral transmucosal fentanyl citrate. *Anesthesiology.* 1991;75:223–229.
213. Christie JM, Simmonds M, Patt R, et al. Dose-titration, multicenter study of oral transmucosal fentanyl citrate for the treatment of breakthrough pain in cancer patients using transdermal fentanyl for persistent pain. *J Clin Oncol.* 1998;16:3238–3245.
214. Farrar JT, Cleary J, Rauck R, et al. Oral transmucosal fentanyl citrate: randomized, double-blinded, placebo-controlled trial for treatment of breakthrough pain in cancer patients. *J Natl Cancer Inst.* 1998;90:611–616.
215. Coluzzi PH, Schwartzberg L, Conroy JD, et al. Breakthrough cancer pain: A randomized trial comparing oral transmucosal fentanyl citrate (OTFC) and morphine sulfate immediate release (MSIR). *Pain.* 2001;91:123–130.
216. Zeppetella G, Ribeiro MD. Opioids for the management of breakthrough (episodic) pain in cancer patients. *Cochrane Database Syst Rev.* 2006:CD004311.
217. Darwish M, Kirby M, Jiang JG, et al. Bioequivalence following buccal and sublingual placement of fentanyl buccal tablet 400 microg in healthy subjects. *Clin Drug Investig.* 2008;28:1–7.
218. Eichman JD, Robinson JR. Mechanistic studies on effervescent-induced permeability enhancement. *Pharm Res.* 1998;15:925–930.
219. Darwish M, Tempero K, Kirby M, et al. Relative bioavailability of the fentanyl effervescent buccal tablet (FEBT) 1,080 pg versus oral transmucosal fentanyl citrate 1,600 pg and dose proportionality of FEBT 270 to 1,300 microg: A single-dose, randomized, open-label, three-period study in healthy adult volunteers. *Clin Ther.* 2006;28:715–724.
220. Darwish M, Kirby M, Robertson P, et al. Absorption of fentanyl from fentanyl buccal tablet in cancer patients with or without oral mucositis: A pilot study. *Clin Drug Investig.* 2007;27:605–611.
221. Blick SK, Wagstaff AJ. Fentanyl buccal tablet: In breakthrough pain in opioid-tolerant patients with cancer. *Drugs.* 2006;66:2387–2393;discussion 2394-5.
222. Portenoy RK, Taylor D, Messina J, et al. A Randomized, Placebo-controlled Study of Fentanyl Buccal Tablet for Breakthrough Pain in Opioid-treated Patients With Cancer. *Clin J Pain.* 2006;22:805–811.
223. Slatkin NE, Xie F, Messina J, et al. Fentanyl buccal tablet for relief of breakthrough pain in opioid-tolerant patients with cancer-related chronic pain. *J Support Oncol.* 2007;5:327–334.
224. Davis MP. Buprenorphine in cancer pain. *Support Care Cancer.* 2005;13:878–887.

225. Evans HC, Easthope SE. Transdermal buprenorphine. *Drugs.* 2003;63:1999–2010.
226. Sittl R. Transdermal buprenorphine in the treatment of chronic pain. *Expert Rev Neurother.* 2005;5:315–323.
227. Muriel C, Failde I, Mico JA, et al. Effectiveness and tolerability of the buprenorphine transdermal system in patients with moderate to severe chronic pain: A multicenter, open-label, uncontrolled, prospective, observational clinical study. *Clin Ther.* 2005;27:451–462.
228. Otton SV, Schadel M, Cheung SW, et al. CYP2D6 phenotype determines the metabolic conversion of hydrocodone to hydromorphone. *Clin Pharmacol Ther.* 1993;54:463–472.
229. Homsi J, Walsh D, Nelson KA, et al. A phase II study of hydrocodone for cough in advanced cancer. *Am J Hosp Palliat Care.* 2002;19:49–56.
230. Walsh SL, Nuzzo PA, Lofwall MR, et al. The relative abuse liability of oral oxycodone, hydrocodone and hydromorphone assessed in prescription opioid abusers. *Drug Alcohol Depend.* 2008;98:191–202.
231. Fiellin DA. Treatment of adolescent opioid dependence: no quick fix. *JAMA.* 2008;300:2057–2059.
232. Wu LT, Pilowsky DJ, Patkar AA. Non-prescribed use of pain relievers among adolescents in the United States. *Drug Alcohol Depend.* 2008;94:1–11.
233. Rodriguez RF, Castillo JM, Castillo MP, et al. Hydrocodone/acetaminophen and tramadol chlorhydrate combination tablets for the management of chronic cancer pain: A double-blind comparative trial. *Clin J Pain.* 2008;24:1–4.
234. Jacox A, Carr DB, Payne R. New clinical-practice guidelines for the management of pain in patients with cancer. *N Engl J Med.* 1994;330:651–655.
235. Levy MH. Pharmacologic management of cancer pain. *Semin Oncol.* 1994;21:718–739.
236. Susce MT, Murray-Carmichael E, de Leon J. Response to hydrocodone, codeine and oxycodone in a CYP2D6 poor metabolizer. *Prog Neuropsychopharmacol Biol Psychiatry.* 2006;30:1356–1358.
237. Ereshefsky L, Riesenman C, Lam YW. Antidepressant drug interactions and the cytochrome P450 system. The role of cytochrome P450 2D6. *Clin Pharmacokinet.* 1995;29(Suppl 1):10–18.
238. Sindrup SH, Arendt N-L, Brosen K, et al. The effect of quinidine on the analgesic effect of codeine. *Eur J Clin Pharmacol.* 1992;42:587–591.
239. Sindrup SH, Brosen K. The pharmacogenetics of codeine hypoalgesia. *Pharmacogenetics.* 1995;5:335–346.
240. Gourlay GK. Advances in opioid pharmacology. *Support Care Cancer.* 2005;13:153–159.
241. Eckhardt K, Li S, Ammon S, et al. Same incidence of adverse drug events after codeine administration irrespective of the genetically determined differences in morphine formation. *Pain.* 1998;76:27–33.
242. Mikus G, Trausch B, Rodewald C, et al. Effect of codeine on gastrointestinal motility in relation to CYP2D6 phenotype. *Clin Pharmacol Ther.* 1997;61:459–466.
243. Schmidt H, Vormfelde SV, Walchner-Bonjean M, et al. The role of active metabolites in dihydrocodeine effects. *Int J Clin Pharmacol Ther.* 2003;41:95–106.
244. Schmidt H, Vormfelde S, Klinder K, et al. Affinities of dihydrocodeine and its metabolites to opioid receptors. *Pharmacol Toxicol.* 2002;91:57–63.
245. Edwards JE, McQuay HJ, Moore RA. Single dose dihydrocodeine for acute postoperative pain. *Cochrane Database Syst Rev.* 2000:CD002760.
246. Collins SL, Edwards JE, Moore RA, et al. Single dose dextropropoxyphene, alone and with paracetamol (acetaminophen), for postoperative pain. *Cochrane Database Syst Rev.* 2000:CD001440.
247. Barkin RL, Barkin SJ, Barkin DS. Propoxyphene (dextropropoxyphene): A critical review of a weak opioid analgesic that should remain in antiquity. *Am J Ther.* 2006;13:534–542.
248. Afshari R, Maxwell S, Dawson A, et al. ECG abnormalities in co-proxamol (paracetamol/dextropropoxyphene) poisoning. *Clin Toxicol (Phila).* 2005;43:255–259.
249. Ulens C, Daenens P, Tytgat J. Norpropoxyphene-induced cardiotoxicity is associated with changes in ion-selectivity and gating of HERG currents. *Cardiovasc Res.* 1999;44:568–578.
250. Minami K, Uezono Y, Ueta Y. Pharmacological aspects of the effects of tramadol on G-protein coupled receptors. *J Pharmacol Sci.* 2007;103:253–260.
251. Raffa RB, Friderichs E, Reimann W, et al. Complementary and synergistic antinociceptive interaction between the enantiomers of tramadol. *J Pharmacol Exp Ther.* 1993;267:331–340.
252. Leppert W, Luczak J. The role of tramadol in cancer pain treatment—a review. *Support Care Cancer.* 2005;13:5–17.
253. Gan SH, Ismail R, Wan Adnan WA, et al. Impact of CYP2D6 genetic polymorphism on tramadol pharmacokinetics and pharmacodynamics. *Mol Diagn Ther.* 2007;11:171–181.
254. Teppema LJ, Nieuwenhuijs D, Olievier CN, et al. Respiratory depression by tramadol in the cat: Involvement of opioid receptors. *Anesthesiology.* 2003;98:420–427.
255. Barnung SK, Treschow M, Borgbjerg FM. Respiratory depression following oral tramadol in a patient with impaired renal function. *Pain.* 1997;71:111–112.
256. Rowbotham MC, Twilling L, Davies PS, et al. Oral opioid therapy for chronic peripheral and central neuropathic pain. *N Engl J Med.* 2003;348:1223–1232.
257. Sindrup SH, Andersen G, Madsen C, et al. Tramadol relieves pain and allodynia in polyneuropathy: A randomised, double-blind, controlled trial. *Pain.* 1999;83:85–90.
258. Wilder-Smith CH, Schimke J, Osterwalder B, et al. Oral tramadol, a mu-opioid agonist and monoamine reuptake-blocker, and morphine for strong cancer-related pain. *Ann Oncol.* 1994;5:141–146.
259. Marinangeli F, Ciccozzi A, Aloisio L, et al. Improved cancer pain treatment using combined fentanyl-TTS and tramadol. *Pain Pract.* 2007;7:307–312.
260. Boureau F, Legallicier P, Kabir-Ahmadi M. Tramadol in post-herpetic neuralgia: A randomized, double-blind, placebo-controlled trial. *Pain.* 2003;104:323–331.
261. Harati Y, Gooch C, Swenson M, et al. Double-blind randomized trial of tramadol for the treatment of the pain of diabetic neuropathy. *Neurology.* 1998;50:1842–1846.
262. Cherny NI, Portenoy RK. Cancer pain management. Current strategy. *Cancer.* 1993;72:3393–3415.
263. Meuret G, Jocham H. Patient-controlled analgesia (PCA) in the domiciliary care of tumour patients. *Cancer Treat Rev.* 1996;22(Suppl A):137-40.
264. Patt RB. PCA: Prescribing analgesia for home management of severe pain. *Geriatrics.* 1992;47:69–72.
265. Swanson G, Smith J, Bulich R, et al. Patient-controlled analgesia for chronic cancer pain in the ambulatory setting: A report of 117 patients. *J Clin Oncol.* 1989;7:1903–1908.
266. Enting RH, Oldenmenger WH, van der Rijt CC, et al. A prospective study evaluating the response of patients with unrelieved cancer pain to parenteral opioids. *Cancer.* 2002;94:3049–3056.
267. Mao J, Price DD, Mayer DJ. Mechanisms of hyperalgesia and morphine tolerance: A current view of their possible interactions. *Pain.* 1995;62:259–274.
268. Gorman AL, Elliott KJ, Inturrisi CE. The d- and l- isomers of methadone bind to the non-competitive site on the N-methyl-D-aspartate (NMDA) receptor in rat forebrain and spinal cord. *Neurosci Lett.* 1997;223:5–8.
269. Rapp SE, Egan KJ, Ross BK, et al. A multidimensional comparison of morphine and hydromorphone patient-controlled analgesia. *Anesth Analg.* 1996;82:1043–1048.
270. Woodhouse A, Hobbes AF, Mather LE, et al. A comparison of morphine, pethidine and fentanyl in the postsurgical patient-controlled analgesia environment. *Pain.* 1996;64:115–121.
271. Coda BA, O'Sullivan B, Donaldson G, et al. Comparative efficacy of patient-controlled administration of morphine, hydromorphone, or sufentanil for the treatment of oral mucositis pain following bone marrow transplantation. *Pain.* 1997;72:333–346.
272. Coda B, Tanaka A, Jacobson RC, et al. Hydromorphone analgesia after intravenous bolus administration. *Pain.* 1997;71:41–48.
273. Dunbar PJ, Chapman CR, Buckley FP, et al. Clinical analgesic equivalence for morphine and hydromorphone with prolonged PCA. *Pain.* 1996;68:265–270.
274. Hug CC Jr, Murphy MR, Rigel EP, et al. Pharmacokinetics of morphine injected intravenously into the anesthetized dog. *Anesthesiology.* 1981;54:38–47.
275. Scholz J, Steinfath M, Schulz M. Clinical pharmacokinetics of alfentanil, fentanyl and sufentanil. An update. *Clin Pharmacokinet.* 1996;31:275–292.

276. Sjogren P, Jonsson T, Jensen NH, et al. Hyperalgesia and myoclonus in terminal cancer patients treated with continuous intravenous morphine. *Pain*. 1993;55:93–97.
277. Christrup LL. Morphine metabolites. *Acta Anaesthesiol Scand*. 1997;41:116–122.
278. Eisele JH Jr, Grigsby EJ, Dea G. Clonazepam treatment of myoclonic contractions associated with high-dose opioids: Case report. *Pain*. 1992;49:231–2.
279. Sjogren P, Jensen NH, Jensen TS. Disappearance of morphine-induced hyperalgesia after discontinuing or substituting morphine with other opioid agonists. *Pain*. 1994;59:313–316.
280. Bruera E, Lawlor P. Cancer pain management. *Acta Anaesthesiol Scand*. 1997;41:146–153.
281. Drexel H, Dzien A, Spiegel RW, et al. Treatment of severe cancer pain by low-dose continuous subcutaneous morphine. *Pain*. 1989;36:169–176.
282. Bruera E, Brenneis C, Michaud M, et al. Use of the subcutaneous route for the administration of narcotics in patients with cancer pain. *Cancer*. 1988;62:407–411.
283. Kerr IG, Sone M, Deangelis C, et al. Continuous narcotic infusion with patient-controlled analgesia for chronic cancer pain in outpatients. *Ann Intern Med*. 1988;108:554–557.
284. Waldmann CS, Eason JR, Rambohul E, et al. Serum morphine levels. A comparison between continuous subcutaneous infusion and continuous intravenous infusion in postoperative patients. *Anaesthesia*. 1984;39:768–771.
285. Moulin DE, Kreeft JH, Murray Parsons N, et al. Comparison of continuous subcutaneous and intravenous hydromorphone infusions for management of cancer pain. *Lancet*. 1991;337:465–468.
286. Roy SD, Flynn GL. Solubility and related physicochemical properties of narcotic analgesics. *Pharm Res*. 1988;5:580–586.
287. Paix A, Coleman A, Lees J, et al. Subcutaneous fentanyl and sufentanil infusion substitution for morphine intolerance in cancer pain management. *Pain*. 1995;63:263–269.
288. Nelson KA, Glare PA, Walsh D, et al. A prospective, within-patient, crossover study of continuous intravenous and subcutaneous morphine for chronic cancer pain. *J Pain Symptom Manage*. 1997;13:262–267.
289. Stuart-Harris R, Joel SP, McDonald P, et al. The pharmacokinetics of morphine and morphine glucuronide metabolites after subcutaneous bolus injection and subcutaneous infusion of morphine. *Br J Clin Pharmacol*. 2000;49:207–214.
290. Hays H. Hypodermoclysis for symptom control in terminal care. *Can Fam Physician*. 1985;31:1253.
291. Kaiko RF, Foley KM, Grabinski PY, et al. Central nervous system excitatory effects of meperidine in cancer patients. *Ann Neurol*. 1983;13:180–185.
292. Fuller RW, Snoody HD. Inhibition of serotonin uptake and the toxic interaction between meperidine and monoamine oxidase inhibitors. *Toxicol Appl Pharmacol*. 1975;32:129–134.
293. Goldstein DJ, Meador-Woodruff JH. Opiate receptors: Opioid agonist-antagonist effects. *Pharmacotherapy*. 1991;11:164–167.
294. Jemal A, Siegel R, Ward E, et al. Cancer statistics, 2007. *CA Cancer J Clin*. 2007;57:43–66.
295. NIH State-of-the-Science Statement on symptom management in cancer: Pain, depression, and fatigue. *State Sci Statements*. 2002;19:1–29.
296. Joranson DE, Gilson AM, Dahl JL, et al. Pain management, controlled substances, and state medical board policy: A decade of change. *J Pain Symptom Manage*. 2002;23:138–147.
297. Agency for Health Care Policy and Research. Management of cancer pain guideline overview. Agency for Health Care Policy and Research Rockville, Maryland. *J Natl Med Assoc*. 1994;86:571–573, 634.
298. American Academy of Pain Medicine. The use of opioids for the treatment of chronic pain. A consensus statement from the American Academy of Pain Medicine and the American Pain Society. *Clin J Pain*. 1997;13:6–8.
299. American ociety fAnesthesiologists Practice guidelines for cancer pain management. A report by the American Society of Anesthesiologists Task Force on Pain Management, Cancer Pain Section. *Anesthesiology*. 1996;84:1243–1257.
300. Federation of State Medical Boards. Model policy for the use of controlled substances for the treatment of pain. *J Pain Palliat Care Pharmacother*. 2005;19:73–78.
301. Adams NJ, Plane MB, Fleming MF, et al. Opioids and the treatment of chronic pain in a primary care sample. *J Pain Symptom Manage*. 2001;22:791–796.
302. Arnold RM, Han PK, Seltzer D. Opioid contracts in chronic non-malignant pain management: Objectives and uncertainties. *Am J Med*. 2006;119:292–296.
303. Fishman SM, Bandman TB, Edwards A, et al. The opioid contract in the management of chronic pain. *J Pain Symptom Manage*. 1999;18:27–37.
304. Jacobson PL, Mann JD. The valid informed consent-treatment contract in chronic non-cancer pain: Its role in reducing barriers to effective pain management. *Compr Ther*. 2004;30:101–104.
305. Katz N, Fanciullo GJ. Role of urine toxicology testing in the management of chronic opioid therapy. *Clin J Pain*. 2002;18:S76-82.
306. Tellioglu T. The use of urine drug testing to monitor patients receiving chronic opioid therapy for persistent pain conditions. *Med Health R I*. 2008;91:279–280, 282.
307. Michna E, Jamison RN, Pham LD, et al. Urine toxicology screening among chronic pain patients on opioid therapy: frequency and predictability of abnormal findings. *Clin J Pain*. 2007;23:173–179.
308. Fleming MF, Davis J, Passik SD. Reported lifetime aberrant drug-taking behaviors are predictive of current substance use and mental health problems in primary care patients. *Pain Med*. 2008;9:1098–1106.
309. Turk DC, Swanson KS, Gatchel RJ. Predicting opioid misuse by chronic pain patients: A systematic review and literature synthesis. *Clin J Pain*. 2008;24:497–508.
310. Bruera E, Macmillan K, Hanson J, et al. The cognitive effects of the administration of narcotic analgesics in patients with cancer pain. *Pain*. 1989;39:13–16.
311. Poole JC, Jahr JS. Opiate receptors: A review of analgesic properties and pharmacological side effects. *J La State Med Soc*. 1992;144:106–108.
312. Deutsch SI, Weizman A, Goldman ME, et al. The sigma receptor: A novel site implicated in psychosis and antipsychotic drug efficacy. *Clin Neuropharmacol*. 1988;11:105–119.
313. Musacchio JM. The psychotomimetic effects of opiates and the sigma receptor. *Neuropsychopharmacology*. 1990;3:191–200.
314. Smith MT, Watt JA, Cramond T. Morphine-3-glucuronide—a potent antagonist of morphine analgesia. *Life Sci*. 1990;47:579–585.
315. DeStoutz ND, Bruera E, Suarez A-M. Opioid rotation for toxicity reduction in terminal cancer patients. *J Pain Symptom Manage*. 1995;10:378–384.
316. Thomas Z, Bruera E. Use of methadone in a highly tolerant patient receiving parenteral hydromorphone. *J Pain Symptom Manage*. 1995;10:315–317.
317. Walsh TD. Prevention of opioid side effects. *J Pain Symptom Manage*. 1990;5:362–367.
318. Bruera E, Miller MJ, Macmillan K, et al. Neuropsychological effects of methylphenidate in patients receiving a continuous infusion of narcotics for cancer pain. *Pain*. 1992;48:163–166.
319. Bruera E, Brenneis C, Paterson AH, et al. Use of methylphenidate as an adjuvant to narcotic analgesics in patients with advanced cancer. *J Pain Symptom Manage*. 1989;4:3–6.
320. Jamison RN, Schein JR, Vallow S, et al. Neuropsychological effects of long-term opioid use in chronic pain patients. *J Pain Symptom Manage*. 2003;26:913–921.
321. Fishbain DA, Cutler RB, Rosomoff HL, et al. Can patients taking opioids drive safely? A structured evidence-based review. *J Pain Palliat Care Pharmacother*. 2002;16:9–28.
322. Chapman SL, Byas-Smith MG, Reed BA. Effects of intermediate- and long-term use of opioids on cognition in patients with chronic pain. *Clin J Pain*. 2002;18:S83-90.
323. Vainio A, Ollila J, Matikainen E, et al. Driving ability in cancer patients receiving long-term morphine analgesia. *Lancet*. 1995;346:667–670.
324. Galski T, Williams JB, Ehle HT. Effects of opioids on driving ability. *J Pain Symptom Manage*. 2000;19:200–208.
325. Byas-Smith MG, Chapman SL, Reed B, et al. The effect of opioids on driving and psychomotor performance in patients with chronic pain. *Clin J Pain*. 2005;21:345–352.
326. Clemons M, Regnard C, Appleton T. Alertness, cognition and morphine in patients with advanced cancer. *Cancer Treat Rev*. 1996;22:451–468.
327. Bruera E, Schoeller T, Montejo G. Organic hallucinosis in patients receiving high doses of opiates for cancer pain. *Pain*. 1992;48:397–399.
328. Minzenberg MJ, Carter CS. Modafinil: A review of neurochemical actions and effects on cognition. *Neuropsychopharmacology*. 2008;33:1477–1502.

329. Webster L, Andrews M, Stoddard G. Modafinil treatment of opioid-induced sedation. *Pain Med.* 2003;4:135–140.
330. Angst MS, Koppert W, Pahl I, et al. Short-term infusion of the mu-opioid agonist remifentanil in humans causes hyperalgesia during withdrawal. *Pain.* 2003;106:49–57.
331. Tilson HA, Rech RH, Stolman S. Hyperalgesia during withdrawal as a means of measuring the degree of dependence in morphine dependent rats. *Psychopharmacologia.* 1973;28:287–300.
332. Laulin JP, Maurette P, Corcuff JB, et al. The role of ketamine in preventing fentanyl-induced hyperalgesia and subsequent acute morphine tolerance. *Anesth Analg.* 2002;94:1263–1269, table of contents.
333. Mao J. Opioid-induced abnormal pain sensitivity: Implications in clinical opioid therapy. *Pain.* 2002;100:213–217.
334. Chen L, Malarick C, Seefeld L, et al. Altered quantitative sensory testing outcome in subjects with opioid therapy. *Pain.* 2009;143:65–70.
335. Ossipov MH, Lai J, King T, et al. Antinociceptive and nociceptive actions of opioids. *J Neurobiol.* 2004;61:126–148.
336. Ossipov MH, Lai J, Vanderah TW, et al. Induction of pain facilitation by sustained opioid exposure: relationship to opioid antinociceptive tolerance. *Life Sci.* 2003;73:783–800.
337. Zhao M, Joo DT. Subpopulation of dorsal horn neurons displays enhanced N-methyl-D-aspartate receptor function after chronic morphine exposure. *Anesthesiology.* 2006;104:815–825.
338. Angst MS, Clark JD. Opioid-induced hyperalgesia: A qualitative systematic review. *Anesthesiology.* 2006;104:570–587.
339. Arner S, Rawal N, Gustafsson LL. Clinical experience of long-term treatment with epidural and intrathecal opioids—a nationwide survey. *Acta Anaesthesiol Scand.* 1988;32:253–259.
340. Collett BJ. Opioid tolerance: The clinical perspective. *Br J Anaesth.* 1998;81:58–68.
341. Foley KM. Controversies in cancer pain. Medical perspectives. *Cancer.* 1989;63:2257–2265.
342. Collin E, Poulain P, Gauvain-Piquard A, et al. Is disease progression the major factor in morphine 'tolerance' in cancer pain treatment? *Pain.* 1993;55:319–326.
343. Chu LF, Angst MS, Clark D. Opioid-induced hyperalgesia in humans: molecular mechanisms and clinical considerations. *Clin J Pain.* 2008;24:479–496.
344. Ram KC, Eisenberg E, Haddad M, et al. Oral opioid use alters DNIC but not cold pain perception in patients with chronic pain—new perspective of opioid-induced hyperalgesia. *Pain.* 2008;139:431–438.
345. Zhao M, Joo DT. Enhancement of spinal N-methyl-D-aspartate receptor function by remifentanil action at delta-opioid receptors as a mechanism for acute opioid-induced hyperalgesia or tolerance. *Anesthesiology.* 2008;109:308–317.
346. Mika J. Modulation of microglia can attenuate neuropathic pain symptoms and enhance morphine effectiveness. *Pharmacol Rep.* 2008;60:297–307.
347. Joly V, Richebe P, Guignard B, et al. Remifentanil-induced postoperative hyperalgesia and its prevention with small-dose ketamine. *Anesthesiology.* 2005;103:147–155.
348. Gardell LR, King T, Ossipov MH, et al. Opioid receptor-mediated hyperalgesia and antinociceptive tolerance induced by sustained opiate delivery. *Neurosci Lett.* 2006;396:44–49.
349. Reznikov I, Pud D, Eisenberg E. Oral opioid administration and hyperalgesia in patients with cancer or chronic nonmalignant pain. *Br J Clin Pharmacol.* 2005;60:311–318.
350. Fillingim RB, Doleys DM, Edwards RR, et al. Clinical characteristics of chronic back pain as a function of gender and oral opioid use. *Spine.* 2003;28:143–150.
351. Mercadante S, Ferrera P, Villari P, et al. Hyperalgesia: An emerging iatrogenic syndrome. *J Pain Symptom Manage.* 2003;26:769–775.
352. Wilson GR, Reisfield GM. Morphine hyperalgesia: A case report. *Am J Hosp Palliat Care.* 2003;20:459–461.
353. Gillman PK. Monoamine oxidase inhibitors, opioid analgesics and serotonin toxicity. *Br J Anaesth.* 2005;95:434–441.
354. Karunatilake H, Buckley NA. Serotonin syndrome induced by fluvoxamine and oxycodone. *Ann Pharmacother.* 2006;40:155–157.
355. Isbister GK, Bowe SJ, Dawson A, et al. Relative toxicity of selective serotonin reuptake inhibitors (SSRIs) in overdose. *J Toxicol Clin Toxicol.* 2004;42:277–285.
356. Lawrence KR, Adra M, Gillman PK. Serotonin toxicity associated with the use of linezolid: A review of postmarketing data. *Clin Infect Dis.* 2006;42:1578–1583.
357. Boyer EW, Shannon M. The serotonin syndrome. *N Engl J Med.* 2005;352:1112–1120.
358. Gillman PK. Serotonin syndrome: history and risk. *Fundam Clin Pharmacol.* 1998;12:482–491.
359. Raffa RB. A novel approach to the pharmacology of analgesics. *Am J Med.* 1996;101:40S-46S.
360. Ailawadhi S, Sung KW, Carlson LA, et al. Serotonin syndrome caused by interaction between citalopram and fentanyl. *J Clin Pharm Ther.* 2007;32:199–202.
361. Rang ST, Field J, Irving C. Serotonin toxicity caused by an interaction between fentanyl and paroxetine. *Can J Anaesth.* 2008;55:521–525.
362. Kapur S, Zipursky RB, Jones C, et al. Cyproheptadine: A potent in vivo serotonin antagonist. *Am J Psychiatry.* 1997;154:884.
363. Gillman PK. The serotonin syndrome. *N Engl J Med.* 2005;352:2454–2456;author reply 2454-6.
364. Bernard SA, Bruera E. Drug interactions in palliative care. *J Clin Oncol.* 2000;18:1780–1799.
365. Das PK, Warkentin DI, Hewko R, et al. Serotonin syndrome after concomitant treatment with linezolid and meperidine. *Clin Infect Dis.* 2008;46:264–265.
366. Hachem RY, Hicks K, Huen A, et al. Myelosuppression and serotonin syndrome associated with concurrent use of linezolid and selective serotonin reuptake inhibitors in bone marrow transplant recipients. *Clin Infect Dis.* 2003;37:e8-11.
367. Richards S, Umbreit JN, Fanucchi MP, et al. Selective serotonin reuptake inhibitor-induced rhabdomyolysis associated with irinotecan. *South Med J.* 2003;96:1031–1033.
368. Steinberg M, Morin AK. Mild serotonin syndrome associated with concurrent linezolid and fluoxetine. *Am J Health Syst Pharm.* 2007;64:59–62.
369. MacDonald N, Der L, Allan S, et al. Opioid hyperexcitability: The application of alternate opioid therapy. *Pain.* 1993;53:353–355.
370. Anderson R, Saiers JH, Abram S, et al. Accuracy in equianalgesic dosing. conversion dilemmas. *J Pain Symptom Manage.* 2001;21:397–406.
371. Gammaitoni AR, Fine P, Alvarez N, et al. Clinical application of opioid equianalgesic data. *Clin J Pain.* 2003;19:286–297.
372. Mercadante S. Opioid rotation for cancer pain: rationale and clinical aspects. *Cancer.* 1999;86:1856–1866.
373. Pereira J, Lawlor P, Vigano A, et al. Equianalgesic dose ratios for opioids. a critical review and proposals for long-term dosing. *J Pain Symptom Manage.* 2001;22:672–687.
374. Thomsen AB, Becker N, Eriksen J. Opioid rotation in chronic non-malignant pain patients. A retrospective study. *Acta Anaesthesiol Scand.* 1999;43:918–923.
375. Ashby MA, Martin P, Jackson KA. Opioid substitution to reduce adverse effects in cancer pain management. *Med J Aust.* 1999;170:68–71.
376. Indelicato RA, Portenoy RK. Opioid rotation in the management of refractory cancer pain. *J Clin Oncol.* 2002;20:348–352.
377. Mercadante S, Casuccio A, Fulfaro F, et al. Switching from morphine to methadone to improve analgesia and tolerability in cancer patients: A prospective study. *J Clin Oncol.* 2001;19:2898–2904.
378. Moryl N, Santiago-Palma J, Kornick C, et al. Pitfalls of opioid rotation: substituting another opioid for methadone in patients with cancer pain. *Pain.* 2002;96:325–328.
379. Hunt G, Bruera E. Respiratory depression in a patient receiving oral methadone for cancer pain. *J Pain Symptom Manage.* 1995;10:401–404.
380. Reyes-Gibby CC, Aday LA, Todd KH, et al. Pain in aging community-dwelling adults in the United States: non-Hispanic whites, non-Hispanic blacks, and Hispanics. *J Pain.* 2007;8:75–84.
381. Dores RM, Lecaude S, Bauer D, et al. Analyzing the evolution of the opioid/orphanin gene family. *Mass Spectrom Rev.* 2002;21:220–243.
382. Niederberger E, Geisslinger G. Proteomics in neuropathic pain research. *Anesthesiology.* 2008;108:314–323.
383. Reymond MA, Schlegel W. Proteomics in cancer. *Adv Clin Chem.* 2007;44:103–142.
384. Shui HA, Ho ST, Wang JJ, et al. Proteomic analysis of spinal protein expression in rats exposed to repeated intrathecal morphine injection. *Proteomics.* 2007;7:796–803.

385. Belfer I, Wu T, Kingman A, Krishnaraju RK, et al. Candidate gene studies of human pain mechanisms: methods for optimizing choice of polymorphisms and sample size. *Anesthesiology.* 2004;100:1562–1572.
386. Ali Z, Raja SN, Wesselmann U, et al. Intradermal injection of norepinephrine evokes pain in patients with sympathetically maintained pain. *Pain.* 2000;88:161–168.
387. Bie B, Pan ZZ. Presynaptic mechanism for anti-analgesic and antihyperalgesic actions of kappa-opioid receptors. *J Neurosci.* 2003;23:7262–7268.
388. Zubieta JK, Heitzeg MM, Smith YR, et al. COMT val158met genotype affects mu-opioid neurotransmitter responses to a pain stressor. *Science.* 2003;299:1240–1243.
389. Bodnar RJ, Klein GE. Endogenous opiates and behavior: 2005. *Peptides.* 2006;27:3391–3478.
390. Kieffer BL, Gaveriaux-Ruff C. Exploring the opioid system by gene knockout. *Prog Neurobiol.* 2002;66:285–306.
391. Waldhoer M, Bartlett SE, Whistler JL. Opioid receptors. *Ann Rev Biochem.* 2004;73:953–990.
392. Lotsch J, Geisslinger G. Are mu-opioid receptor polymorphisms important for clinical opioid therapy? *Trends Mol Med.* 2005;11:82–89.
393. Carroll L, Voisey J, van Daal A. Gene polymorphisms and their effects in the melanocortin system. *Peptides.* 2005;26:1871–1885.
394. Kraus J, Borner C, Giannini E, et al. Regulation of mu-opioid receptor gene transcription by interleukin-4 and influence of an allelic variation within a STAT6 transcription factor binding site. *J Biol Chem.* 2001;276:43901–43908.
395. Ikeda K, Ide S, Han W, et al. How individual sensitivity to opiates can be predicted by gene analyses. *Trends Pharmacol Sci.* 2005;26:311–317.
396. Lichtermann D, Franke P, Maier W, et al. Pharmacogenomics and addiction to opiates. *Eur J Pharmacol.* 2000;410:269–279.
397. Campa D, Gioia A, Tomei A, et al. Association of ABCB1/MDR1 and OPRM1 gene polymorphisms with morphine pain relief. *Clin Pharmacol Ther.* 2008;83:559–566.
398. Reyes-Gibby CC, Shete S, Rakvag T, et al. Exploring joint effects of genes and the clinical efficacy of morphine for cancer pain: OPRM1 and COMT gene. *Pain.* 2007;130:25–30.
399. Gough AC, Smith CA, Howell SM, et al. Localization of the CYP2D gene locus to human chromosome 22q13.1 by polymerase chain reaction, in situ hybridization, and linkage analysis. *Genomics.* 1993;15:430–432.
400. Johansson I, Yue QY, Dahl ML, et al. Genetic analysis of the interethnic difference between Chinese and Caucasians in the polymorphic metabolism of debrisoquine and codeine. *Eur J Clin Pharmacol.* 1991;40:553–556.
401. Kasai S, Hayashida M, Sora I, et al. Candidate gene polymorphisms predicting individual sensitivity to opioids. *Naunyn Schmiedebergs Arch Pharmacol.* 2008;377:269–281.

CHAPTER 20 ■ MEDICATION MISUSE AND SUBSTANCE ABUSE

MANAGEMENT OF THE PATIENT MISUSING MEDICATIONS

Prescription opioid abuse, as indicated by several large-scale epidemiological databases (eg, National Household Survey on Drug Abuse, Drug Abuse Warning Network), is increasing in the United States. Prescription drug abuse has become prevalent in the United States and, unlike the pattern of abuse observed with illicit drugs such as heroin, which is heavily localized to the inner cities of very large metropolitan areas, it is most prevalent in rural, suburban, and small- to medium-sized urban areas.[1]

In our practice, we have established a clear difference in the management of the patient who misuses medications and those who use illicit substances. We define misuse as the nonprescription use of prescribed medications in stabilized pain complaint, diversion of prescribed medications, unauthorized use of legal recreational substances, and/or use of illegal recreational substances. Components contributing to misuse behaviors include:

1. Prescription noncompliance
2. Treatment noncompliance
3. Communication noncompliance
4. Insufficient/inadequate support system
5. Vocational/recreational issues
6. Hostility toward providers

The various categories of misuse are listed in Table 20.1. Potential indicators of risk for misuse are previous documentation of misuse/addiction on the patient record; anecdotal reports by referring clinician or medical record indicators of potential issues; patient report of substance abuse/addiction; independent reports of abuse/addiction (eg, from family or friends); supporting data which includes issues with housing status, support system status, vocational/recreational status, strong medication biases, and emotional instability; psychological comorbidity (eg mood disturbance, cognitive dysfunction); frequent missed appointments; issues with staff abuse (verbal or physical).

If misuse of medications is suspected, the nature of the pain complaint should be reassessed and checked for appropriate diagnosis and stability. The nature of the misuse should be determined and a verbal warning should be given where appropriate. A clinic appointment with the prescriber should be scheduled and an independent verifier (spouse, significant other) should also attend. At this appointment, a report on medication use (patient's understanding of the purpose of the medication and the pattern of use) should be determined. A family member's verification of the medication use should be obtained with some account of the patient's current level of functioning. The pain complaint should be documented and tracked carefully. From the prescriber's perspective, the indication for the medication(s) in question should be reviewed and justified according to the patient's medical condition. If appropriate, a urine toxicology screen should be considered. In certain circumstances, particularly if the pattern of misuse (with early prescription refills), a pill count should be considered in the patient's presence. Interventional options for continued medication misuse are listed in Table 20.2.

If patients' behaviors become unmanageable, discharge from the clinic should be considered. In particular,

TABLE 20.1
CATEGORIES OF MEDICATION MISUSE

Category	Behavior
Abuse	Intentional use other than as prescribed; seeking effects other than medically intended
Inappropriate use	Unintentional use other than as prescribed
Diversion	Selling, loaning, trading, sharing
Addiction	Continued and escalating use despite consequences; drug craving; compulsive use; loss of control (including inability to reduce use despite pain intensity reduction)

TABLE 20.2
INTERVENTIONAL OPTIONS FOR PATIENTS MISUSING PRESCRIPTION MEDICATIONS

1. Provide careful instruction regarding treatment goal.
2. Provide careful instruction regarding medication use and purpose.
3. Provide clear guidelines regarding use of recreational substances.
4. Simplify regimen.
5. Limit number of pills per prescription.
6. Schedule frequent visits with prescriber (minimum monthly visits until stable).
7. Schedule frequent follow-up in-person visits with Clinic nurse.
8. Perform random urine toxicology screens.
9. Perform random counting of pills or patches.
10. Impose independent verification as condition of continued care.
11. Enlist family assistance in medication storage and dispensing.
12. Use a signed opioid contract.

TABLE 20.3

PROCEDURES FOR PATIENT DISCHARGE FROM MEDICAL CARE

1. Provide patient with repeated documented warnings of possible discharge if there is ongoing failure to comply
2. Sign opioid agreement (copy to patient and to medical record)
3. Schedule return visit to explain reasons for discharge and outline method of discharge
4. Instruct patient to seek alternative provider
5. If patient fails to obtain alternative provider, implement tapering schedule of Pain Clinic-prescribed medications
6. Contact Risk Management and inform of impending discharge

continued care of the patient becomes impossible if the patient's behavior risks harm to self or to others; if there is evidence of physical or continued verbal abuse; or if the patient fails to follow instructions despite repeated warnings. In the event of termination of care, we recommend following the procedures listed in Table 20.3. A copy of our opioid agreement is shown in Appendix F.

Dealing with substance abuse and opioid misuse can greatly complicate management of the patient with pain associated with cancer. The clinician caring for such a patient must adopt a proactive position and remain alert for potential problems. Certainly, it is not ethical to deny patients treatment for pain due to cancer just because of a history of substance abuse. On the other hand, patients who are actively noncompliant with medication management must be controlled by decisive actions and effective procedures and policies.

OPIOID ABUSE-DETERRENT TECHNOLOGIES

Abuse and diversion of prescription opioids have a detrimental effect on individual and public health. Comparing poison center data, it appears that hydrocodone is the most commonly abused drug.[2] The nonmedical use of opioids appears to be predictable based on potency and extent of prescriptive use. Dasgupta et al.,[3] using data from the Drug Abuse Warning Network (DAWN), evaluated the major prescription opioids and the association between prescriptive medical use in kilograms and reported morbidity, as measured by a ratio between the two. The ratio was similar for the intermediate-potency opioids (hydrocodone, methadone, oxycodone, and morphine) but was much lower for low-potency opioids (codeine, meperidine, pentazocine, and propoxyphene) and much greater for high-potency opioids (hydromorphone and fentanyl). When the drugs were adjusted by potency (relative to morphine), the rates of reported morbidity per kilogram of morphine equivalent opioid in prescriptive usage were similar among the opioids. This represents a serious problem given the large number of legitimate prescriptions written in the United States. Joranson et al.[4] noted that, from 1990 to 1996, there were increases in medical use of morphine (59%), fentanyl (1168%), oxycodone (23%), and hydromorphone (19%), and a decrease in the medical use of meperidine (35%). During 1997 through 2002, total use of oxycodone increased by 403% and fentanyl by 227%.[5] This increase in oxycodone consumption appears to have been influenced by the introduction of OyxContin in 1996. From this data, Gilson et al.[5] concluded that the increased medical use of several different opioids was associated with increased abuse. The increased number of prescriptions written for hydrocodone and oxycodone between 1995 and 2004 was associated with similar increases in nonmedical use and the number of emergency department (ED) visits during this time period.[6]

Some abuse of opioids is predictable because of their abuse liability, their availability for medical purposes, criminal demand for drugs of abuse, and imperfect control systems. Opioids may be ingested whole, crushed and then ingested, crushed and then snorted, or injected intravenously after extraction from the tablet or capsule. Currently available formulations for such drugs are designed for oral administration but do not include mechanisms to prevent or retard improper methods of administration such as chewing, injection, and snorting.

An additional serious clinical problem has arisen when therapeutic doses of sustained release opioids are taken with alcohol (ethanol). The problem was discovered with a once-a-day sustained release formulation of hydromorphone (Palladone capsules). In 2005, Palladone capsules were withdrawn from the market in the United States and Canada due to dose-dumping when coingested with alcohol. Patients consuming 240 mL of 40% ethanol had a sixfold average increase in peak blood levels of hydromorphone.

Opioids, particularly modified-release preparations, can be tampered with in many ways.[7] Several pharmaceutical strategies have been proposed to deter the abuse of sustained release formulations of opioid analgesics. These strategies include formulations that contain a sequestered opioid antagonist or aversive agent which is released only upon product tampering (eg, crushing, extraction) and formulations that deter abuse by resisting crushing and drug extraction with the use of common solvents.

Abuse deterrent technology research is currently focused in the following areas:

1. Deterrent packaging
   a. RFID (radio frequency identification) protection
      Reliable RFID technology has the potential to make copying of medications extremely difficult.
   b. Tamper-proof bottles
2. Physical design (in the form of matrices, gels, beads, osmotic pumps, bioerodible hydrogels, implants, etc.)
   a. Difficult to crush
   b. Difficult to extract
3. Aversive component (make use of toxic components which are only released if the formulation is crushed or otherwise tampered with)
   a. Capsaicin—burning sensation
   b. Ipecac—emetic
   c. Bitrex—bitter taste
   d. Niacin—flushing
4. Pharmacologic (unaltered state opioid antagonist is not released)

a. Bioavailable agonist with sequestered antagonist
  b. Prodrugs (require enzymatic cleavage in the gastrointestinal (GI) tract for the active metabolite to be produced)
5. Combination mechanisms
  a. Pharmacologic and physical

Several drugs (Embeda, Remoxy) are currently under consideration by the Food and Drug Administration (FDA). Embeda is extended-release morphine with sequestered naltrexone. After oral ingestion, naltrexone remains sequestered in the pellet core while passing through the GI tract without significant absorption. If the Embeda capsule is crushed, chewed, or dissolved, naltrexone is released, potentially significantly reducing the euphoric effect of the opioid. Remoxy is a long-acting oxycodone gelatin capsule. It has a sticky, high-viscosity capsule formulation making it difficult to inject or snort. Freezing or physically crushing Remoxy does not appear to trigger a significant release of its content of oxycodone. Submerging Remoxy in high-proof alcohol or water for hours at a time appeared to release just a fraction of its oxycodone.

In order to better predict which patients are more likely to misuse opioids, clinicians should assess risk before for prescribing opioids, with frequent reassessments during treatment. The Screener and Opioid Assessment for Patients with Pain (SOAPP) assesses family and personal history of substance abuse, history of legal problems, craving for prescription medication, nicotine dependence, and mood swings (Appendix C).[8] A score of 7 or higher is considered positive. Patients typically answer the SOAPP questionnaire at initial assessment and once more at 6-month follow-up. In order to monitor current aberrant drug-related behavior, a brief, self-reporting questionnaire, Current Opioid Misuse Measure (COMM) was developed (Appendix D). Initial studies by Butler et al.[9] show some promise for this instrument.

PRESCRIPTION DRUG ABUSE

As noted, prescription drug abuse is increasing throughout the United States. Much of the information available on prescription drug abuse is not directly related to cancer patients with pain. However, as increasing numbers of patients survive cancer or have longer survival times than previously, issues related to long-term opioid use in the nonmalignant chronic pain patient may become applicable to the long-term cancer pain survivor. Joranson et al.[4] evaluated the proportion of drug abuse related to opioids use and the trends in medical use and abuse of five opioids (fentanyl, hydromorphone, meperidine, morphine, and oxycodone) between 1990 and 1996. The authors concluded that a trend of increasing medical use of opioids to treat pain did not appear to contribute to increases in opioid abuse. In a reassessment of this situation during the period of 1997 to 2002, the same group noted that the increase in medical use of opioids was a growing public health problem and should be addressed by identifying the causes and sources of diversion, without interfering with legitimate medical practice and patient care.[5]

The consumption of therapeutic opioids in the United States increased from 74 mg per person in 1997 to 329 mg per person in 2006, a 347% increase. During the same period, the therapeutic use of methadone increased by 1129% mg/person and oxycodone by 899% mg/person.[10] Americans, constituting only 4.6% of the world's population, have been consuming 80% of the global opioid supply, and 99% of the global hydrocodone supply, as well as two thirds of the world's illegal drugs.[10] Retail sales of opioid medications have increased from a total in 1997 of 50.7 million grams of commonly utilized opioids (including methadone, oxycodone, fentanyl base, hydromorphone, hydrocodone, morphine, meperidine, and codeine) to 115.3 million grams in 2006, an overall increase of 127% with increases ranging from 196% for morphine, 244% for hydrocodone, 274% for hydromorphone, 479% for fentanyl base, 732% for oxycodone, to 1177% for methadone.[10]

In 2001, the Substance Abuse and Mental Health Services Administration (SAMHSA) estimated that over 11 million people have taken prescription-type drugs for nonmedical uses at least once in their lifetime, almost four times greater than in the 1980s. This rise in prescription nonmedical use includes teenagers and young adults.[11] Various programs collect data on prescription opioid abuse and misuse, including the National Survey on Drug Use and Health (NSDUH) and the Drug Abuse Warning Network (DAWN). DAWN, initiated in 1988, is a national data system that collects information about ED visits that are related to substance abuse. The number of mentions of psychotropic drugs during a drug-related visit is the key endpoint for this system. DAWN defines drug abuse as "nonmedical use of a substance for psychic effect, dependence, suicide attempt/gesture, or the use of prescription drugs in a manner that is inconsistent with the accepted medical practice."

Hughes et al.[2] used data from poison centers as a real-time, geographically specific, surveillance system for prescription opioid abuse and compared data from DAWN. Poison center rates of abuse and misuse were highest for hydrocodone at 3.75 per 100,000 population, followed by oxycodone at 1.81 per 100,000 population with significant regional variations. DAWN ED data showed a similar pattern of abuse with most mentions involving hydrocodone and oxycodone. In both poison center and DAWN data, young adults are the most likely to manifest drug abuse.

There is a complex relationship between the therapeutic use of opioids and other psychotherapeutics and the consequences of escalating care, abuse, and nonmedical use of these substances. Superimposed on this relationship is the influence of illegal recreational substance use. Although the prevention of drug abuse is an important societal goal, it should not override and hinder patients' ability to receive appropriate health care. For many patients, opioids, when used appropriately, are the most effective way to treat pain, and often the only treatment option that provides significant relief. When deciding on opioid prescription, physicians should decide if opioids are indicated in the management of the patient's pain complaint, as not all pain complaints can be treated effectively with opioids. Physicians should also ask patients about their previous and current histories of alcohol and other drug use. Attention should also be paid to a family history of addiction. Patients with histories of substance use, mental health problems, or both should receive special attention and comanagement from pain management and/or addiction specialists when possible. Appropriate treatment of coexisting mental health disorders should be considered part of successful pain management.

Oxycodone Abuse

Annual consumption of oxycodone has increased 42-fold in the United Kingdom and threefold in the United States from 1999 to 2003.[12] Oxycodone abuse has been a continuing problem in the United States since the early 1960s. The large amount of oxycodone (10 to 160 mg) present in controlled release formulations (OxyContin) renders these products highly attractive to opioid abusers and doctor-shoppers. Oxycodone appears to be abused for its euphoric effects. Zacny and Gutierrez[13] characterized the subjective and psychomotor effects of oxycodone in non drug-abusing volunteers and noted that the subjective effects were dose related. Although oxycodone produced abuse liability-related subjective effects, it also produced unpleasant effects. Peak liking and drug-wanting ratings were increased by all doses of oxycodone, and trough ratings of liking (dislike) were lower in the 20-mg and 30-mg oxycodone conditions. Cognitive and psychomotor impairment were obtained with the higher doses of oxycodone.

OxyContin is abused either as intact tablets or by crushing or chewing the tablet and then swallowing, snorting or injecting. Cicero et al.[1] noted that prescription drug abuse was a prevalent problem in the United States between 2002 and 2004, that OxyContin was the prevalent prescription opioid abused, and that most OxyContin abusers (>87%) had extensive current and past histories of substance abuse. There is some suggestion that the marketing of OxyContin contributed to its abuse by minimizing its abuse potential to prescribing physicians.

Products containing oxycodone in combination with acetaminophen or aspirin are also abused orally. According to the Florida Department of Law Enforcement, oxycodone was found in 5.6% (716) of the total drug-related deaths in Florida in 2005. Based on the toxicology reports, oxycodone was cited as a causative drug in 340 deaths. The manner of oxycodone deaths cited included accidental (65%), suicide (16%), natural (13%), and undetermined (4%). Abuse of oxycodone is most frequently seen in conjunction with the abuse of other drugs, although fatalities have been reported with oxycodone alone.[14] Although OxyContin tablets are safe and effective when taken intact and as recommended by the manufacturer for the treatment of moderate to severe, ongoing pain, abusers have discovered that crushing the tablets defeats the controlled-release mechanism and makes much of the oxycodone immediately available, which can then be ingested or administered by intranasal or intravenous routes, sometimes with fatal outcome. When combined with opioids, self-administration of other depressant drugs can substantially increase the likelihood of a fatal outcome.[15] The 2001 DAWN mortality report noted that 89% of deaths involving heroin/morphine also had mentions of at least one other drug. Similar findings were also reported for other opioid analgesics such as methadone, codeine, oxycodone, and hydrocodone. In 2001 alone, multidrug episodes were reported 56% of the time.[16] Between 1997 and 2001, oxycodone mentions increased 276%. Cone et al.[14] reported on the role of oxycodone in 1,243 mortality cases collected from an oxycodone postmortem database from 23 states. Only 30 (3.3%) of the drug abuse cases involved oxycodone as the single reported chemical entity; of these, 12 cases had OxyContin identified as a source of oxycodone. Of the 919 drug abuse cases, the vast majority (N = 889, 97%) were multiple drug abuse deaths in which there was at least one other plausible contributory drug in addition to oxycodone. The most prevalent drug combinations were oxycodone in combination with benzodiazepines, alcohol, cocaine, other narcotics, marijuana, or antidepressants.

Certain sectors of the population seem to be especially vulnerable to the nonmedical use of drugs, including adolescents, college students, individuals with known psychiatric disorders, the elderly, and patients with undertreated pain. Reasons for use include inadvertent use, self-medication, "experimentation," and abuse or dependence. Some authors suggest that medical prescription is a common source[17] and others suggest that the main sources are illicit and include family, friends, and others.[18] The current evidence suggests that although oxycodone is abused for nonmedical reasons, it does not appear to have properties uniquely different from other opioids to merit additional concern about its abuse potential.

Methadone Maintenance and Opioid Detoxification

Opioid addiction is a chronic relapsing disorder that is associated with significant social and health consequences, including high levels of unemployment, criminal activity, reliance on social services, blood-borne infections, and a high prevalence of concurrent psychiatric disorders.[19] Treatment is aimed at a reduction in risks associated with substance abuse including relapses to opioid and polysubstance use and promoting psychosocial adjustment.[20] Chronic heroin abusers suffer endogenous opioid deficiency because of down-regulation of opioid production, which creates an overwhelming craving.[21] As a replacement option, methadone is intended to eliminate the euphoric effect of heroin, the abstinence symptoms associated with withdrawal, and cravings associated with chronic use of heroin.

Methadone maintenance treatment is a long-term opioid replacement therapy introduced in 1965 and is considered an effective and accepted intervention for opioid dependence.[22] Buprenorphine is also an effective intervention for use in the maintenance treatment of heroin dependence, but may be less effective than methadone delivered at adequate dosages.[23] Methadone is an orally effective, long acting medication and should be compatible with normal performance in vocational activities.[24] Methadone maintenance is used in the short term for detoxification purposes and also as long-term treatment which allows complete social and personal rehabilitation and prevents the health damages related to drug use.[25] Despite clinical effectiveness, patient satisfaction with treatment varies.[26] When providing opioids for treatment of drug addiction, monitoring is necessary to track individual patient progress and to minimize the potential public health impact of diverted drugs. Maintenance treatment typically takes place in highly structured and regulated specialty programs. Once a therapeutic dose is achieved, patients frequently can be maintained for many years with the same dose.

Methadone dosages ranging from 60 to 100 mg/day are more effective than lower dosages in retaining patients and in reducing use of heroin and cocaine during treatment.[22] Doses as low as 20 mg may improve treatment retention, but higher doses are often necessary to suppress illicit drug use.[27] The minimal effective dose is usually 50 mg, but some individuals need much larger doses.[28-29] Opioid dependent patients with Axis I psychiatric comorbidity may need significantly higher methadone doses. Treatment is usually initiated with 25 to 30 mg of methadone once daily. The dose is gradually titrated in 5- to 10-mg increments per day to a dose range of 60 to 120 mg, which usually provides relief from abstinence symptoms, generally without perceptible sedation effects. Cancer pain specialists are reminded that treating drug addiction requires a federal license and is not legal for physicians without this endorsement.

Tapering off opioids may also be considered in addicted patients. In opioid detoxification programs, a patient is taken off the drug either abruptly or gradually in order to eliminate physical dependence with the minimum of discomfort from withdrawal symptoms. Detoxification has repeatedly shown substantially poorer outcomes than methadone maintenance.[30] Detoxification by itself is not an effective treatment for dependence.[31] In a review of ultra-rapid detoxification for opioids, the limited efficacy of this approach even at 3-month follow-up was found to contrast strongly with the long-term efficacy of methadone stabilization treatment.[32] In a study by Sees et al.,[33] patients who were stable while receiving methadone maintenance had significant declines in heroin use, needle-related HIV risk behaviors, and drug-related crime. However, methadone stabilization is not the total solution to the problem of opioid dependence and addiction. Cocaine use, sex-related HIV risk behaviors, employment problems, and family problems persisted, and more than 50% of patients in both groups used heroin at least once during any given month of treatment.

Although untreated alcohol or benzodiazepine withdrawal is potentially more dangerous, opioid withdrawal causes intensely disturbing symptoms. Withdrawal symptoms begin 3 to 6 hours after the last use of heroin, but they may not begin for a number of days after abrupt discontinuation of methadone. Following cessation of a short half-life opioid, symptoms reach peak intensity within 2 to 4 days, with most of the obvious physical withdrawal signs no longer observable after 7 to 14 days. Opioid withdrawal is rarely life-threatening or associated with significant aberrations of mental state. However, completion of withdrawal is difficult for most people. Symptoms include GI tract distress (diarrhea and cramping), marked anxiety, irritability, insomnia, pathognomonic skin piloerection, and an influenza-like syndrome characterized by rhinorrhea, lacrimation, and myalgias. This syndrome may last 5 to 10 days. In addition, a protracted abstinence phase may last for months and is characterized by asthenia, depression, and hypotension.[34]

Methadone in tapering doses can be used for the management of opioid withdrawal.[35] The severity of opiate withdrawal symptoms is related to the pretreatment opioid dose.[36] Methadone can be tapered by 10% to 20% per day for inpatients after an initial day or two of stabilization. For outpatients, the dose is tapered 5% to 10% per week. Clonidine may also be considered for non–opioid-based detoxification. One mechanism underlying opioid withdrawal is noradrenergic hyperactivity. Use of α-2 adrenergic agonists acting centrally can moderate the symptoms of noradrenergic hyperactivity. Clonidine in initial doses of 0.1 to 0.2 mg every 4 hours with careful monitoring of blood pressure eliminates most commonly reported withdrawal symptoms. Some symptoms, such as anxiety and myalgias, are less responsive to clonidine and may require the concomitant use of benzodiazepines and/or nonsteroidal anti-inflammatory drugs (NSAIDs). Clonidine may shorten the detoxification period to 1 to 2 weeks.[37] Adverse effects are most severe for the few days of peak withdrawal when maximal doses of clonidine are administered. Aside from hypotension, the adverse effects more commonly associated with clonidine are drowsiness, fatigue, lethargy and dry mouth. Clinically, hypotension is the most significant adverse effect and can be adequately managed by limiting doses and reducing the dose of medication according to blood pressure changes.[38]

Ultra-rapid detoxification is a variant that is performed with the patient under general anesthesia during 24 hours. Because the patient is anesthetized during the acute phase of withdrawal, he or she does not consciously experience the unpleasant acute opioid withdrawal syndrome. Most of the rapid protocols use clonidine along with an opioid antagonist, as well as adjuvant benzodiazepines and antiemetics to treat the withdrawal syndrome. However, the effectiveness and safety of anesthesia-assisted detoxification have been questioned. Although detoxification under anesthesia accelerates the detoxification procedure, there is a lack of randomized clinical trials evaluating its effectiveness compared to traditional detoxification procedures and a lack of data on long-term abstinence.[39] A systematic review noted a lack of evidence to support this approach.[32] Safety concerns have also been raised.[40-41] Naltrexone may also be used in the pharmacological treatment of relapse prevention and may be helpful especially in highly motivated patients.[42] Unfortunately, this method has not been validated for different patient populations.[43] The setting for detoxification is also debatable. Unfortunately, there is very limited data to guide the clinician about the outcomes or cost-effectiveness of inpatient or outpatient approaches to opioid detoxification.[44]

Suboxone Therapy

Buprenorphine is a schedule III, μ-opioid partial agonist with a greater margin of safety than full agonists and a less intensive withdrawal.[45-46] As a partial agonist, it can substitute for other opioids and suppress opioid withdrawal at low doses. It was originally marketed for parenteral treatment of acute pain. One of buprenorphine's advantages is its long duration of action, allowing it to be dosed daily.

Buprenorphine (Subutex) and combined buprenorphine and naloxone (Suboxone) are currently the only agents approved by the FDA for the office-based treatment of opioid dependence. Two sublingual tablet formulations have been developed for detoxification and maintenance treatment of opioid dependence, and these preparations were approved by the FDA in October, 2002. Before 2002, treatment options for addicts had included detoxification using clonidine or methadone or methadone maintenance treatment. Short-term taper with buprenorphine in heroin addicts resulted in better treatment compliance compared to patients treated with clonidine.[47] Continuing treatment with buprenorphine-naloxone also improved outcome compared with short-term detoxification.[48] In addition, medication type (buprenorphine-naloxone versus clonidine) was the single best predictor of treatment retention and treatment success, regardless of treatment setting.[49]

Like methadone, buprenorphine can be abused, although the abuse potential appears to be low.[50] In Finland, buprenorphine (Subutex) is the most abused opioid.[51] To deter abuse, a combination sublingual tablet (Suboxone) was developed that contains buprenorphine and naloxone (Narcan) in a 4:1 ratio. Naloxone in this formulation discourages patients from crushing and injecting the tablets but does not affect its efficacy if taken sublingually, as directed. Sublingual naloxone has poor bioavailability, but, if the combination tablets are injected, the effect of naloxone predominates, precipitating withdrawal symptoms in opioid-dependent patients. Proper maintenance therapy with buprenorphine or buprenorphine-naloxone suppresses withdrawal symptoms in patients dependent on opioids and replaces tolerance to parenterally administered opioids.[52] Buprenorphine should be started when patients are experiencing mild to moderate withdrawal symptoms. This can be as soon as 4 hours after the last use of a short-acting opioid such as heroin or as late as 48 hours or more after taking a long-acting opioid such as methadone or slow-release oxycodone. The initial dose is typically buprenorphine 4 mg sublingually. After a period of clinical assessment (usually 4 to 12 hours), an additional 2 to 4 mg of buprenorphine is often needed to ameliorate withdrawal symptoms. Subsequent dosing should be increased over 3 or 4 days to achieve a total maintenance dosage of buprenorphine of 8 to 32 mg daily, usually in divided doses given twice a day or four times a day. Maintenance treatment with buprenorphine is designed to reduce or eliminate cravings for opioids, prevent withdrawal symptoms from emerging, and deter the use of other opioids by blocking their effects. Discontinuation of therapy usually requires gradual dose reduction (eg, reducing the daily dose by 2 mg every week). Federal regulations mandate that physicians who wish to use buprenorphine for the treatment of addiction complete a specialized training course.

MANAGEMENT OF SUBSTANCE ABUSE ISSUES

Substance abuse presents a complex set of physical, psychological, and social issues that always complicates cancer treatment and pain management. Patients who are actively abusing illicit drugs, alcohol, or prescription drugs pose clinical problems distinct from patients in drug-free recovery and those in methadone maintenance programs. In some cases, compliance with treatments for cancer may be so poor that the substance abuse actually shortens life expectancy by preventing the effective administration of oncologic therapy. Outcomes may also be altered by the use of drugs in a manner that negatively interacts with therapy or predisposes patients to other serious morbidity.

It is difficult to define substance abuse and addiction in cancer patients, since the terminology has been developed from addict populations without medical illness. By definition, the use of an illicit drug, or the use of a prescription drug without a medical indication, is abuse. Any drug that is used in a compulsive manner or continually used despite harm to the user or others also merits consideration of a diagnosis of addiction. Because drug-taking norms are not clearly known for prescription medications used for legitimate medical purposes, there is less certainty about the behaviors that could be characterized as aberrant. Various definitions of abuse that include the phenomena related to physical dependence or tolerance are not applicable to patients who receive potentially abuseable drugs for legitimate medical purposes. A true addiction is only one of several possible explanations, but is more likely with certain behaviors. The diagnosis of pseudoaddiction should also be considered if the patient is reporting distress related to unrelieved symptoms. Pseudoaddiction is an iatrogenic syndrome resulting from inadequate pain management. As a result, patients engage in relief-seeking behaviors as though they are drug-seeking. The relief-seeking behaviors promptly resolve upon institution of effective analgesic therapy. Behaviors such as aggressively complaining about the need for higher doses or occasional unilateral drug escalations may be indications that the patient's pain is undermedicated. Impulsive drug use may also indicate the existence of another psychiatric disorder, diagnosis of which may have therapeutic implications. When a patient is diagnosed with cancer, an appropriate definition of addiction is that it is a behavioral disorder characterized by the compulsive use of a substance resulting in physical, psychological, or social harm to the user and continued use despite that harm.[53]

Substance abuse issues have been considered to be rare in a cancer patient setting.[54] However, the reason for the apparently low frequency of diagnosis of alcoholism and drug addiction among cancer patients is probably underdiagnosis.[55] The magnitude of substance abuse in the United States practically guarantees the likelihood that those who manage pain in cancer patients will have to deal with this problem. Nearly one third of the population of the United States has used illicit drugs, and an estimated 6% to 27% have a substance abuse problem of some type.[56-59] Because of the prevalence of substance abuse and the association between drug abuse and some types of cancer, problems related to abuse and addictions are encountered in palliative care settings. The abuse of prescription opioids has grown rapidly since the mid-1980s and is now as frequent as the abuse of cocaine.[60] Between 1999 and 2002, the number of opioid poisonings on death certificates increased 91.2%; heroin and cocaine poisonings increased 12.4% and 22.8%, respectively.[61] Paulozzi[62] measured the role of opioids in drug abuse–related deaths in 28 metropolitan areas from the Drug

Abuse Warning Network (DAWN). The number of reports of opioids increased 96.6% from 1997 to 2002; methadone, oxycodone, and unspecified opioid analgesics accounted for 74.3% of the increase. The increase in deaths involving methadone reflected the increase in methadone used as an analgesic rather than methadone used in narcotics treatment programs. Oxycodone reports increased 727.8% (from 72 to 596 reports). By 2002, opioids were noted more frequently as a cause of accidental death than were heroin or cocaine.

There is a high risk of recidivism for drug abuse and addiction. The risk of relapse is higher because of the stress associated with cancer and the ready availability of centrally-acting drugs. Complete prevention of relapses may be impossible in such a setting. If there is a general understanding that compliance and abstinence are not realistic, conflicts with staff in terms of management goals may be reduced. The goal of team management should be the creation of a structure for therapy that includes sufficient social/emotional support and limit-setting to contain the harm done by relapses and to render them less frequent. Severe substance-use disorder and comorbid psychiatric diagnoses may prevent a small subgroup of patients from complying with the requirements of oncologic therapy. In such circumstances, clinicians must reestablish limits on multiple occasions and attempt to develop an increasing variety and intensity of supports. In the population of patients with cancer and substance abuse, pain and symptom management often is complicated by multiple medical, psychosocial, and administrative problems. A team approach can be very useful in addressing these problems and avoiding provider burn-out. The most effective team may consist of an oncologist, a physician with expertise in pain/palliative care, nurses, social workers, and, if possible, a mental health professional with expertise in addiction medicine. Frequent team meetings and consultations with other clinicians may be needed. Ultimately, appropriate expectations must be clarified and failing therapy modified.

Illicit drug use, actual or suspected misuse of prescribed medications, or actual substance use disorders are among the most serious difficulties in the clinical setting, and can impair pain management. Opioid misuse can complicate chronic pain management, and the nonmedical use of opioids is a growing public health problem. Despite the benefits of opioid therapy, a subset of patients using opioids in the long-term may exhibit problematic opioid use. Problems associated with use include behaviors such as seeking prescriptions from multiple prescribers, forging prescriptions, preoccupation with obtaining more opioids despite evidence of adequate relief of pain, and unsanctioned dose escalations. Abuse of prescription opioids is escalating, commensurate with the number of prescriptions.[63] Katz and Fanciullo determined that the rates of opioid misuse in chronic pain ranged from 20% to 40%.[64] Early and proper identification along with careful monitoring for signs of opioid misuse, abuse, and addiction in chronic pain patients is essential. Portenoy suggested that forging prescriptions, stealing or borrowing drugs, frequently losing prescriptions, and resisting changes to medication, despite adverse side effects, are more predictive of opioid misuse than aggressive complaining about the need for more drugs, drug hoarding, and unsanctioned dose escalations or other forms of noncompliance; the latter three may be indicative of poorly controlled pain[65] (Table 20.4). However, Wasan et al.[66] found that physicians only judged 13.9% of chronic pain patients prescribed opioids as having aberrant drug behaviors, when approximately 50% had positive urine toxicology screens for illicit drugs, and 8.7% had no evidence of any opioids in their urine samples. Some providers rely on informal patient self-reports of medication use to determine whether the patients are engaging in inappropriate behaviors. However, when self-reports were compared with urine tests, up to 50% of substance abusers report falsely.[67] Urine toxicology screens are the "gold standard" for detecting substance use, yet it may not be cost-effective to routinely screen all patients with urine toxicology.

TABLE 20.4
ABERRANT DRUG BEHAVIORS PREDICTING A SUBSTANCE ABUSE DISORDER

Selling prescription drugs
Forging prescriptions
Stealing drugs
Injecting oral formulations
Obtaining prescription drugs from nonmedical sources
Concurrently abusing alcohol or other illicit drugs
Escalating doses on multiple occasions or failing to comply with the prescribed regimen despite warnings
"Losing" prescribed medication on multiple occasions
Repeatedly seeking prescriptions from other clinicians or from emergency room without informing the original prescribing clinician
Evidence of deteriorating ability to function (eg, work, family, social) that appears related to drug use

(From Jaffe J. Opiates: Clinical Aspects. In: Lowinson J, Ruiz P, Millman R, eds. *Substance abuse: a comprehensive text*. Baltimore: Williams & Wilkins, 1997:563–590.)

Variables such as reported family history of substance abuse, past problems with drugs or alcohol, and a history of legal problems can be useful in predicting problems with opioid use.[68] Sullivan et al.[69] reported that depressive, anxiety, and drug abuse disorders were associated with increased use of regular opioids in the general population and that depressive and anxiety disorders were more common and more strongly associated with prescribed opioid use than drug abuse disorders.

All patients who are prescribed potentially abuseable drugs should be monitored for the development of aberrant drug-related behaviors. The need for this monitoring is especially important in patients who have a remote or current history of substance or alcohol abuse. If there is a high level of concern about such behaviors, monitoring may require relatively frequent visits as well as regular assessment of significant others who can provide observations about patients' drug use.

Urine toxicology screening may be used to diagnose or monitor substance abuse in a variety of clinical settings. The analysis can be used to detect prescription medications (opioids, benzodiazepines, amphetamines, barbiturates), illegal substances (heroin, cocaine, marijuana), and nonillicit substances of abuse (eg, alcohol). Passik et al.[54] retrospectively reviewed 111 cancer patients treated at a tertiary-care cancer center who had received urine toxicology screening for suspected drug abuse. Fifty-six of the 111 patients had evidence of one or more illicit drugs, a prescription medication that had not been ordered, or alcohol; 50 patients had negative screens. The likelihood of a positive screen was higher if the patient had human immunodeficiency virus (HIV) infection (100% vs. 46.6%) or was undergoing treatment for chronic nonmalignant pain (100% vs. 43.9%). Documentation of the urine toxicology screen in the medical record was infrequent: 37.8% of the charts listed no reason for obtaining the test and the ordering physician could not be identified in 29% of the records. Eighty-nine percent of the records did not contain a subsequent mention of the result of the screen. These results suggest that as state regulations that protect physicians' prescribing of opioids for pain place the onus upon the prescriber to monitor abuse, more systematic utilization of urine toxiciology results is important, along with follow-up documentation for changes in management.

If urine toxicology screening is incorporated into a cancer pain management treatment plan, the clinician should clearly document who is ordering the test and why. Informed consent should be obtained from the patient before testing. Furthermore, there should be clear discussion of the results and their perceived interpretation (addiction, self-medication, and so on) and their impact on clinical decisions and subsequent management. Finally, additional plans for follow-up and subsequent screening should be outlined.

We do not do routine toxicology screening on all our patients. Special screening is required for patients we consider to be "at risk" (see "Indicators for Misuse of Medications" earlier in this chapter). If a urine sample is obtained, the patient's urine temperature is tested (should be approximately body temperature) and the sample verified by measuring urine creatinine (>20 mg/dL). All our samples are tested by gas chromatography/mass spectrometry (GCMS), and if we are trying to identify a specific opioid, we indicate that opioid on the request form. A sample that proves positive for illicit substances such as heroin, cocaine, or methamphetamine results in a mandatory clinic appointment for discussion of the results and treatment implications.

In our clinical practice, we frequently encounter issues relating to marijuana, cocaine, methamphetamine, and alcohol abuse. It is not unusual for patients to ask our advice regarding the use of marijuana for medical reasons. Illicit drug use, particularly with cocaine and methamphetamine, is problematic in the cancer patient with pain who is undergoing active treatment for disease. Many of these patients require ongoing therapy with opioids for pain control. There are no national guidelines or standards for opioid prescription in this situation, yet it violates federal Drug Enforcement Agency (DEA) regulations to prescribe opioids for a known substance abuser. Importantly, the needs of our patients for pain control in a safe environment must be carefully considered. In an effort to manage these most difficult of patients, we address the salient issues associated with these substances.

MEDICAL MARIJUANA

Cannabis has known medicinal significance for thousands of years. It is obtained from the plant *Cannabis sativa*. Cannabis is also known as hemp. *Marijuana* describes the dried cannabis flowers and leaves which are smoked, and *hashish* refers to blocks of cannabis resin, which can be eaten. The medical use of cannabis (this refers to herbal therapy, synthetic tetrahydrocannabinol (THC), and cannabinoids) is legal only in a limited number of countries, including Canada, Belgium, Austria, the Netherlands, the United Kingdom, Spain, Israel, Finland, and a number of U.S. states. In the United States, marijuana is regulated as a Schedule I controlled substance and its use is prohibited under federal law. The U.S. Food and Drug Adminstration does not support the use of (smoked) marijuana for medical purposes, stating that no sound scientific studies, animal or human data support its safety or efficacy. Twelve U.S. states have passed legislative actions making (medical) cannabis available upon a physician's recommendation.[70] Therapeutic use of cannabis and cannabis-based medicines raises safety concerns for patients, clinicians, policy-makers, insurers, researchers and regulators. Wang et al.[71] noted that the short-term use of existing medical cannabinoids appeared to increase the risk of nonserious adverse events. The risks associated with long-term use were poorly characterized in published clinical trials and observational studies. High-quality trials of long-term exposure are required to further characterize safety issues related to the use of medical cannabinoids.

Reported benefits from cannabinoids include analgesic, antiemetic, antioxidative, neuroprotective, and anti-inflammatory activity, as well as modulation of glial cells and tumor growth regulation.[72] Both the users and those who advocate medicinal cannabis claim favorable effects for the treatment of refractory neurological symptoms, pain associated with multiple sclerosis (MS) or spinal cord injury,[73] chronic neuralgic pain, AIDS-related anorexia,[74] HIV-medication-induced nausea and vomiting, Crohn disease,[75] and Gilles de la Tourette syndrome. In oncology, beneficial effects have been reported for cancer-associated anorexia, (delayed) chemo- or radiotherapy-induced nausea, and vomiting.[76] In addition, palliative effects reported included treatment of insomnia,[77] mood elevation, appetite stimulation,[78] and pain relief.[73]

The use of cannabinoids in cancer has been extensively reviewed.[77,79] When cannabis is smoked, THC is absorbed into the bloodstream after several minutes via the lungs; by contrast, when taken orally it takes 1 to 3 hours to enter the bloodstream. After smoking, THC is metabolized first in the lungs and then in the liver. The metabolite 9-carboxy-THC, which is not psychoactive, is detectable in blood several minutes after smoking cannabis. Slightly more potent than THC, 11-hydroxy-THC is a metabolite that crosses the blood-brain barrier more rapidly, and which is found in very low concentrations in the blood after smoking and at higher concentrations after oral use. THC and its metabolites account for most of the psychoactive effects of cannabis.

In our practice, when asked by patients to consider the authorization of marijuana for medical reasons, we determine the appropriateness of use on an individual basis. In addition, we determine if there are potential adverse effects from the use of marijuana (eg, smoke inhalation in an immunocompromised patient). Assuming there are medical reasons for use and there are no contraindications to use, the patient is asked to sign a consent form to assume risks for medical marijuana (Appendix G). If the patient chooses to use marijuana, we strongly suggest third-party (spouse or partner endorsement of appropriateness of use and lack of potential drug interactions or adverse effects. The indications for medical use of marijuana are documented in the medical record and a physician form of authorization for medical marijuana use is completed (Appendix H).

COCAINE ABUSE

Cocaine, or benzoylmethylecgnine, is an ester of benzoic acid and methylecognine. It is a naturally occurring substance found in the leaves of the *Erythroxylum coca* plant. The plant is endogenous to South America, Mexico, Indonesia, and the West Indies. Peoples of ancient civilizations used the coca leaves for religious and ceremonial reasons. In 1884, it was used as the first anesthetic. By the late 19th century, cocaine was widely used for its analgesic properties to include nerve block anesthesia, epidural, and spinal anesthesia. As an ester-type local anesthetic, cocaine blocks voltage-gated sodium channels in the neuronal membrane. Cocaine exhibits its vasoconstrictive action therapeutically by inhibiting local reuptake of norepinephrine. The ester link is rapidly hydrolyzed by plasma cholinesterases, which contributes to cocaine's short half-life. Cocaine alkaloid is extracted from leaves and then converted to cocaine hydrochloride ("coke") using hydrochloric acid. This white powder is usually insufflated but can also be dissolved in water and injected. Cocaine hydrochloride is dissolved in water, mixed with a strong base, and heated. Cocaine base is extracted by the addition of an organic solvent. Free base will dry into a hard rock upon evaporation. Crack cocaine is then usually smoked out of a glass pipe.

Cocaine exhibits profound central nervous system (CNS) and cardiovascular toxicity. Cocaine blocks the reuptake of catecholamines (dopamine, norepinephrine) and serotonin. Increased serotonergic activity can result in seizures and may be involved in the addiction and reward effects of cocaine. Excessive dopamine activity may cause the majority of CNS symptoms, both the euphoric and the toxic effects. CNS symptoms include euphoria, increased self-confidence and alertness at lower doses, and aggressiveness, disorientation, and hallucinations at higher doses. Repetitive use of cocaine results in the depletion of the dopamine stores. This can result both in an intense craving for cocaine and in what is referred to as a "washed-out" syndrome. Cocaine can also affect the hypothalamus and cause hyperthermia. Cocaine is also known to cause vasoconstriction, which can result in hypertension, cerebrovascular accident (CVA), cardiac ischemia, and end-organ and tissue infarcts. Cocaine is also a CYP3A4 substrate, and a strong CYP2D6 inhibitor. Drugs that inhibit CYP3A4 may increase cocaine toxicity (eg, azole antifungals, propofol) and cocaine may increase toxicity of CYP2D6 substrates (eg, amphetamines, tricyclic antidepressants, and certain opioids, including codeine/hydrocodone/oxycodone).

Cocaine may be administered by insufflation (snorting), intravenous injection, smoking, ingestion, or mucousal application. The half-life of cocaine is approximately 0.7 to 1.5 hours and most of the administered dose is eliminated within a few hours. Cocaine and its major metabolite, benzoylecgonine, may be detected in urine, blood, saliva, and meconium. Benzoylecgonine may be detected in urine up to 3 days after last drug usage by enzyme-multiplied immunoassay technique or gas chromatography/mass spectrometry and up to 7 days by radioimmunoassay. It may be detected up to 10 days following chronic heavy daily usage.

Abuse of cocaine can be extremely dangerous. It causes acute and chronic disease affecting multiple systems, including the central nervous, cardiovascular, respiratory, gastrointestinal, renal, and endocrine. Crack lung has been described in patients with acute pulmonary syndromes after inhaling freebase cocaine.[80] Patients may present with a combination of fever, chest pain, dyspnea, hypoxemia, diffuse alveolar infiltrates that may be persistent, and respiratory failure. Varied effects of the drug occur, with inter- and intraindividual variation dependent on the amount of the drug taken, the route of abuse, nutritional status, gender, whether used alone or in combination with other drugs, and whether previous exposure has occurred. Cocaine is capable of causing significant morbidity or mortality on single or repeated use. It is a very dangerous recreational drug, particularly because of increasing availability. Cocaine generally causes euphoria, but also may produce agitation, anxiety, panic, and psychosis. Complications associated with intranasal cocaine use may mimic other diagnoses including Wegener granulomatosis, nasal lymphoma, and necrotizing granulomatous vasculitis.[81-84]

In 2004, more than 3% of people over the age of 12 in the United States used cocaine and/or methamphetamine.[85] A substantial number of addicted users eventually gain the desire but lack the ability to stop using the drug. There are significant societal and health-related problems from cocaine abuse. Cocaine users often present in acute crises and require a service capable of responding to their needs. The majority of individuals seeking treatment smoke crack, and are likely to be multiple drug users. Cocaine abuse may inhibit the response to imatinib in chronic myelogenous leukemia (CML) patients.[86] Lifetime substance abuse or dependence appears to have an adverse association with survival after bone marrow transplant when other clinical factors are equal.[87]

Treatments for cocaine addiction are complex and must address a variety of problems. Treatments for cocaine and crack cocaine users typically involve counseling, the use of antidepressants and, rarely, substitute prescribing. Behavioral interventions can be helpful but only in a limited number of users. Currently, there are no approved medications to treat this disorder. Pharmacologic treatments for stimulant users are few and largely ineffective. Some evidence suggests that dual dopamine/serotonin release agents may be useful for the treatment of cocaine and other stimulant abuse.[88] Aripiprazole (Abilify) is an atypical antipsychotic that is a partial agonist at D_2 receptors and may attenuate the effects of dextroamphetamine that are associated with the abuse of stimulants.[89] Conjugate vaccines for cocaine abuse are in development.[85] Both phase I and II trials have been completed using a cholera toxin B conjugated cocaine preparation.[90-91]

METHAMPHETAMINE ABUSE

Abuse of the psychostimulant methamphetamine is a major worldwide epidemic, and recent trends indicate an alarmingly widespread increase across all segments of the U.S. population, including increased use among adolescents.[92] Amphetamine-type substances are the second most-widely abused drugs after cannabis, and not only do the characteristics of methamphetamine use vary by region around the world, they also vary within the North American region.[60]

Methamphetamine, a stimulant colloquially known as "crystal meth," "crank," "ice," "chalk," or "Tina," is a highly addictive substance that can be snorted, smoked, ingested orally or rectally, and injected. It is a methyl derivative of amphetamine, and is a powerful psychostimulant that directly affects the autonomic nervous system and CNS even when taken in small amounts. Methamphetamine induces the release of monoamine transmitters through nonexocytotic mechanisms, involving both their redistribution from synaptic vesicle sites into the cytoplasm and their reverse transport through the plasma membrane uptake carriers.[93-94] In the brain, a primary action of methamphetamine is to elevate the levels of extracellular monoamine neurotransmitters (dopamine, serotonin, norepinephrine) by promoting their release from the nerve ending. It produces memory and recall impairments in humans.[95]

Methamphetamine is a cationic molecule with potent sympathetic and CNS action[96] that is an analog of amphetamine.[94] Although both molecules are very similar, methamphetamine is more highly lipophilic, crosses the blood-brain barrier more readily, and is therefore more potent than its parent compound.[97] Crystal methamphetamine is a smokeable, crystalline solid form of methamphetamine. To a recreational drug user, the advantage of the smokeable form of methamphetamine over the oral form is the very rapid and intense "high." The type of stimulant most used has shifted from nonmedical use of pharmaceutical amphetamine to use of powder methamphetamine and then to the use of "ice" (a crystallized chunk of amphetamine that makes for a more intense reaction).[60] The production of methamphetamine is difficult to control because it can be made from chemicals that are contained in everyday products ranging from cleaning fluids to over-the-counter medications. The majority of subsequent precursor diversion initiatives have targeted ephedrine and pseudoephedrine as chemicals that convert readily to methamphetamine, and which are widely available as decongestant medications.

Following oral administration, peak methamphetamine concentrations are seen in 2.6 to 3.6 hours and the mean elimination half-life is 10.1 hours (range: 6.4 to 15 hours). The amphetamine metabolite peaks at 12 hours. Following intravenous injection, the mean elimination half-life is slightly longer (12.2 hours). Methamphetamine is metabolized to the active metabolite amphetamine and the inactive metabolites p-OH-amphetamine and norephedrine.

Short-term effects of methamphetamine include an initial "rush," increased energy, a general sense of well-being, and decreased appetite, which typically lasts 6 to 8 hours. Acute effects of methamphetamine result in excitation with increased alertness, highly focused attention, motivation, confidence, mood, energy, and decreased appetite.[98] Persons under the influence of acute ingestion of methamphetamine can appear excessively talkative, excited, agitated, aggressive, restless, and may be observed performing repetitive meaningless tasks. Extended use may result in psychological symptoms which include persistent anxiety, paranoia, insomnia, auditory hallucinations, delusions, psychotic or violent behavior, and homicidal or suicidal thinking.[99] Behavioral signs may include unprovoked violent behavior, and poor coping abilities. Additional signs of chronic use include high blood pressure, pronounced fatigue, malnutrition, involuntary movement disorders, sexual dysfunction, weight loss, nose bleed from intranasal ingestion, and dental problems. Acute and chronic effects of methamphetamine can severely impact the cardiovascular system. Chronic CNS hyperstimulation can cause headaches. "Meth mouth" is characterized by widespread tooth decay and tooth loss, advanced tooth wear and fracture, and oral soft tissue inflammation and breakdown.[100]

Adverse effects of methamphetamine include restlessness, insomnia, hyperthermia, and possibly convulsions. Long-term use can lead to addiction, paranoia, mood disturbances, agitation, psychosis, and cognitive impairment. Discontinuation often results in a withdrawal syndrome which includes dysphoria, fatigue, sleep disturbances, and increased appetite. Withdrawal is characterized more by psychiatric symptoms than physical symptoms. With chronic users, symptoms of withdrawal may persist for over 12 months.[97] Abuse is associated with a wide range of psychological, medical, and social problems. Use is associated with risky and antisocial behaviors, including other illicit drug use.[101] The profoundly addictive properties of methamphetamine are directly related to its reinforcing effects, mediated by the rapid and sustained increases in monoamine (primarily dopamine) neurotransmission immediately following its ingestion.

The complex interaction between psychic, environmental, and behavioral factors makes methamphetamine dependence a difficult disorder to treat. Complicating recovery are the severe withdrawal symptoms that include severe anhedonia and depression, as well as intense cravings for the drug. Treatment of dependence combines cognitive, behavioral, and psychological approaches. There are no Food and Drug Administration (FDA)-approved medications for the treatment of methamphetamine dependence. Modafinil (200 mg/day) may be useful in reducing methamphetamine use in selected methamphetamine-dependent patients.[102]

ALCOHOL ABUSE

Excessive drinking is associated with acute medical complications, chronic diseases, reproductive problems, nutritional deficiencies, psychological problems, and injuries. The presence of other medical conditions is especially true for patients with head and neck cancer, who are likely to have significant tobacco and alcohol use.[103] Epidemiological studies have demonstrated a positive association between alcohol consumption and an increased risk for breast cancer and suggest even moderate alcohol consumption leads to a significantly increased risk.[104] The National Institute on Alcohol Abuse and Alcoholism (NIAAA) estimated that the prevalence of alcohol dependence in the United States is 5%, but up to three of every ten adults drink alcohol at levels associated with adverse health and social consequences.[105] Alcohol-related morbidity and mortality occur at drinking levels below those typically associated with alcohol abuse or dependence.[106-107]

Various diseases, including hypertension, stroke, cardiomyopathy, cirrhosis, chronic pancreatitis, brain atrophy, osteoporosis, various types of cancer (including liver, oral, throat, larynx, esophagus, and probably breast and colon), gastroesophageal reflux, esophagitis, peptic ulcers, pancreatitis, and seizures are associated with excess alcohol use. In addition, excessive alcohol uses causes mental health and social problems. Certain medications including opioids, antidepressants, antihistamines, anti-epileptic drugs, and sedative/hypnotics interact harmfully with alcohol.

Screening for unhealthy alcohol use is helpful and clinicians should question patients on the average weekly number of alcoholic drinks. In a primary care setting, a single screening question, "How many times in the past year have you had x or more drinks in a day?," where $x = 5$ for men and 4 for women, and a response of >1 is considered positive, was predictive of unhealthy alcohol use.[108] The CAGE questionnaire is a four-item screening test that is better at identifying alcohol dependence than lower levels of problem drinking or binge drinking[109] (Appendix N). Patients who report at least 1 heavy drinking day (5 drinks for men and 4 drinks for women) are at-risk drinkers and require further assessment and counseling about safe drinking levels. Clinicians should screen all patients annually to determine their level of alcohol consumption and to advise them on safe drinking levels (<2 drinks per day for men younger than 65 years and <1 drink per day for women and men 65 years and older). Binge drinking (>4 drinks per occasion for men and >3 drinks per occasion for women) also indicates risky alcohol use. At-risk drinking may be considered as drinking at levels that can lead to diverse physical, psychological, and social consequences; alcohol abuse disorders are characterized by continued drinking despite adverse consequences.

Screening patients can be difficult because of patient denial and misreporting of alcohol use. Alcohol biomarkers are useful to supplement patient self-report and provide more objective evidence on alcohol use. Laboratory tests, such as γ-glutamyl transferase, aspartate aminotransferase, alanine aminotransferase, and mean corpuscular volume alone do not accurately detect alcohol problems.[110] Percentage of carbohydrate deficient transferrin (CDT) is the only laboratory marker approved by the FDA to detect chronic heavy drinking. Measurement of CDT can reveal alcohol-related changes in the serum transferrin glycosylation pattern. CDT is a more alcohol-specific indicator than liver-function tests.[111] The CDT test incorporates fractions of total transferrin. However, this marker is confounded by liver disease.[112] Persons who drink more than 40 to 60 g of ethanol per day often have a CDT level of more than 2.5%.[113] The test is most sensitive in men between the ages of 30 and 60 years and is less sensitive in women and episodic drinkers.[114-117]

Comorbid conditions such as other recreational drug use and psychiatric disorders frequently occur in patients with alcohol problems. About one half of women and 33% of men with a history of alcohol use disorders have at least 1 other psychiatric disorder.[118] Untreated alcohol dependence can intensify depression and increase the likelihood of suicide and other self-destructive behavior.[119] Individuals with alcohol dependence are at increased risk for developing dependence on illicit and prescription drugs.[120]

For patients who misuse alcohol but are not alcohol dependent, the goal of treatment is to decrease alcohol consumption to safe levels. If patients cannot moderate alcohol intake, they should abstain from alcohol. For patients with alcohol abuse and dependence, various psychological counseling strategies and drugs (eg, naltrexone, disulfiram) may be effective. The ultimate goal of treatment is abstinence. Benzodiazepines are first-line therapy for patients who require pharmacologic prophylaxis or treatment for alcohol withdrawal. Haloperidol can treat agitation and hallucinations. Withdrawal symptoms generally begin 6 to 24 hours after the intake of alcohol is substantially reduced or stopped. Minor withdrawal may peak at about 36 hours, whereas major withdrawal may peak at 50 hours and last up to 5 days. Delirium tremens is characterized by fever, profound confusion, and hallucinations and usually occurs before the second to third day of abstinence. Treatment of minor withdrawal consists of supportive care and possibly medications, whereas treatment of major withdrawal requires medication and possibly hospitalization. A 10-item Clinical Institute Withdrawal Assessment Scale for Alcohol Revised (CIWA) can be used to measure symptom severity and provide guidance for treatment.[121]

Concomitant alcohol use is an issue or contraindicated for many drugs due to the potential for pharmacokinetic (eg, altered clearance) or pharmacodynamic (eg, effects on the CNS) interactions. Alcohol enhances the effects of opioids on the CNS and even moderate drinking may pose a risk of potential drug–drug interaction.[122] Unintended, rapid drug release in a short period of time of the entire amount or a significant fraction of the drug contained in a modified release dosage form is often referred to as "dose dumping." Dose dumping is a serious concern with controlled release preparations. Generally dose-dumping is observed to arise from a compromise of the release-rate-controlling mechanism. Some modified-release oral dosage forms contain drugs and excipients that exhibit higher solubility in ethanolic solutions compared to water. Such products can be expected to exhibit a more rapid drug dissolution and release rate in the presence of ethanol. Therefore, concomitant consumption of alcoholic beverages along with these products might be expected to have the potential to induce dose dumping. Warnings by regulatory bodies and a product recall by the

FDA have generated much interest in the area of dose dumping from controlled-release opioid analgesic formulations when coingested with alcohol.

Tramadol release from Ultram ER tablets was significantly increased in the presence of ethanol.[123] Dose dumping was not observed when Kadian was taken concomitantly with alcohol.[124] After a pharmacokinetic study in healthy volunteers indicated a potentially fatal interaction between alcohol and hydromorphone hydrochloride extended release capsules (Palladone; Purdue Pharma L.P., Stamford, Conn.), the FDA requested the removal of this opioid from the market. In the study, coingestion of Palladone with 240 mL (8 oz) of 40% (80 proof) alcohol raised peak plasma hydromorphone concentrations approximately sixfold, compared with ingestion with water, with one subject experiencing a 16-fold increase in peak blood level. This study also showed that 8 ounces of 4% alcohol (equivalent to two thirds of a typical serving of beer) could in some subjects result in almost twice the peak plasma hydromorphone concentration than when the drug was ingested with water. Dose dumping may also occur with Avinza. In vitro studies performed by the FDA demonstrated that when Avinza 30 mg was mixed with 900 mL of buffer solutions containing ethanol (20% and 40%), the dose of morphine that was released was alcohol concentration-dependent, leading to a more rapid release of morphine. Single daily dosing of OROS hydromorphone did not result in dose dumping with alcohol.[125] Prolonged release mechanisms appear to remain intact with MS Contin and OxyContin with alcohol ingestion.[126] Nonetheless, alcohol ingestion is a real hazard for patients consuming opioids.

RECOMMENDATIONS

Cocaine and methamphetamine use are problematic for us. With very few exceptions, we do not allow use of these substances. In patients with a history of use or who are actively using these substances, we will do routine urine toxicology analysis for these substances and also GCMS analysis for opioids that we are prescribing. If illicit substances are found, patients will be required to have weekly urine analyses until they are drug free. If a urine analysis is "dirty," a tapering schedule from their prescribed opioids is commenced and patients are warned that opioids will continue to be tapered until they are either off all opioids or they can abstain from illicit drug use. In patients who continue to use illicit substances despite repeated warnings, a referral for appropriate drug treatment is made. In some situations, patients will also be counseled by us that continued use of illicit substances may impact future care of their cancer at our facility. Problematic alcohol use is not frequently encountered in our patient population especially when patients are in active treatment for their disease. It is more frequently encountered when disease is in remission or patients have just been diagnosed with cancer. This is potentially a very dangerous situation, particularly with opioid prescription; continued alcohol use will usually result in a referral for appropriate treatment of this disease or a discontinuation of opioid prescription.

References

1. Cicero TJ, Inciardi JA, Munoz A. Trends in abuse of OxyContin and other opioid analgesics in the United States: 2002–2004. *J Pain.* 2005; 6:662–672.
2. Hughes AA, Bogdan GM, Dart RC. Active surveillance of abused and misused prescription opioids using poison center data: a pilot study and descriptive comparison. *Clin Toxicol (Phila).* 2007; 45:144–151.
3. Dasgupta N, Kramer ED, Zalman MA, et al. Association between non-medical and prescriptive usage of opioids. *Drug Alcohol Depend.* 2006; 82:135–142.
4. Joranson DE, Ryan KM, Gilson AM, Dahl JL. Trends in medical use and abuse of opioid analgesics. *JAMA.* 2000; 283:1710–1714.
5. Gilson AM, Ryan KM, Joranson DE, Dahl JL. A reassessment of trends in the medical use and abuse of opioid analgesics and implications for diversion control: 1997-2002. *J Pain Symptom Manage.* 2004; 28:176–188.
6. Wisniewski AM, Purdy CH, Blondell RD. The epidemiologic association between opioid prescribing, non-medical use, and emergency department visits. *J Addict Dis.* 2008; 27:1–11.
7. Zacny J, Bigelow G, Compton P, et al. College on Problems of Drug Dependence taskforce on prescription opioid non-medical use and abuse: position statement. *Drug Alcohol Depend.* 2003; 69: 215–232.
8. Akbik H, Butler SF, Budman SH, et al. Validation and clinical application of the Screener and Opioid Assessment for Patients with Pain (SOAPP). *J Pain Symptom Manage.* 2006; 32:287–293.
9. Butler SF, Budman SH, Fernandez KC, et al. Development and validation of the Current Opioid Misuse Measure. *Pain.* 2007; 130: 144–156.
10. Manchikanti L, Singh A. Therapeutic opioids: a ten-year perspective on the complexities and complications of the escalating use, abuse, and nonmedical use of opioids. *Pain Physician.* 2008; 11:S63-88.
11. Substance Abuse and Mental Health Services Administration. Results from the 2002 National Survey on Drug Use and Health: National Findings. Studies OoA, ed. Rockville, MD: DHHE 2003A.
12. Reid CM, Martin RM, Sterne JA, et al. Oxycodone for cancer-related pain: meta-analysis of randomized controlled trials. *Arch Intern Med.* 2006; 166:837–843.
13. Zacny JP, Gutierrez S. Characterizing the subjective, psychomotor, and physiological effects of oral oxycodone in non-drug-abusing volunteers. *Psychopharmacology (Berl).* 2003; 170:242–254.
14. Cone EJ, Fant RV, Rohay JM, et al. Oxycodone involvement in drug abuse deaths. II. Evidence for toxic multiple drug-drug interactions. *J Anal Toxicol.* 2004; 28:616–624.
15. Darke S, Zador D. Fatal heroin 'overdose': a review. *Addiction.* 1996; 91:1765–1772.
16. Novak S, Nemeth WC, Lawson KA. Trends in medical use and abuse of sustained-release opioid analgesics: a revisit. *Pain Med.* 2004; 5:59–65.
17. Cicero TJ, Surratt H, Inciardi JA, Munoz A. Relationship between therapeutic use and abuse of opioid analgesics in rural, suburban, and urban locations in the United States. *Pharmacoepidemiol Drug Saf.* 2007; 16:827–840.
18. Carise D, Dugosh KL, McLellan AT, et al. Prescription OxyContin abuse among patients entering addiction treatment. *Am J Psychiatry.* 2007; 164:1750–1756.
19. Elkader AK, Brands B, Dunn E, et al. Major depressive disorder and patient satisfaction in relation to methadone pharmacokinetics and pharmacodynamics in stabilized methadone maintenance patients. *J Clin Psychopharmacol.* 2009; 29:77–81.
20. Corsi KF, Lehman WK, Booth RE. The effect of methadone maintenance on positive outcomes for opiate injection drug users. *J Subst Abuse Treat.* 2009; 37:120–126.
21. Kreek MJ. Opioid receptors: some perspectives from early studies of their role in normal physiology, stress responsivity, and in specific addictive diseases. *Neurochem Res.* 1996; 21:1469–1488.
22. Faggiano F, Vigna-Taglianti F, Versino E, Lemma P. Methadone maintenance at different dosages for opioid dependence. *Cochrane Database Syst Rev.* 2003:CD002208.
23. Mattick RP, Kimber J, Breen C, Davoli M. Buprenorphine maintenance versus placebo or methadone maintenance for opioid dependence. *Cochrane Database Syst Rev.* 2008:CD002207.
24. Dole VP, Nyswander ME, Kreek MJ. Narcotic blockade. 1966. *J Psychoactive Drugs.* 1991; 23:following 232.

25. McLellan AT, Lewis DC, O'Brien CP, Kleber HD. Drug dependence, a chronic medical illness: implications for treatment, insurance, and outcomes evaluation. *JAMA.* 2000; 284:1689–1695.
26. Dyer KR, White JM. Patterns of symptom complaints in methadone maintenance patients. *Addiction.* 1997; 92:1445–1455.
27. Goldstein A. Blind comparison of once-daily and twice-daily dosage schedules in a methadone program. *Clin Pharmacol Ther.* 1972; 13:59–63.
28. Preston KL, Umbricht A, Epstein DH. Methadone dose increase and abstinence reinforcement for treatment of continued heroin use during methadone maintenance. *Arch Gen Psychiatry.* 2000; 57:395–404.
29. Strain EC, Stitzer ML, Liebson IA, Bigelow GE. Dose-response effects of methadone in the treatment of opioid dependence. *Ann Intern Med.* 1993; 119:23–27.
30. Hubbard RL, Rachal JV, Craddock SG, Cavanaugh ER. Treatment Outcome Prospective Study (TOPS): client characteristics and behaviors before, during, and after treatment. *NIDA Res Monogr.* 1984; 51:42–68.
31. Mattick RP, Hall W. Are detoxification programmes effective? *Lancet.* 1996; 347:97–100.
32. O'Connor PG, Kosten TR. Rapid and ultrarapid opioid detoxification techniques. *JAMA.* 1998; 279:229–234.
33. Sees KL, Delucchi KL, Masson C, et al. Methadone maintenance vs 180-day psychosocially enriched detoxification for treatment of opioid dependence: a randomized controlled trial. *JAMA.* 2000; 283:1303–1310.
34. Martin WR, Jasinski DR. Physiological parameters of morphine dependence in man—tolerance, early abstinence, protracted abstinence. *J Psychiatr Res.* 1969; 7:9–17.
35. Amato L, Davoli M, Minozzi S, et al. Methadone at tapered doses for the management of opioid withdrawal. *Cochrane Database Syst Rev.* 2005:CD003409.
36. Glasper A, Gossop M, de Wet C, et al. Influence of the dose on the severity of opiate withdrawal symptoms during methadone detoxification. *Pharmacology.* 2008; 81:92–96.
37. Kleber HD, Riordan CE, Rounsaville B, et al. Clonidine in outpatient detoxification from methadone maintenance. *Arch Gen Psychiatry.* 1985; 42:391–394.
38. Gowing L, Farrell M, Ali R, White J. Alpha2 adrenergic agonists for the management of opioid withdrawal. *Cochrane Database Syst Rev.* 2004:CD002024.
39. Favrat B, Zimmermann G, Zullino D, et al. Opioid antagonist detoxification under anaesthesia versus traditional clonidine detoxification combined with an additional week of psychosocial support: a randomised clinical trial. *Drug Alcohol Depend.* 2006; 81: 109–116.
40. Hamilton RJ, Olmedo RE, Shah S, et al. Complications of ultrarapid opioid detoxification with subcutaneous naltrexone pellets. *Acad Emerg Med.* 2002; 9:63–68.
41. Whittington RA, Collins ED, Kleber HD. Rapid opioid detoxification during general anesthesia: is death not a significant outcome? *Anesthesiology.* 2000; 93:1363–1364.
42. Kirchmayer U, Davoli M, Verster A. Naltrexone maintenance treatment for opioid dependence. *Cochrane Database Syst Rev.* 2003: CD001333.
43. Minozzi S, Amato L, Vecchi S, et al. Oral naltrexone maintenance treatment for opioid dependence. *Cochrane Database Syst Rev.* 2006:CD001333.
44. Day E, Ison J, Strang J. Inpatient versus other settings for detoxification for opioid dependence. *Cochrane Database Syst Rev.* 2005: CD004580.
45. Jasinski DR, Pevnick JS, Griffith JD. Human pharmacology and abuse potential of the analgesic buprenorphine: a potential agent for treating narcotic addiction. *Arch Gen Psychiatry.* 1978; 35: 501–516.
46. Walsh SL, Preston KL, Stitzer ML, et al. Clinical pharmacology of buprenorphine: ceiling effects at high doses. *Clin Pharmacol Ther.* 1994; 55:569–580.
47. Brigham GS, Amass L, Winhusen T, et al. Using buprenorphine short-term taper to facilitate early treatment engagement. *J Subst Abuse Treat.* 2007; 32:349–356.
48. Woody GE, Poole SA, Subramaniam G, et al. Extended vs short-term buprenorphine-naloxone for treatment of opioid-addicted youth: a randomized trial. *JAMA.* 2008; 300:2003–2011.
49. Ziedonis DM, Amass L, Steinberg M, et al. Predictors of outcome for short-term medically supervised opioid withdrawal during a randomized, multicenter trial of buprenorphine-naloxone and clonidine in the NIDA clinical trials network drug and alcohol dependence. *Drug Alcohol Depend.* 2009; 99:28–36.
50. Smith MY, Bailey JE, Woody GE, Kleber HD. Abuse of buprenorphine in the United States: 2003-2005. *J Addict Dis.* 2007; 26: 107–111.
51. Simojoki K, Vorma H, Alho H. A retrospective evaluation of patients switched from buprenorphine (Subutex) to the buprenorphine/naloxone combination (Suboxone). *Subst Abuse Treat Prev Policy.* 2008; 3:16.
52. Montoya ID, Gorelick DA, Preston KL, et al. Randomized trial of buprenorphine for treatment of concurrent opiate and cocaine dependence. *Clin Pharmacol Ther.* 2004; 75:34–48.
53. Rinaldi RC, Steindler EM, Wilford BB, et al. Clarification and standardization of substance abuse terminology. *JAMA.* 1988;259: 555–557.
54. Passik SD, Kirsh KL, McDonald MV, et al. A pilot survey of aberrant drug-taking attitudes and behaviors in samples of cancer and AIDS patients. *J Pain Symptom Manage.* 2000;19:274–286.
55. Bruera E, Moyano J, Seifert L, et al. The frequency of alcoholism among patients with pain due to terminal cancer. *J Pain Symptom Manage.* 1995;10:599–603.
56. Colliver JD, Kopstein AN. Trends in cocaine abuse reflected in emergency room episodes reported to DAWN. Drug Abuse Warning Network. *Public Health Rep.* 1991;106:59–68.
57. Gfroerer J, Brodsky M. The incidence of illicit drug use in the United States, 1962-1989. *Br J Addict.* 1992;87:1345–1351.
58. Kessler RC, McGonagle KA, Zhao S, et al. Lifetime and 12-month prevalence of DSM-III-R psychiatric disorders in the United States. Results from the National Comorbidity Survey. *Arch Gen Psychiatry.* 1994;51:8–19.
59. Regier DA, Shapiro S, Kessler LG, et al. Epidemiology and health service resource allocation policy for alcohol, drug abuse, and mental disorders. *Public Health Rep.* 1984;99:483–492.
60. Maxwell JC, Rutkowski BA. The prevalence of methamphetamine and amphetamine abuse in North America: A review of the indicators, 1992-2007. *Drug Alcohol Rev.* 2008;27:229–235.
61. Paulozzi LJ. Opioid analgesic involvement in drug abuse deaths in American metropolitan areas. *Am J Public Health.* 2006;96: 1755–1757.
62. Paulozzi LJ, Budnitz DS, Xi Y. Increasing deaths from opioid analgesics in the United States. *Pharmacoepidemiol Drug Saf.* 2006;15:618–627.
63. Soderstrom CA, Dischinger PC, Kerns TJ, et al. Epidemic increases in cocaine and opiate use by trauma center patients: Documentation with a large clinical toxicology database. *J Trauma.* 2001;51: 557–564.
64. Katz N, Fanciullo GJ. Role of urine toxicology testing in the management of chronic opioid therapy. *Clin J Pain.* 2002;18:S76-82.
65. Portenoy RK. Opioid therapy for chronic nonmalignant pain: A review of the critical issues. *J Pain Symptom Manage.* 1996;11: 203–217.
66. Wasan A, Fernandez E, Jamison RN, et al. Association of anxiety and depression with reported disease severity in patients undergoing evaluation for chronic rhinosinusitis. *Ann Otol Rhinol Laryngol.* 2007;116:491–497.
67. Cook RF, Bernstein AD, Arrington TL, et al. Methods for assessing drug use prevalence in the workplace: A comparison of self-report, urinalysis, and hair analysis. *Int J Addict.* 1995;30:403–426.
68. Michna E, Ross EL, Hynes WL, et al. Predicting aberrant drug behavior in patients treated for chronic pain: Importance of abuse history. *J Pain Symptom Manage.* 2004;28:250–258.
69. Sullivan MD, Edlund MJ, Steffick D, et al. Regular use of prescribed opioids: Association with common psychiatric disorders. *Pain.* 2005;119:95–103.
70. O'Connell TJ, Bou-Matar CB. Long term marijuana users seeking medical cannabis in California:[2001-2007] Demographics, social characteristics, patterns of cannabis and other drug use of 4117 applicants. *Harm Reduct J.* 2007;4:16.
71. Wang T, Collet JP, Shapiro S, et al. Adverse effects of medical cannabinoids: A systematic review. *CMAJ.* 2008;178:1669–1678.
72. Carter GT, Ugalde V. Medical marijuana: Emerging applications for the management of neurologic disorders. *Phys Med Rehabil Clin N Am.* 2004;15:943–954.

73. Rice AS. Cannabinoids and pain. *Curr Opin Investig Drugs.* 2001; 2:399–414.
74. Gorter R. Management of anorexia-cachexia associated with cancer and HIV infection. *Oncology (Williston Park).* 1991;5:13–17.
75. Massa F, Monory K. Endocannabinoids and the gastrointestinal tract. *J Endocrinol Invest.* 2006;29:47–57.
76. Tramer MR, Carroll D, Campbell FA, et al. Cannabinoids for control of chemotherapy induced nausea and vomiting: quantitative systematic review. *BMJ.* 2001;323:16–21.
77. Walsh D, Nelson KA, Mahmoud FA. Established and potential therapeutic applications of cannabinoids in oncology. *Support Care Cancer.* 2003;11:137–143.
78. Strasser F, Luftner D, Possinger K, et al. Comparison of orally administered cannabis extract and delta-9-tetrahydrocannabinol in treating patients with cancer-related anorexia-cachexia syndrome: A multicenter, phase III, randomized, double-blind, placebo-controlled clinical trial from the Cannabis-In-Cachexia-Study-Group. *J Clin Oncol.* 2006;24:3394–3400.
79. Hall W, Christie M, Currow D. Cannabinoids and cancer: Causation, remediation, and palliation. *Lancet Oncol.* 2005;6:35–42.
80. Forrester JM, Steele AW, Waldron JA, et al. Crack lung: An acute pulmonary syndrome with a spectrum of clinical and histopathologic findings. *Am Rev Respir Dis.* 1990;142:462–467.
81. Alameda F, Fontane J, Corominas JM, et al. Reactive vascular lesion of nasal septum simulating angiosarcoma in a cocaine abuser. *Hum Pathol.* 2000;31:239–241.
82. Chauhan SS, Krishnan J, Heffner DK. Solitary fibrous tumor of nasal cavity in patient with long-standing history of cocaine inhalation. *Arch Pathol Lab Med.* 2004;128:e1-4.
83. Fuchs HA, Tanner SB. Granulomatous disorders of the nose and paranasal sinuses. *Curr Opin Otolaryngol Head Neck Surg.* 2009; 17:23–27.
84. Gertner E, Hamlar D. Necrotizing granulomatous vasculitis associated with cocaine use. *J Rheumatol.* 2002;29:1795–1797.
85. Orson FM, Kinsey BM, Singh RA, et al. Substance abuse vaccines. *Ann N Y Acad Sci.* 2008;1141:257–269.
86. Breccia M, Gentilini F, Alimena G. Cocaine abuse may influence the response to imatinib in CML patients. *Haematologica.* 2007; 92:e41-2.
87. Chang G, Antin JH, Orav EJ, et al. Substance abuse and bone marrow transplant. *Am J Drug Alcohol Abuse.* 1997;23:301–308.
88. Rothman RB, Blough BE, Baumann MH. Dopamine/serotonin releasers as medications for stimulant addictions. *Prog Brain Res.* 2008;172:385–406.
89. Lile JA, Stoops WW, Vansickel AR, et al. Aripiprazole attenuates the discriminative-stimulus and subject-rated effects of D-amphetamine in humans. *Neuropsychopharmacology.* 2005;30:2103–2114.
90. Haney M, Kosten TR. Therapeutic vaccines for substance dependence. *Expert Rev Vaccines.* 2004;3:11–18.
91. Martell BA, Mitchell E, Poling J, et al. Vaccine pharmacotherapy for the treatment of cocaine dependence. *Biol Psychiatry.* 2005; 58:158–164.
92. Shrem MT, Halkitis PN. Methamphetamine abuse in the United States: Contextual, psychological and sociological considerations. *J Health Psychol.* 2008;13:669–679.
93. Fleckenstein AE, Volz TJ, Riddle EL, et al. New insights into the mechanism of action of amphetamines. *Annu Rev Pharmacol Toxicol.* 2007;47:681–698.
94. Sulzer D, Sonders MS, Poulsen NW, et al. Mechanisms of neurotransmitter release by amphetamines: A review. *Prog Neurobiol.* 2005;75:406–433.
95. Belcher AM, Feinstein EM, O'Dell SJ, et al. Methamphetamine influences on recognition memory: Comparison of escalating and single-day dosing regimens. *Neuropsychopharmacology.* 2008;33: 1453–1463.
96. Davidson C, Gow AJ, Lee TH, et al. Methamphetamine neurotoxicity: necrotic and apoptotic mechanisms and relevance to human abuse and treatment. *Brain Res Brain Res Rev.* 2001;36:1–22.
97. Meredith CW, Jaffe C, Ang-Lee K, et al. Implications of chronic methamphetamine use: A literature review. *Harv Rev Psychiatry.* 2005;13:141–154.
98. Cho AK, Melega WP. Patterns of methamphetamine abuse and their consequences. *J Addict Dis.* 2002;21:21–34.
99. Nordahl TE, Salo R, Leamon M. Neuropsychological effects of chronic methamphetamine use on neurotransmitters and cognition: A review. *J Neuropsychiatry Clin Neurosci.* 2003;15:317–325.
100. Curtis EK. Meth mouth: A review of methamphetamine abuse and its oral manifestations. *Gen Dent.* 2006;54:125–129.
101. Iritani BJ, Hallfors DD, Bauer DJ. Crystal methamphetamine use among young adults in the USA. *Addiction.* 2007;102:1102–1113.
102. Shearer J, Darke S, Rodgers C, et al. A double-blind, placebo-controlled trial of modafinil (200 mg/day) for methamphetamine dependence. *Addiction.* 2009;104:224–233.
103. Yung KC, Piccirillo JF. The incidence and impact of comorbidity diagnosed after the onset of head and neck cancer. *Arch Otolaryngol Head Neck Surg.* 2008;134:1045–1049.
104. Hamajima N, Hirose K, Tajima K, et al.. Alcohol, tobacco and breast cancer—collaborative reanalysis of individual data from 53 epidemiological studies, including 58,515 women with breast cancer and 95,067 women without the disease. *Br J Cancer.* 2002; 87:1234–1245.
105. Alcoholism NIoAAa. *Helping patients who drink too much: A clinician's guide.* Public Health Service, 2007.
106. Fiellin DA, Reid MC, O'Connor PG. Outpatient management of patients with alcohol problems. *Ann Intern Med.* 2000;133: 815–827.
107. Reid MC, Fiellin DA, O'Connor PG. Hazardous and harmful alcohol consumption in primary care. *Arch Intern Med.* 1999;159: 1681–1689.
108. Smith PC, Schmidt SM, Allensworth-Davies D, et al. Primary Care Validation of a Single-Question Alcohol Screening Test. *J Gen Intern Med.* 2009.
109. Buchsbaum DG, Buchanan RG, Centor RM, et al. Screening for alcohol abuse using CAGE scores and likelihood ratios. *Ann Intern Med.* 1991;115:774–777.
110. Fiellin DA, Reid MC, O'Connor PG. Screening for alcohol problems in primary care: A systematic review.*Arch Intern Med.* 2000; 160:1977–1989.
111. Helander A, Nordin G. Insufficient standardization of a direct carbohydrate-deficient transferrin immunoassay. *Clin Chem.* 2008; 54:1090–1092.
112. Imbert-Bismut F, Naveau S, Morra R, et al. The diagnostic value of combining carbohydrate-deficient transferrin, fibrosis, and steatosis biomarkers for the prediction of excessive alcohol consumption. *Eur J Gastroenterol Hepatol.* 2009;21:18–27.
113. Helander A, Fors M, Zakrisson B. Study of Axis-Shield new %CDT immunoassay for quantification of carbohydrate-deficient transferrin (CDT) in serum. *Alcohol Alcohol.* 2001;36: 406–412.
114. Anton RF, Lieber C, Tabakoff B. Carbohydrate-deficient transferrin and gamma-glutamyltransferase for the detection and monitoring of alcohol use: results from a multisite study. *Alcohol Clin Exp Res.* 2002;26:1215–1222.
115. Burke V, Puddey IB, Rakic V, et al. Carbohydrate-deficient transferrin as a marker of change in alcohol intake in men drinking 20 to 60 g of alcohol per day. *Alcohol Clin Exp Res.*1998;22:1973–1980.
116. Conigrave KM, Degenhardt LJ, Whitfield JB, et al. CDT, GGT, and AST as markers of alcohol use: The WHO/ISBRA collaborative project. *Alcohol Clin Exp Res.* 2002;26:332–339.
117. Fleming M, Mundt M. Carbohydrate-deficient transferrin: validity of a new alcohol biomarker in a sample of patients with diabetes and hypertension. *J Am Board Fam Pract.* 2004;17: 247–255.
118. Lapham SC, Smith E, C'De Baca J, et al. Prevalence of psychiatric disorders among persons convicted of driving while impaired. *Arch Gen Psychiatry.* 2001;58:943–949.
119. Darke S, Duflou J, Torok M. Toxicology and circumstances of completed suicide by means other than overdose. *J Forensic Sci.* 2009;54:490–494.
120. Sintov ND, Kendler KS, Walsh D, et al. Predictors of illicit substance dependence among individuals with alcohol dependence. *J Stud Alcohol Drugs.* 2009;70:269–278.
121. Sullivan JT, Sykora K, Schneiderman J, et al. Assessment of alcohol withdrawal: The revised clinical institute withdrawal assessment for alcohol scale (CIWA-Ar). *Br J Addict.* 1989;84:1353–1357.
122. Weathermon R, Crabb DW. Alcohol and medication interactions. *Alcohol Res Health.* 1999;23:40–54.
123. Traynor MJ, Brown MB, Pannala A, et al. Influence of alcohol on the release of tramadol from 24-h controlled-release formulations during in vitro dissolution experiments. *Drug Dev Ind Pharm.* 2008;34:885–889.

124. Johnson F, Wagner G, Sun S, et al. Effect of concomitant ingestion of alcohol on the in vivo pharmacokinetics of KADIAN (morphine sulfate extended-release) capsules. *J Pain*. 2008;9:330–336.
125. Sathyan G, Sivakumar K, Thipphawong J. Pharmacokinetic profile of a 24-hour controlled-release OROS formulation of hydromorphone in the presence of alcohol. *Curr Med Res Opin*. 2008;24:297–305.
126. Walden M, Nicholls FA, Smith KJ, et al. The effect of ethanol on the release of opioids from oral prolonged-release preparations. *Drug Dev Ind Pharm*. 2007;33:1101–1111.

CHAPTER 21 ■ SYMPTOM-DIRECTED PAIN MANAGEMENT INTERVENTIONS

When managing cancer pain by interventions, it is important to distinguish between tumor-related pain and nontumor-related pain such as that following treatments (radiation therapy, chemotherapy, surgical resection of tumor). Indeed, many of the pain management issues seen in cancer survivors are similar to those chronic noncancer-pain patients. However, in either situation, it is extremely important to establish a cancer diagnosis and treatment plan for the newly diagnosed cancer patient prior to initiation of any interventional pain management strategy. Failure to do so may result in inappropriate interventions (with associated risks) in these patients.

Clinicians managing terminally ill cancer patients with tumor-related pain generally turn to interventional pain management only after medication management has failed. Failure of therapy exists when the patient considers the pain relief inadequate and cannot obtain further relief without unacceptable side effects. In some situations, the use of an interventional modality can be less invasive and troublesome to the patient than continued aggressive medication management. Interventional strategies should be considered under the following headings: radiation, surgical, pharmacologic, and physical (heat/cold) ablation, and neuraxial therapy. Augmentative modalities for nontumor pain will also be briefly considered.

RADIATION STRATEGIES

The goals of radiation therapy may be considered curative or palliative. The aims of radiation palliation are to allow for a symptom-free period longer than the debilitation associated with curative treatment, prolong useful or comfortable survival, relieve distressing symptoms (eg, pain and obstruction), and avert impending problems (eg, spinal cord compression). Radiation therapy is generally considered a local-regional treatment modality. It has a pivotal role in the treatment of cancer pain caused by bone metastases (see "Focused Management Strategies for Painful Bone Metastases," page 306), epidural neoplasm (see "Management of Epidural Spinal Cord Compression," page 304), and cerebral metastases.[1] Especially when combined with cytotoxic chemotherapy, limited surgical excision, or both, radiation can control disease at the primary site and regional nodes without the need for surgical extirpation, as was frequently used in past years.

Approximately 40% of patients referred for radiation therapy have advanced cancer that does not respond to curative treatment and is accompanied by pain.[2] Rutten et al.[3] evaluated the pain characteristics that help to predict the pain-relieving efficacy of radiation therapy for cancer pain. In a study of 51 patients, they found a significant relationship between pain characteristics (the presence of radiating pain and a low pain score [<35/100] before radiation) and a complete response to palliative radiation therapy. Complete responses to treatment occurred within 21 days of the start of radiation.

Radiation therapy has become a mainstay in the treatment of both primary and metastatic disease of the spine and spinal cord. Although radiation therapy has proven effective in controlling tumors, side effects such as radiation-induced myelitis limit the safely deliverable doses and decrease its efficacy when treating previously irradiated areas. Stereotactic radiosurgery permits high dose treatment while minimizing exposure to surrounding healthy tissues, increasing the safety of initial treatment, and allowing additional radiation of recurrent spinal lesions.

Gerszten et al.[4] reported on the efficacy of Cyberknife treatment on patients with painful metastatic spinal lesions. Axial and radicular pain improved in 74 of 79 patients with a mean radiation treatment dose of 14 Gy. With similar doses for the treatment of painful solitary spinal metastases with or without cord compression, Ryu et al. noted that the median time to pain relief was 14 days and the earliest time of pain relief was within 24 hrs. Complete pain relief occurred in 46%, partial relief in 18.9%, stable symptoms in 16.2%, and relapse of pain at the treated spinal segment was 6.9%. The median duration of pain relief at the treated spine was 13.3 months and the overall pain control rate for one year was 84%

Radiation therapy also has a role in the management of painful, noncancer-related chronic conditions. The Gamma Knife has been used to treat patients with trigeminal neuralgia. Little et al.[5] noted that treatment failed in 33% within 2 years. Thirty-two percent of patients were pain free and off medication and 63% had at least a good outcome at 7 years. When Gamma Knife was used as the primary treatment, 45% of the patients were pain free at 7 years. By contrast, 10% of patients in whom previous treatment had failed were pain free. When needed, salvage therapy with repeat Gamma Knife, microvascular decompression, or percutaneous lesioning was successful in 70%. Posttreatment facial numbness was reported as very bothersome in 5%, most commonly in patients who underwent another invasive treatment. After Gamma Knife, 73% reported that trigeminal neuralgia had no impact on their quality of life.

SURGICAL STRATEGIES

There are a variety of different surgical strategies for symptom-directed interventional tumor pain control (Table 21.1). Simple tumor resection of painful lesions

TABLE 21.1

SURGICAL STRATEGIES FOR SYMPTOM-DIRECTED INTERVENTIONAL TUMOR PAIN CONTROL

Type of Surgery	Specifics/Goal
Tumor resection	Cure
Palliative	Tumor debulking
	Decompression of innervated structures
	Prophylactic and preventative (eg, intramedullary rodding of impending long bone fracture)
Neurosurgical ablative	Cordotomy (open, percutaneous): Lower cervical/thoracic
	High cervical (C1)
	Myelotomy: Commissural punctate
	Dorsal rhizotomy
	Surgical sympathectomy
	Peripheral neurectomy
	Dorsal root entry zone lesions
	Medullary or mesencephalic spinothalamic tractotomy
	Stereotactic mesencephalic spinothalamic
	Tractotomy
	Thalamotomy
	Hypothalamotomy*
	Cingulumotomy
	Cortical gyrectomy*
	Hypophysectomy

*Indicates historical interest only.

(e.g., intra-abdominal tumors or extremity tumors) may result in both resolution of painful lesions and potentially a cure of disease. In patients with advanced disease with evidence of widespread metastatic lesions, surgical resection might still be indicated as part of an effort to palliate symptoms by tumor debulking, decompression of innervated structures, relief of obstruction, or prevention such as intramedullary rodding of impending long bone fractures.

Although limb salvage has replaced amputation in the primary treatment of diseases such as sarcoma, recurrent or persistent disease remains a challenging problem. Pain, fracture, and significant neurologic impairment may accompany primary, recurrent, or metastatic tumors of the major joints. Palliative hemipelvectomy, forequarter amputation, and hip, knee, or shoulder disarticulation for the palliation of pain and symptomatic malignancy have been described as methods of improving quality of life. These procedures are relatively reliable, and may provide excellent pain relief in select groups of patients.

SURGICAL MANAGEMENT OF METASTATIC SPINAL LESIONS

Surgical intervention plays an important role in the comprehensive care of patients with metastatic spinal lesions. Metastatic disease involving the axial skeleton is a common source of morbidity in patients suffering from various primary malignancies (Fig. 21.1). Adult patients with cancers of the lung, breast, and prostate are most likely to be affected. The thoracic region of the spine is involved in approximately 70% of cases.

Multiple surgical options exist for the treatment of spinal metastases; selection is based upon the patient's general condition, spinal stability, evidence of spinal cord and nerve root compression, pain, and tumor sensitivity to radiation and chemotherapy. Surgical approaches to the spine with metastatic disease include laminectomy, posterior decompression, posterolateral decompression via the pedicle, posterior instrumentation, anterior decompression, and anterior instrumentation. Sometimes a combined anterior and posterior procedure is indicated. Intraoperative radiation with shielding of the spinal cord has also been described.[6] Surgery is indicated particularly when the primary tumor is relatively radioresistant, current or previous radiotherapy has failed, or the origin of the lesion cannot be determined. Surgical intervention is also favored when neurologic deficits or intractable axial spinal pain are caused by tumor-related spinal instability or pathological fracture that results in retropulsed bone and disc material. Surgery has multiple potential benefits, including protection of the nervous system, stabilization of the spine, reduction of pain, and the ability to obtain a tissue sample for diagnosis.

Only 20% of spinal metastases involve the lumbar spine. The lumbar spine has several unique features that can potentially complicate successful regional decompression and stabilization, including the large size and high weight-bearing demand of the lumbar vertebral bodies, the transition between the kyphotic rib-fixated thoracic spine to a more mobile lordotic lumbar spine, and the restricted access to the lower lumbar segments because of the presence of the pelvic ring. The lumbar nerve roots also innervate muscles that play critical roles in ambulation and cannot be routinely sacrificed to enhance posterolateral access to the vertebral bodies as may be done in the thoracic spine. Also unique is the direct extension of retroperitoneal malignancies into this region of the spine.

Holman et al.[7] demonstrated that when surgical procedures are used for lesions exclusively involving the lumbar spine, significant and lasting reduction in pain due to tumor-related spinal instability, as well as improvement in neurologic status and restoration of ambulatory function, can result. Although the authors concluded that the risk of surgery-related complications was significant, it was also comparable with that obtained in studies involving cervical and thoracic lesions. The indications for surgery in patients with lumbar lesions are similar to those for patients with disease in other spinal regions. Impending or progressive neurologic deficits because of neural compression are not unusual.

Ibrahim et al.[8] reported on a multicenter study of 223 patients referred for surgery for metastatic spine diseases. Surgical therapies were effective in improving quality of life through better pain control and improved sphincter control; these patients also survived longer than those who did not get surgery. As the authors remarked, spinal surgery is not a treatment for the systemic cancer, it is a method of prolonging life and improving the quality of life.

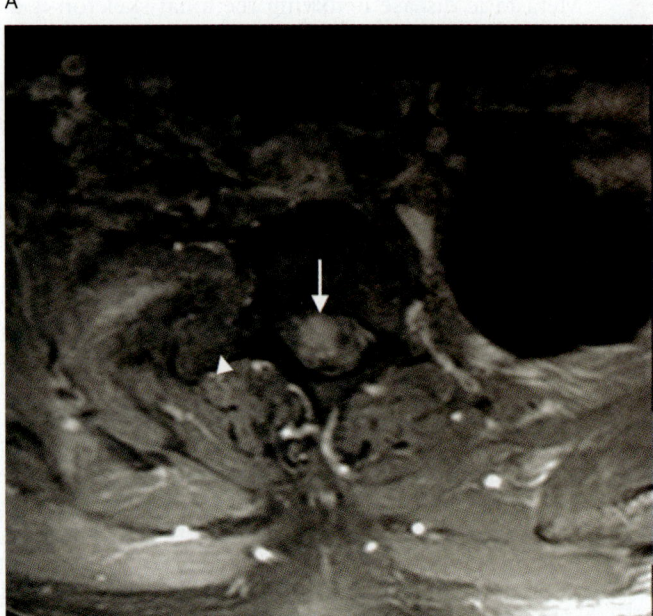
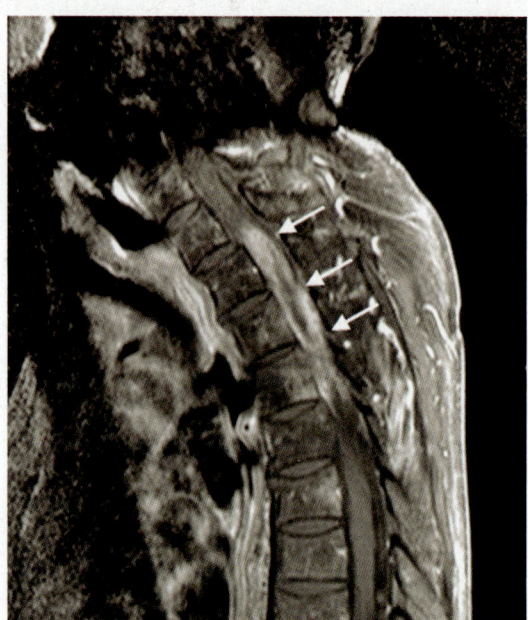

FIGURE 21.1 A 76-year-old man with metastatic mesothelioma. He was evaluated for persistent right chest wall pain after thoracotomy for a pleural mesothelioma. MRI (**A**) (axial T1, fat suppressed, post contrast) shows inoperable intramedullary enhancement *(arrow)* with paraspinal transforaminal involvement *(arrow head)*. Sagittal MRI (**B**) shows intramedullary enhancement from T1 through T3 *(arrows)*. This patient was evaluated for surgical decompression but was deemed not to be a surgical candidate because of the intramedullary location of the tumor. MRI, Magnetic resonance imaging.

NEUROSURGICAL PROCEDURES

Ablative neurosurgical procedures have been used for several hundred years in the attempt to treat pain associated with cancer.[9] The early operations were mainly peripheral neurectomies, but advances in anesthesia made subsequent intracranial and intraspinal procedures possible. The growth of the basic neurologic sciences that began in the late 19th century led to new surgical procedures based upon anatomical pathways. Most of the important clinical developments in ablative neurosurgery occurred in the first half of the 20th century, culminating in the publication of *Pain: Its Mechanisms and Neurosurgical Control* in 1955 by White and Sweet.[10] Several more recent textbooks reviewing ablative neurosurgical procedures for pain are also available.[11–13]

The use of ablative neurosurgical procedures in the management of pain associated with cancer has been sharply curtailed in the past 30 years. The factors responsible for this include:

1. More aggressive care of the underlying malignant disease, eliminating some of the causes of pain
2. Major advances in the use of oral opioids and adjunctive medications for control of pain associated with cancer
3. More accurate reporting of operative morbidity and mortality and long-term follow-up of surgical patients
4. The development of implanted electrical stimulators for pain relief
5. Most significantly, the development of neuraxial medication delivery systems that have dramatically reduced the number of patients requiring ablative surgery for effective pain relief

By contrast, improvements in the science and art of neurologic surgery have made certain procedures safer and more readily available. Advances in the quality of imaging studies and improved anesthetic techniques have also played a significant role. The surgical microscope, improved lesion-making apparatus, neuronavigation, and endoscopic procedures have all brought new possibilities to the surgeon.

Surgical results will be optimized when the surgeon is a member of a comprehensive interdisciplinary team caring for the patient with cancer and pain.[14] Effective communication between the team members and the patient are a necessity if good surgical decisions are to be made. In general, the patient should have a life expectancy of greater than 3 months if an open (surgical) ablative operation is planned. Percutaneous ablative procedures are wiser for those with less than a 3-month life expectancy. Furthermore, the patient must have reasonable bleeding and clotting parameters (International Normalized Ratio [INR] <1.5, adequate platelet counts) and must be able to resist infection and heal the wound. Special care needs to be exercised if the surgical procedure involves a region of skin that has been previously treated with radiation therapy. The technical skill and experience of the neurosurgeon is an outcome factor that should not be overlooked. Surgeons who rarely perform operations for pain, particularly those requiring stereotactic approaches, cannot be expected to have the high success rates and low complication rates described in the literature by those who have performed hundreds of similar operations.

An important issue that accompanies a surgical procedure to alleviate pain is the management of the patient who is receiving large amounts of opioids at the time a surgical procedure is elected. It is not warranted to require the patient to reduce or cease opioids before surgery. Such a patient will be very opioid tolerant, and the personnel involved in the perioperative care must be prepared to deal with this issue. If the operation successfully alleviates the preoperative pain, the patient's need for opioids may be dramatically reduced and a previously well-tolerated dose may now lead to significant side effects, including respiratory depression and oversedation. If such events are anticipated, a careful taper of opioids should be planned accordingly.

The neurosurgeon's contribution to the management of pain associated with cancer includes more than ablative surgery. Neuromodulation by means of implanted electrical stimulators and drug delivery to the cerebrospinal fluid via implanted catheters and pumps is also useful. All aspects of neuraxial medications are discussed in "Neuraxial Analgesia," Chapter 22 and will not be covered in this section. Electrical stimulation is discussed in "Neuromodulatory Treatments for Pain Associated with Cancer," later in this chapter.

Peripheral Neurectomy

Peripheral neurectomy involves cutting a nerve distal to the dorsal root, external to the spine or cranium. The role of peripheral neurectomy in the management of pain due to cancer is very limited.[15] The theoretical advantages are the ease of surgery, complete denervation in the distribution of the cut nerve, and, that a preoperative nerve block with a local anesthetic will accurately reveal the extent of denervation and whether or not pain relief can be expected from the operation. The disadvantages of a peripheral neurectomy include the loss of all sensory modalities in the denervated region, the loss of motor function if the nerve to be cut is mixed, the re-innervation that will occur because of both peripheral and central sprouting, and the potential for growth of the neoplasm to go beyond the denervated region and lead to pain recurrence.

Surgical intercostal neurectomy may be useful in a patient with chest wall neoplasm too frail to undergo dorsal rhizotomy. The loss of intercostal muscle function in the denervated region is usually inconsequential. Denervation of abdominal segments may result in muscle weakness that produces an asymmetrical abdominal protuberance that the patient may find painful and embarrassing. Neurectomies in the extremities are usually unwise because of the paresis that ensues. Cranial rhizotomies are usually a better choice than neurectomies for pain due to cancer. Peripheral neurectomies can also lead to a painful neuroma or denervation pain; both can be difficult to manage.

Surgical Sympathectomy

Sympathectomy involves excision or cauterization of the paravertebral sympathetic chain and associated ganglia or their peripheral branches. Surgical sympathectomy plays a limited role in the management of pain secondary to cancer. Nociceptive afferents from the viscera travel in the sympathetic chains and vagus nerve and may be surgically interrupted. Splanchniectomy may be part of an abdominal operation and can provide relief of visceral-mediated pain. However, this is a formidable surgical procedure by itself that can usually be much more easily accomplished with neurolytic agents that are percutaneously administered.

Some of the pains associated with cancer are not nociceptive but arise from nerve injury by the neoplasm, surgery, or radiation therapy. This component of neuropathic pain may respond to sympathectomy. Therefore, if the patient's pain persists after somatic blocks or ablative surgery, sympathetic block is warranted to ascertain if the pain can be eliminated. If so, a sympathectomy should be considered.[16] In addition to the traditional older methods for an open sympathectomy, there are now endoscopic and percutaneous methods of achieving sympathectomy. Neurolytic sympathetic blocks are probably a better choice than open sympathectomy in the cancer pain patient.

Dorsal Rhizotomy

A rhizotomy is a surgical procedure to cut nerve roots. Because most peripheral nociceptive impulses are conveyed through a mixed somatic nerve to the spinal cord via the dorsal root, dorsal rhizotomy was the most commonly performed operation for pain relief in the first 75 years of the 20th century. As better clinical trials with longer follow-ups were reported, the popularity of dorsal rhizotomy waned. This was initially because of the development of cordotomy and then the use of intraspinal opioids. The advantages of dorsal rhizotomy include: All modalities of sensation but no motor function is lost in the denervated area, large areas can be denervated by cutting many adjacent dorsal roots, and nerve blocks can be used to determine the required extent of denervation. The disadvantages include the fact that one cannot totally denervate an extremity without losing useful function, a laminectomy is required for each root to be cut, and sprouting, both peripheral and central, may cause pain relief to be temporary. This operation is particularly useful for thoracic and abdominal wall pain but it will not interrupt or attenuate visceral pain. From a practical perspective, it is always necessary to section two roots above and two roots below the region of pain to get reliable pain relief that may last for the duration of the patient's life. This can lead to the need for very extensive laminectomies if an open procedure is contemplated.

Percutaneous dorsal rhizotomies have particular utility in the patient with pain due to cancer. This strategy does put at risk the artery that accompanies the dorsal root; particularly in the lower thoracic region this can lead to spinal cord infarction. Sacral rhizotomy via a laminectomy at S2 and epidural ligation of all the nerve roots in the cauda equina can effectively alleviate pelvic pain in the patient who has already had urinary and fecal diversionary procedures.[17]

It is unclear whether or not resection of the dorsal root ganglion adds to the likelihood of success for dorsal rhizotomy.[18] Most of this controversy relates to patients with lumbar rhizotomy for failed back surgery syndrome and cannot be extrapolated to patients with pain due to cancer. Ganglionectomy is frequently followed by a transient dysesthetic pain syndrome in the denervated area and patients should be warned of this. Ganglionectomy is an extradural procedure and the risk of cerebrospinal fluid (CSF) leak is far less than after intradural rhizotomy.

Cranial rhizotomy may be useful in patients with head and neck cancer that has not been controlled by other means. The traditional procedure has been a posterior fossa approach to the trigeminal, nervus intermedius, and glossopharyngeal and upper vagal nerves accompanied by section of the dorsal roots of C2 and C3 (there is no dorsal root of C1). Such an operation produces complete anesthesia of the face and pharynx and can only be done unilaterally. It can provide significant pain relief (75% success rate) in appropriately selected patients for the duration of the cancer patient's life. Unfortunately, many patients with advanced head and neck cancers have extensive tumor involvement which overlaps dermatomal segments that reduces the likelihood of successful pain relief with single nerve cranial rhizotomy.

Cordotomy

A cordotomy involves an incision or Radio Frequency (RF) lesion made in the anterolateral quadrant of the spinal cord to interrupt the axons of the spinothalamic tract (Fig. 21.2). Cordotomy was the most commonly performed operation for cancer pain before the advent of intraspinal opioids. The advantages of cordotomy are that only pain and temperature sensation are abolished contralateral to the lesion in the spinal cord, commencing three segments below the level incised. This means that the level of the operation can be tailored to the region of pain. Motor loss is not expected and touch and position sense remain intact. The disadvantages include the tendency of the pain relief to fade after a year or so, the fact that bilateral lesions can lead to impairment of bladder function, and that bilateral high cervical cordotomy can lead to Ondine Curse, the failure to breath when the patient is asleep.[19] Cordotomy can be performed at the upper thoracic level for lower half of the body pains and at the high cervical level for pains below C5. Percutaneous cordotomy is performed at the C1-2 level and offers the possibility of surgical pain relief in a patient too debilitated to withstand an open procedure.[20] A computed tomography (CT)-guided method has been developed that lowers the risks of an inappropriate lesion site. For most cancer pain patients, percutaneous C1-2 cordotomy is the procedure of choice, although bilateral lesions do have significant risks to both bladder function and loss of CO_2 responsiveness. The quality of pain relief is identical with both the open and percutaneous operations. Raslan[21] described the use of percutaneous CT-guided radiofrequency ablation of upper cervical spinal cord pain pathways in the treatment of cancer-related pain. Fifty-one patients with cancer-related body or face pain were treated with computed tomography-guided radiofrequency ablation of the spinothalamic tract or trigeminal tract nucleus in the upper cervical region of the spinal cord. Forty-one patients underwent a unilateral cervical cordotomy, and ten patients underwent a trigeminal tractotomy–nucleotomy (TR-NC). Patients with somatic pain on one side of the body reaching to the midline and below dermatome C5 and patients with visceral pain restricted to one side of the body not reaching the midline were offered cervical cordotomy. Patients with somatic pain involving one side of the face, tongue, or inner mouth were offered the option of TR-NC. Forty-one patients underwent cervical cordotomy at C1-2 level, and ten patients underwent TR-NC also at the C1-2 level. The results from these procedures are shown in Table 21.2.

Postoperatively, 98% of the patients were Grade I or II, which was categorized as a successful procedure. At 1 month postoperatively, 98% of the patients remained Grade I or II, which decreased to 80% at 6 months follow-up. One patient, who was Grade III at 1-month follow-up, dropped to Grade IV at 3 months follow-up and died before the 6-month follow-up contact. Despite two patients having only one lesion performed and the procedure halted, results in terms of pain relief in the first 3 months were not affected and most likely reflect the effect of a single lesion. No complications related to the procedures used were observed. No change in motor strength was recorded in any patient. No patient developed sleep apnea. There were no permanent or serious

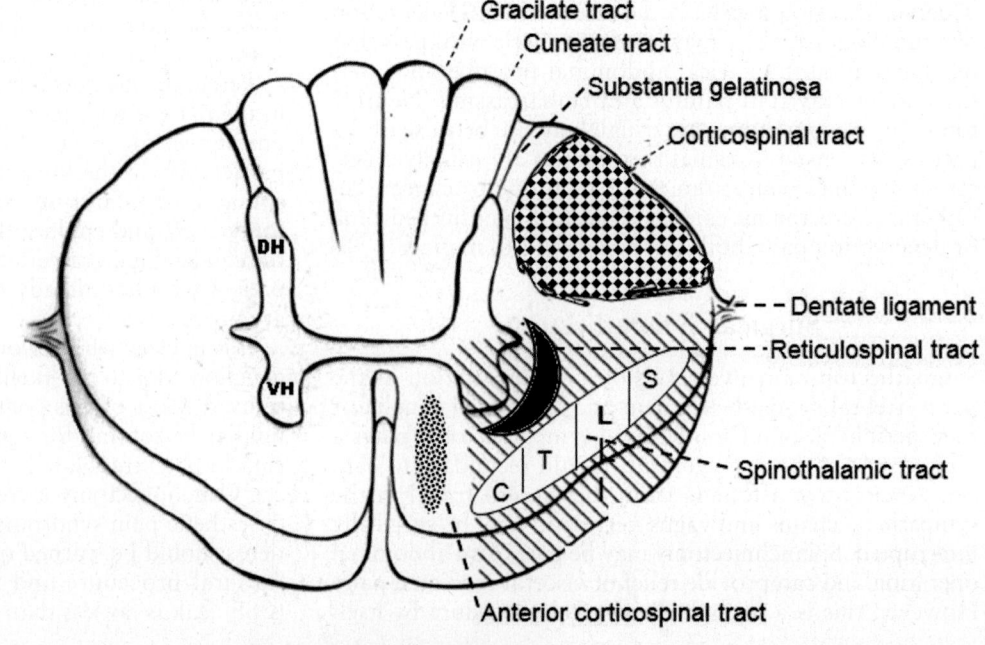

FIGURE 21.2 Anatomic representation of cordotomy at lower cervical/upper thoracic level. The spinothalamic tract lies in the anterolateral quadrant and is laminated with the sacral fibers being most dorsal and the cervical fibers most ventral. The reticulospinal tract lies medial to the spinothalamic tract and includes fibers related to bladder function. DH, Dorsal horn; VH, ventral horn. (Modified from Raslan AM. Percutaneous computed tomography-guided radiofrequency ablation of upper spinal cord pain pathways for cancer-relate pain. Neurosurgery, 2008;62(3 Supp 11):226–233. Reprinted with permission.)

TABLE 21.2
PERCUTANEOUS RADIOFREQUENCY CORDOTOMY AND TRIGEMINAL TRACTOTOMY FOR RELIEF OF INTRACTABLE CANCER PAIN

Scale	Pain	Immediate Postoperative	6 Months Postoperative
I	No pain	41 (80.4%)	16 (32%)
II	Partial satisfactory pain relief	9 (17.6%)	24 (48%)
III	Partial nonsatisfactory pain relief	1 (2%)	7 (14%)
IV	Same, no change in pain	0 (0%)	3 (6%)
V	Worse pain	0 (0%)	0 (0%)
Total		51 (100%)	50 (100%)*

*One patient died by 6-month follow-up evaluation. (Modified from Raslan AM. Percutaneous computed tomography-guided radiofrequency ablation of upper spinal cord pain pathways for cancer-related pain. *Neurosurgery*. 2008;62:226–233; discussion 233–234.)

complications such as respiratory depression and/or weakness in this series. Complications were transient and not severe. Hypotension occurred in three cases (two cordotomies and one TR-NC). All patients responded to treatment with 24-hour parenteral fluid administration and were discharged without event. Headache was reported in four patients (three cordotomies and one TR-NC). All were treated with analgesics and fluids for 48 hours and discharged without event. Dysesthesia occurred in two patients undergoing cordotomy and persisted in one patient for 3 days and in the other for 2 weeks, which completely resolved by the first month follow-up assessment.

Most other large series reveal an 80% success rate in cancer patients, although those who survive for several years may lose the cordotomy effect. Failure to get initial pain relief almost always means that the cordotomy lesion was not large enough or that it was not far enough above the source of pain. Midline or bilateral pain from the pelvis is better treated with a midline myelotomy than bilateral cordotomies.

Myelotomy

Myelotomy for pain is an operation to incise the spinal cord in the dorsal midline so as to transect the decussating spinothalamic fibers and/or damage the visceral afferent tract that ascends in the deep medial dorsal columns. On the basis of these novel pathways, midline myelotomy (either commissural or punctate), has been developed as treatment of visceral pain. Midline myelotomy has the advantage of producing bilateral pain relief from a single incision in the spinal cord. At first, this operation was thought to provide pain relief by sectioning the decussating spinothalamic fibers. However, the studies of Willis et al. and the clinical observations of Hitchcock have indicated that there is a visceral afferent tract that travels in the deep midline of the dorsal columns.[22] The axons of this pathway ascend in the ipsilateral dorsal column and terminate in the nucleus gracilis from where the nociceptive input is transmitted to the contralateral ventral posterolateral thalamus. This tract probably explains the observation that pain relief can be found in regions of the body below the level of pain and temperature loss. A midline myelotomy, whether longitudinal or punctate, has a very low risk of impairing motor function, although some proprioceptive losses in the lower extremities are not rare after this procedure. The procedure requires a low thoracic laminectomy and the duration of pain relief may not be more than a year in many patients.

Hwang et al.[23] reported on the use of a punctate midline myelotomy at the T3 vertebral level in a small number of patients with visceral pain associated with hepatobiliary or pancreatic cancer. Although only six patients were studied, their results suggest some use of this technique in the management of severe pain for these particular cancers. In an experimental animal model, Chang[24] reported on the use of a high cervical punctate midline myelotomy for intractable visceral pain due to abdominal or pelvic cancers. Similarly, Hitchcock[25] described a high cervical midline myelotomy that produced pain relief without sensory loss, but few have replicated his findings.[12] Nauta et al.[26] performed a punctate midline myelotomy in six cancer patients with intractable refractory visceral pain and noted good pain relief with significant opioid reductions postprocedure.

Dorsal Root Entry Zone Lesions

Dorsal root entry zone (DREZ) lesions require destroying the central projections of nociceptive afferents where they enter the spinal cord. DREZ were first performed by Nashold in 1975, although Sindou described sectioning the lateral root fibers going to the Lissauer tract in 1972. In North America, the Nashold strategy has been the most commonly utilized. This operation has the advantages of producing complete sensory loss in the segments incised, has a long-lasting effect, does not produce any motor loss, and is most effective for neuropathic pain states. Its disadvantages include requiring a laminectomy for each level to be lesioned, risk to spinal cord function with ipsilateral motor and dorsal column function loss (about 10% of patients), and being a major operation with significant surgical stress. The lesion in the root entry zone can be made with a radiofrequency electrode, a laser, or a knife. In the management of pain due to cancer, it is not clear that this operation is any better than dorsal rhizotomy, which certainly has less risk of spinal cord dysfunction.

An analogous operation can be performed on the descending trigeminal nucleus and root entry zone in the medulla to treat chronic pain in the face and pharynx; this is much more commonly used for neuropathic pains than those due to cancer.[27] Only pain and temperature sensation is lost; corneal anesthesia does not ensue. The operation can be performed bilaterally if necessary.

Medullary or Mesencephalic Spinothalamic Tractotomy

This is an open operation with direct visualization of the brain stem and the localization of a lesion in the spinothalamic tract by anatomic features. This permits a higher section of the spinothalamic tract and a higher level of analgesia that includes the cervical region. The operation has been most frequently performed for cancer pain involving the shoulder and neck on the opposite side of the body. The success rate has been around 50% with a 15% complication rate, and the pain relief often does not last for more than a year.[28] This is a major surgical procedure and is rarely performed today; stereotactic surgical procedures and aggressive use of opioids have superseded this operation.

Stereotactic Mesencephalic Spinothalamic Tractotomy

Open mesencephalic tractotomy had a much-too-high neurologic complication rate; in 1962 Spiegel and Wycis described stereotactic mesencephalic tractotomy. This operation has been widely used and is known to yield a 50% to 80% success rate; however, most patients will again report pain after a year or so.[29] The operative mortality is 5% to 10%, and about 20% of patients complain of transient dysesthesias or oculomotor disturbances. This operation is aimed at sectioning the spinothalamic fibers and adjacent spinoreticular fibers. A limited number of neurosurgeons are comfortable performing stereotactic lesions for pain. The surgical stress and morbidity are low; this operation does have utility for cancer pain patients. The pain is relieved on the opposite side of the body from the tractotomy and bilateral lesions can be made for bilateral pain. Head and neck as well as body pains can be controlled by mesencephalic tractotomy, as the trigeminal and spinal noxious afferent thalamic fibers are adjacent to each other.

Thalamotomy

This operation destroys a target area in the thalamus. A panoply of thalamic sites have been the target for stereotactic relief of pain. The results have been highly variable, certainly in part because of the different targets and lesion sizes (Table 21.3). The major issue with all of the sites has been the transient pain relief; good results do not often last more than 1 year. Producing a lesion in the thalamus by radiofrequency current, cryoprobe, or radiosurgery (Gamma Knife) may have significant side effects if the lesion is not precisely located in the desired area. Modern magnetic resonance imaging (MRI) scanning and neuronavigation equipment have reduced the risk of target errors.

Lesions in the ventrocaudal nuclei produce the loss of all sensory modalities as well as pain and for this reason

TABLE 21.3

SITE OF THALAMOTOMY FOR PAIN RELIEF

Ventrocaudal nucleus
Thalamolaminar region (medial thalamotomy)
Pulvinar
Dorsomedian nucleus
Anterior nuclei

they are not optimal for most patients. Lesions in the medial thalamus or pulvinar have been more useful as they only produce pain relief without sensory loss. Lesions in the anterior nuclei seem to resemble cingulumotomy in producing abatement of suffering rather than pain. Many other regions have been targeted, but the reported case series are small and results not reliable. Thalamotomy utilizing the Gamma Knife to avoid any surgical procedure is probably going to be used more in coming years.[30]

Hypothalamotomy

This operation has rarely been performed and the true long-term results are unknown. It does not have a place in the current neurosurgical armamentarium.

Cingulumotomy

Bilateral lesions are made in the mesial frontal lobes to interrupt the cingulum bundles. This operation was first performed by Foltz and White in 1962.[29] Large series of patients have been carefully studied and the clinical results are well established. The principle of this operation is to disconnect the limbic structures that process affective states from the spinothalamic afferents that transmit pain sensations. The short-term success rate for patients with cancer is about 80%; good data on long-term outcomes is sparse but we know there is some drop off.[30] Cingulumotomy does not alter sensation in any way. Patients report that they still have pain but that it does not cause them to suffer. It clearly does not alter cognition or judgment. Originally performed through bilateral frontal burr holes with radiofrequency lesions, it is now possible to perform cingulumotomy using stereotactic radiosurgery (Gamma Knife) and avoid any surgical procedure.

Cortical Gyrectomy

Shortly after World War II, resections of the postcentral and even precentral gyri were reported to be useful in the management of pain on the opposite side of the body. Follow-up reports and larger case series did not reveal many long-term good results; this operation is not performed today in the pursuit of pain relief.[31]

Hypophysectomy

The recognition that some cancers were endocrine dependent led to the idea that hypophysectomy might remove the trophic hormones and retard tumor growth and dissemination. The initial procedures were performed sub-frontally via an open craniotomy. Then, innovative techniques such as transecting the pituitary stalk while preserving the gland, the use of stereotaxis to make a lesion within the pituitary fossa, and the injection of alcohol via a transsphenoidal route broadened the use of this operation. It was also recognized that endocrine sensitivity was not required for the patient to obtain pain relief; nor was tumor regression. Pain relief may start very rapidly after pituitary destruction. Significant complications including partial diabetes insipidus in 75.5%, and CSF leaks in 11.3% after transsphenoidal microsurgical hypophysectomy were reported in one series.[32] Stereotactic radiosurgery (Gamma Knife) has greatly reduced the morbidity associated with pituitary operations. Approximately 70% of patients with disseminated cancer will gain significant pain relief for 3 months up to 1 year from this operation, no matter how the lesion in the gland is made.[32] Hormone replacement therapy is usually required. The mechanism of pain relief is not understood. Pituitary ablation may have some utility for the disseminated cancer pain patient who has failed opioid therapy by oral and intrathecal routes.[33]

PHARMACOLOGIC AND PHYSICAL (HEAT/COLD) ABLATIVE MODALITIES

The pharmacologic and physical ablative modalities involve blocking nociceptive transmission, primarily by neurolytic injections and the application of heat or cold directly to nervous tissue or tumor. Neurolysis uses chemicals (typically phenol or alcohol) or heat (radiofrequency) or cold (cryoablation) to interrupt nociceptive pathways and thereby achieve pain relief. Targeted ablation of discrete tumor masses may eliminate or debulk tumor size and indirectly cause pain relief by this mechanism.

Chemical Neurolysis

Historically, a large number of agents have been used for chemical neurolysis. Some of these agents have included hypertonic cold saline solution, chlorocresol, ammonium salt solutions, osmic acid, and glycerol. Osmic acid is an aqueous solution of osmium tetroxide, which is an oxidizing agent with a high affinity for lipids and coagulate proteins. Following contact with organic substances, osmic acid is rapidly reduced to stable lower oxides and becomes inert. Osmic acid in a 1% aqueous solution has been used successfully for chemical synovectomy in patients with chronic knee synovitis.[34] Glycerol is a neurolytic agent found endogenously, and may act as a membrane stabilizing agent by inhibition of ectopic impulse generation at the site of nerve injury.[35] The neurophysiologic mechanism of glycerol neurolysis appears to be a nonspecific conduction block of large and small fibers, which is established within minutes of its application. Anhydrous glycerol application on normal nerves showed a rapid loss of C-fiber conduction within 5 minutes of application; after 10 to 30 minutes, a complete conduction block in all fiber types was produced.[35] Glycerol may damage thin unmyelinated fibers (C fibers), small-diameter (AΔ fibers), and large-diameter (Aβ) myelinated fibers. Morphological studies have demonstrated glycerol-induced damage of large-diameter myelinated fibers,[36] as well as damage of both small myelinated/unmyelinated and large myelinated fibers.[37-38] Electrophysiologic studies have suggested nonselective damage of small myelinated/unmyelinated and large myelinated fibers[35] and more selective damage of large myelinated fibers.[38] Absolute glycerol in volumes not exceeding 0.3 mL has been used in the treatment of trigeminal neuralgia.[39] Most of these agents are not easily available. Clinicians now use phenol or alcohol for chemical neurolysis.

Phenol (carbolic acid) is a neurolytic agent with local anesthetic properties. It is soluble in water to a maximum ratio of 1:15; consequently, at room temperature, a concentration of 6.7% cannot be exceeded for aqueous phenol. Commonly, 1-g amounts of phenol crystals are sterilized and stored in light-opaque 20-mL containers. Clinicians can add either water for injection to produce aqueous phenol or glycerin to produce hyperbaric solutions. Solutions of phenol are prepared by dissolving phenol crystals in saline, distilled sterile water, glycerin, or radiocontrast agents. When injected near motor nerves, phenol can produce flaccid paralysis and might also cause systemic complications, such as nausea and vomiting, central nervous system (CNS) stimulation, cardiovascular depression, and cardiac arrhythmias.[40] The ideal concentration of phenol for neurolytic treatment is not precisely defined but varies from 3% to 10%. Motor weakness, anterior and posterior root damage, and direct cord injury were noted in primates following epidural administration of 0.5 mL of 3% phenol.[41] A concentration of 12% produces the maximal axonotomic effect.[42] Concentrations >5% cause protein denaturation.

Alcohol (ethyl alcohol) concentrations greater than 35% are needed to produce neurolysis.[43] Its administration is associated with a burning sensation. Ethyl alcohol is commercially available as a colorless solution and can be easily injected through small-bore needles. A concentration of 40% alcohol seems to be equivalent to 3% phenol as a neurolytic agent.[44] Neurolysis is achieved by dehydration, with extraction of cholesterol, phospholipids, and cerebrosides, and precipitation of mucoproteins. This results in sclerosis of nerve fibers and the myelin sheath. There is nonselective destruction of nervous tissue by precipitation of cell membrane proteins and the extraction of lipid compounds, resulting in demyelination and subsequent Wallerian degeneration. By contrast with the action of phenol, alcohol often spares the Schwann cell tube which implies that the axon may regenerate over its former course. Chua and Kong[45] reported on the effect of alcohol neurolysis of the sciatic nerve for the treatment of hemiplegic knee flexor spasticity. Eight patients underwent neurolysis with 50% to 100% alcohol (mean concentration was 66.3%). The authors noted that all patients had improvement in terms of reduction of spasticity with minimal side effects (no patient had associated painful dysesthesias with injection) and beneficial effects lasted at least 6 months.

Thermal Neurolysis

Thermal ablation involves energy sources with either heat (radiofrequency, laser, microwave) or cold (cryoablation).

Radiofrequency (RF) ablation implies the use of coagulation induction from all electromagnetic energy sources with frequencies less than 900 kHz; most devices function in the range 375 to 500 kHz.[46] Rosomoff described the use of radiofrequency ablation for pain relief in 1965.[47] He perfected the use of radiofrequency to perform a percutaneous C1-2 cordotomy. This obviated the need for a laminectomy to perform an open cordotomy and brought the potential of pain relief to patients too ill or infirm to undergo a formal surgical procedure. Radiofrequency ablation is also used extensively for the treatment of various nontumor-related chronic pain complaints, including trigeminal neuralgia and pain of spinal origin (low back, radicular, and mechanical). Pulsed RF treatment is supposedly safer than conventional RF and therefore should be preferred if preliminary data are validated. In pulsed RF, the output of the generator is interrupted. The usual pattern is 2 cycles of 20 ms each of active cycle. This offers the advantage that a generator output of normal intensity can be used during the active phase of the duty cycle. The passive phase is inserted to enable the heat washout to take away the heat that has been formed during the active cycle. The pulsing characteristic of the duty cycle supposedly does not have any biologic effect by itself. Van Boxem et al.[48] commented on the use of pulsed RF for the management of spinal pain (nontumor associated) and concluded that the role of RF denervation needed further study particularly for the management of cervicogenic headache.

Laser ablation implies the use of light energy for ablation. Cryoneurolysis is a method of destroying neural tissues by the application of very low temperatures. The freezing of tissue with rapid thawing leads to disruption of cellular membranes and induces cell death.[49] In the two main types of systems, argon gas and either gas or liquid nitrogen are used. Temperatures are measured either at the tip of the cryoprobe or in the handle. Most have a built-in nerve stimulator for localization of nerves. The nerve stimulator allows a frequency choice for sensory (100 Hz) or motor (2 Hz) responses. Current probes range in size from 1.4 to 2 mm. The 2.0-mm probe forms a 5.5-mm ice ball, whereas the 1.4-mm probe forms a 3.5-mm ice ball. At 10°C, larger myelinated fibers stop conducting, but all nerve fibers stop conducting at −20°C. The extent and duration of the effect is a function of the degree of freezing obtained and the length of time of exposure. Long-term pain relief from nerve freezing occurs because ice crystals create vascular damage to the vasa nervorum which produces severe endoneural edema. Endoneural fluid pressure increases about 20 mm within 90 minutes of the cryolesioning. Changes in the elastic properties of the perineurium cause a decrease in extracellular fluid pressure within 24 hours, which increases again and then reaches a plateau about 6 days postlesion. This ultimately causes Wallerian degeneration but leaves the myelin sheath and endoneurium intact.[50] The Schwann cell basal lamina is spared and ultimately provides the structure for regeneration.

Thermal Tumor Ablation

Modalities for thermal tumor ablation include the use of both heat and cold. Both these modalities will be discussed.

Radiofrequency Tumor Ablation

Radiofrequency ablation is a form of high-temperature thermal therapy that induces coagulation necrosis by heating tissue to temperatures near 100°C. Above 50°C to 60°C, tissue denatures and cells die. During the application of RF energy, a high frequency alternating current moves from the tip of an electrode into the tissue surrounding that electrode. As the ions within the tissue attempt to follow the change in the direction of the alternating current, their movement results in frictional heating of the tissue (Fig. 21.3). As the temperature within the tissue becomes elevated beyond 60°C, cells begin to die, resulting in a region of necrosis surrounding the electrode.

Developments in the technology and techniques of ablation as well as in image guidance have allowed application of this treatment to different parts of the body and are being used for cure, debulking, and palliation of different tumor types. Radiofrequency ablation has been applied to a broad spectrum of primary tumors and locations, including liver, kidney, pancreas, adrenal, breast, and lung tumors[51] and for the treatment of primary bone tumors such as osteoid osteomas.[52] In addition, radiofrequency ablation has also been used for pain relief associated with bone and soft tissue metastases.[53] Radiofrequency ablation is technically straightforward and can be performed by using standard image-guided biopsy skills, with light sedation, as an outpatient procedure. Unlike surgery, ablation can be repeated many times without additional difficulty or morbidity. The equipment to perform radiofrequency ablation is relatively inexpensive and can be guided by ultrasound, computed tomography (CT), or magnetic resonance imaging (MRI).

Percutaneous, image-guided, in situ tumor ablation with a thermal energy source, such as an RF, laser, or microwave source, is a promising technique for the treatment of focal malignant disease. These techniques allow the destruction of tumors without the need for removal by a more invasive surgical procedure. RF ablation has been used for the treatment of a variety of neoplasms, including osteoid osteoma; hepatocellular carcinoma (HCC); renal

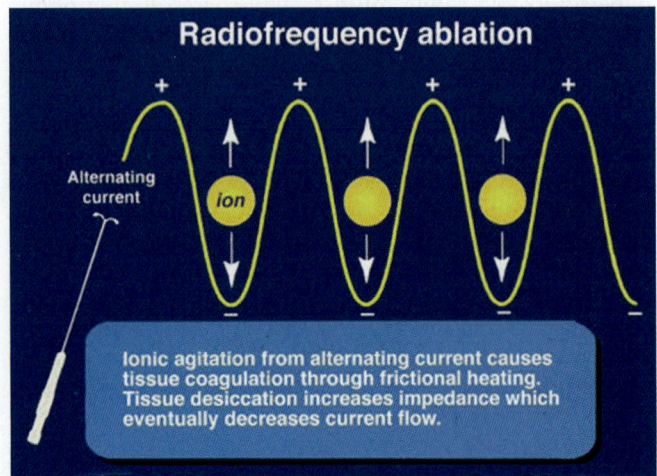

FIGURE 21.3 Alternating electrical current is passed across the electrode array at the tip of the radiofrequency needle, resulting in ionic agitation and heating in the tissue surrounding the electrode array. (From Curley SA. Radiofrequency ablation of malignant liver tumors. *Oncologist*. 2001;6:14–23. With permission from AlphaMed Press, Inc.)

cell carcinoma; hyperfunctioning parathyroid adenoma; and hepatic, cerebral, and retroperitoneal metastases from a variety of primary tumors. The procedures are generally performed by using 14- to 21-gauge partially insulated electrodes placed with imaging guidance (CT, MRI, or ultrasound) into the tumor to be ablated. When attached to an appropriate RF generator, RF current is emitted from the noninsulated portion (ie, exposed tip) of the active electrode, and the current attempts to find the path to ground. RF ablation can be performed with either monopolar or bipolar techniques; monopolar techniques are more commonly used for tumor ablation. When a monopolar technique is used, a large dispersive electrode (grounding pad) is usually placed on the patient's thigh. When a bipolar technique is used, a second (passive or ground) electrode is placed within 5 cm of the active electrode. With either approach, current passing through tissue from the active electrode leads to ion agitation, which is converted by means of friction into heat. The process of cellular heating induces almost immediate and irreparable cellular damage, which leads to coagulation necrosis. Because ion agitation, and thus, tissue heating, is greatest in areas of highest current density (ie, closest to the active electrode tip), necrosis is limited to a relatively small volume of tissue surrounding the RF electrode. The single most important determinant of tissue heating (and thus, the extent of coagulation necrosis that is achievable) is RF current density. The greater the current density surrounding the needle electrode, the more energy is deposited in tissue and the more tissue can be heated to lethal temperatures. If too much energy is applied too rapidly, however, biologic tissues can be heated to temperatures greater than their boiling point. This in turn results in gas production, charring, and cavitation, which lead to increased circuit impedance and thus limit further energy application. Several approaches have been used, including the use of hooked needle electrodes, perfusion-cooled electrodes, multielectrode arrays, and clustered needle electrodes and the development of algorithms for pulsed energy delivery.

In situ tumor ablation is virtually always performed with imaging guidance. Currently, ultrasound is most commonly used for guidance in probe placement, owing to its flexibility, widespread availability, relatively low cost, and real-time imaging capabilities. RF ablation can also be performed with CT or MR imaging guidance; however, the static nature of CT and the complexity of the MR imaging environment have limited their use. The development of CT fluoroscopic systems may result in a larger role for CT in the future.

Because some metastatic tumors will involve the vertebral body and paraspinal region, and because RF heating at around 45°C is cytotoxic to the spinal cord and peripheral nerves,[54–56] the temperature effects of RF heating on the adjacent thecal sac contents must be considered before RF ablation of spinal or paraspinal tumors.[57] In patients with extensive osteolysis with no intact cortex between tumor and spinal cord or nerve roots, RF ablation may not be an option because of the potential of thermal injury to adjacent neural tissue.[57] With tumors in close proximity to the thecal sac, a remote temperature sensor may offer a prudent margin of safety because the procedure could then be terminated if deleterious temperature rises are observed adjacent to nervous tissue (Fig. 21.4).

Cryoprobe Tumor Ablation

Cryoablation is performed by using a closed cryoprobe that is placed on or inside a tumor. The freezing and thawing process leads to cell death and reduction in tumor bulk. This can lead to pain reduction by relieving compression on innervated structures and by destroying nerves within the tumor itself. The effects, both injurious and beneficial, of cold on tissue have been known for some time. The therapeutic uses of cold water and ice applications for diverse illnesses and injuries, including wounds, infections, and ulcerations, have continued as part of the regimen to relieve pain, prevent swelling, and reduce fever. This use of low temperatures can be termed cryotherapy, which describes, in a broad sense, the therapeutic uses of cold. For the most part, cryosurgery has been used for treatment of nonresectable cancers, especially those which are metastatic from cancers primary in the colon and rectum. Cryoablation has also been used for intercostal nerve ablation. The addition of ultrasound guidance for this technique may be beneficial in allowing visualization of the pleura, thus helping to avoid the potential complication of pneumothorax associated with this procedure[58] (Fig. 21.5).

Spinal Neurolysis

Both intradural (especially in the cauda equina) or extradural (at the spinal foramina) blocks or denervations introduce lesions at the nerve root level. Techniques employed include injections of phenol or alcohol, electrodes for radiofrequency or cryoablation destruction.

Spinal neurolysis may be an effective method for pain control in cancer patients with limited life expectancy, who have nociceptive pain covering 2 or 3 dermatomes (especially in sacral, perineal, and thoracic areas), and in patients who are severely compromised or who have absent bladder and/or bowel function (Fig. 21.6). Intrathecal neurolysis with small volumes of alcohol or phenol requires careful positioning to place the affected sensory nerve root uppermost (for alcohol) or in the most dependent position (for phenol). Patient movement during or shortly after injection can spread the drug to other dermatomes or to motor roots. The popularity of spinal neurolysis has waned with the increasing use of neuraxial infusion therapy. Randomized, prospective studies on the effects of spinal neurolysis on pain relief are lacking. Indeed, much of the published data in this area lacks uniform patient selection, inadequately reports preblock analgesic therapy, inconsistently evaluates outcome, and inadequately follows up patients for the long-term. Based on the studies available, good pain relief may be anticipated in approximately 51% of appropriately selected patients, moderate pain relief in 23%, and poor relief in 26%.[59–60] Gerbershagen[61] showed that the success rate of intrathecal alcohol neurolysis declined with repeated injections with approximately 60% of patients obtaining some relief with the first block, 30% with a second block, 8% with a third block, and 3% with more than three blocks. Papo and Visca[59] reported on the use of phenol for subarachnoid rhizotomy in 290 cancer patients. They reported good results (pain free until death) in 40%, and fair results (reduced analgesic requirements or temporary complete relief) in 35%. Patients with pain localized to

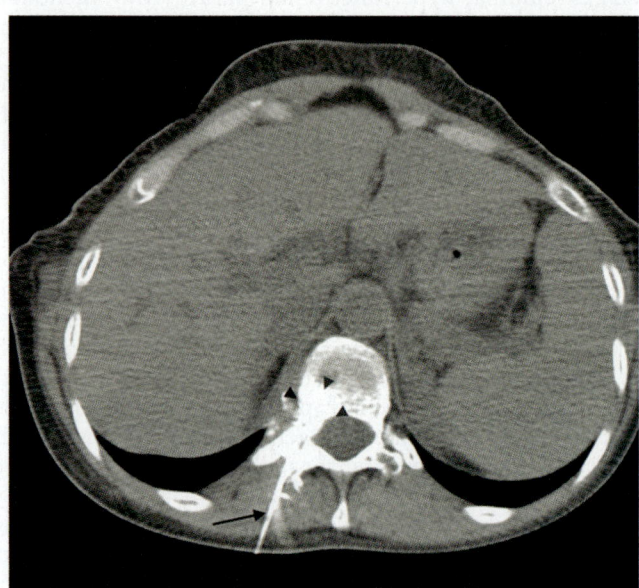

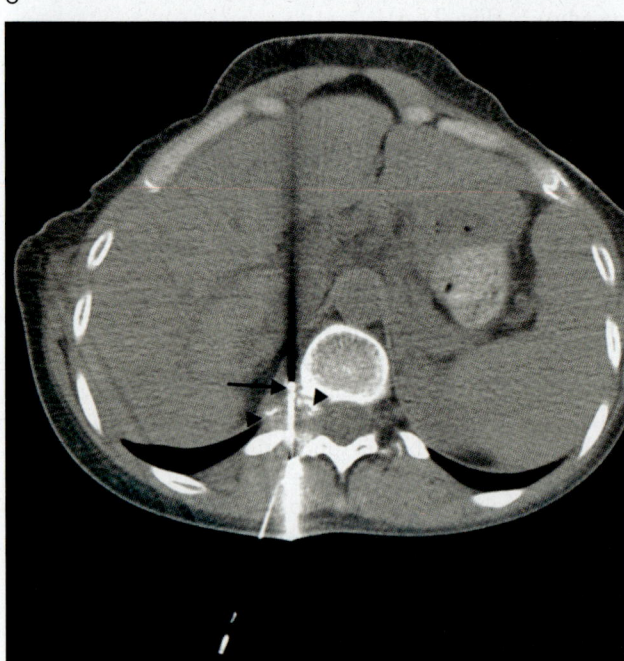

FIGURE 21.4 A 50-year-old woman with metastatic breast cancer to the right T12/L1 paraspinal region. Patient had severe right paraspinal and flank pain not relieved with large doses of oral opioids and gabapentin. PET CT (**A**) shows area of increased uptake *(arrow)* in the right paraspinal area with nerve root involvement. Patient was scheduled for RF ablation under CT guidance. Because of proximity to the thecal sac, a temperature probe was placed at the T12 paraspinal level (**B**). The temperature probe was placed in close proximity to the T12 foramen *(black arrow)*. A 2-cm lesion was placed at the same level. When ablation was started, the temperature probe immediately indicated temperatures in the region of 41°C. Because of concerns of cord damage, RF ablation was abandoned and a decision was made to proceed with chemical neurolysis with aqueous phenol 10%. Before injection of phenol, 0.5 cc of contrast was injected through the temperature probe, which confirmed contrast spread in tumor outside the epidural space *(black arrow heads)*. Phenol 10% 1 cc was then injected. After completion of this injection, the RF needle was reinserted directly into the tumor (**C**). The tip of the probe is shown in the tumor *(black arrow)*. Again, 0.5 cc of contrast was injected, which showed good contrast spread throughout the tumor *(black arrows)*. Aqueous phenol 10% 0.5 cc was then injected. 24 hours after the procedure, the patient reported significant improvement in her pain and also reported a band of numbness in her right flank. PET, Positron-emission tomography; CT, computed tomography; RF, radiofrequency.

sacral dermatomes had the best results. Swerdlow[60] reviewed 13 reports of the results of phenol and alcohol rhizotomies and found good relief of pain in about 60% of patients. In reviewing results of his own patients, he found that pain relief lasted less than 2 months in half the patients and less than 1 month in 25%. Complications lasting longer than a week occurred in 15%.

Slatkin and Rhiner[62] described the use of neurolytic saddle blocks with phenol in four patients with intractable pain. The target location of pain in these patients was rectal/vaginal, perineal/buttocks, penis, and scrotum/penis. Phenol 6% to 10% in glycerin in volumes varying from 0.6 mL to 1 mL was injected at either L5/S1 or L4/5. All patients experienced at least 50% pain relief with reductions in opioid use varying from 17% to 94%. None of the phenol injections was associated with any unexpected adverse effects. Because of its hyperbaricity relative to cerebrospinal fluid (CSF) and intrinsic anesthetic effects, phenolglycerin has become the neurolytic agent of choice for most spinal neurolytic blocks (Fig. 21.7). These qualities are of particular value in the performance of intrathecal saddle blocks where correct patient positioning allows hyperbaric phenol to pool dorsally, thereby maximizing neurolysis of the sensory roots. The most common complications of phenol saddle blocks are temporary paresis of bladder or rectal function, and leg weakness. Each of these complications is concentration dependent, being seen more commonly at higher concentrations of phenol, eg, 10% to 15%.[63] Gerbershagen reported an absence of motor dysfunction using a 0.75 mL dose of phenol 5% to 10%.[61] The technique for neurolytic saddle block requires patients to be placed in a seated position with posterior

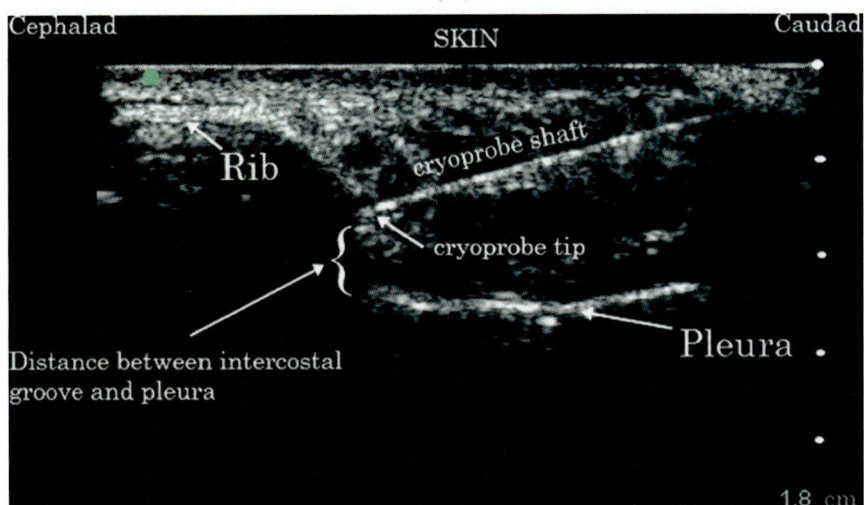

FIGURE 21.5 Ultrasound guidance for intercostal cryoablation. The needle tip is visible and placed at the intercostal groove, within the internal intercostal muscle. (Reused with permission from Byas-Smith MG, Gulati A. Ultrasound-guided intercostal nerve cryoablation. *Anesth Analg.* 2006; 103:1033–1035.)

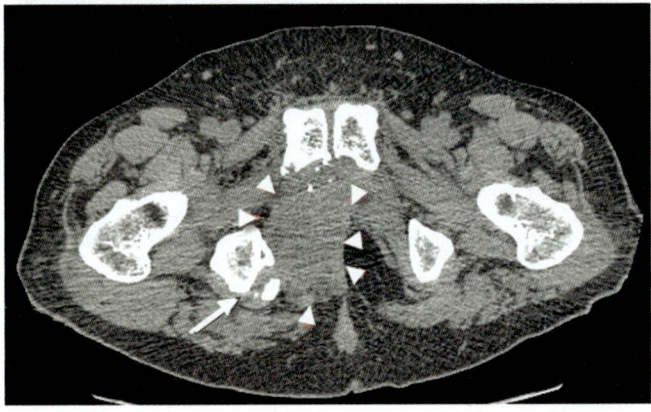

FIGURE 21.6 CT scan of a 59-year-old man with recurrent epithelioid sarcoma of the pelvis with metastasis to the lung and perirectal region. *Arrow heads* show large perirectal mass in pelvis. Patient had severe right buttock/perineal pain because of tumor involvement of right ischial tuberosity *(arrow)*. Because of the tumor location, the patient was unable to put weight on his right buttock region and sit comfortably for periods beyond 30 seconds. Patient underwent a neurolytic saddle block with phenol 5% in glycerin 1.0 mL, which resulted in excellent pain relief for more than 1 year (direct weight bearing on right buttock, unlimited sitting tolerance) with no associated side effects. CT, Computed tomography.

tilt at approximately a 45-degree angle. A lumbar puncture is performed as caudally as possible at the most suitable interspace. The phenol-glycerin solution is drawn up into a 1-mL syringe. Because of the high viscosity of the phenol-glycerin solution, a 22-gauge needle is typically used for injection. Once CSF flow is obtained, the spinal needle bevel is turned caudally and free flow of CSF is confirmed. An initial injection of 0.2 to 0.3 mL is made. Once the injection is completed, the spinal needle stylet is replaced and the patient is asked to report changes in the ability to move his/her ankle and foot. After 15 minutes, an additional incremental injection of 0.2 mL is made. Patients should report the onset of numbness or pain relief in the saddle area. Unilateral numbness should prompt a change in position favoring the less numb side. Each incremental injection should be repeated after a minimum period of 15 minutes. A total volume of 1.0 mL should generally not be exceeded in one session. After completion of injection, the needle is flushed with preservative free normal saline and the patient should remain seated upright for a period of approximately 1 hour.

A

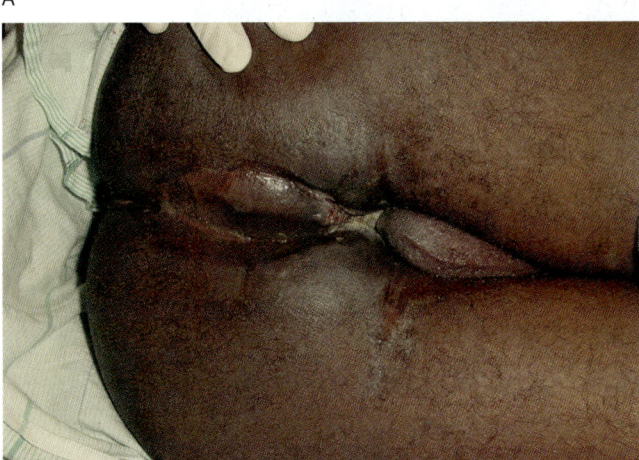

B

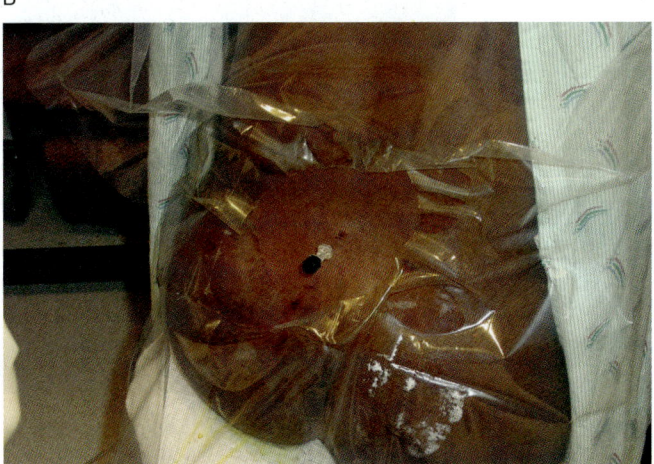

FIGURE 21.7 A 35-year-old HIV-positive man with intractable perianal pain secondary to a squamous cell carcinoma. The patient is lying on his left side (**A**). The patient was unable to sit for periods greater than 30 seconds. He had a functioning colostomy and was continent of urine. (**B**) A neurolytic saddle block was performed with phenol 10% in glycerin at the L4/5 interspace in the sitting position. He received incremental doses of 0.2 mL of phenol to a final volume of 1.0 mL. During the block, the patient's sitting tolerance improved, and 20 minutes after the block, he reported complete resolution of his pain.

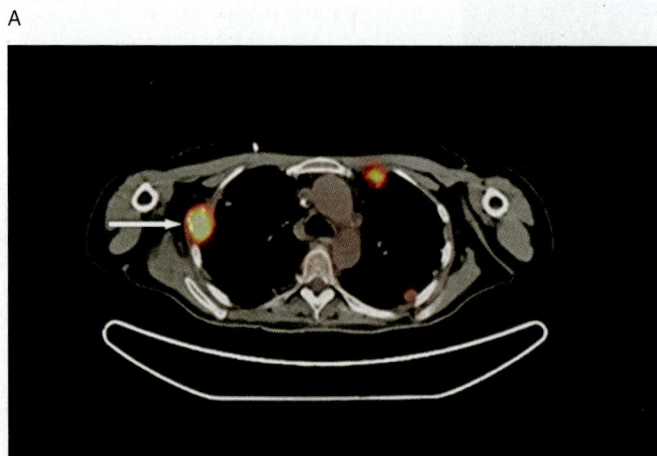
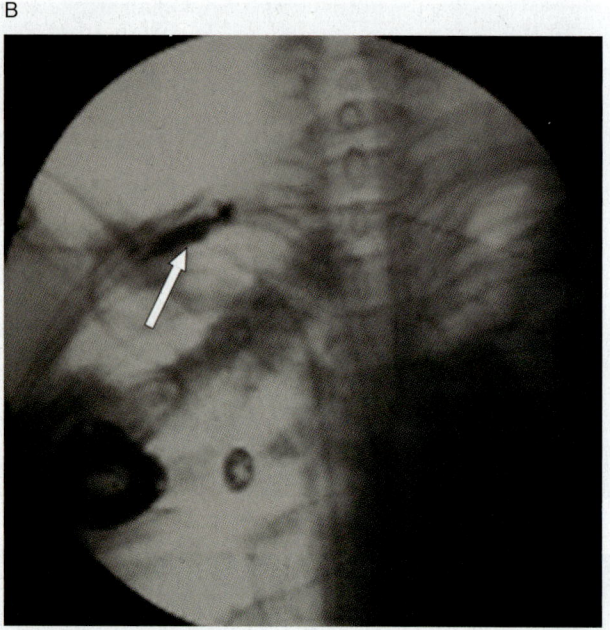

FIGURE 21.8 A: PET CT scan of 42-year-old woman with known metastatic leiomyosarcoma to the chest wall. Scan shows increased fludeoxyglucose activity at the level of the right third rib with abutment onto the lung *(arrow)*. **B:** Patient was successfully treated with posterolateral neurolytic intercostal blocks at ribs 2, 3, and 4 using 3 cc aqueous phenol 5% at each level. Figure shows contrast spread in the second intercostal space before injection of neurolytic solution. PET, Positron-emission tomography; CT, computed tomography.

Other Procedures

Intercostal neurolysis is usually indicated for metastatic disease involving the chest wall or ribs (Figs. 21.8 and 21.9). Autonomic nervous system blocks for visceral pain, although often overlooked, can prove quite effective. In general, these blocks should be considered *analgesic adjuvants* and not definitive pain relief treatment. These procedures should allow patients to lower drug dosages and thereby reduce side effects, or to experience better pain relief from current dosages in order to improve their quality of life. It is inappropriate to promise patients permanent relief, since their disease may progress and spread.

Celiac Plexus Block

The celiac plexus, originating from the sympathetic fibers of the thoracic splanchnic nerves, contains preganglionic splanchnic afferent fibers, parasympathetic preganglionic fibers from the phrenic and vagus nerves, and postganglionic sympathetic fibers, both efferent and afferent. It is the principal area for abdominal visceral nociceptive

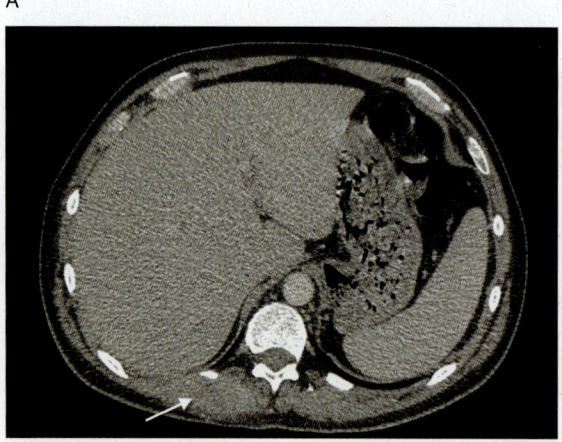
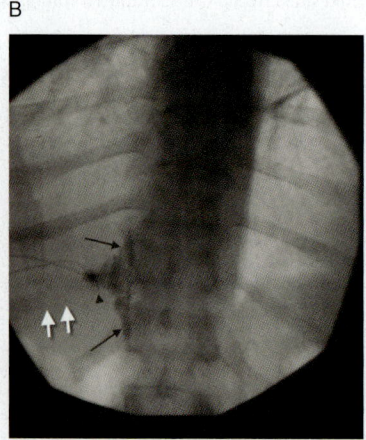

FIGURE 21.9 A 49-year-old man with recurrent sarcoma complaining of intractable right paraspinal pain. Patient recently underwent surgical resection of a large paraspinal mass in the right upper lumbar region with 12th rib resection and adjunctive radiation treatment. Unfortunately, the mass recurred with involvement of the 11th rib *(arrow)*. **A:** Patient underwent a neurolytic intercostal/paravertebral block with aqueous phenol 5% in the region of the 11th rib because of proximity of the mass to the midline posteriorly. **B:** Position of the needle (arrow head) inferiorly to the 11th rib, with injection of contrast material spreading in the right paravertebral space. *Black arrows* indicate spread of contrast. *White arrows* show obvious tumor infiltration of the 11th rib posteriorly (compare with 11th rib on left).

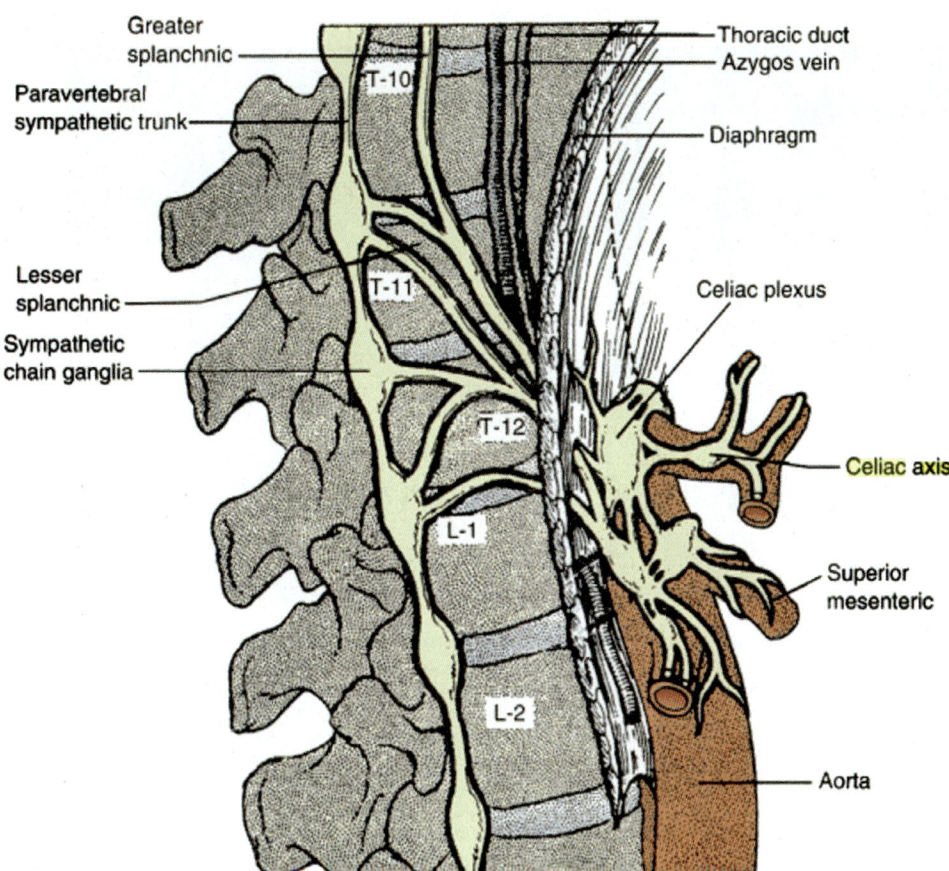

FIGURE 21.10 Anatomy of celiac plexus. (Reused with permission from Mulroy MF, et al. *A practical approach to regional anesthesia*. 4th ed. Philadelphia: Lippincott Williams & Wilkins, 2009).

transmission. Nociceptive impulses originating from all the abdominal viscera (pancreas, liver, stomach, intestine proximal to transverse colon, renal pelvis, proximal ureter, and gallbladder) are carried by visceral nerve fibers that pass through the celiac plexus and thoracic splanchnic nerves. The celiac plexus surrounds the axis of the celiac artery and overlaps the aorta at this level (Fig. 21.10). The plexus varies anatomically in relation to the vertebral column from the bottom of T12 to the middle of L2.[64] The plexus is not a separate and distinct structure, but rather a dense network of ganglia around the aorta between celiac and superior mesenteric artery. It has a more consistent anatomic relationship with the celiac artery. It lies in areolar tissue behind the stomach, pancreas, and omental bursa; retroperitoneal in front of the aorta and crura of the diaphragm, and between the adrenal glands.

Interruption of nociceptive input at the level of either the celiac plexus or the thoracic splanchnic nerves is a potentially effective means of visceral pain control (Fig. 21.11). Preblock, CT scanning is useful to define retroperitoneal anatomy, extent of tumor spread, and the vertebral relationship for the origin of the celiac artery. De Cicco et al.[65] suggest that when the celiac area is free from anatomic distortions and the single-needle neurolytic celiac plexus block technique is used, the needle tip should be positioned cephalad to the celiac artery to achieve a wider neurolytic spread. It appears that only a complete (four-quadrant) neurolytic spread in the celiac area can guarantee long-lasting analgesia. When the celiac area is free from anatomic alterations and a single-needle precrural approach is chosen, the needle tip position in relation to the celiac artery may be critical. For pain associated with pancreatic tumors, differentiation of pancreatic tumor located in the head or in the tail and body of the gland usually is important because of variation in clinical picture of the symptoms, characteristic of pain, spread of the tumor, and even treatment strategy.[66–69] Rykowski and Maciej[70] assessed the effectiveness and duration of pain relief after neurolytic celiac plexus block (NCPB) in pancreatic cancer pain specifically for tumor localization and for different stages of cancer growth. The authors concluded that unilateral transcrural celiac plexus neurolysis provided effective pain relief in 74% of patients with pancreatic cancer pain. Neurolysis was more effective in cases with tumor involving the head of the pancreas. In the cases with advanced tumor proliferation, regardless of the technique used, the analgesic effects of NCPB were not satisfactory.

For tumor-related visceral intra-abdominal pain, varying reports of success are associated with NCPB. Eisenberg et al.[71] performed a meta-analysis of the efficacy and safety of NCPB for cancer pain. Twenty-one studies were retrospective, one was prospective, and two were randomized and controlled. Sixty-three percent of cancer types were pancreatic in origin and 37% were nonpancreatic. A bilateral posterior approach with volumes varying from 15 to 50 mL of 50% to 100% alcohol was the most common technique. Nonradiological guided NCPB was performed in 32%; guidance was by CT in 28%, radiograph in 34%, fluoroscopy in 5%, or ultrasound in <1%. Good to excellent pain relief resulted

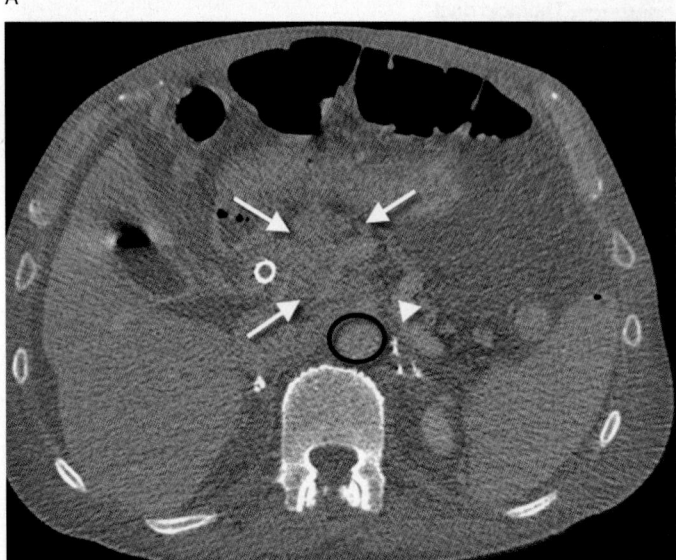
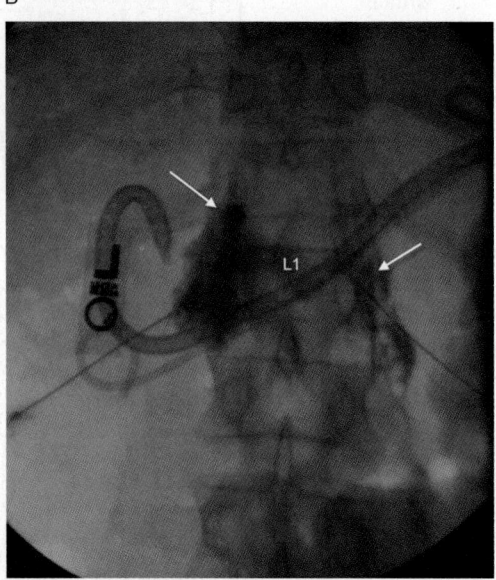

FIGURE 21.11 A 63-year-old man with metastatic pancreatic cancer, complaining of severe epigastric pain not well controlled with fentanyl patches 200 μg/hr q48 hrs. Patient had previously undergone an endoscopic ultrasound-guided neurolytic celiac plexus block that failed to relieve his pain. **A:** CT scan of abdomen shows extensive tumor *(arrows)* involving the celiac plexus between the celiac artery and superior mesenteric artery preventing neurolysis of plexus via the anterior approach. Aorta is outlined with *black circle*. Patient underwent a successful bilateral thoracic splanchnic neurolytic block for pain control (**B**). Fluoroscopic image shows bilateral needle placement at upper third of L1 vertebral body. Contrast inject shows bilateral paravertebral spread *(arrows)*. CT, Computed tomography.

in 89% during the first 2 weeks after NCPB. Long-term follow-up beyond 3 months revealed persistent benefit. Partial to complete pain relief continued in approximately 90% of patients alive at 3 months post-NCPB and in 70% to 90% until death even if beyond 3 months post-NCPB. Patients with pancreatic cancer responded similarly to those with other intra-abdominal malignancies. Common adverse effects were transient, including local pain (96%), diarrhea (44%), and hypotension (38%); complications occurred in 2%. This analysis suggests that NCPB has long-lasting benefit for 70% to 90% of patients with pancreatic and other intra-abdominal cancers, regardless of the technique used, that adverse effects are common but transient and mild, and that severe adverse effects are uncommon.

Polati et al.[72] compared the efficacy of NCPB to pharmacological management in a randomized, prospective, double blind trial of 24 patients with pancreatic cancer. Immediately after the block, patients reported significant pain relief compared with those who received only pharmacological management ($P < .05$), but long-term results did not differ between the two groups. NCPB was associated with a reduction in analgesic drug administration and drug-related adverse effects, and was considered an effective tool in the treatment of pancreatic cancer pain. Wong et al.[73] studied the effect of NCPB on pain relief, quality of life (QoL), and survival in patients with unresectable pancreatic cancer. One hundred patients were randomly assigned to receive either NCPB or systemic analgesic therapy alone with a sham injection. The type of block performed in this study was standardized to a bilateral splanchnic nerve block at L1 vertebral level with 10 mL absolute alcohol injected through each needle. Pain intensity was lower for NCPB over time ($P = .01$). However, opioid consumption ($P = .93$), and frequency of opioid adverse effects were not significantly different between groups. In the first 6 weeks, fewer NCPB patients reported moderate or severe pain (pain intensity rating of ≥5 out of 10) versus opioid-only patients (14% versus 40%, $P = .005$). At 1 year, 16% of NCPB patients and 6% of opioid-only patients were alive but survival did not differ significantly between groups. In this study, both NCPB and optimized systemic analgesic therapy alone provided effective pain relief, with NCPB providing significantly better pain relief, but NCPB had no effect on opioid consumption, QoL, or survival. These results suggest that application of a pain management protocol (optimal systemic analgesic therapy), with or without NCPB, can maintain pain intensity in the "mild" category over time in most patients, even those with advanced disease. NCPB may be considered an efficacious adjunctive analgesic therapy, but a key intervention is the implementation of an aggressive pain management protocol with opioids used throughout the course of disease.

Unfortunately, NCPB is associated with both minor and major complications. Documented side effects and complications from celiac plexus block include myofascial back pain,[71] hypotension,[71-72] intravascular injection,[74] damage to the artery of Adamkiewicz[75-76] with a subsequent anterior spinal artery syndrome,[77] paraplegia[78-79] secondary to either a spinal with a neurolytic solution or the spinal artery syndrome,[80] retroperitoneal pain,[81] reversible paraplegia,[82] infection,[83] loss of anal and bladder sphincter function,[79] mild or persistent diarrhea,[71,84] retroperitoneal fibrosis,[85] pleural effusion,[86] chylothorax,[87] neurologic injury (footdrop),[88] intradiscal injection,[89] and aortic pseudoaneurysm.[83] Other possible problems include discogenic backache, spinal or epidural spread of injected solution, postdural puncture headache, piercing of renal parenchymal tissue, pneumothorax, L1 and/or L2 neuralgia, lumbar plexus block, psoas muscle injection, spasm and/or damage to the celiac artery, intra-bowel injection, bleeding into the peritoneal cavity or retroperitoneum, and thrombosis of any pierced vessels.

Davies[79] determined the incidence of major complications following NCPB. In 2,730 neurolytic blocks performed from 1986 to 1990, the overall incidence of major complications (paraplegia, bladder and bowel dysfunction) was 1 per 683 procedures. A number of other authors suggest that the incidence of a catastrophic sequela after NCPB to be in the region of 1.0% to 2.0%.[71,90–91] Eisenberg et al.[71] quote a 1% incidence of neurological complications, defined as lower extremity weakness, paresthesia, epidural anesthesia, and lumbar puncture, although it is difficult to determine the incidence of any particular complication. Unilateral paralysis due to spread of neurolytic solution to the lumbar plexus,[92] and bilateral paresis due to subarachnoid injection have been reported.[93] Galizia and Lahiri[94] presented a case of total bilateral sensory and motor loss in a L1-5 distribution immediately after celiac plexus block. Cherry and Lamberty[78] also reported paraplegia two hours after an alcohol injection. They speculated that the cause of the paraplegia was an anterior spinal artery syndrome caused by lumbar artery ischemia due to spasm. Anterior spinal artery syndrome due to anterior spinal artery ischemia results in a predominantly motor lesion, since the anterior two thirds of the spinal cord, including the anterior horn cells, is supplied almost exclusively by the anterior spinal artery. The loss of pain and temperature sense, intact fine touch and position sense, and lower extremity paralysis are characteristic. Spinal cord ischemia most likely results from thrombosis or spasm of the artery of Adamkiewicz, usually located on the left of the spine between vertebrae T8 and L4, which supplies the lower two thirds of the spinal cord.[76] Paraplegia has been reported with each percutaneous method regardless of the use of radiologic guidance. There are even reports of paraplegia following surgical neurolysis.[95]

Transcrural and transaortic techniques attempt to minimize the neurological complications occasionally reported with the retrocrural approach (Fig. 21.12). Singler[96] and Hilgier and Rykowski[97] reported using the transcrural approach in 41 patients, with transient diarrhea as a side effect in some patients. In 148 patients who received the transaortic approach,[98–100] transient orthostatic hypotension and diarrhea occurred as the main side effects in some. However, Kaplan et al.[101] reported on a case of aortic dissection as a complication of transaortic celiac plexus block. Sett and Taylor[83] reported the development of a traumatic pseudoaneurysm following the procedure. Naveira et al.[102] described the presence of an atheromatous plaque as a cause of resistance to needle passage during a transaortic celiac plexus block under CT guidance. Although the incidence of major vascular complications following this approach is largely undetermined, translumbar aortography, which punctures the lumbar aorta, has a mortality of 0.05%, with 27% of fatalities resulting from aortic dissection and aneurysm rupture,[103] yielding an incidence of 1.35 per 10,000 procedures.

Some authors have recommended the use of CT scanning, guided by a radiologist, as a method of reducing or eliminating the morbidity associated with celiac neurolysis[104] (Fig. 21.13). However, one can surmise that not all

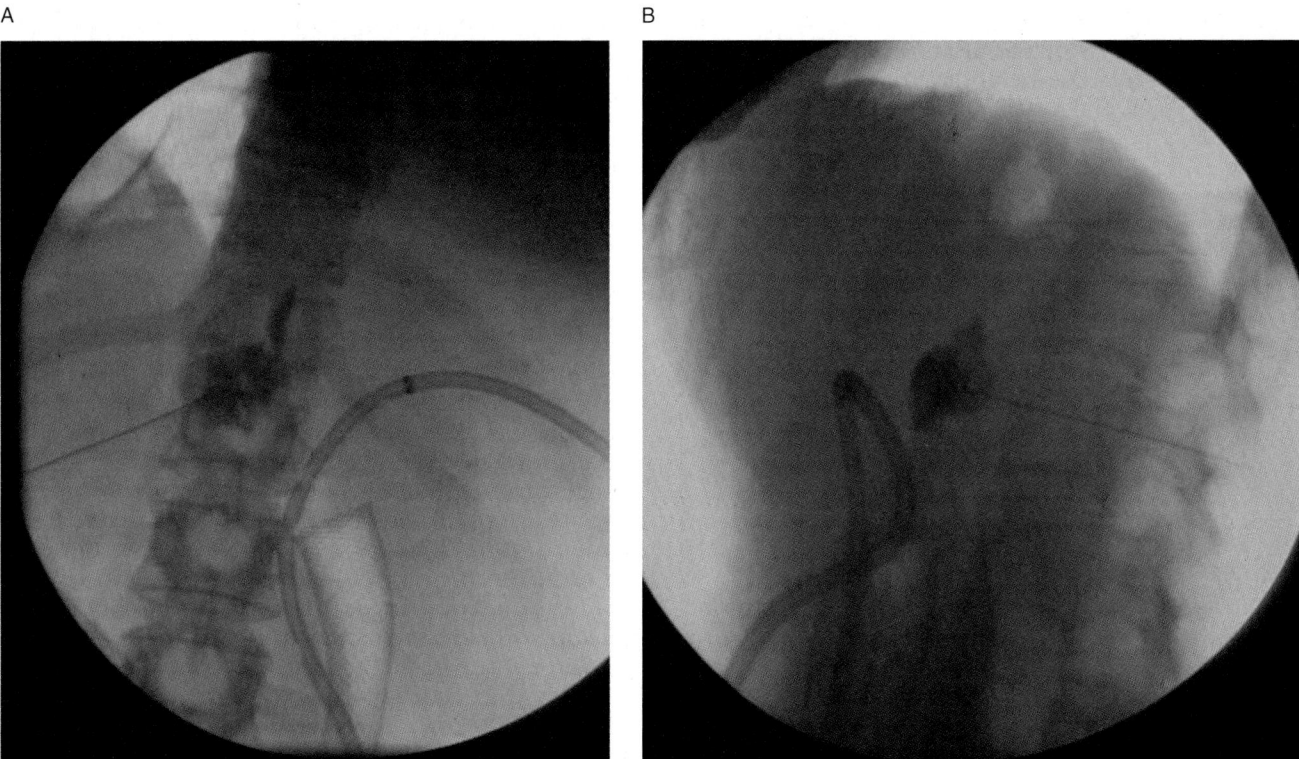

FIGURE 21.12 A 58-year-old woman with intractable tumor-related visceral pain from metastatic colon cancer. A CT scan of abdomen revealed metastatic lesion in the head of the pancreas abutting the second part of the duodenum. A transaortic neurolytic celiac plexus block was performed for pain relief. Fluoroscopic images anteroposterior (**A**) and lateral (**B**) show good retroperitoneal contrast spread in the midline at the level of the upper third of L1 vertebral body. CT, Computed tomography.

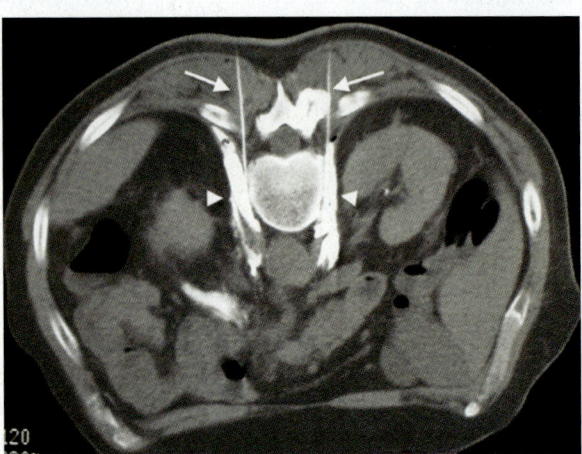

FIGURE 21.13 A 55-year-old man with intractable abdominal pain secondary to pancreatic cancer. A CT-guided left-sided transcrural approach **(A)** failed to demonstrate adequate periaortic contrast spread presumably secondary to tumor encroachment *(arrow)*. Because of this, the block was converted to a bilateral splanchnic nerve block **(B)**. Axial CT shows bilateral needle placement *(arrows)* at level of L1 with good contrast spread in the retrocrural space *(arrow heads)*. CT, Computed tomography.

adverse events from celiac plexus blocks were reported, regardless of the approach used. The only truly accurate determination of complication rates associated with celiac plexus blocks will be through a mandatory central registry of all procedures.

The development of endoscopic ultrasound (EUS) has allowed real-time access to the celiac axis using a short needle via an anterior approach.[105] Linear array endosonographic imaging from the posterior lesser curve of the gastric fundus allows identification of the aorta. Targeting the celiac plexus is based on the position of the celiac plexus relative to the position of the celiac trunk (Fig. 21.14). Color Doppler ultrasonography is used to confirm the vascular nature of the structures. A 22-gauge needle is inserted under EUS guidance immediately adjacent and anterior to the lateral aspect of the aorta at the level of the celiac trunk. Michaels and Draganov[106] suggest that EUS guided celiac plexus block/neurolysis is simple to perform and avoids serious complications such as paraplegia or pneumothorax that are associated with the posterior approach. However, reports evaluating the efficacy and safety of EUS celiac plexus neurolysis are limited and claims of improved safety associated with EUS NCPB need to be interpreted with caution.

Because of the accuracy of lesions produced by radiofrequency ablation, there has been growing interest in the use of this technique for neurolysis of splanchnic nerves as it offers the potential of accurate nerve destruction ablation with a predictable ablative lesion that is well circumscribed and controlled. Another advantage of RF ablation is that it has an immediate effect, unlike alcohol and phenol, which may be delayed. When cells are heated above 45°C, cellular proteins denature and cell membranes lose their integrity as their lipid components melt. The size and shape of the necrotic RF lesion is dependent on the probe gauge, length of the exposed tip, probe temperature and the duration of treatment. Garcea et al.[107] and Raj[108] described the technique of bilateral percutaneous splanchnic nerve RF ablation. With the patient in the prone position and using fluoroscopy, the T12 vertebral body is identified and a 14-gauge, 5-cm extracath needle inserted. The stylet is removed and a 15-cm, 20-gauge curved RF needle with a 15-mm lesion tip is inserted. The tip of the curved needle should face laterally until it passes the intervertebral foramen. Then the tip can be turned medially once it reaches the lateral surface of the vertebral body. The needle should be positioned at the junction of anterior one third and posterior two third of the lateral side of the T11 or T12 vertebral body (Figs. 21.15 and 21.16). Fluoroscopy should ensure that the needle stays posterior to the aorta and anterior to the foramen. The needle should remain retrocrural and this position should be confirmed by contrast injection. The needle is aspirated and if no fluid is obtained, further oblique views are taken to confirm correct positioning of the needle. Before RFA splanchnic lesioning, impedance is

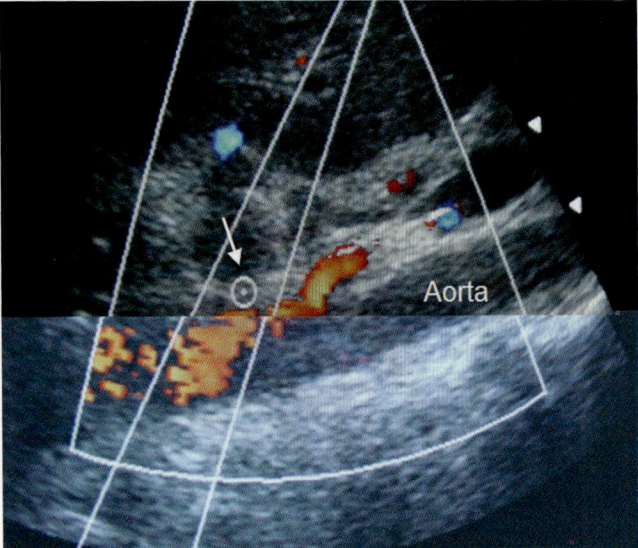

FIGURE 21.14 A 58-year-old man with pancreatic cancer. A neurolytic celiac plexus block was performed via the anterior approach under ultrasound guidance. The aorta is shown in longitudinal view. Color flow shows the celiac axis take-off from the aorta and the target area for needle placement is shown *(arrow)* at the base of the celiac artery take-off.

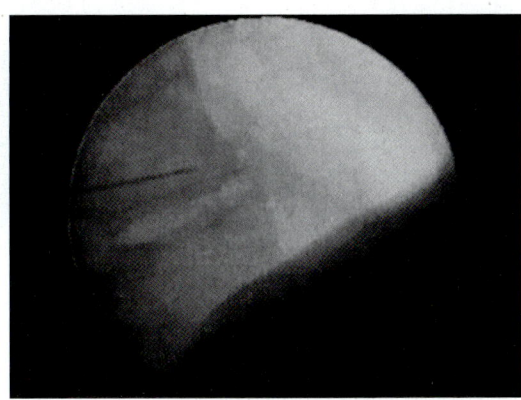

FIGURE 21.15 Lateral image of radiofrequency needle against T12 body

noted below 250 ohms, and motor and sensory test stimulation are undertaken using 2 Hz (to 2 V) and 50 to 100 Hz (to 1 V), respectively. On sensory stimulation the correct patient response is a sensation in the epigastric region. If stimulation is in a girdle-like fashion around the chest wall, the needle should be moved more anteriorly. Motor stimulation is conducted to ensure that no contraction of the intercostal muscles is observed. If both these responses are satisfactory, then RF ablation is undertaken. After test stimulation, 2 to 5 mL of local anesthetic with triamcinolone 40 mg is injected to reduce lesioning discomfort and reduce the occurrence of neuritis. The RF lesion is produced at 80°C for 90 seconds. A second lesion at the same settings is done by turning the needle 180 degrees.

Superior Hypogastric Plexus Block

Pelvic pain associated with cancer arises from visceral involvement, from tumor extension to the muscles and bones of the pelvic wall, and from nerve involvement. Visceral pain may be a significant feature of advanced stage cancers of the pelvis such as cervical, bladder, prostate, and rectum. Relief of pain from pelvic organ nociception is possible because afferent fibers innervating these structures travel in the sympathetic nerves, trunks, ganglia, and rami. The superior hypogastric plexus is situated in the retroperitoneum, bilaterally extending from the lower third of the fifth lumbar vertebral body to the upper third of the first sacral vertebral body (Fig. 21.17). The plexus innervates the pelvic viscera via the hypogastric nerves and inferior hypogastric plexuses. It is embedded in the subserous fascia between the bifurcation of the common iliac arteries and divides into two trunks at the lower third of L5 to the upper third of S1. It supplies the visceral innervation to most of the pelvic structures, descending colon, rectum, and internal genitalia except the ovaries and fallopian tubes.

A surgeon can divide the superior hypogastric plexus (presacral neurectomy) either at laparotomy[109] or at laparoscopy.[110] Various nonsurgical approaches to the

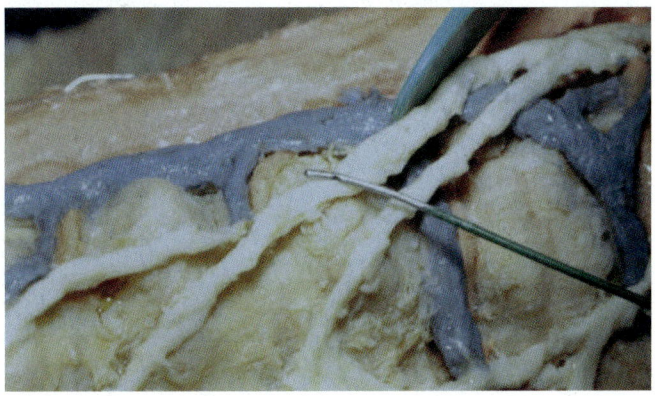

FIGURE 21.16 A 15-mm active-tip radiofrequency needle for lesioning the splanchnics at T11-T12 placed over the splanchnic nerves in a cadaver. (From Raj PP, Sahinler B, Lowe M. Radiofrequency lesioning of splanchnic nerves. *Pain Pract.* 2002;2:241–247. Reprinted with permission from Wiley-Blackwell.)

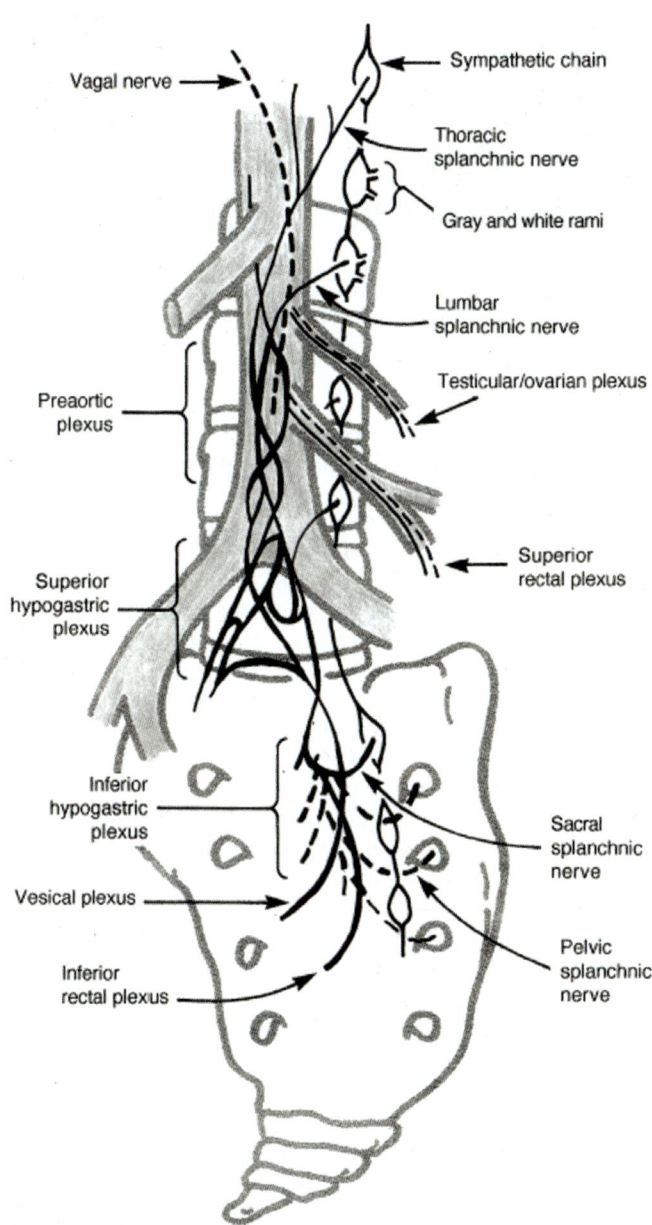

FIGURE 21.17 Superior hypogastric plexus. The plexus is a retroperitoneal structure below the aortic bifurcation. It receives fibers from the lumbar splanchnic nerves. Distally, the hypogastric nerves arise from the plexus which supply the inferior hypogastric plexus. (From Bosscher H. Blockade of the superior hypogastric plexus block for visceral pelvic pain. *Pain Pract.* 2001;1:162–170. Reprinted with permission of Wiley-Blackwell.)

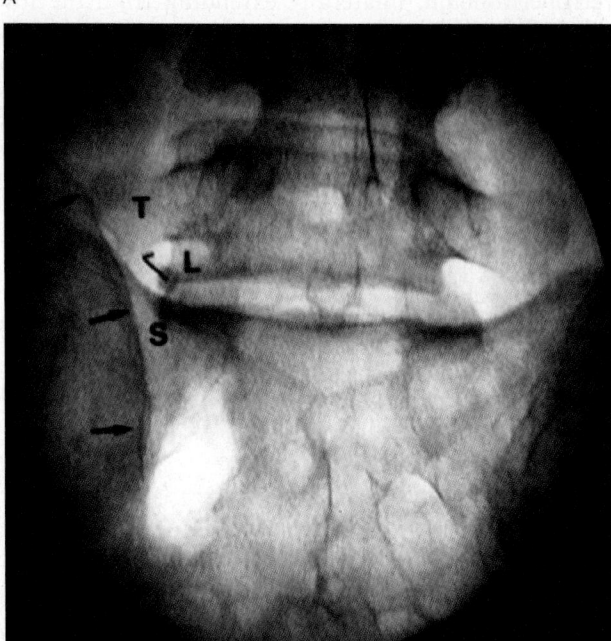 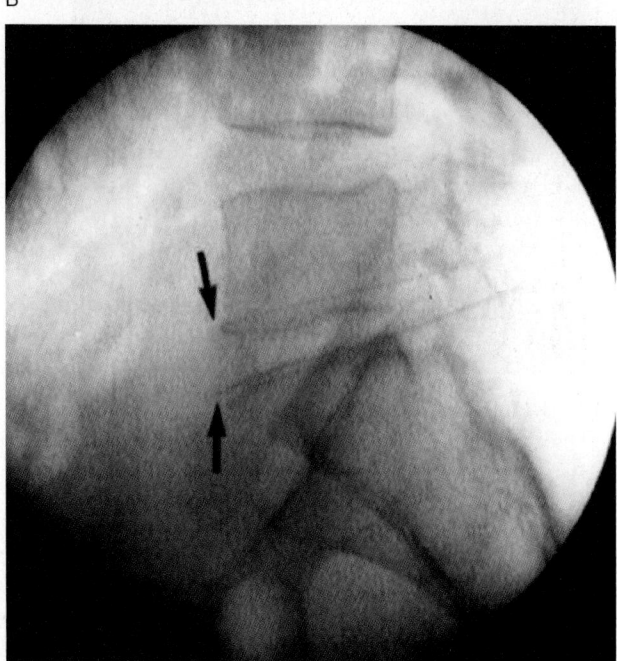

FIGURE 21.18 Superior hypogastric plexus block. Posterior approach. Anteroposterior view of the L5/S1 junction is shown (**A**). There is a window between the L5 transverse process *(T)*, the sacral ala *(S)*, and the anterolateral margin of the L5 vertebral body *(L)*. The iliac crest is just lateral to the window *(arrows)*. Final needle position is shown on the lateral view (**B**). Both needles are just anterior to the L5/S1 junction *(arrows)*. (Reused with permission from Stevens DS, Balatbat GR, Lee FM. Coaxial imaging technique for superior hypogastric plexus block. *Reg Anesth Pain Med.* 2000;25:643–647.)

plexus are also possible. Plancarte et al.[111] used a bilateral percutaneous phenol nerve block approach for the management of intractable pelvic visceral pain. This technique involves a two-needle posterior approach using fluoroscopic guidance. However, proper needle localization can be difficult using the posterior approach because of bony obstacles such as the sacral ala and the transverse process of L5 (Fig. 21.18). An alternative fluoroscopic approach was described by Kanazi et al.[112] With this technique, the patient is placed in the supine position with 15 degrees of Trendelenburg. Using fluoroscopy guidance, the L5 vertebral body is identified. A skin wheal is raised 2 to 3 cm inferior to the umbilicus, and the subcutaneous tissue is infiltrated using 0.5% lidocaine with a 25-gauge, 1.25-inch needle. A 22-gauge, 6-inch needle is inserted in the midline perpendicular to the floor until it contacts the caudad two thirds of the L5 vertebral body. The needle is then aspirated to check for intra-arterial or venous puncture. Radiopaque solution (5 to 10 mL) is injected, and the spread of the dye is confirmed in posteroanterior (PA) and lateral radiographic views (Fig. 21.19).

Alternative approaches advocated include a single-needle CT-guided anterior approach[113] and two-needle posterior transdiscal.[114] Ina et al.[115] advocated the deliberate passage of needles through the L5-S1 disc (transdiscal approach) for patients with difficult anatomy, and reported on the safe and successful use of this technique in eight patients. Gamal et al.[114] also reported on the advantages of a transdiscal approach for superior hypogastric plexus block in pelvic cancer pain. Erdine et al.[116] described this approach. For this approach, the patient was placed in the prone position with a pillow beneath the iliac crest to facilitate opening of the interdiscal space. The L_5-S_1 interdiscal space was identified under fluoroscopy with the fluoroscope directed in an oblique fashion and angled 15 to 25 degrees to obtain the best image of the disc. The entry point was approximately 5 to 7 cm from

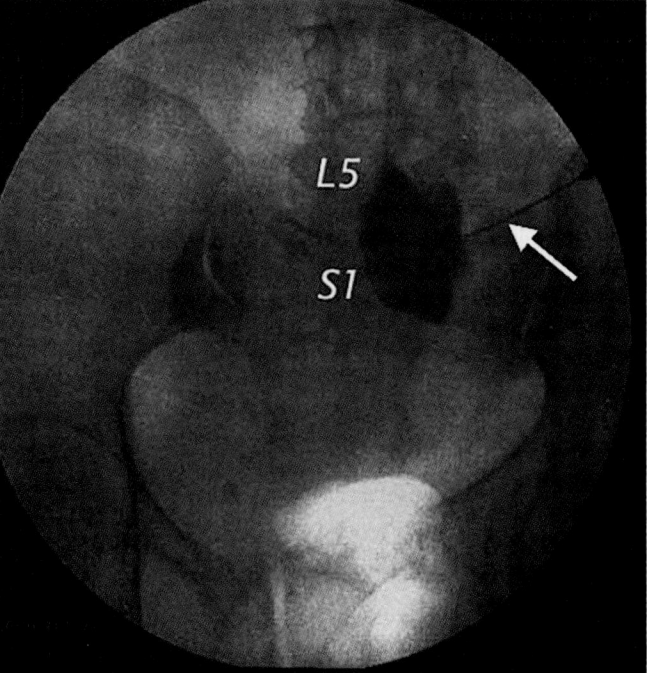

FIGURE 21.19 Superior hypogastric plexus block. Transdiscal approach. The entry point is 5 to 7 cm from the midline *(arrow)*. After disc entry, the needle is advanced until loss of resistance is felt, indicating the needle has passed through the L5/S1 disc. (Reused with permission from Gamal G, Helaly M, Labib YM. Superior hypogastric block: Transdiscal versus classic posterior approach in pelvic cancer pain. *Clin J Pain.* 2006;22:544–547.)

the midline. After local anesthetic infiltration of the skin and the subcutaneous tissues with 2% lidocaine, a 22-gauge, 10-cm needle was introduced by tunnel vision lateral to the inferior aspect of the facet joint. The needle was advanced through the disc. While the disc was entered, 0.5 mL of radiopaque iohexol solution was administered to verify needle position within the disc by lateral and anteroposterior views. The needle was then advanced further under lateral fluoroscopic control, and a 5-mL syringe with saline was attached for loss of resistance. When the needle passes outside the L5-S1 interdiscal space, 3 mL of iohexol was administered to verify its final position. Cephazolin 50 mg in 1mL was administered intradiscally to prevent discitis. One gram of cephazolin as a prophylactic antibiotic is also given intravenously 30 minutes before the procedure. For CT-guided blocks, a series of contiguous scans, or a short spiral scan, was performed starting from the L3-L4 interspace down to S1 to locate the aortic bifurcation. A 10 cm, 20-gauge needle is introduced, using a guide system and biopsy calculation software included in the CT scanner, which permits calculation of the lateral shift and the needle angulation needed for accurate placement of the needle. The tip of the needle is positioned in the midline, anteriorly to the left iliac vein and just below the aortic bifurcation. When the needle tip is in the precalculated position, 1 mL of contrast medium (300 mg/mL) is injected, and a series of scans is obtained to verify the needle position and check contrast spreading before introducing the neurolytic solution (Fig. 21.19). An alternative anterior approach using fluoroscopy was described by Kanazi et al.[112] Patients were placed in the supine position and 15 degrees Trendelenburg. Using fluoroscopy, the L5 vertebral body was identified. A skin wheal was raised 2 to 3 cm inferior to the umbilicus, and the subcutaneous tissue was infiltrated using 0.5% lidocaine with a 25-gauge, 1.25-inch needle. A 22-gauge, 6-inch needle was inserted in the midline perpendicular to the floor until it contacted the caudad two thirds of the L5 vertebral body. The needle was then aspirated to check for intra-arterial or venous puncture. Radiopaque solution (5 to 10 mL) was injected, and the spread of the dye is confirmed in PA and lateral radiographic views (Fig. 21.20).

The superior hypogastric plexus block offers a practical, minimally invasive alternative for controlling cancer pain associated with tumor extension into the pelvic viscera. An incomplete block may occur in patients with retroperitoneal disease, due to limited spread of phenol.[117] Despite the use of a unilateral needle insertion under CT guidance,[118] the results are sometimes less favorable than those obtained with bilateral needle placement because of the bilateral distribution of pelvic pain.[119] De Leon-Casasola et al.[117] evaluated the efficacy and safety of the block in 26 patients with extensive gynecologic, colorectal, or genitourinary cancer who suffered uncontrolled, incapacitating pelvic pain. Neurolysis was carried out under fluoroscopy with bilateral needle placement and injection of 8 mL of 10% phenol on each side. Criteria for success of the block were a decrease in visual analog score (VAS) of at least 70% or pain intensity rating of less than 3 out of 10 during the first 2 weeks after the block, and a decrease in oral opioid requirements of at least 30% with disappearance of bothersome side effects 2 weeks after the block. All patients reported a VAS of 10/10 before the block, despite oral opioid therapy. Mean use of morphine before the first neurolytic block in all patients was 953 ± 722 mg/day with a median of 780 mg/day (range: 80 to 2780 mg/day). Postprocedure patients in the success group demonstrated significantly less daily oral intake of morphine than patients in the failure group (736 ± 633 vs. 1443 ± 703 mg/day, $P = .02$).[117] Sixty-nine percent of patients had satisfactory pain relief (VAS <4/10). Fifty-seven percent of these patients had satisfactory relief after one block, the remaining 12% after a second block. Thirty-one percent had moderate pain control (VAS: 4 to 7 out of 10) after 2 blocks and received supplementary neuraxial analgesia therapy. Both groups of patients experienced significant reductions in oral opioid therapy after the neurolytic blocks. Patients who had a good response during a 6-month follow-up period required no additional blocks. There were no intraoperative complications such as bladder puncture or retroperitoneal hematomas. Two patients had transvascular neurolytic blocks without problems. There were no long-term complications, such as urinary or fecal incontinence.

Neurolytic superior hypogastric plexus blocks are useful for patients with intractable visceral pelvic pain and appear to have a low incidence of side effects or complications. However, many diseases of the pelvis also involve the pelvic side wall and other somatic structures at the time of diagnosis, thus limiting the usefulness of the block.

A

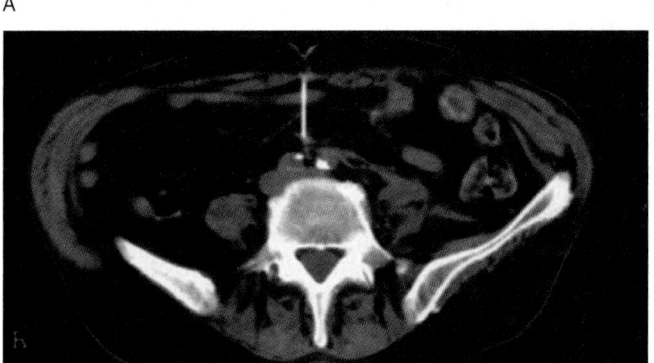

B

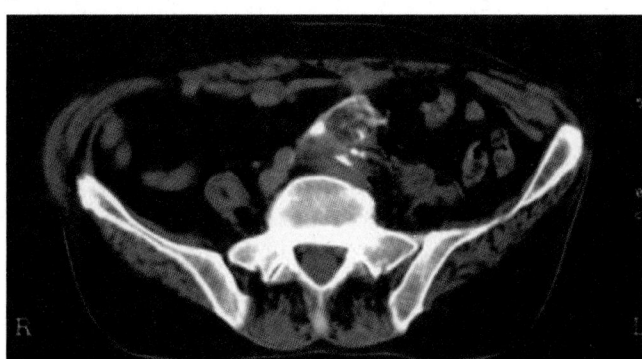

FIGURE 21.20 CT scans show anterior superior hypogastric plexus block. **A:** Needle tip is located just caudal to the aortic bifurcation. **B:** Scan shows the correct spread of the neurolytic solution around the common iliac vessels. CT, Computed tomography. (Reused with permission from Cariati M, De Martini G, Pretolesi F, et al. CT-guided superior hypogastric plexus block. *J Comput Assist Tomogr.* 2002;26: 428–31.)

NEUROMODULATORY TREATMENTS FOR PAIN ASSOCIATED WITH CANCER

Neuromodulative approaches to the nervous system are either electrical or pharmacologic. Electrical modulation is most commonly used for various noncancer-related pain syndromes, including failed back surgery syndrome (FBSS), complex regional pain syndrome (CRPS), neuropathic pain, angina, and ischemic limb pain. Intraspinal delivery of medications (both opioids and local anesthetics) is used to treat both nociceptive and neuropathic pain problems. Medication infusion has emerged as a major resource in cancer pain management, whereas electrical stimulation plays a relatively minor role. Much of the growing interest in infusion therapy results from improved technology for continuous infusion, using epidural, intrathecal, or intracerebroventricular catheters connected to external infusion pumps, subcutaneous injection reservoirs, or implanted programmable infusion pumps. Neuraxial medication infusions are discussed in detail in "Neuraxial Analgesia," Chapter 22.

Electrical Stimulation For The Relief Of Pain Associated With Cancer

Electrical stimulation of skin, peripheral nerves, spinal cord, deep brain structures, and motor cortex have all been utilized in the treatment of pain associated with cancer; some successes have been reported with all of these stimulation sites, but properly conducted clinical trials are few. These stimulation strategies are not uniformly available and wide variation in their use is common.

Transcutaneous Skin Stimulation

Stimulation of the skin is a noninvasive treatment strategy that has been utilized for millennia. Modern electronics simplifies the use of this technique. Transcutaneous skin stimulation is commonly known as transcutaneous electrical nerve stimulation (TENS), as well as transcutaneous electrical stimulation and transcutaneous nerve stimulation. TENS has been in common use for 40 years in the United States, and units can be rented for evaluation and then purchased if treatment is successful. In general, electrodes are applied to the skin in the region of pain and stimulation undertaken for prolonged periods. Side effects rarely occur, and most are related to skin irritation from the electrodes and conductive gel; frequently moving the electrodes usually solves this problem. Although there are many case series and individual case reports, a recent systematic review of the literature found only two adequate randomized controlled trials with 64 participants and stated that the effectiveness of TENS could not be determined for relief of cancer pain.[120–122] This is true of TENS for other types of pain as well. Unfortunately, the responses to different sources of pain (eg, local infiltration, bone metastasis, neuropathic pains associated with radiation or chemotherapy) are unknown. However, because this treatment strategy is relatively inexpensive, very safe, and noninvasive,[123] it should not be overlooked as a nonpharmacologic intervention that could be beneficial for some patients.[124]

Transcutaneous electroanalgesia (TSE) is an unproven method of electrical stimulation that uses electrodes placed over the spine and operates at a higher frequency than traditional TENS. With TSE stimulation, there is no sensory stimulation. Robb et al[121] compared the effectiveness of TENS with TSE and placebo in 41 women with chronic pain following breast cancer treatment. In this study, neither form of electrical stimulation was more effective than placebo.

Peripheral Nerve Stimulation

There are only small case series or individual case reports describing the use of implanted peripheral nerve stimulators for pain associated with cancer. No one manufactures electrodes specifically designed for peripheral nerves, and most interventionalists who utilize this strategy adapt spinal cord stimulation electrodes for peripheral nerve stimulation (PNS), a less than optimal solution. We are not aware of current usage to treat pains associated with cancer, although it clearly had been tried when implanted stimulators first became available.[125] PNS is most commonly used for neuropathic pain in the distribution of a single major nerve.

Spinal Cord Stimulation

Spinal cord stimulation (SCS) has been utilized in the treatment of various chronic pain states since the 1970s. In spite of widespread utilization, properly conducted clinical trials are few and far between, and there has been little discussion of the use of SCS in patients with pains associated with cancer. Almost 30 years ago, a review of the world's literature revealed a total of 51 cases of cancer pain patients treated with dorsal column stimulation and commented upon the lack of reported trials.[125] This remains the case to date, although the technology for SCS has significantly improved in both reliability and efficacy. SCS requires that an electrode be placed in the epidural space dorsal to the spinal cord and that it is connected to a device that generates electricity and is implanted beneath the skin. Electrodes can be percutaneously inserted or implanted under direct vision by laminotomy. Pulse generators today are battery operated and may be rechargeable. New technology is developing continually and makes SCS easier to perform and more efficacious, although usually at greater cost.

There are no reviews of the use of SCS for the treatment of cancer pain. Most of the studies relate to low back pain, complex regional pain syndrome, neuropathic pain, vascular disease, and angina. However, patients with cancer may develop neuropathic pains related to chemotherapy or radiation therapy and tumor invasion of nerves. Such patients may be candidates for spinal cord stimulation, as discussed by Hamid[126] and Cata.[127] Other pain symptoms (generally ischemic in origin) that are seen in cancer patients may also be amenable to SCS.[128–129] Neuropathic pain of any etiology may be treated successfully by SCS. When medications fail, SCS may be considered. However, if the patient has tumor involvement of the epidural space, electrodes cannot be safely implanted through that region because of the risk of epidural hemorrhage and separation of the electrode from the dura by tumor.

Deep Brain Stimulation

Deep brain stimulation (DBS) for the relief of chronic pain has been used since the 1950s but is no longer as popular as it was 25 years ago.[130] Indeed, it is not Food and Drug Administration-approved in the United States. It is clear that there are two quite distinct targets: the lateral thalamus-internal capsule region and the periventricular/periaqueductal grey (PVG/PAG). Stimulation in the lateral thalamus/internal capsule region produces paresthesiae, just like SCS) or PNS. The patient must perceive the paresthesiae in the region of pain to obtain pain relief. This site works best for neuropathic pain states. PVG/PAG stimulation does not produce paresthesiae and seems to work better for nociceptive pains, such as those secondary to cancer. The electrodes are implanted stereotactically under local anesthesia; after a trial period with externalized leads, the system can be internalized with implantation of the pulse generator, usually just below the clavicle on the upper chest wall. Many patients have both nociceptive and neuropathic components of their pain; electrodes at both sites may be required for optimal pain relief.

Today, the consensus is that deep brain stimulation for pain relief should be an end-of-the-road treatment, to be used when all else has failed. Review of the published series suggests that nociceptive pains have about a 70% success rate, whereas neuropathic pains have, at best, a 50% long-term success rate.[130] Pains due to cancer seem to respond like other nociceptive pains. Good results may fade over several years. Patients need to realize that complete pain relief is rarely obtained; 50% relief is considered a good result.

Motor Cortex Stimulation

Motor cortex stimulation (MCS) is a pain-relieving procedure in development; conclusions about efficacy and duration of effect are not yet possible, in spite of enthusiastic reports by its developers and early proponents.[131] An electrode is placed in the epidural space over the motor cortex as localized by functional imaging or neuronavigation and connected to an implanted pulse generator. Complications have been very infrequent; the issues are long-term efficacy and types of pain that can be treated. It appears to be useful for central pain states such as poststroke pain or trigeminal denervation pains, but we can find no reports of its use in cancer pain patients.[132] Because MCS is not FDA-approved in the United States, most of the information on its utility comes from abroad.

References

1. Lippitz BE, Kraepelien T, Hautanen K, et al. Gamma knife radiosurgery for patients with multiple cerebral metastases. *Acta Neurochir Suppl.* 2004;91:79–87.
2. Hoegler D. Radiotherapy for palliation of symptoms in incurable cancer. *Curr Probl Cancer.* 1997;21:129–183.
3. Rutten EH, Crul BJ, van der Toorn PP, et al. Pain characteristics help to predict the analgesic efficacy of radiotherapy for the treatment of cancer pain. *Pain.* 1997;69:131–135.
4. Gerszten PC, Ozhasoglu C, Burton SA, et al. CyberKnife frameless stereotactic radiosurgery for spinal lesions: Clinical experience in 125 cases. *Neurosurgery.* 2004;55:89–98;discussion 98–99.
5. Little AS, Shetter AG, Shetter ME, et al. Long-term pain response and quality of life in patients with typical trigeminal neuralgia treated with gamma knife stereotactic radiosurgery. *Neurosurgery.* 2008;63:915–923;discussion 923–924.
6. Kondo T, Hozumi T, Goto T, et al. Intraoperative radiotherapy combined with posterior decompression and stabilization for non-ambulant paralytic patients due to spinal metastasis. *Spine.* 2008;33:1898–1904.
7. Holman PJ, Suki D, McCutcheon I, et al. Surgical management of metastatic disease of the lumbar spine: Experience with 139 patients. *J Neurosurg Spine.* 2005;2:550–563.
8. Ibrahim A, Crockard A, Antonietti P, et al. Does spinal surgery improve the quality of life for those with extradural (spinal) osseous metastases? An international multicenter prospective observational study of 223 patients. *J Neurosurg Spine.* 2008;8:271–278.
9. Loeser JD. Ablative neurosurgical operations – introduction. In: Loeser JD, ed. *Bonica's management of pain*, 3rd ed. Philadelphia: Lippincott, 2000:2007–2010.
10. White J, Sweet W. *Pain: Its mechanisms and neurosurgical control.* Springfield, Illinois: C.C. Thomas, 1955.
11. Burchiel KJ. *Surgical management of pain.* New York: Theime, 2002.
12. Gybels JM, Sweet WH. *Neurosurgical treatment of persistent pain.* Basel: Karger, 1989.
13. North RB, Levy RM. *Neurosurgical management of pain.* New York: Springer-Verlag, 1996.
14. Loeser JD. Neurosurgical approaches to palliative medicine. In: Doyle D, Hanks GW, MacDonald N, eds. *Oxford Textbook of Palliative Medicine*, 1st ed. Oxford: Oxford University Press, 1993:221–229.
15. Loeser JD, Swain WH, Tew JMJ, et al. Neurosurgical operations involving peripheral nerves. In: Bonica JJ, ed. *The management of pain in clinical practice*, 2nd ed. Philadelphia: Lea and Febiger, 1990:2044–2066.
16. Hardy RW, Bay JW. Surgery of the sympathetic nervous system. In: Schmidek HH, Sweet WH, eds. *Operative neurosurgical techniques*, 3rd ed. Philadelphia: Saunders, 1995:1637–1646.
17. Uchida K, Kobayashi S, Yayama T, et al. Metastatic involvement of sacral nerve roots from uterine carcinoma: A case report. *Spine J.* 2008;8:849–852.
18. Wilkinson HA, Chan AS. Sensory ganglionectomy: Theory, technical aspects, and clinical experience. *J Neurosurg.* 2001;95:61–66.
19. Sweet WH, Poletti CE. Operations in the brain stem and spinal canal, with an appendix on open cordotomy. In: Wall PD, Melzack R, eds. *Textbook of pain*, 3rd ed. Edinburgh: Churchill Livingstone, 1994:1113–1135.
20. Tasker RR. Percutaneous Cordotomy. In: Schmidek HH, Sweet WH, eds. *Operative neurosurgical techniques*, 3rd ed. Philadelphia: Saunders, 1995:1595–1611.
21. Nauta HJ, Westlund KN, Willis WD. Midline myelotomy. In: Burchiel K, ed. *Surgical management of pain.* New York: Theime, 2002:714–731.
22. Hwang SL, Lin CL, Lieu AS, et al. Punctate midline myelotomy for intractable visceral pain caused by hepatobiliary or pancreatic cancer. *J Pain Symptom Manage.* 2004;27:79–84.
23. Chang DS, Lin CL, Lieu AS, et al. High cervical midline punctate myelotomy in the management of visceral pain in the mouse. *Kaohsiung J Med Sci.* 2003;19:159–162.
24. Hitchcock E. Stereotactic cervical myelotomy. *J Neurol Neurosurg Psychiatry.* 1970;33:224–230.
25. Raslan AM. Percutaneous computed tomography-guided radiofrequency ablation of upper spinal cord pain pathways for cancer-related pain. *Neurosurgery.* 2008;62:226–233.
26. Nauta HJ, Soukup VM, Fabian RH, et al. Punctate midline myelotomy for the relief of visceral cancer pain. *J Neurosurg.* 2000;92:125–130.
27. Gorecki JP, Little KM. Brainstem ablative procedures. In: Follett KA, ed. *Neurosurgical pain management.* Philadelphia: Elsevier, 2004:190–193.
28. Frank F, Fabrizi AP, Gaist G. Stereotactic mesencephalic tractotomy in the treatment of chronic cancer pain. *Acta Neurochir (Wien).* 1989;99:38–40.

29. Tasker RR. Stereotactic Surgery. In: Wall PD, Melzack R, eds. *Textbook of pain,* 3rd ed. Edinburgh: Churchill Livingstone, 1994: 1137–1157.
30. Young RF. Ablative brain operations for chronic pain. In: Loeser JD, ed. *Bonica's management of pain,* 3rd ed. Philadelphia: Lippincott, 2000:2048–2065.
31. White J, Sweet WH. *Pain and the neurosurgeon.* Springfield, Illinois: C.C. Thomas, 1969.
32. Tindall GT, Payne NS, Nixon DW. Transsphenoidal hypophysectomy for disseminated carcinoma of the prostate gland. Results in 53 patients. *J Neurosurg.* 1979;50:275–282.
33. Hayashi M, Taira T, Chernov M, et al. Gamma knife surgery for cancer pain-pituitary gland-stalk ablation: A multicenter prospective protocol since 2002. *J Neurosurg.* 2002;97:433–437.
34. Bessant R, Steuer A, Rigby S, et al. Osmic acid revisited: Factors that predict a favourable response. *Rheumatology (Oxford).* 2003; 42:1036–1043.
35. Burchiel KJ, Russell LC. Glycerol neurolysis: Neurophysiological effects of topical glycerol application on rat saphenous nerve. *J Neurosurg.* 1985;63:784–788.
36. Lunsford LD, Bennett MH, Martinez AJ. Experimental trigeminal glycerol injection. Electrophysiologic and morphologic effects. *Arch Neurol.* 1985;42:146–149.
37. Hara H, Kobayashi S. Glycerol injection to the rat trigeminal nerve: histological and immunohistochemical studies. *Acta Neurochir (Wien).* 1992;119:111–114.
38. Rengachary SS, Watanabe IS, Singer P, et al. Effect of glycerol on peripheral nerve: An experimental study. *Neurosurgery.* 1983;13: 681–688.
39. Eide PK, Stubhaug A. Relief of trigeminal neuralgia after percutaneous retrogasserian glycerol rhizolysis is dependent on normalization of abnormal temporal summation of pain, without general impairment of sensory perception. *Neurosurgery.* 1998;43:462–472.
40. Superville-Sovak B, Rasminsky M, Finlayson MH. Complications of phenol neurolysis. *Arch Neurol.* 1975;32:226–228.
41. Katz JA, Sehlhorst S, Blisard KS. Histopathologic changes in primate spinal cord after single and repeated epidural phenol administration. *Reg Anesth.* 1995;20:283–290.
42. Iggo A, Walsh EG. Selective block of small fibres in the spinal roots by phenol. *Brain.* 1960;83:701–708.
43. Labat G, Greene MB. Contribution to modern method of diagnosis and treatment of so-called sciatic neuralgias. *Am J Surg.* 1931; 11:435.
44. Moller JE, Helweg-Larsen J, Jacobsen E. Histopathological lesions in the sciatic nerve of the rat following perineural application of phenol and alcohol solutions. *Dan Med Bull.* 1969;16:116–119.
45. Chua KS, Kong KH. Alcohol neurolysis of the sciatic nerve in the treatment of hemiplegic knee flexor spasticity: Clinical outcomes. *Arch Phys Med Rehabil.* 2000;81:1432–1435.
46. Goldberg SN, Dupuy DE. Image-guided Radiofrequency Tumor Ablation: Challenges and Opportunities—Part I. *J Vasc Interv Radiol.* 2001;12:1011–1126.
47. Rosomoff HL, Brown CJ, Sheptak P. Percutaneous radiofrequency cervical cordotomy: Technique. *J Neurosurg.* 1965;23:639–644.
48. Van Boxem K, van Eerd M, Brinkhuize T, et al. Radiofrequency and pulsed radiofrequency treatment of chronic pain syndromes: The available evidence. *Pain Pract.* 2008;8:385–393.
49. Rubinsky B, Lee CY, Bastacky J, et al. The process of freezing and the mechanism of damage during hepatic cryosurgery. *Cryobiology.* 1990;27:85–97.
50. Myers RR, Powell HC, Heckman HM, et al. Biophysical and pathological effects of cryogenic nerve lesion. *Ann Neurol.* 1981;10: 478–485.
51. Hadjicostas P, Malakounides N, Varianos C, et al. Radiofrequency ablation in pancreatic cancer. *HPB (Oxford).* 2006;8:61–64.
52. Callstrom MR, Charboneau JW. Percutaneous ablation: safe, effective treatment of bone tumors. *Oncology (Williston Park).* 2005;19: 22–26.
53. Belfiore G, Tedeschi E, Ronza FM, et al. Radiofrequency ablation of bone metastases induces long-lasting palliation in patients with untreatable cancer. *Singapore Med J.* 2008;49:565–570.
54. Froese G, Das RM, Dunscombe PB. The sensitivity of the thoracolumbar spinal cord of the mouse to hyperthermia. *Radiat Res.* 1991;125:173–180.
55. Letcher FS, Goldring S. The effect of radiofrequency current and heat on peripheral nerve action potential in the cat. *J Neurosurg.* 1968;29:42–47.
56. Yamane T, Tateishi A, Cho S, et al. The effects of hyperthermia on the spinal cord. *Spine.* 1992;17:1386–1391.
57. Dupuy DE, Hong R, Oliver B, et al. Radiofrequency ablation of spinal tumors: Temperature distribution in the spinal canal. *AJR Am J Roentgenol.* 2000;175:1263–1266.
58. Byas-Smith MG, Gulati A. Ultrasound-guided intercostal nerve cryoablation. *Anesth Analg.* 2006;103:1033–1035.
59. Papo I, Visca A. Phenol subarachnoid rhizotomy for the treatment of cancer pain: A personal account of 290 cases. In: Bonica JJ, Ventafridda V, eds. *Advances in pain research and therapy, Vol. 2.* New York: Raven Press, 1979:339–346.
60. Swerdlow W. Subarachnoid and extradural neurolytic neurolytic blocks. In: Bonica JJ, Ventafridda V, eds. *Advances in pain research and therapy, Vol. 2.* New York: Raven Press, 1979:325–327.
61. Gerbershagen HU. Neurolysis. Subarachnoid neurolytic blockade. *Acta Anaesthesiol Belg.* 1981;32:45–57.
62. Slatkin NE, Rhiner M. Phenol saddle blocks for intractable pain at end of life: report of four cases and literature review. *Am J Hosp Palliat Care.* 2003;20:62–66.
63. Ischia S, Luzzani A, Ischia A, et al. Subarachnoid neurolytic block (L5-S1) and unilateral percutaneous cervical cordotomy in the treatment of pain secondary to pelvic malignant disease. *Pain.* 1984;20: 139–149.
64. Ward EM, Rorie DK, Nauss LA, et al. The celiac ganglia in man: Normal anatomic variations. *Anesth Analg.* 1979;58:461–465.
65. De Cicco M, Matovic M, Balestreri L, et al. Single-needle celiac plexus block: Is needle tip position critical in patients with no regional anatomic distortions? *Anesthesiology.* 1997;87:1301–1308.
66. Lillemoe KD, Cameron JL, Kaufman HS, et al. Chemical splanchnicectomy in patients with unresectable pancreatic cancer. A prospective randomized trial. *Ann Surg.* 1993;217:447–455.
67. Lillemoe KD, Sauter PK, Pitt HA, et al. Current status of surgical palliation of periampullary carcinoma. *Surg Gynecol Obstet.* 1993; 176:1–10.
68. Ventafridda GV, Caraceni AT, Sbanotto AM, et al. Pain treatment in cancer of the pancreas. *Eur J Surg Oncol.* 1990;16:1–6.
69. Warshaw AL, Fernandez-del Castillo C. Pancreatic carcinoma. *N Engl J Med.* 1992;326:455–465.
70. Rykowski JJ, Hilgier M. Efficacy of neurolytic celiac plexus block in varying locations of pancreatic cancer: Influence on pain relief. *Anesthesiology.* 2000;92:347–354.
71. Eisenberg E, Carr DB, Chalmers TC. Neurolytic celiac plexus block for treatment of cancer pain: A meta-analysis. *Anesth Analg.* 1995;80:290–295.
72. Polati E, Finco G, Gottin L, et al. Prospective randomized double-blind trial of neurolytic coeliac plexus block in patients with pancreatic cancer. *Br J Surg.* 1998;85:199–201.
73. Wong GY, Schroeder DR, Carns PE, et al. Effect of neurolytic celiac plexus block on pain relief, quality of life, and survival in patients with unresectable pancreatic cancer: A randomized controlled trial. *JAMA.* 2004;291:1092–1099.
74. Benzon HT. Convulsions secondary to intravascular phenol: A hazard of celiac plexus block. *Anesth Analg.* 1979;58:150–151.
75. Woodham MJ, Hanna MH. Paraplegia after coeliac plexus block. *Anaesthesia.* 1989;44:487–489.
76. De Conno F, Caraceni A, Aldrighetti L, et al. Paraplegia following coeliac plexus block. *Pain.* 1993;55:383–385.
77. Bowen Wright RM. Precautions against injection into the spinal artery during coeliac plexus block [letter]. *Anaesthesia.* 1990;45: 247–248.
78. Cherry DA, Lamberty J. Paraplegia following coeliac plexus block. *Anaesth Intensive Care.* 1984;12:59–61.
79. Davies DD. Incidence of major complications of neurolytic coeliac plexus block. *J R Soc Med.* 1993;86:264–266.
80. Van Dongen RT, Crul BJ. Paraplegia following coeliac plexus block. *Anaesthesia.* 1991;46:862–863.
81. Gimenez A, Martinez-Noguera A, Donoso L, et al. Percutaneous neurolysis of the celiac plexus via the anterior approach with sonographic guidance. *AJR Am J Roentgenol.* 1993;161:1061–1063.
82. Jabbal SS, Hunton J. Reversible paraplegia following coeliac plexus block. *Anaesthesia.* 1992;47:857–858.
83. Sett SS, Taylor DC. Aortic pseudoaneurysm secondary to celiac plexus block. *Ann Vasc Surg.* 1991;5:88–91.
84. Dean AP, Reed WD. Diarrhoea—an unrecognised hazard of coeliac plexus block. *Aust N Z J Med.* 1991;21:47–48.
85. Pateman J, Williams MP, Filshie J. Retroperitoneal fibrosis after multiple coeliac plexus blocks. *Anaesthesia.* 1990;45:309–310.

86. Fujita Y, Takaori M. Pleural effusion after CT-guided alcohol celiac plexus block. *Anesth Analg.* 1987;66:911–912.
87. Fine PG, Bubela C. Chylothorax following celiac plexus block. *Anesthesiology.* 1985;63:454–456.
88. Brown DL. A retrospective analysis of neurolytic celiac plexus block for nonpancreatic intra-abdominal cancer pain. *Reg Anesth.* 1989;14:63–65.
89. Noda J, Umeda S, Mori K, et al. Disulfiram-like reaction associated with carmofur after celiac plexus alcohol block. *Anesthesiology.* 1987;67:809–810.
90. Lieberman RP, Waldman SD. Celiac plexus neurolysis with the modified transaortic approach. *Radiology.* 1990;175:274–276.
91. Brown DL, Moore DC. The use of neurolytic celiac plexus block for pancreatic cancer: Anatomy and technique. *J Pain Symptom Manage.* 1988;3:206–209.
92. Thompson GE, Moore DC, Bridenbaugh LD, et al. Abdominal pain and alcohol celiac plexus nerve block. *Anesth Analg.* 1977;56:1–5.
93. Smith RC, Davidson NM, Ruckley CV. Hazard of chemical sympathectomy. *Br Med J.* 1978;1:552–553.
94. Galizia EJ, Lahiri SK. Paraplegia following coeliac plexus block with phenol. Case report. *Br J Anaesth.* 1974;46:539–540.
95. Hayakawa J, Kobayashi O, Murayama H. Paraplegia after intraoperative celiac plexus block. *Anesth Analg.* 1997;84:447–448.
96. Singler RC. An improved technique for alcohol neurolysis of the celiac plexus. *Anesthesiology.* 1982;56:137–141.
97. Hilgier M, Rykowski JJ. One needle transcrural celiac plexus block. Single shot or continuous technique, or both. *Reg Anesth.* 1994;19:277–283.
98. Feldstein GS, Waldman SD, Allen ML. Loss of resistance technique for transaortic celiac plexus block [letter]. *Anesth Analg.* 1986;65:1092–1093.
99. Ischia S, Luzzani A, Ischia A, et al. A new approach to the neurolytic block of the coeliac plexus: The transaortic technique. *Pain.* 1983;16:333–341.
100. Ischia S, Ischia A, Polati E, et al. Three posterior percutaneous celiac plexus block techniques. A prospective, randomized study in 61 patients with pancreatic cancer pain. *Anesthesiology.* 1992;76:534–540.
101. Kaplan R, Schiff-Keren B, Alt E. Aortic dissection as a complication of celiac plexus block. *Anesthesiology.* 1995;83:632–635.
102. Naveira FA, Speight KL, Rauck RL. Atheromatous aortic plaque as a cause of resistance to needle passage during transaortic celiac plexus block. *Anesth Analg.* 1996;83:1327–1329.
103. Hessel SJ. Complications of angiography and other catheter procedures. In: Abrams H, ed. *Angiography: vascular and interventional radiology.* Boston: Little, Brown, 1983:1041–1055.
104. Moore DC. Neurolytic celiac plexus block: Can paraplegia and death after neurolytic celiac plexus block be eliminated? [letter]. *Anesthesiology.* 1996;84:1522–1523.
105. Levy MJ, Wiersema MJ. Endoscopic ultrasound-guided pain control for intra-abdominal cancer. *Gastroenterol Clin North Am.* 2006;35:153–165.
106. Michaels AJ, Draganov PV. Endoscopic ultrasonography guided celiac plexus neurolysis and celiac plexus block in the management of pain due to pancreatic cancer and chronic pancreatitis. *World J Gastroenterol.* 2007;13:3575–3580.
107. Garcea G, Thomasset S, Berry DP, et al. Percutaneous splanchnic nerve radiofrequency ablation for chronic abdominal pain. *ANZ J Surg.* 2005;75:640–644.
108. Raj PP, Sahinler B, Lowe M. Radiofrequency lesioning of splanchnic nerves. *Pain Pract.* 2002;2:241–247.
109. Lee RB, Stone K, Magelssen D, et al. Presacral neurectomy for chronic pelvic pain. *Obstet Gynecol.* 1986;68:517–521.
110. Chen FP, Soong YK. The efficacy and complications of laparoscopic presacral neurectomy in pelvic pain. *Obstet Gynecol.* 1997;90:974–977.
111. Plancarte R, Amescua C, Patt RB, et al. Superior hypogastric plexus block for pelvic cancer pain. *Anesthesiology.* 1990;73:236–239.
112. Kanazi GE, Perkins FM, Thakur R, et al. New technique for superior hypogastric plexus block. *Reg Anesth Pain Med.* 1999;24:473–476.
113. Cariati M, De Martini G, Pretolesi F, et al. CT-guided superior hypogastric plexus block. *J Comput Assist Tomogr.* 2002;26:428–431.
114. Gamal G, Helaly M, Labib YM. Superior hypogastric block: Transdiscal versus classic posterior approach in pelvic cancer pain. *Clin J Pain.* 2006;22:544–547.
115. Ina H, Kobyashi MD, Imai S, et al. A new approach to the superior hypogastric plexus block: Trans-vertebral disc (L5-S1) technique. *Reg Anesth.* 1992;17 (suppl):123.
116. Erdine S, Yucel A, Celik M, et al. Transdiscal approach for hypogastric plexus block. *Reg Anesth Pain Med.* 2003;28:304–308.
117. de Leon-Casasola OA, Kent E, Lema MJ. Neurolytic superior hypogastric plexus block for chronic pelvic pain associated with cancer. *Pain.* 1993;54:145–151.
118. Waldman SD, Wilson WL, Kreps RD. Superior hypogastric plexus block using a single needle and computed tomography guidance: Description of a modified technique. *Reg Anesth.* 1991;16:286–287.
119. De Leon-Casasola OA, Plancarte-Sanchez R, Patt RB, et al. Superior hypogastric plexus block using a single needle and computed tomography guidance [letter]. *Reg Anesth.* 1993;18:63.
120. Robb KA, Bennett MI, Johnson MI, et al. Transcutaneous electric nerve stimulation (TENS) for cancer pain in adults. *Cochrane Database Syst Rev.* 2008:CD006276
121. Robb KA, Newham DJ, Williams JE. Transcutaneous electrical nerve stimulation vs. transcutaneous spinal electroanalgesia for chronic pain associated with breast cancer treatments. *J Pain Symptom Manage.* 2007;33:410–419.
122. Searle RD, Bennett MI, Johnson MI, et al. Transcutaneous electrical nerve stimulation (TENS) for cancer bone pain. *J Pain Symptom Manage.* 2009;37:424–428.
123. Ventafridda V, Sganzerla EP, Fochi C, et al. Transcultaneous nerve stimulation in cancer pain. In: Bonica JJ, Ventafridda V, eds. *Advances in pain research and therapy.* New York: Raven Press, 1979:509–515.
124. Chabal C. *Transcutaneous electrical nerve stimulation.* 3rd ed. Philadelphia: Lippincott, 2000.
125. Loeser JD. Dorsal column and peripheral nerve stimulation for relief of cancer pain. In: Bonica JJ, Ventafridda V, eds. *Advances in pain research therapy.* New York: Raven Press, 1979:499–507.
126. Hamid B, Haider N. Spinal cord stimulator relieves neuropathic pain in a patient with radiation-induced transverse myelitis. *Pain Pract.* 2007;7:345–347.
127. Cata JP, Cordella JV, Burton AW, et al. Spinal cord stimulation relieves chemotherapy-induced pain: A clinical case report. *J Pain Symptom Manage.* 2004;27:72–78.
128. Tiede JM, Ghazi SM, Lamer TJ, Obray JB. The use of spinal cord stimulation in refractory abdominal visceral pain: Case reports and literature review. *Pain Pract.* 2006;6:197–202.
129. Ting JC, Fukshansky M, Burton AW. Treatment of refractory ischemic pain from chemotherapy-induced Raynaud's syndrome with spinal cord stimulation. *Pain Pract.* 2007;7:143–146.
130. Rezai AR. Deep brain stimulation for chronic pain. In: Burchiel K, ed. *Surgical management of pain.* New York: Thieme, 2002:565–574.
131. Meyerson B, Linderoth B. Intracerebral and motor cortex stimulation. In: Loeser JD. *Bonica's management of pain.* 3rd ed. Philadelphia: Lippincott, 2000:1877–1889.
132. Lima MC, Fregni F. Motor cortex stimulation for chronic pain: Systematic review and meta-analysis of the literature. *Neurology.* 2008;70:2329–2337.

CHAPTER 22 ■ NEURAXIAL ANALGESIA

The ability to administer neuraxial medications has revolutionized oncology pain management in appropriately selected patients.[1–3] In particular, patients with pain refractory to systemic medication who were previously treated with ablative or neurodestructive procedures are now managed with neuraxial analgesia. As a result, the use of neurolytic and ablative procedures in cancer pain management has significantly declined. Neuraxial analgesia will often allow patients to improve their quality of life and to reduce dosage in their current drug regimens[4] or to derive greater pain relief from their equivalent doses.[5] The risks of neuraxial analgesia are not zero, but they are less than those accompanying ablative and neurodestructive interventions.

Neuraxial analgesia means drug administration within the spinal canal. The modality involves the injection or infusion of medications into the intrathecal space (also known as the subarachnoid space) or epidural space (Fig. 22.1). The epidural space is located within the spinal canal between the dura and connective tissues covering the vertebrae and ligamentum flavum. Most of the epidural space is filled with fat and does not contain free fluid, unlike the intrathecal space, which contains cerebrospinal fluid (CSF), spinal cord, and nerve roots. The epidural space also contains mixed nerves, because they travel to and from the spinal cord to innervated structures. Medications injected into the epidural space are effective locally on mixed nerves (local anesthetics), may traverse intrathecally and be effective on the spinal cord (primarily hydrophilic opioids such as morphine), or are absorbed systemically in the epidural vascular system and have distant effects (lipophilic opioids such as fentanyl). The intrathecal space, by contrast, is fluid-filled and refers to the area between the arachnoid and pia mater of the brain and spinal cord that contains CSF. The spinal cord is surrounded by three meninges: the dura mater, arachnoid, and pia (Fig. 22.2). The arachnoid and pia, also called the leptomeninges, are separated by the intrathecal space, which contains CSF, arteries and veins, and nerve roots. CSF has an important role in the distribution and elimination of intrathecal medications. It is formed mainly in the choroid plexus of the brain, circulates in the subarachnoid space, and is resorbed into the venous blood through arachnoid villi and through the ependymal lining of the ventricles. In humans, the volume of CSF is replaced three or four times each day at a rate of 0.3–0.4 mL/min. Clinically, the intrathecal space is entered after puncture of the dura mater and free flow of CSF is obtained. Various medications can be injected intrathecally (Table 22.1). These medications act on nerve roots/rootlets (local anesthetics), or bind to synaptic and axonal neuroreceptors in the dorsal horn of the spinal cord, such as μ-receptors (opioids),

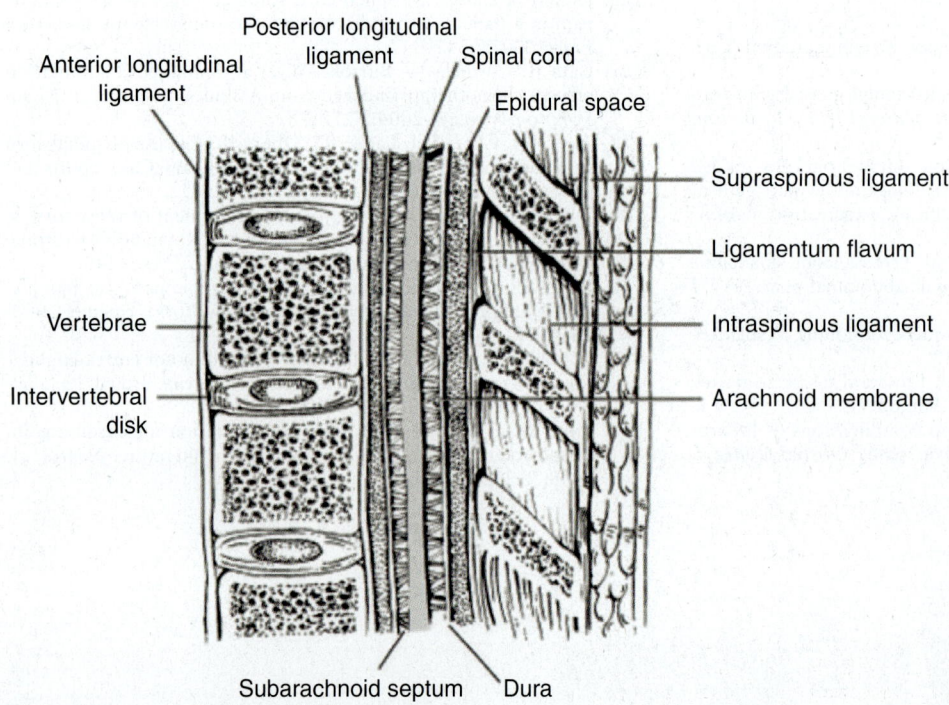

FIGURE 22.1 Anatomy of the epidural and intrathecal space. (From Morgan, G, Mikhail M and Murray M. Clinical Anesthesiology [ital]. 4th ed., p. 292. New York: McGraw Hill Professional. Copyright McGraw Hill Companies, Inc., 2006.)

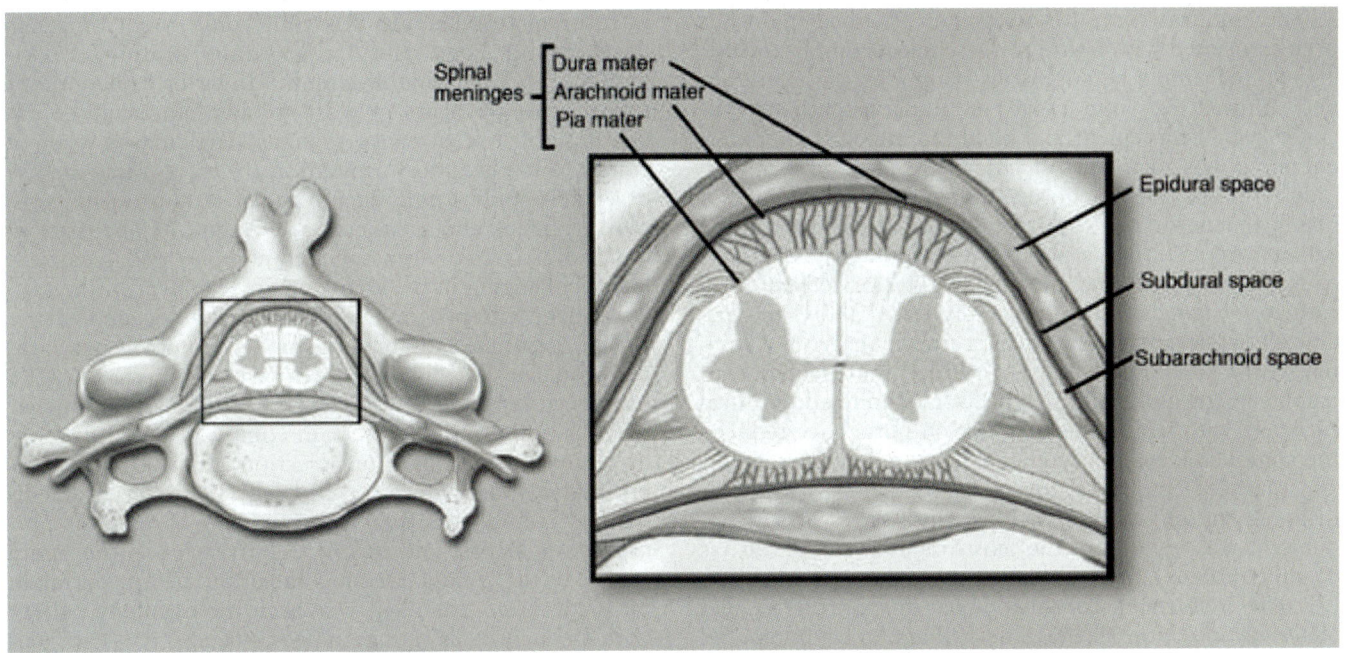

FIGURE 22.2 Location of spinal meninges, epidural space, and intrathecal space. (Reused with permission from Marie Dauenheimer, CMI; Ghafoor VL, et al. Intrathecal drug therapy for long-term pain management. *Am J Health Syst Pharm*. 2007;64:2447–2461.)

calcium channels (calcium channel blockers), or on gamma-aminobutyric acid (GABA) receptors (baclofen, midazolam), where they modulate nociceptive processes.

The clinical effects of neuraxial medications are influenced usually by the position of the catheter tip[6] and by the space in which the catheter is placed (epidural vs. intrathecal). Different systems are available to deliver neuraxial medications by continuous infusion. These systems may involve externalized spinal catheters, subcutaneous reservoirs, or implanted infusion pumps (constant rate or programmable).[7] Although such delivery systems have come into widespread use, particularly for the management of chronic nonmalignant pain, the overall use of long-term intrathecal and epidural opioid administration has been less for cancer pain.

TABLE 22.1

MEDICATIONS USED FOR NEURAXIAL (EPIDURAL, INTRATHECAL) INFUSION

Medication Class	Epidural	Intrathecal
Local anesthetic	Bupivacaine Ropivacaine	Bupivacaine
Opioids	Morphine Hydromorphone Fentanyl Meperidine	Morphine Hydromorphone Sufentanil Meperidine
α-2 agonists	Clonidine	Clonidine
N-type calcium channel blocker		Ziconotide
Antispasmodics		Baclofen
Gamma-aminobutyric acid agonist		Midazolam

CHOICE OF SPINAL DELIVERY SYSTEM

A variety of neuraxial delivery systems are available.[7] The patient's diagnosis, pain pattern, life expectancy, and the cost of the pain therapy modality have traditionally influenced the selection of a specific drug delivery system. Ever since Behar et al.[8] first reported on the use of epidural morphine for the treatment of cancer pain, pain management specialists have been looking for a means to overcome the technical problems that can arise during long-term treatment with neuraxial medications. Prominent among these issues is the development of a robust and reliable system of drug administration that is relatively free from complications. Some of the potential complications include leakage and occlusion, catheter dislodgment, infection, and pain on injection or infusion. Attempts to reduce these problems have included tunneling of catheter to the flank or the anterior abdominal wall or implantation of a subcutaneous injection port located on the patient's anterior chest wall.

Infusion systems may be considered for short-term or long-term administration. The systems commonly used for short-term (usually less than 1 month) are percutaneously inserted into the epidural or intrathecal space without tunneling. Long-term systems are either subcutaneously tunneled and externalized or fully implanted. Fully-implanted systems may have a subcutaneous injection port, an implanted reservoir for continuous infusion at a fixed rate, or a programmable infusion system utilizing a battery powered motor-driven pump. New delivery system technology is in development that will obviate the need for a motor and its high power consumption, thereby reducing replacement costs and surgical risks.

The epidural route for treatment of cancer pain has been associated with a variety of technical complications.[9] The use of simple percutaneous temporary catheters has been limited. Advantages of percutaneous catheters include ease of placement and ability to attach to an external pump. Disadvantages include the risk of infection with long-term use, lack of dose stability, a high incidence of displacement of the catheter, and fibrosis around the catheter tip resulting in pain on injection and loss of efficacy. A two-piece silicone-rubber exteriorized epidural catheter system described by DuPen et al.[10] allows for specific spinal–level location of the catheter tip from a lumbar entry site and does help reduce the incidence of displacement and pain on injection. Tunneled epidural catheters with subcutaneous injection ports have reduced the complication rate accompanying simple percutaneous and tunneled epidural catheters, particularly for catheter dislodgment and early infections.[9] In a series of 313 patients, it was noted that the most frequent complications of subcutaneous injection ports were pain on injection (12.0% incidence), occlusion of the portal system (10.9%), infection (8.1%) and leakage of administered medication such that it did not all reach the epidural space (2.1%).[11] Possible disadvantages of these systems include the need for skin puncture with each delivery system use and the increased cost of the system.

The intrathecal route is more efficient and potentially less expensive than epidural delivery for the treatment of refractory cancer pain.[12] Advantages of intrathecal administration include better distribution of medication to the target site and enhanced pain relief.[13] Concerns about externalized intrathecal catheters focus around potentially higher risks of complications (particularly meningitis, CSF fistula, and CSF hygroma) compared to epidural catheters. Clinicians who use the intrathecal route have tended to avoid percutaneously inserted, subcutaneously tunneled, "open" or externalized catheters, preferring a totally implanted system that might reduce the likelihood of these complications. However, such concerns appear to be largely unfounded,[14] particularly with appropriate care of the system.

Fully implanted systems, especially if programmable, are the most convenient for long-term treatment with intrathecal opioids. At this time, only Medtronic has developed a Food and Drug Administration (FDA)-approved programmable pump. However, concomitant use of other medications with opioids significantly complicates the use of these systems particularly when it comes to medication formulation (often requires the use of a compounding pharmacist) and dose adjustment (complex regimens and protocols are required). The issue of dose adjustments and associated complexities is particularly challenging in the changing environment of the cancer patient with progressive disease and associated pain.

The use of implantable infusion technology is not without problems; complication rates varying from 5% to 15% have been reported.[11,15–18] Overall, these systems appear to offer a lower risk of certain complications (infection, displacement, and pain on injection) than other systems but may also introduce specific delivery system problems (battery failure, pump torsion, overfilling of reservoir, programming errors, and so on).[19] Furthermore, the pump cannot be safely implanted in a radiation therapy portal. In our experience, the ideal system in the oncology patient with frequently changing analgesic needs is an externalized, implanted, intrathecal system connected to an external pump and managed at home through a home infusion company. Expensive hardware is avoided; home care has been dependable and safe in our environment.

CHOICE OF NEURAXIAL MEDICATION

The efficacy of neuraxial opioid therapy for both chronic nonmalignant pain and cancer pain is well documented but it has its limitations (*vide infra*).[20] Stearns et al.[21] proposed an algorithmic approach to intrathecal drug delivery for the management of cancer pain. Medications suggested for use included various opioids, bupivacaine, baclofen, clonidine, droperidol, ketamine, and midazolam. Table 22.2 lists our recommendations for intrathecal drug delivery. Intrathecal morphine has a long safety record and is the only μ agonist approved by the FDA for long-term administration. At this time, no drugs other than morphine, ziconotide, and baclofen are

TABLE 22.2

RECOMMENDED MEDICATION DOSES AND CONCENTRATIONS FOR INTRATHECAL THERAPY

Drug	Standard Concentration	Maximum Recommended Compounded Concentration	Typical Starting Daily Dose	Maximum Dose/Day
Baclofen	50 μg/mL, 0.5 mg/mL, 2 mg/mL	2 mg/mL	100 μg	~2000 μg
Bupivacaine	0.25%, 0.5%, 0.75%	40 mg/mL	48 mg	300 mg
Clonidine	100 μg/mL, 500 μg/mL	2 mg/mL	50 μg	1.5 mg
Fentanyl	50 μg/mL	6000 μg/mL	~100 μg	~1500 μg
Hydromorphone		10 mg/mL	0.25 mg	4 mg
Morphine	10 mg/mL, 25 mg/mL	30 mg/mL	1 mg (opioid tolerant), 0.5 mg (opioid naive)	15 mg
Sufentanil	50 μg/mL	50 μg/mL	1 μg (opioid tolerant), 0.1 μg (opioid naive)	15 μg
Ziconotide	25 μg/mL, 100 μg/mL	2 mg/mL	1.4 μg	19 μg

FDA-approved for intrathecal use. Local anesthetics have been used with increasing frequency for refractory pain control but have limitations, particularly with regards to lower extremity function and bladder/bowel control. Baclofen, although safe and approved for long-term use by the FDA, has little effect in pain management, unless pain is associated with spasticity, and should not be tried for other pain-related complaints. The usefulness of clonidine is unclear, and its effects on the circulatory system may be unpredictable and difficult to manage.[22] Ziconotide is FDA-approved for intrathecal use but its side effects have been problematic. Long-term use of unapproved medications intrathecally should be considered experimental as their safety profiles are unproven by this route of administration, in spite of widespread use in nonmalignant pain states. In light of recent associations of intrathecal medications with granuloma formation,[23-24] patients who require high-dose or high-concentration intrathecal opioid therapy and those who receive drugs or admixtures not approved for intrathecal use should be monitored closely for signs of an extra-axial mass or catheter malfunction.[24]

NEURAXIAL OPIOID THERAPY

Intractable cancer pain has been routinely treated with the neuraxial (intrathecal or epidural) infusion of opioids for more than a quarter-century. Spinal and supraspinal sites are the areas at which intrathecal or epidural morphine injections are effective.[25] Initial reports indicated high efficacy and few complications or side effects.[26-30] At that time, many believed that the solution to intractable pain was in hand and widespread application awaited only the development of suitable long-term delivery systems.[31] Subsequently, additional case series and surveys made it clear that neuraxial administration of opioids was not risk free,[32] that tolerance to neuraxial opioids could be as big a problem as tolerance to oral or systemic opioids,[33-35] and that not all patients with pain from cancer experienced good pain relief with neuraxial opioids.[18,36-37] The failure rate of epidural and intrathecal opioids in cancer pain can be as high as 30%.[38-39] Techniques of drug delivery also seemed to play a role in outcomes. Gourlay et al[40] reported that bolus dosing of neuraxial opioids resulted in less tolerance than a continuous infusion. On the other hand, Hassenbusch et al.[41] reported that chronic epidural morphine infusions were associated with very little tolerance development. As the field of neuraxial opioids developed, it became clearer that there were distinct differences between epidural and intrathecal administration, some related to drug pharmacokinetics, others to anatomy and technique advances and that the intrathecal route was better suited to treatment at home by continuous infusion than the epidural route.[42] Route of administration is now recognized as a critical factor for neuraxial opioid administration.

Epidural Administration

Although the objective of epidural administration is to affect pain relief by altering spinal cord dorsal horn synaptic transmission, there is some systemic absorption by all epidurally-administered drugs, including opioids.[43] One of the most important factors governing the spinal bioavailability of epidurally-administered opioids is their ability to redistribute out of the epidural space and into surrounding tissues. The kinetics of drug movements among epidural, intrathecal, and plasma compartments are complex, and the epidural and intrathecal spaces cannot be viewed simply as two compartments separated by a single barrier.[44] CSF and plasma pharmacokinetics of opioids do not parallel their epidural pharmacokinetics and the hydrophobic character of opioids governs multiple aspects of their lumbar epidural pharmacokinetics. A significantly larger proportion of the epidural dose of morphine reaches the CSF than is the case for any of the other more lipid-soluble opioids.[44]

The utility of each drug to be administered epidurally must be determined by studying whether the observed analgesia is due to selective action on the spinal dorsal horn or is related to systemic uptake of the drug and effects upon sites other than the spinal cord, such as the brain or peripheral nerves. Obviously, combinations of these two effects are likely for many opioids. Morphine is the standard drug against which all others are compared for efficacy and side effects. It was the first opioid administered into the epidural space that was active on the dorsal horn. Studies have shown conclusively that it produces analgesia by its actions on the dorsal horn of the spinal cord.[45] Subsequent studies have shown that highly lipophilic opioids, such as fentanyl, sufentanil, or alfentanil are inappropriate for epidural administration because of their rapid systemic uptake and effects outside of the spinal dorsal horn.[46-50]

Reports documenting the use of different opioids in the epidural space are now available; morphine is clearly the drug of choice for the majority of patients for this application. However, the long-term superiority to systemically administered drugs has been debated. In 1989, Sjogren reported no significant differences between oral and epidural routes of administration in long-term treatment of 14 cancer patients when pain relief, sedation, and reaction times were assessed.[51] Hassenbusch et al. studied the efficacy and safety of continuous epidural morphine administration in 69 patients with cancer pain in the midline abdomen/pelvis or lower extremities who did not respond adequately to systemic opioid treatment.[52] The detailed characteristics of the pain syndromes were not described for each patient. An epidural catheter was placed for evaluation of efficacy of morphine: 60% of this group reported good pain relief and had an internalized catheter and Infusaid pump (a pump with a fixed infusion rate) implanted. Before the administration of epidural drug, the patients reported a visual analog scale (VAS) of 8.6 ± 0.3. One month after implantation of the catheter and pump, the VAS scores were 3.8 ± 0.4 ($P < .001$). Long-term benefits were described: 80% of the implanted patients reported satisfactory pain relief (at least a 30% reduction from preimplant VAS levels) at 3 and 6 month reevaluation. Also, the systemic opioid requirements were significantly decreased compared to preimplantation levels: by 79% at 1 month and 64% at 9 months. Some tolerance was seen: the mean epidural dose was 20.7 ± 2.6 mg/day 1 month after implantation and rose to 49.3 ± 9.9 mg/day 9 months after initiation of this treatment strategy. This study had a very low complication rate and reported no instances of respiratory depression, epidural infection, meningitis, epidural scarring, or catheter failure. This was one of the seminal studies that demonstrated good long-term results with epidural morphine infusion in patients with pain from cancer.

By contrast, other studies have revealed a much higher failure rate with morphine.[38-39] Nine years' experience with epidural morphine in 146 cancer pain patients was reported by Samuelsson et al.[53] The mean treatment time for each patient was 92 days and epidural opioids were the sole pain treatment in 53% of patients. They reported that the mean dose of epidural morphine was 18 mg/day with a range of 6 to 120 mg/day. At the termination of this treatment strategy, the mean daily dose was 69 mg/day with a range of 2 to 540 mg/day. Absence of an initial satisfactory response to epidural morphine was noted in 25 patients. Withdrawal from initially successful therapy was observed in 27 patients; an additional nine patients experienced catheter failures and five reported drug-related reasons for termination of epidural morphine. Those most likely not to respond to epidural morphine were patients with neuropathic pain states, those with movement-induced incident pain, those with visceral pain and those with painful cutaneous ulcerations.

Our review of the literature and our own experiences suggest that epidural opioid administration is not likely to be a successful long-term therapy for pain associated with cancer, particularly if it is the sole analgesic therapy. The major issue is the development of fibrosis around the epidural catheter that impedes drug delivery and results in local pain at the time of injection.[54] Tolerance does occur, but it is not usually an unmanageable problem. Maintenance of the catheter in a favorable position can also be a problem. We strongly prefer intrathecal administration of drugs in setting of cancer pain, as we believe it a more reliable method of drug delivery and it does not, in our hands, have increased risks.

Intrathecal Administration

Intrathecal drug delivery offers significant advantages for pain relief over epidural administration of opioids. These include: uniform drug distribution within the CSF (as long as highly lipophilic drugs are not used), superior efficacy of pain relief, relative absence of systemic effects at clinically useful intrathecal doses, ease and certainty of catheter insertion by CSF aspiration or contrast agent injection, and lower reported incidence of complications. As in the epidural space, the behavior of opioids in the intrathecal space is governed largely by their lipid solubility. Hydrophobic opioids have a very large apparent volume of distribution compared with that of more hydrophilic opioids.[55] Rapid elimination of hydrophobic opioids from the CSF results in very limited rostral spread in CSF. In addition, the bioavailability of these opioids at spinal cord sites more rostral than the site of administration is also very limited. This explains why delayed respiratory depression is observed clinically with morphine but not with fentanyl or sufentanil.

The ratio of intrathecal dosing to oral dosing is approximately 1 to 300, thereby significantly reducing the systemic opioid exposure. Implanted catheters and pumps can be used to infuse any opioid in aqueous solution, including morphine, hydromorphone, methadone, meperidine, fentanyl, and sufentanil. The intrathecal delivery route has been the subject of numerous reports with somewhat differing conclusions.[2,15,18,36,52,56-64] Most of these reports describe significant pain relief from intrathecal opioids, but this literature suffers from many deficiencies and a complete picture of the use of this technology is often difficult to ascertain. Few studies have defined pain relief in a prospective fashion using standardized instruments. Some studies have described a few patients who manifested no pain relief to intrathecal opioids in spite of often astronomical increments in dosing.[60,63,65-66] In most cases we do not know if this was a failure of the delivery system or a pain that did not respond to opioid treatment. The actual rate of patients with cancer pain not responsive to intrathecal opioids is not known, but it is certainly not zero. Nor do we know with any precision the efficacy of intrathecal opioids for the relief of cancer pain.

A useful study by Paice[60] contrasted the pain relief from intrathecal opioids in patients with cancer and non-malignant diseases. The best results were seen in patients with cancer pain of somatic origin. However, when compared to non–cancer pain patients, the average initial dose of opioid was higher in the patients with cancer. Whereas the average dose used by cancer patients rapidly increased and then reached a plateau, non–cancer patients seemed to exhibit a more gradual but constant dose increase over long periods of use. This study contrasted with that of Yaksh and Onofrio[64] who studied the changes in morphine infusion dosing in 130 cancer pain patients and reported that the initial average dose of 4.8 ±0.4 mg/day increased to 21 ± 9 mg/day after 1 year of therapy. Plummer's study in 1991[11] indicated wide variations in the dose requirements to adequately control cancer pain. They indicated that the type of pain also played a significant role in the response to intrathecal opioids, similar to what was reported above for epidural opioids. Long-term intrathecal morphine infusions were studied by Gestin et al.[67] in 50 patients with advanced cancer and pain. The average infusion lasted 142 (range: 7 to 584) days and the mean starting dose was 2.5 (range: 0.4 to 8.3) mg/day; this increased to a mean final dose of 9.2 (range: 1 to 94) mg/day. The average dose was 5.4 (range: 1 to 23) mg/day and all the patients were said to have satisfactory pain relief. One interesting report suggested that methadone given intrathecally produced pain relief inferior to that seen with morphine, even with doses ten times the equivalent of morphine.[68]

Adverse Effects of Neuraxial Opioid Therapy

The adverse effects of systemic morphine are well described in the medical literature. Neuraxial administration of this drug results in a similar range of side effects, despite the more limited distribution of the drug in the body. Some of these side effects are temporary, normally lasting for the first several days after initiation of therapy and then resolving; others are more enduring.[69] In a retrospective study of 82 patients receiving long-term opioid therapy for noncancer-pain, Winkelmuller and Winkelmuller[70] reported the most frequent side effects as constipation (50%), disturbance of micturition (42.7%), and nausea (36.6%). These occurred early in the course of therapy and responded to appropriate medication. Some patients experienced a loss of libido or amenorrhea for the first 6 to 8 months of therapy, but these side effects proved self-limiting to most patients and disappeared after 12 to 14 months of therapy. In most series, common problems associated with intrathecal opioid therapy have included nausea, vomiting, pruritus, urinary retention, and constipation. Less common adverse events have been respiratory depression and opioid-induced hyperalgesia. Less frequently recognized by clinicians are problems associated with endocrine abnormalities (in particular, sexual dysfunction) and edema.

Abs et al.[71] reported on the endocrine consequences of long-term intrathecal opioid use and noted that, in patients receiving intrathecal opioids, the majority of men and all women developed hypogonadotropic hypogonadism, about 15% developed central hypocorticism, and about 15% developed growth hormone (GH) deficiency. In this study of 73 patients (29 men and 44 women; mean age, 49.2 ± 11.7 year) receiving intrathecal opioids, the mean duration of opioid treatment was 26.6±16.3 months and the mean daily dose of morphine was 4.8 (3.2 mg). Decreased libido or impotency was present in 23 of 24 men receiving opioids. Serum testosterone level was less than 9 nmol/L in 25 of 29 men and was significantly lower than that in the control group ($P < .001$). The free androgen index was below normal in 18 of 29 men and was significantly lower than that in the control group ($P < .001$). The serum luteinizing hormone (LH) level was less than 2 U/L in 20 of 29 men and was significantly lower than that in the control group ($P < .001$). Serum follicle-stimulating hormone (FSH) was comparable in both groups. Decreased libido was present in 22 of 32 women receiving opioids. All 21 premenopausal women developed either amenorrhea or an irregular menstrual cycle, with ovulation in only one. Serum LH, estradiol, and progesterone levels were lower in the opioid group. In all 18 postmenopausal women, significantly decreased serum LH ($P < .001$) and FSH ($P = .012$) levels were found. The 24-hour-urinary free cortisol excretion was below 20 microg/day in 14 of 71 opioid patients and was significantly lower than that in the control group ($P = .003$). The peak cortisol response to insulin-induced hypoglycemia was below 180 μg/L in 9 of 61 opioid patients and was significantly lower than that in the nonopioid group ($P = .002$). The insulin-like growth factor I standard deviation (SD) score was below −2 SD in 12 of 73 opioid patients and was significantly lower than that in the control group ($P = .002$). The peak growth GH response to hypoglycemia was below 3 μg/L in 9 of 62 subjects and was significantly lower than that in the control group ($P = .010$). Thyroid function tests were normal. No other metabolic disturbances were noted, apart from significantly decreased high-density lipoprotein cholesterol levels ($P = .041$) and elevated total/high density lipoprotein cholesterol ratio ($P = .008$) in the opioid group compared to the control group. Supplementation with gonadal steroids improved sexual function in most patients.

Water retention and peripheral edema caused by intrathecal opioids can be problematic, resulting in limitations of physical activity and the production of lymphedema, ulcerations, and hyperpigmentation of the skin.[72] Cephalad migration of opioids within the CSF and interaction with opioid receptors in the posterior pituitary gland with the release of vasopressin may explain opioid-induced fluid retention.[69] We have had patients whose fluid retention was so profound that their intrathecal opioids had to be discontinued.

Catheter-tip inflammatory-like masses or granulomas have been attributed to implanted intrathecal catheters used for long-term pain management (Fig. 22.3).[24] The first case was reported by North et al. in 1991.[73] Drug that precipitates from solution can cause an inflammatory mass and mimic a tumor in the subarachnoid space.[74] Preliminary experimental evidence suggests that dural mast cell activation and subsequent release of inflammatory mediators (such as cytokines and histamine) are responsible for catheter tip inflammatory mass lesions.[23,75] Cases have occurred in patients receiving commercially prepared preservative-free morphine sulfate alone, as well as formulations of hydromorphone and morphine sulfate alone or in combinations with other analgesics and local anesthetics prepared by compounding pharmacies. The incidence of granuloma formation has been estimated to be 0.04% after 1 year of therapy, increasing to 1.15% after 6 years of therapy.[76] We suspect that the actual rate of granuloma formation is significantly higher; many cases have probably not been reported to central data banks and smaller granuloma may not be clinically apparent. High CSF drug levels of opioids, and in particular, drug concentration infused rather than absolute dose have been implicated as the cause of the inflammatory masses.[77] Yaksh et al.[78] noted 30% of granulomas developed in patients receiving less than 10 mg/day; 40% were using morphine concentrations of less than 25 mg/mL. Many of these patients were receiving drug mixtures, which may also be a key factor in granuloma formation.

Symptoms and signs consistent with inflammatory masses include diminished or loss of drug (analgesic) effect, new-onset radicular and back pain, and associated spinal cord neurologic deficits. Overt findings may include changes in the patient's baseline neurologic condition, such as motor weakness (including gait difficulties), sensory loss (including proprioceptive loss), hyper- or hypoactive lower extremity reflexes, and any evidence of bowel or bladder sphincter dysfunction.[79] Imaging with a gadolinium-enhanced magnetic-resonance imaging (MRI) or computed tomography (CT) myelogram confirms the diagnosis. Plain MRI or CT scan or x-ray is of no value in establishing this diagnosis. Clinical evaluation based solely on the development of neurologic symptoms or decreasing analgesic efficacy alone in the absence of specific imaging studies lacks sufficient sensitivity to exclude the presence of catheter-associated masses.[80] Subtle prodromal symptoms and signs may include diminishing analgesic effects (loss of previously satisfactory pain relief) and remarkable or unusual increases in the patient's underlying pain. Some patients may manifest frequent dose escalations in the attempt to recapture analgesic effects. In other cases, dose escalations and sizable drug boluses reduce the patient's pain only temporarily or to a lesser degree than previous experience predicted. Gradual, insidious neurologic deterioration weeks or months after the

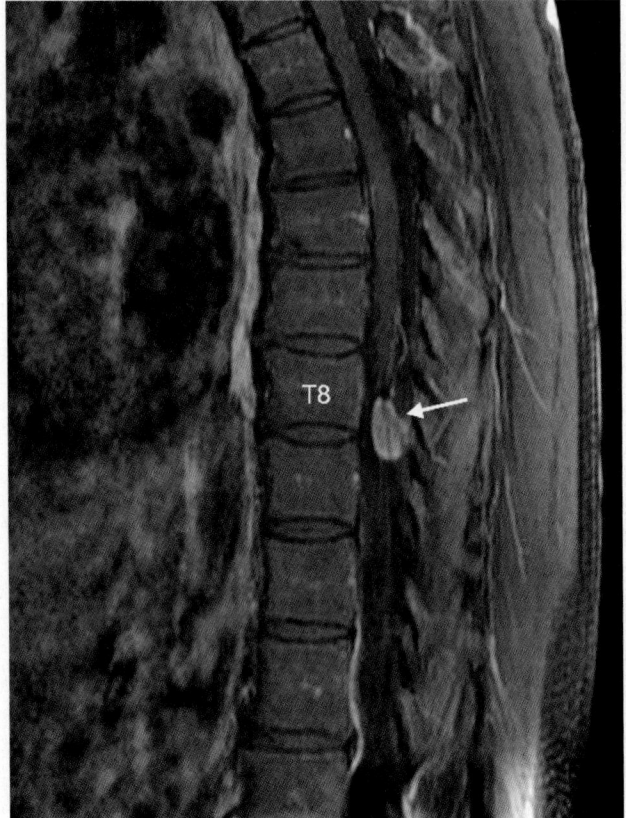
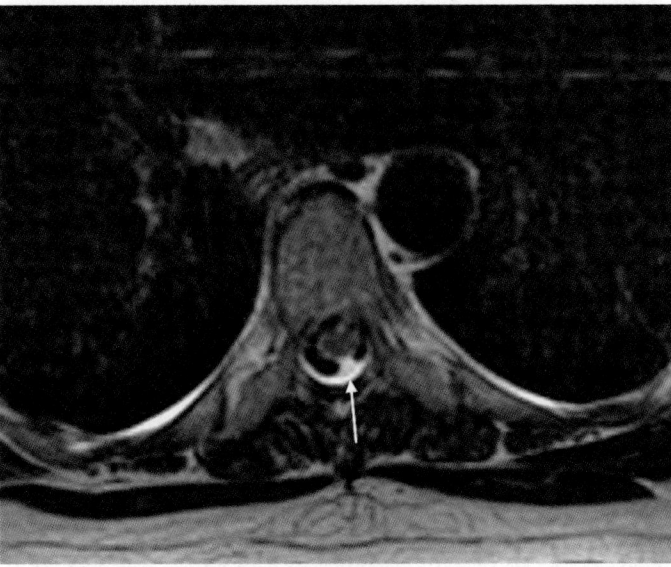

FIGURE 22.3 A 51-year-old woman who received an intrathecal catheter (tip T8/9) for failed back syndrome. Four years later, patient presented with severe radicular back pain at T8 level. Sagittal MRI (T1, fat suppressed, post gadolinium) shows a granuloma at T8 level (**A**) *(arrow)*. Axial MRI (**B**) shows the granuloma dorsal to the cord *(arrow)*. The catheter was surgically removed with gradual resolution of symptoms. MRI, Magnetic resonance imaging.

appearance of subjective symptoms was the most common clinical course before the onset of myelopathy or cauda equina syndrome.[24] Catheter tip granuloma formation is a potential neurologic disaster and must be considered as an emergent problem in any patient who manifests new symptoms and signs of pain or spinal cord dysfunction.

Escalating doses of intrathecal morphine may prove problematic because of increased risk for hyperalgesia and myoclonus.[57] Opioid-induced hyperalgesia is a pronociceptive phenomenon that can occur with acute or chronic opioid administration. This paradoxical effect is likely due to the opioid effects on a variety of cellular targets including N-methyl-D-aspartic acid (NMDA) receptors, spinal glutamate transporters, and protein kinase C[81-82] and does not appear to be an opioid-receptor mediated event.[83] Ibuki et al.[84] demonstrated the increased content of excitatory amino acid neurotransmitter in spinal cord tissue with intrathecal morphine administration. Sakurada et al.[83] suggests that nociception associated with high-dose intrathecal morphine may mediated by morphine-3-glucuronide. Opioid-induced hyperalgesia is discussed extensively in Chapter 19.

Bolus Versus Continuous Infusion of Opioids

The optimal method of delivery of neuraxial opioids (bolus vs. continuous infusion) is unclear. Controversies exist regarding the development of tolerance, differences in quality of pain relief, and duration of effect between the two modalities of administration. The behavior of opioids when administered as a slow continuous infusion is different from single injection bolus.[43] As a slow infusion, the concentration of morphine is limited to a short distance from the point of administration. This implies that the CSF is a very poorly mixed compartment. By contrast, a single bolus injection of intrathecal morphine has a prolonged and extensive neuraxial effect.[85]

Clinical effectiveness of intermittent bolus and continuous infusion of epidural opioids may not differ. In a study of 28 patients with severe cancer pain, these modalities were compared.[40] The mean duration of treatment was 169 (range: 6 to 537) days for continuous infusion patients and 140 (range: 28 to 378) days for repeated bolus doses. Both treatment modalities provided adequate pain control and the modalities were judged equally effective. Rauck et al.[86] evaluated the efficacy and safety of an intrathecal bolus delivery system of morphine in 119 cancer patients with cancer pain refractory to systemic opioids or uncontrollable opioid-related side effects. Pain relief, reduction in systemic opioid use, and reduction in opioid-related complications were evaluated together as a measure of overall success over a 16-month period. Patients were eligible if they had pain from cancer or cancer therapies or experienced pain that could only be controlled at doses that caused intolerable side effects. In addition, patients were enrolled if they had a life expectancy of 4 months or greater. Although not reported directly, it appears that there were only nine patients remaining in the study by month 16. The median starting bolus was 1 mg of morphine and the median average daily dose was 1.8 mg/day.

Median bolus size and median average daily dose increased steadily to 2.5 mg and 5.1 mg/day, respectively, at 4 months. Average numeric analog scale pain decreased from 6.1 to 4.2 at 1 month and was maintained through month 7 ($P < .01$) and through month 13 ($P < .05$). Systemic opioid use was significantly decreased throughout the study ($P < .01$). The majority of patients in this present study decreased their overall opioid requirements by greater than 50% when using intrathecal opioids; many discontinued systemic use entirely. There was a pronounced decrease in the incidence of opioid-related side effects with intermittent intrathecal dosing compared to previous systemic dosing. Overall success (>50% reduction in numeric VAS pain score, use of systemic opioids, or opioid complication severity index) was reported in 83%, 90%, 85%, and 91% of patients at months 1, 2, 3, and 4, respectively. The most commonly recorded complications were sleep disorders, daytime drowsiness, constipation, and nausea. Frequency and severity of sleep disorder, daytime drowsiness, urinary retention, and constipation were significantly improved by 1 month, and five of the eight complications were significantly improved at 4 months.

Tolerance to the antinociceptive effect of morphine is well established in most mammals.[87] Tolerance occurs for a number of reasons, including previous opioid exposure, changes in pain modality or intensity, and psychological factors. However, in patients with cancer, it may be difficult to determine the precise reason for dose increase because of the often progressive nature of the disease and associated increase in pain. Systemic morphine via repeated subcutaneous injections can result in substantial tolerance within 3 days.[87] By contrast, tolerance develops more slowly to morphine at localized spinal sites.[35,88–89] Animal studies with chronic intrathecal catheters and continuous infusion of morphine over a period of days demonstrate a dose-dependent antinociception that declines over the infusion interval implying the development of opioid tolerance.[90] Tolerance produced by morphine infusion is dependent on an increase in local phosphorylating activity by protein kinase C in the dorsal horn of the spinal cord.[91] Human studies of repeated intrathecal or epidural morphine administration have produced conflicting results. Ventafridda et al.[18] observed a rapid loss of effectiveness of 1 mg of morphine during a 3- to 5-day sequence of once-daily intrathecal injections in cancer patients. In a retrospective study of the doses of morphine administered intrathecally by chronic infusion in a population of 163 patients (130 patients had pain that was metastatic in origin) treated by 19 physicians, Yaksh and Onofrio[64] reported a time-dependent increase from 4.8 ± 0.4 mg/day at week 1 (n = 130) to 16 ± 4 mg at 24 weeks (n = 33) and to 21 ± 9 mg at 52 weeks (n = 10). However, 48% of patients infused for periods in excess of 3 months showed less than a twofold increase in dose by 3 months. In a series of 35 patients treated with continuous intrathecal morphine (mean = 5.4 months) for intractable cancer pain, Penn and Paice[61] reported that the occurrences of tolerance were infrequent and could be managed effectively. A retrospective review of 159 patients with refractory cancer pain treated with daily boluses of intrathecal morphine demonstrated only a moderate increase in intrathecal opioid dose that did not limit the patients' ability to obtain adequate relief.[92]

The mean follow-up period was 95 days (range: 5 to 909 days), the mean starting dose of intrathecal morphine was 2.69 mg (range: 1 to 7.5 mg), and the mean terminal dose was 7.82 mg (range: 1 to 80 mg).

In summary, these studies suggest that, although tolerance to the effect of spinal morphine may develop in the cancer patient, tumor progression is much more likely to increase opioid requirements in a patient with opioid-responsive pain.

Assessment of Long-Term Efficacy of Neuraxial Opioids

The long-term benefits of epidural and intrathecal opioid therapy for cancer pain have been difficult to objectively assess for many reasons:

1. The criteria for treatment success are often vague and frequently vary between reports. There have been no standardized outcomes criteria.
2. The patient selection criteria for initiation of neuraxial opioid therapy have varied widely. In some centers, neurologists or oncologists are primarily responsible for pain management. They may be more content with systemic analgesics and more conservative with invasive measures than pain management specialists. They may refer patients for consideration of neuraxial therapies late in the course of the illness, when metastases have already become widespread, nociceptive inputs are high, and tolerance can be a significant problem. Frequently, such patients require supplementary local anesthetics for pain control; opioids alone are inadequate. By contrast, other centers, where pain management specialists have primary responsibility of cancer pain management, may initiate spinal therapy at an early stage, possibly even when systemic therapy may be equally if not more effective.
3. Cancer patients frequently have more than one type or location of pain, and the outcomes data are not specifically related to an identified pain site or type.
4. Meaningful statistical inferences cannot be made from the data as presented.

Some patients who experience inadequate pain relief and/or intolerable side effects from systemic opioids can obtain pain relief without side effects with intrathecal or epidural administration of the same or different drugs. There will be additional patients who never experience adequate pain relief with neuraxial opioids (so called "treatment failures"—*vide infra*). Different types of pain in patients with cancer may respond differentially to spinal opioids.[93] Arner and Arner[94] studied the differential effects of epidural morphine in patients with cancer pain. They utilized intermittent bolus doses of morphine in 55 patients with different patterns of cancer pain (daily dose range: 4 to 480 mg; dose interval range: 3 to 12 hours). Twenty-eight of the 55 patients (51%) became pain free. Another 21 patients were completely relieved of one of two pain types, whereas other coexisting pain types were either unaffected or only partially relieved. Six patients reported no pain relief. Continuous pain originating from deep somatic structures led to the best outcomes with epidural morphine. Continuous visceral pain or intermittent somatic pain originating from such things as a pathologic fracture, led to less predictable outcomes. Pains that were cutaneous in origin, thought to be neuropathic, or secondary to intestinal obstruction rarely responded. Coexisting pains that were not related to the underlying malignancy were not alleviated at all in ten patients. This study and others[53] suggested that there was some predictability for pain relief based upon the character of the pain after treatment with epidural morphine.

Summary of Neuraxial Opioid Use in Cancer Pain

Current knowledge on the use of spinal opioids in cancer-related pain allows us to make the following generalizations, based upon the literature and our own experience of cancer patients with pain:

1. It is common to see a slow increase in mean daily opioid dose requirements in many patients, often at a rate that doubles every few months. Some patients may escalate their dose requirements even more rapidly, particularly in the terminal phase of their disease.[95]
2. Dose escalation tends to be slower with intrathecal than epidural administration systems. This may relate to the tendency for fibrosis to occur around epidural catheters.[16]
3. The escalation of dose over time tends to be slower in patients receiving continuous infusions as opposed to intermittent bolus injections.[96] This may be related to the more rapid development of tolerance when spinal opioid receptors are exposed intermittently to high opioid doses.
4. Higher spinal opioid doses are required for pain that is neuropathic in origin than for somatogenic pain.[94] Opioid requirements for visceral pain are usually intermediate between neuropathic and somatic. There is no type of pain that never or always responds to neuraxial opioids.
5. Incident pain (occurring with activity) is difficult to control with neuraxial opioids.[86]
6. Higher systemic opioid requirements before implementation of spinal opioids are associated with higher neuraxial requirements.[97]
7. Many cancer pain patients who have not obtained pain relief with systemic opioids eventually demonstrate little benefit from epidural or intrathecal opioids. Although pain relief is adequate in 45% to 90% of patients with initiation of intraspinal opioid therapy, dose escalation and increased need for supplemental oral opioid therapy occur commonly over the first few months of therapy.[18,36,64,94,96] Van Dongen et al.[98] noted that 33% of patients failed intrathecal morphine therapy (after intrathecal therapy started because of failure of epidural therapy) and required the addition of bupivacaine for improved pain control.
8. Before the widespread use of intrathecal opioids, the most commonly utilized ablative procedure for pain from cancer was cordotomy. This operation was originally done via a laminectomy, but in the late 20th century percutaneous methods for cervical cordotomy were developed. The long-term results for pain relief after cordotomy (there are only case series, not cohort studies or high quality trials) appear to be better than those for neuraxial opioids and the quality of pain relief also seems superior. Of course, the initial complication rate was also higher for cordotomy. However, health care is largely a social convention; today, there are very few cordotomies performed for cancer pain in the United States and neuraxial opioids are the standard when oral or parenteral medications are inadequate.

Intracerebroventricular Opioids

It is possible to deliver opioids directly into the cerebral ventricles using an intracerebroventricular (ICV) catheter attached to a subcutaneous reservoir. A neurosurgeon is required for catheter placement. Morphine sulfate has been the most commonly administered drug; it has a dramatic increase in potency in the ICV route when compared to intrathecal or epidural infusions. The ICV route may affect supraspinal pathways for analgesia that are not accessible to spinally administered opioids.[99] ICV morphine doses have been reported from 50 to 700 µg/day.[100–101] The most commonly utilized drug administration system consists of a battery-driven infusion pump, implanted subcutaneously in the anterior abdominal or chest wall, and connected by subcutaneous tubing to the ventricular catheter that delivers the drug into the lateral ventricle.

Another administration strategy has been to connect the ICV catheter to an Ommaya reservoir and utilize intermittent percutaneous drug injections. ICV injections appear to last significantly longer than intraspinally administered drug. Some patients have been reported to obtain excellent pain relief via an implanted ventricular catheter connected to a subcutaneous Ommaya reservoir with 1 to 2 injections per day.[15] ICV drug delivery is particularly useful in head and neck cancer pain. Its use has also been reported in patients who initially manifested a favorable response to intraspinal infusions of opioids and subsequently development tolerance and were nearing the end of life. ICV injections or infusions manifest similar safety and side effects to intraspinal infusions, with the exception that an increased risk of respiratory depression exists during the first 3 days of therapy.[15]

Some refractory head and neck cancer pains do not respond to spinal opioids but will respond to ICV opioids. By contrast, pains below the waist are more amenable to spinal drug administration. Ballantyne et al.[102] performed a meta-analysis of 1,587 cancer patients, comparing ICV to the more commonly performed epidural and intrathecal opioid administration. All patients included had intractable cancer pain that had not adequately responded to systemic treatment. This study showed that sedation and confusion was observed in 4% to 5% of patients receiving ICV therapy. Pruritus, urinary retention, and persistent nausea occurred more frequently with spinal administration than with ICV therapy. Patients receiving ICV morphine required an initial dose of 0.25 to 2.0 mg/day. Onset of pain relief occurred in 2 to 30 minutes, and the typical duration of pain relief after a single dose was 12 to 48 hours. Tolerance seemed to be less of a problem than with either epidural or intrathecal therapy. Dose escalation was very gradual (the average increase in daily dosage was 0.375 mg/month). In a subsequent study,

Ballantyne et al.[103] reported on 72 uncontrolled trials in cancer patients assessing ICV (13 trials, 337 patients), epidural catheters (31 trials, 1343 patients), and subarachnoid catheters (28 trials, 722 patients). These uncontrolled studies suggested excellent pain relief in 73% of ICV patients compared with 72% of those with epidural and 62% of those with subarachnoid catheters. Unsatisfactory pain relief was infrequent in all three treatment groups. Side effects, commonly persistent nausea, persistent and transient urinary retention, transient pruritus, and constipation occurred more frequently in patients with epidural and subarachnoid catheters. On the other hand, respiratory depression, sedation, and confusion were more common with ICV. The incidence of major infection when implanted pumps were used with epidural and subarachnoid catheters was zero. Reported complications with ICV therapy were less than with epidural or subarachnoid catheters. ICV administration of opioids should be considered in patients with head and neck cancer pain that does not respond adequately to intraspinal delivery of drug.

INTRATHECAL THERAPY WITH BUPIVACAINE AND MORPHINE

The use of neuraxial opioids with local anesthetic agents is well established for postoperative pain management.[104–108] Bupivacaine-induced adverse effects including sensory deficits, motor complaints (especially lower-extremity impairment), bladder/bowel dysfunction, and signs of autonomic dysfunction led to concerns about these effects that have limited the consideration of this modality for home care in cancer patients. We now know that this form of neuraxial therapy can be safely administered in the outpatient setting. The safety and efficacy of long-term epidural bupivacaine-opioid infusion in 68 patients with cancer pain refractory to epidural opioids alone has been demonstrated.[109] The majority of these patients experienced pain relief with little or no sympathetic or sensorimotor impairment after the first 24 hours with bupivacaine concentrations of varying from 0.125% to 0.25%, and could receive management at home or in chronic care settings without the need for rehospitalization. Transient postural hypotension during the first 24 hours occurred in only 9% of patients and was easily managed with close monitoring and fluid therapy during initiation of therapy.

The number of patients who will require neuraxial therapy with local anesthetics in addition to opioids is unknown. Reasons for selection of patients vary and therapy can be started before systemic opioid therapy has been optimized. The usual indications for intrathecal bupivacaine and morphine therapy are progressive pain not responding to opioid therapy or unacceptable opioid-related side effects in patients who have satisfactory pain control. Clinicians should also distinguish the need for intrathecal therapy over epidural. Certain tumor-related pain problems predictably are less likely to respond to epidural analgesia.[13] These include mucocutaneous ulcers, pain caused by body movements as a result of fracture, edematous swelling and/or ischemia of an extremity, and neuropathic pain from plexus infiltration. In these situations, the administration of intrathecal morphine (IT-morphine) alone does not appear to offer any significant advantages.[95] Different sites of drug action and synergistic effects of bupivacaine and morphine are also important for refractory pain problems.[110] IT-bupivacaine with its predilection for unmyelinated axons could contribute to the clinical efficacy by blocking slow, "burning" pains[111] which may not respond to morphine alone.

In addition, the combination may delay the occurrence of tolerance to IT-morphine because of the smaller doses and the added analgesic effects of bupivacaine. The route of administration is also important and favors the intrathecal over epidural route.[13] Better and more predictable drug distribution to the required area is probably the primary reason why intrathecal medications are more effective. Distribution of effect after epidural injection of local anesthetics varies widely and may only be partially predicted based upon known factors.[112] Epidural anesthesia has an unpredictable extent and duration. Differences in the surface area of the lumbosacral dura, epidural fat volume, and epidural venous plexus velocity might explain the variability in the extent and duration of epidural anesthesia.[113] Cranial spread of lumbar epidural anesthesia is more extensive than caudad spread.[114] Block of the fifth lumbar and first sacral segments by anesthetics is often delayed or incomplete[115] and may be related to the large size of these nerve roots.[116] This is obviously problematic in cancer patients complaining of radicular pain in these distributions. Intrathecal administration at the appropriate level will result in a more predictable effect. For all the reasons enumerated above, we prefer intrathecal to epidural drug administration for the relief of cancer pain.

Mechanism of Intrathecal Drug Distribution

The importance of intrathecal volumes, versus that of the concentrations and doses, for the intensity and spread of spinal analgesia during chronic infusions of IT-morphine and bupivacaine is still unclear. Kroin et al.[117] could not demonstrate any advantage in placing the catheter tip at more rostral locations, such as at the midthoracic or cervical cord when using hydrophilic drugs for pain relief. Van Zundert et al.[118] demonstrated that a constant 70-mg dose of subarachnoid lidocaine delivered in a 0.5%. 1%, 2%, 5%, or 10% solution produced the same pinprick level of analgesia, degree of motor block, and duration of spinal anesthesia. Wagemans et al.[63] measured the pH of CSF in a patient receiving high doses of intrathecal morphine who failed to demonstrate either motor or sensory block after injection of 75 mg of lidocaine 5%. This patient's CSF pH fell outside the physiologic range at 7.19 (normal range: 7.27 to 7.37), suggesting a possible explanation for the decreased activity of the local anesthetic. Kroin et al.[119] noted an absence of ataxia at IT-bupivacaine doses of 0.4 to 0.5 mg/hour in dogs. The human CSF volume is approximately 10 times that of a dog. Therefore, one might reasonably assume that doses of bupivacaine up to 3 mg/hour are safe in patients without evidence of neurologic deficit. When patients have neurologic deficits due to nerve damage or polyneuropathies, it is appropriate to reduce doses substantially (0.5 to 1.0 mg/hour) to avoid causing motor disturbances.

The location of the infusion catheter tip relative to the targeted spinal cord segments is critical because of the limited capacity for CSF to distribute drugs away from the catheter tip. It is important to understand the mechanism of intrathecal drug delivery when administered as a slow intrathecal infusion. Human and animal studies of intrathecal drug distribution have been conducted as single bolus injections made at relatively rapid injection rates of tens of milliliters per minute.[120] However, infusion pumps used for the delivery of intrathecal morphine and bupivacaine deliver drug at much lower rates, sometimes as low as a few microliters per day. Bernards[120] characterized the distribution of baclofen and bupivacaine within the CSF and spinal cord at very low infusion rates in a pig model.[120] Bupivacaine concentration, when infused at 20 μL/hour, differed significantly between the anterior and posterior halves of the spinal cord and as a function of distance from the site of administration (Figs. 22.4 and 22.5). For both bupivacaine and baclofen, most of the drug recovered in the CSF and spinal cord was found within 1 cm of the site of administration. In the same experiment, a faster infusion rate of 1000 μL/hour imparted slight forward motion to the injectate with slightly better drug distribution. This suggests that there is poor mixing within the CSF and that drug distribution with slow continuous infusion is very limited. Of interest, baclofen, a more hydrophilic drug than bupivacaine, in bolus doses or infused at 1000 μL/hour distributed between the anterior and posterior spinal cord, but did not do so at infusion rates of 20 μL/hour. Hydrophilic drugs may have better distribution at bolus doses or higher infusion rates within the CSF.

The primary mechanisms responsible for drug movement within the CSF are Brownian motion (slight effect), kinetic energy imparted by the act of injection (slight effect when infused at slow rates), and CSF motion itself. Drug will move in the CSF as long as it is suspended in CSF, and its distribution will be limited only by the rate and extent of CSF motion. Motion of CSF is driven by cyclic expansion and contraction of the CSF vasculature during cardiac systole and diastole. The magnitude of motion is greatest in the upper cervical regions and decreases with distance from the cranial vault, becoming negligible at the level of the cauda equina.[120] Spinal CSF motion is also divided into three distinct channels, medioventral, dorsomedial, and lateral.[121] These channels are distinct by the timing and magnitude of CSF oscillation. Within a given channel, the timing and magnitude of CSF motion is highly variable, with some areas along the cord devoid of either rostral or caudad motion. Also circumferential motion is not present between anterior and posterior sides of the spinal cord, presumably because of anatomical barriers (dentate ligament and spinal nerve roots) traversing

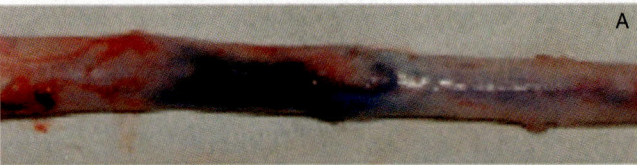
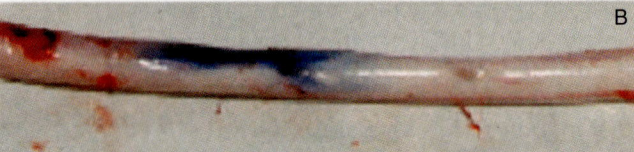
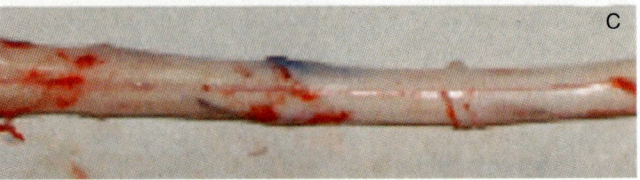

FIGURE 22.5 Photographs of approximately 3-cm-long section of spinal cord in which methylene blue was added to drug infusion (20 μL/hour for 8 hours). There is heavy staining of the posterior segment of the spinal cord adjacent to the tip of the infusion catheter (**A**), minimal staining of the lateral surface of the spinal cord (**B**), and no visible staining of the anterior surface of the spinal cord (**C**). (Reused with permission from Bernards CM. Cerebrospinal fluid and spinal cord distribution of baclofen and bupivacaine during slow intrathecal infusion in pigs. *Anesthesiology.* 2006;105:169–178.)

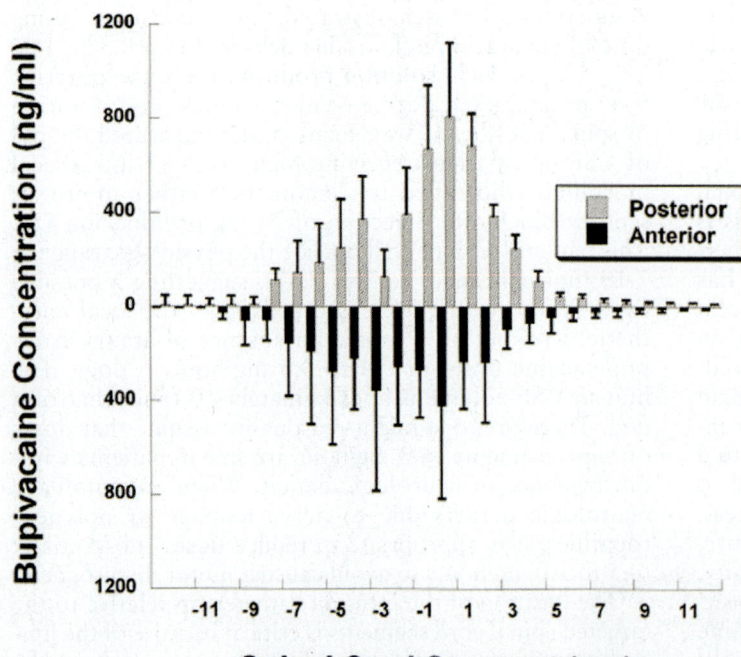

FIGURE 22.4 Average bupivacaine concentration in spinal cord specimens. Bupivacaine concentration differed significantly between the anterior and posterior halves of the spinal cord and as a function of distance from the site of administration. (Reused with permission from Bernards CM. Cerebrospinal fluid and spinal cord distribution of baclofen and bupivacaine during slow intrathecal infusion in pigs. *Anesthesiology.* 2006;105:169–178.)

TABLE 22.3
FACTORS LIMITING NET MOVEMENT WITHIN THE CEREBROSPINAL FLUID

Factor	Effect
Cardiac cycle	Propels CSF in opposite directions during each cycle
CSF pulse wave	The more caudad from foramen magnum, the smaller the pulse wave
Regional	Some areas are devoid of motion (at least sometimes)
Anatomical	Most CSF motion occurs in rostrocaudal axis, not circumferentially

CSF, Cerebrospinal fluid.

the lateral subarachnoid space. Factors limiting net CSF movement are summarized in Table 22.3. Placement of the infusion catheter tip at a precise level within the CSF is critical, especially if low infusion rates are utilized.

Clinical Efficacy of Intrathecal Local Anesthetics with Morphine

A number of clinical studies support the use of intrathecal bupivacaine and morphine for severe, intractable pain. Two reports, published in 1990 and 1991, first described the benefits of this approach in cases of refractory cancer pain.[12-13] Nitescu et al.[12] compared the efficacy of epidural and intrathecal pain treatment with morphine and bupivacaine in 25 patients with severe, multifocal cancer pain, where epidural administration of morphine and bupivacaine failed to provide acceptable pain relief. Both epidural and intrathecal catheter systems consisted of open, subcutaneously tunneled catheters. Fifteen patients had infradiaphragmatic pain, and ten had both infra- and supradiaphragmatic pain. The investigators assessed consecutive epidural and intrathecal periods (2 to 174 days, median: 50 days; 1 to 305 days, median: 37 days, respectively) in terms of daily analgesic dosages giving acceptable pain relief and quality of life expressed as sleeping hours and walking/daily activities. They placed both epidural and intrathecal catheters using a midline approach at between T11 and L5 vertebral levels. Eleven patients received preservative-free morphine solutions 0.2 to 2.0 mg/mL and the other 14 received morphine with preservatives in solutions of 10 mg/mL. Bupivacaine 2.5 to 5.0 mg/mL, diluted or not with isotonic saline, was added to morphine until concentrations judged to be suitable with respect to the daily dosages and volumes were obtained. Epidural solutions were administered as intermittent injections 2 to 6 times per day, for a total of 1,242 treatment days (range per patient: 2 to 174 days; median: 50 days). All patients receiving intrathecal treatment began with intermittent injections given 1 to 15 times/day (mean: 3; median: 2), and continued in 18 patients. In seven patients, the initial, intermittent administration continued until termination of treatment by continuous infusion of morphine, with or without bupivacaine. The combined, intermittent and continuous treatment duration ranged from 1 to 305 days (median: 37 days). Eleven patients received treatment at home for 7 to 125 days (median: 46 days). With intrathecal treatment, the total opioid consumption and the daily doses of spinal morphine and bupivacaine decreased significantly both at the start of treatment and for the 6-month follow-up period. Intrathecal treatment provided more satisfactory pain relief, and because of lower daily doses and volume, proved to be more suitable for treatment at home than epidural treatment. Sjoberg et al.[13] reported on the applicability of long-term (1-305, median = 23, days) intrathecal bupivacaine and morphine in 52 patients with complex "refractory" cancer pain. Particular consideration was given to the dosages, concentrations, volumes, and proportions of the drugs, and to side effects and complications that they could attribute to the long-term administration of bupivacaine. The investigators estimated efficacy from the daily dosage (intraspinal and total opioids, and intraspinal bupivacaine), scores of nonopioid analgesic and sedative consumption, gait and daily activities, and amount and pattern of sleep. Intrathecal treatment began with a test dose of 1 to 6 mg of morphine (median: 2) and 1.0 to 12.5 mg bupivacaine (median: 4.5), given in a volume of 1.0 to 8.0 mL (median: 4). Intrathecal daily volumes ranged from 1 to 114 mL and increased with the duration of the intrathecal treatment, the median values being about three times higher at 6 months (30 mL) than at 2 days after the start (9 mL). Eighty-five percent of patients obtained continuous and acceptable pain relief (VAS: 0 to 2 out of 10 vs. pretrial: 7 to 10 out of 10), 60% of them with daily doses of IT-bupivacaine of 1.5 mg/hour. Temporary, moderate, or severe "breakthrough" pain (VAS: 3 to 8), not always relieved by escalating intrathecal treatment, was experienced in eight patients (15%). Higher IT-bupivacaine doses (>60 to 305 mg/day), not always giving acceptable pain relief, were necessary in 13 patients (25%) with deafferentation pain in spinal cord, or plexus (brachial, lumbosacral), or celiac plexus, or from large, ulcerated mucocutaneous tumors. By combining IT-bupivacaine with IT-morphine, it was possible to use relatively low IT-morphine doses (10 to 25 mg/day during the first 2 months of treatment) in more than half of the patients. intrathecal treatment significantly decreased the total (all routes) opioid consumption and significantly improved sleep, gait, and daily activities. For the whole period of observation (6 months), the intrathecal treatment was assessed as adequate in 3.8%, good in 23.1%, very good in 59.6%, and excellent in 13.5% of the cases. Adverse effects of the IT-bupivacaine (paresthesia, paresis, gait impairment, urinary retention, anal sphincter disturbances, and orthostatic hypotension) did not occur with doses of 2.5 to 3.0 mg/hour (approx. 60 to 70 mg/day). Paresthesia in patients at bolus doses exceeding 1.25 mg was sometimes experienced as very unpleasant. Two patients who experienced paresthesia refused to continue IT-bupivacaine therapy for fear of becoming paralyzed. Because of this, the authors suggested an upper limit of the incremental dose of IT-bupivacaine per demand of 1.25 mg. With IT-bupivacaine infusion, most of the patients did not complain of unpleasant paresthesias at doses up to 3 mg/hour. Paresis and gait impairment usually did not occur with infusion doses (3 mg/hour). The incidence of early urinary retention was 27%. Late urinary retention appeared consistently at daily dose of bupivacaine greater than 60 mg/day.

Subsequent to this report, a number of other studies have confirmed the efficacy of IT-morphine/bupivacaine combinations for the treatment of severe, refractory cancer pain.[95,98,122–129] These reports demonstrate that intrathecal therapy is both efficacious and safe for long-term administration and that local anesthetic may be administered safely throughout the neuraxis.

In a follow-up study from the 1991 report, Sjoberg et al.[126] tested the clinical efficacy of a constant infusion of 0.5 mg/mL morphine plus 4.75 mg/mL bupivacaine (morphine:bupivacaine approximately 1:10), given through externalized intrathecal catheters to 53 patients. They obtained satisfactory pain relief, defined as VAS scores of 0 to 2 vs. 6 to 10 in the preintrathecal stage, with relatively low daily doses of intrathecal morphine (median: 6 mg). Daily intrathecal volumes (median: 10 mL) were low, whereas the daily dose of intrathecal bupivacaine was relatively high (median: 50 mg). Side effects attributable to intrathecal bupivacaine occurred in the forms of late urinary retention (33%), paresthesias (41%), paresis/gait impairment (33%), and occasional episodes of orthostatic arterial hypotension (1.8%). Appelgren et al.[123] reported on continuous intracisternal and high cervical intrathecal bupivacaine analgesia in refractory head and neck pain (see "Novel Techniques with Intrathecal Therapy," page 294). Mercadante et al.[129] prospectively evaluated the clinical response to intrathecal morphine and levobupivacaine in 45 opioid-tolerant advanced-cancer patients who had failed multiple, systemic opioid trials. Subcutaneous catheters with ports were placed in either the lumbar or thoracic level corresponding to the most painful dermatome. Most patients had somatic pain due to bone metastases (29 patients); 16 patients had mixed pain syndromes with a prevalent neuropathic component. Initial intrathecal morphine doses were calculated from the previous opioid consumption using an oral-intrathecal ration of 100:1. Initial levobupivacaine doses were 12.5 mg/day and the combination of morphine and levobupivacaine was infused at a rate of 2 mL/hour. If pain was inadequately controlled, the dose of levobupivacaine was increased to 25 mg/day before increasing the daily intrathecal dose of morphine. Average doses of intrathecal morphine at the time of death was 19.7 mg/day (13.5-25.9) with an opioid escalation index of 0.19 mg/day. Average local anesthetic dose at the time of death was 54.4 mg/day (33.5 to 75.4). Mean survival time was 71 days (95% confidence interval [CI]: 41–101).

Table 22.4 provides our guidelines for starting intrathecal therapy with the combination of morphine and bupivacaine in patients with refractory cancer pain. Many of our patients have a temporary percutaneous epidural catheter placed at an appropriate level before the decision to utilize a permanent intrathecal catheter. This usually results in adequate pain control as we plan and schedule elective intrathecal catheter placement. Before surgical placement, an estimate of the required level for placement of the intrathecal catheter tip is made, based on the patient's predominant pain location and on review of appropriate imaging showing relevant pathology. We usually use an initial solution of bupivacaine 0.5% mixed

TABLE 22.4

GUIDELINES FOR INITIATING INTRATHECAL BUPIVACAINE/MORPHINE THERAPY

1) Place intrathecal catheter tips at the appropriate anticipated segment of maximum pain input (particularly with thoracic and cervical pain). For pain that is predominantly:
    a) distal lower extremity (L5/S1), catheter tips should be placed cauded at approximately the L5 vertebral level.
    b) proximal lower extremity (L2, L3), catheter tips should be placed at T12/L1 vertebral level
    c) sacral area, place catheter tips at approximately T12 vertebral level.
    d) perineal, place catheter tip at L4 vertebral level.
    e) pelvic (T10-L1), catheter tip should be placed at T10 vertebral level.
    f) mid-to-upper abdomen, catheter tip should be placed at approximately T7 vertebra level.
2) Always use double filters with externalized systems (see below)
3) Titrate IT-dosage individually:
    a) For opioid tolerant patients, start with morphine (200 μg/mL) and relatively high bupivacaine (0.5 mg/mL) concentrations at volume rates of 0.4 mL/hour.
    b) On starting therapy, bolus with 1 mL of the combined solution.
    c) If using PCIA, set the incremental dose per demand at or below 2.5 mg of IT-bupivacaine (0.2 mL q30 min).
4) Be prepared to use higher IT-bupivacaine doses (per hour) in patients with deafferentation pain from the spinal cord, brachial or lumbosacral plexus, pain from celiac plexus, ischemic and colicky pain, and smarting pain from large, ulcerated mucocutaneous tumors.
5) Limit the daily dose of IT-morphine <15 mg to avoid the possibility of opioid-induced myoclonus and hyperalgesia.
6) Lower extremity motor impairment and/or bowel/bladder dysfunction will depend on daily bupivacaine dose and location of intrathecal catheter tip. Patients are greatest risk for these side effects are those with pre-existing neurologic deficits (sensory or motor) and low-lying catheters (L5 vertebral level). In these patients, deficits may not be seen with daily intrathecal bupivacaine doses <10 mg/day.
7) Treat opioid withdrawal independently of IT-morphine doses.
8) Adjust the dosages as necessary. The effects of dose changes may be slow in onset (up to 24 hours for morphine effects).

IT, Intrathecal; PCIA, patient-controlled intrathecal analgesia.

with preservative-free morphine 200 µg/mL at an infusion rate of 0.4 mL/hour. This relatively high bupivacaine concentration will result in motor impairment in the lower extremities in most patients, but we do this deliberately to achieve satisfactory pain control immediately after catheter placement. If patients do not have indwelling urinary catheters before implantation, we will place a catheter as patients frequently develop urinary retention with this concentration of bupivacaine. If there is inadequate effect from the bupivacaine, we bolus the patient with 0.2 mL of the infusate and increase the rate by 0.2 mL/hour. This may be repeated hourly until there is adequate distribution of local anesthetic (as judged by patient reporting of adequate pain relief and/or appropriate sensory dermatomal changes to testing). This opioid concentration is also acceptable and does not usually result in significant side effects (even with concomitant use of systemic opioids) as most patients are opioid tolerant before catheter placement. Twenty-four hours after implantation, if the patient's tumor-associated pain is satisfactorily controlled and the patient is experiencing bupivacaine-induced lower-extremity motor impairment, we reduce the bupivacaine concentration by 0.05% to 0.1% and maintain the infusion rate to obtain optimal function while maintaining adequate pain relief. Typically, we maintain the same morphine dose, particularly if the patient is not having opioid-related side effects.

We strongly believe that infection risk can be reduced by using a double-filter system. With such a double-filter system, there is significant dead space (often more than 7 mL) within the external infusion system and concentration change effects may not be obvious for a considerable period of time (sometimes up to 24 hours) if the filters and tubing are not changed at the time of the concentration change. After obtaining the new solution for infusion, new filters are placed and the external system purged with the new infusate to the external catheter. The new external system is then attached to the intrathecal catheter using sterile precautions. The infusion is then restarted at the previous rate. If the patient is not experiencing significant lower-extremity motor impairment but is having undesirable numbness in the lower extremities with adequate pain control, we will typically reduce the bupivacaine concentration to 0.4% initially. Depending on the degree of impairment or adequacy of pain control, bupivacaine doses may reduce by further increments of 0.1% or 0.05%. If motor impairment is profound in the lower extremities and pain control is adequate, we will reduce the bupivacaine concentration to 0.3% instead of 0.4%, in an effort to more quickly restore function. The time interval for these dosing changes is typically 24 to 48 hours, until function is deemed satisfactory or pain control becomes compromised. Our ultimate goal is to find the lowest dose of bupivacaine that will allow adequate function (defined on an individual patient basis) with optimal pain relief. With daily doses of bupivacaine greater than 10 mg/day, many patients will have urinary difficulties. Continuous indwelling urinary catheters have a significant associated infection risk, and we prefer intermittent catheterization. Patients are instructed to self-catheterize 3 to 4 times per day on a scheduled basis while the intrathecal catheter is in use. Some patients do regain urinary control with effective pain-relieving dosing of bupivacaine.

Neurotoxicity of Intrathecal Local Anesthetics

The advantages of neuraxial drug delivery are well defined in cancer pain.[20] For pain relief, only morphine and ziconotide are FDA-approved; the use of other medications for intrathecal management are off-label and may have risks that are not well defined. In 2005, a polyanalgesic consensus conference provided recommendations for intrathecal drug delivery for the management of cancer pain.[21] The recommended (based only on what was used by the participants) drugs used in combination included opioids (morphine, hydromorphone, fentanyl, sufentanil, meperidine, buprenorphine), local anesthetics (bupivacaine, ropivacaine, tetracaine), clonidine, baclofen, midazolam, neostigmine, adenosine, ketorolac, droperidol, ketamine, gabapentin, and octreotide. The authors noted that some patients may require six adjuvants to control pain at the end of life. In a commentary on these recommendations, Penn[130] recommended that any medications except morphine (or hydromorphone), bupivacaine, ziconitide, and clonidine not be used, because the safety profiles of these other medications have not been established for intrathecal use. In addition, he noted that baclofen, although safe, has little effect on pain, and time should not be wasted trying it. Compounding pharmacists can produce any combination of medications in high concentrations. The risk of toxicities associated with intrathecal medication use may be increased now that more clinicians are using various combinations of medications in high concentrations. As an example of this potential, we review here the current safety profile of local anesthetics as it related to neurotoxicity.

In 1985, Ready et al.[131] reported on the neurotoxic effects of local anesthetics in rabbits. They noted that concentrations of local anesthetics used clinically did not produce persistent neurologic effects but lidocaine and tetracaine in high concentrations (far exceeding those clinically used) produced extensive irreversible neurologic injury and histologic changes. Spinal cord or nerve root toxicity may manifest itself as histologic, physiologic, or behavioral/clinical derangements after exposure to a spinal drug. Neurohistopathology may be classified as neural injury, gliosis, or damage to the myelin sheath, and also describes inflammatory changes and involvement of the arachnoid cell layers. Physiologic neurotoxicity of spinal drugs includes changes in spinal cord blood flow, disruption of the blood–brain barrier, and changes in the electrophysiology of impulse conduction. Behavioral and clinical signs of neurotoxicity include pain, motor and sensory deficits, and bowel and bladder dysfunction.[132] Yamashita et al.[133] studied the histopathologic effect of 2% tetracaine, 10% lidocaine, 2% bupivacaine, and 2% ropivacaine in an animal experiment. These concentrations are 2 to 4 times as large as those used clinically. Histopathologic changes observed were vacuolation in the white matter confined within the dorsal funiculus and chromatolytic damage of motor neurons, with round cytoplasm and laterally placed nuclei predominantly in the ventral horn. Vacuolation in the dorsal funiculus in the tetracaine and lidocaine groups were significantly worse than in the bupivacaine and ropivacaine groups. Preferential damage to nerve roots after intrathecal administration of local anesthetics has been demonstrated in other animal studies.[134-135] In situ rat sciatic nerve experiments with solutions of 3% chloroprocaine, 1% tetracaine, 2% lidocaine, or 0.75% bupivacaine applied exteriorly to the epineurium have produced significant endoneurial edema.[136] Electron microscopy of these preparations revealed abnormal mast cells, Schwann cell injury, and axonal dystrophy. Further studies with the same model found that histologic evidence of nerve injury correlated well with both anesthetic potency and concentration.[137] For example, 0.5 mL of 10% procaine produced severe nerve injury, whereas 1 mL of 5% procaine did not. Increasing concentrations and doses of hyperbaric bupivacaine solutions (1% and 2% in 10% dextrose) was associated with nerve tissue damage, which did not occur with hypobaric (same concentrations in water) solutions.[138] Histopathologic changes were observed in the proximal portion of the posterior root at its entry to the spinal cord and to nearby posterior white matter in rats injected with 5% bupivacaine, 20% lidocaine, and 10% lidocaine.[139] Electron microscopic examination showed widespread degeneration of both the myelin sheaths and axons in severely injured areas such as the proximal portion of the posterior root in the rats treated with 20% lidocaine. Axonal degeneration with the almost-intact myelin sheath in mildly injured areas was mainly observed in rats treated with less than 10% lidocaine and 5% bupivacaine. The histopathologic characters of neurotoxicity caused by lidocaine and bupivacaine were virtually identical. Lesions caused by both drugs spread from the posterior roots (entry zone) just at the entry into the spinal cord, to the posterior white matter. The lesions were likely caused by axonal degeneration. The histologic damage caused by lidocaine and bupivacaine appears to involve the sensory system but not the motor system. The incidence and severity of the lesions are quite different between lidocaine and bupivacaine groups; lesions induced by lidocaine were more widely distributed and more severe than those induced by bupivacaine at concentrations of equivalent potency. Moreover, at higher concentrations, lidocaine produced sensory impairment and persistent hindlimb limitation, whereas bupivacaine did not.

Clinically used concentrations of lidocaine (5% as a single bolus or continuous infusion),[140] and tetracaine (1% single repeated bolus injections)[141] are associated with potentially severe neurotoxicity, although the long-term intrathecal infusion of usual clinical concentrations of bupivacaine 0.5% was not associated with obvious neurotoxicity.[123] Several cases studies have reported on persistent neurologic symptoms after uncomplicated intrathecal hyperbaric bupivacaine 0.5% injections.[142-144] In the case of lidocaine, the important variable is not the concentration administered, but rather the perineural concentration of lidocaine. In laboratory experiments showing increased toxicity with increased concentration administered, the concentration administered and perineural concentration were linearly related.[145] In histopathologic, electrophysiologic, behavioral, and neuronal cell models, lidocaine and tetracaine seem to have a greater potential for neurotoxicity than bupivacaine at clinically relevant concentrations.[132] Li et al.[146] noted that continuous infusion of 0.5% bupivacaine, 1.5% lidocaine, and 2% 2-chloroprocaine at 100 μL/hour for 24 hours resulted in neuronal vacuolation that was more intense with lidocaine and 2-chloroprocaine than bupivacaine. However, different neuropathologic studies have demonstrated the clinical safety of long-term infusion of intrathecal bupivacaine and morphine at usual clinical doses.[126,147-148] Of course, toxicity issues in patients with normal life expectancies are mitigated by the shorter life expectancies of cancer patients. This is particularly true when pain relief is needed in the preterminal or terminal epochs of a patient with cancer. In such situations, the long-term toxicity effects become irrelevant.

ALTERNATIVE NEURAXIAL DRUGS

Some patients may not respond to intrathecal bupivacaine/morphine combinations or may experience function-limiting side effects, particularly with local anesthetic use. In this situation, adjuvant agents can be considered.

Clonidine

Clonidine, originally developed as an α-2 adrenergic agonist for the treatment of hypertension, was noted to produce pain relief after epidural administration in patients with chronic pain.[149] There are several reasons to consider neuraxial clonidine for intractable cancer pain. Clonidine is a centrally acting α-2 adrenergic agonist with established analgesic effects[150-151] and has synergistic effects with both spinal opioids[152-153] and spinal local anesthetics.[154-155] Like opioid receptors, there is a high density of α-2 adrenoreceptors in the superficial dorsal horn of the spinal cord.[156] α-2 adrenoreceptor activation blocks transmission of noxious sensory information at the level of the spinal cord by both pre- and postsynaptic mechanisms.[157-159] Clonidine's analgesic activity is mediated through pre- and postsynaptic α-2 receptors localized in the superficial layers of the spinal dorsal horn. It is a potent antinociceptive agent. Systemic, spinal, and supraspinal effects of clonidine have been reported; the antinociceptive effects of clonidine are probably mediated via spinal and supraspinal sites of action.[160] Cholinergic transmission at the spinal cord level is related to α-2 adrenergic agonist-mediated analgesia.[161-162] Intrathecal α-2 adrenergic agonists increase the CSF concentration of acetylcholine[162] and nicotinic and muscarinic receptors may play an important role in clonidine-evoked antinociception.[163-164] Clonidine has been administered orally, transdermally, intravenously, epidurally, and intrathecally for the treatment of a variety of pain problems including labor pain, surgical pain, and chronic pain.[165] As the site of action for the antinociceptive properties of clonidine is predominantly the spinal cord, spinal delivery may be the most effective.[166] In 1996, the FDA approved administration of clonidine (Duraclon) by continuous epidural infusion as an adjunctive therapy with neuraxial opioids for the treatment of pain in cancer patients who are tolerant or unresponsive to neuraxial opioids alone. Clonidine can be used in combination with opioids, potentiating their analgesic effects without the development of tolerance.[167] It should be noted that the FDA did not approve intrathecal administration of clonidine.

The physician using clonidine for long-term neuraxial infusion should be aware of unique challenges associated with this drug and method of administration. The benefits obtained for pain relief are offset by a dose-dependent sedation and hemodynamic changes. Rebound systemic hypertension (systolic blood pressure readings to values greater than 200 mm Hg) can be observed with abrupt cessation of the neuraxial infusion of clonidine.[22] If abrupt cessation of neuraxial clonidine occurs, the patient should be treated with oral clonidine, initially with a dose of 0.2 mg, then 0.1 mg every hour until the patient's blood pressure is satisfactorily controlled or a total of 0.8 mg has been given. Of interest, clonidine decreases blood pressure after epidural administration by actions in the spinal cord,[168–169] brainstem,[170] and periphery.[171] The hypotensive action of clonidine is counteracted at larger doses by a peripheral vasoconstrictive action. Similar degrees of hypotension are observed from epidural and intrathecal clonidine injection.[172] Although clonidine can clearly reduce sympathetic nervous system activity by a spinal action,[168] which would result in greater potency of intrathecal than epidural injection to reduce blood pressure, clonidine can also decrease sympathetic nervous system activity after systemic redistribution to peripheral and brain sites. This systemic redistribution of clonidine is the likely reason for the similar degree of hypotension with the two routes of administration.

Epidural

Epidural clonidine produces analgesia by a spinal mechanism in patients after surgery and in those with cancer pain,[173] and it appears to be an effective treatment for severe cancer pain in patients in whom other treatments fail.[174] For this reason, clonidine is an effective analgesic when administered intraspinally but a poor analgesic when administered systemically.[175] An epidural bolus injection of clonidine 150 μg has a T_{max} of 60 ±7 minutes and the C_{max} was 228 ±56 ng/mL.[176] The long plasma elimination half-life of clonidine (approximately 14 hours following epidural administration) suggests the potential for plasma accumulation with continuous epidural infusion.[177] However, Boswell et al.[167] demonstrated that clonidine did not accumulate in the plasma compartment during prolonged (14-day) continuous infusion in cancer patients.

Clinical experience with neuraxial clonidine largely comprises postoperative analgesia studies, although Eisenach[174] has reported on its long-term use in cancer pain. This and other clinical studies[178–180] suggest that intrathecal and epidural clonidine in combination with other agents such as opioids or local anesthetics can be a suitable treatment for intractable cancer pain. The pivotal trial, which led to approval by the FDA, studied the efficacy of epidural clonidine in 85 patients with cancer who continued to have either severe pain despite large systemic or epidural doses of opioids or who were experiencing therapy-limiting side effects from opioids.[174] Patients were randomized to receive either epidural clonidine 30 μg/hour or a placebo in a double blind, multicenter study. All patients received rescue medication (epidural morphine) by patient-controlled analgesia (PCA). Patients' primary pain was considered neuropathic in nature in 42% and nonneuropathic in 58%. Successful pain relief (defined as a decrease in either morphine use of VAS scores) was more common with epidural clonidine (45%) than with placebo (21%) and was particularly prominent in those patients with neuropathic pain (56% vs. 5%). The onset of side effects from epidural clonidine occurred early in treatment, without any delayed onset effects. Blood pressures remained approximately the same level as baseline in the placebo group but decreased by approximately 10 mm Hg in the clonidine group and were a serious complication in 2 patients. This fixed dose of clonidine was effective in the subgroup with neuropathic, but not with somatic pain. For patients in the nonneuropathic pain groups, the likelihood of success was similar for each treatment group regardless of whether the pain was characterized as visceral or somatic, which suggests that the addition of clonidine in the treatment of such conditions does not confer additional benefit over epidural opioids.

Intrathecal

Given clonidine's lipophilicity (similar to fentanyl), one would expect its neuraxial effects to be more pronounced and selective after intrathecal rather than epidural administration. As predicted by its high lipid solubility, clonidine's analgesic effects following neuraxial administration of bolus doses are of short duration; therefore, sustained pain relief can be achieved only with continuous infusion.[181]

Clinically, intrathecal clonidine appears much more potent than epidural clonidine in the treatment of acute pain (ratio approximately 8:1 to 10:1), but only slightly more potent in the treatment of chronic, especially neuropathic pain (<2:1).[172] Typical clinical doses of intrathecal clonidine are 30 to 150 μg, if given by bolus injection, and 8 to 400 μg/day by continuous infusions, usually in combination with morphine.

A number of clinical reports document the efficacy of intrathecal clonidine for intractable cancer pain.[179–180,182] Hassenbusch et al.[165] studied the effects of intrathecal clonidine administered by implanted programmable pumps. Clonidine monotherapy was initiated at 1 μg/hour and escalated to a maximum dose of 40 μg/hour. Thirty-one patients were enrolled; six with active cancer and 29 with nonmalignant pain that was predominantly neuropathic in origin. The six cancer patients suffered from cancer and radiation therapy effects on brachial or lumbosacral plexuses. During the dose titration phase, one patient died from advanced malignant disease. The dose titration phase consisted of the initiation of clonidine at infusion rates of 0.1 μg/hour (2.4 μg/day) for each patient and, using the programmability of the pump, increased every 12 hours to reach a final rate of 0.7 μg/hour (16.8 μg/day) at the end of 6 days. Further dose-escalation stages, still using small incremental increases every 12 hours, were repeated with clonidine doses reaching a potential maximum of 50 μg/hour (1200 μg/day) during the titration stages. In the later part of the study, the potential maximum was lowered to 40 μg/hour (960 μg/day) because no additional analgesia was observed between 40 and 50 μg/hour. Each patient continued through the study dose-escalation stages until intolerable side effects developed or the maximum dose rate of 40 μg/hour was reached, with dose escalations occurring automatically unless the patient reported intolerable side effects. Of the remaining 30 patients, 22 had successful dose-titration phases. Seven patients failed the titration phase because of inability to obtain at least 50% pain/symptom relief without intolerable side effects. The side effects in these seven patients were symptomatic systemic hypotension; unacceptable confusion although 70% of these patients experienced adequate pain relief; headaches; and malaise and lethargy. Systemic hypotension was seen most often at clonidine doses of 325 to 650 μg/day. Hypotension first appeared at doses in the lower end of this range as postural systolic hypotension, but increased with higher dose rates to hypotension even while recumbent. Of the remaining 22 patients, 13 (59%) had long-term successful pain relief with follow-up periods ranging from 6.3 to 44 months (median: 16.7 months). While receiving clonidine, two patients died from metastatic end-stage cancer and one from a cause unrelated to clonidine infusion or cancer. These patients also had adequate pain relief from intrathecal clonidine until death (range: 6.3 to 16.7 months, median: 9.7 months). Nine patients were unable to obtain long-term satisfactory pain relief, either because of inadequate pain relief or intolerable side effects. At 6 months, 77.3% (17/22) of patients with success in the dose-titration phase had continued good pain relief with intrathecal clonidine. Fifty-nine percent (59%) of the patients successful in the dose titration stage (42% of all patients considered) were considered long-term successes.

Ackerman et al.[183] also reported on the efficacy of intrathecal clonidine or clonidine/opioid combinations in a mixed pain population of complex reginal pain syndrome, neuropathic pain, and cancer pain. All 15 patients had neuropathic pain disorders or mixed nociceptive/neuropathic pain problems in which the neuropathic component was predominant. Five patients were deemed trial failures. Ten of the 15 patients had significant pain relief with IT-clonidine and continued on clonidine at daily doses ranging from 75 μg/day to 944 μg/day. Patients were maintained on clonidine unless pain recurred despite dose escalation of clonidine, at which time an opioid was added to the intrathecal infusion. Eight patients received IT-clonidine in combination with IT-opioid medications. Seven of these had failed IT-clonidine alone; the eighth had previously failed IT-opioid and had clonidine added to his existing IT-opioid therapy. Three received hydromorphone (200 to 8000 mg/day) and four morphine (0.15 to 15 mg/day) with clonidine. Four patients then failed 2-drug therapy (duration 6 to 21 months). Two continued with intrathecal clonidine/hydromorphone (duration 19 to 29 months) and 1 with clonidine/ morphine (duration 21 months). After initiation of intrathecal clonidine, one patient reported good relief with clonidine/morphine until his death 5 months later. In this population, intrathecal clonidine was of limited utility for most patients. It may be of benefit for subset(s) of patients, but duration of relief was typically less than 18 months.

In summary, intrathecal clonidine is relatively safe and usually well tolerated. As monotherapy for pain complaints that are predominantly neuropathic in origin, it does not provide consistent pain relief. When clonidine is used in combination with IT-opioids, relatively few patients (approximately 20%) obtain adequate pain relief.

Neostigmine

Cholinergic mechanisms are involved in the control of nociceptive input in the central nervous system and both muscarinic and nicotinic cholinergic receptors are located in the spinal cord dorsal horn.[184–185] Animal models demonstrate that IT-neostigmine produces dose-dependent antinociception at the muscarinic and to a lesser degree at the nicotinic receptors.[186] IT-neostigmine also produces an antagonism on touch-evoked allodynia at the spinal level in a rat model of neuropathic pain.[187] IT-neostigmine probably inhibits the metabolism of spinally released acetylcholine while increasing the concentration of acetylcholine in CSF which acts on spinal muscarinic and nicotinic receptors.[188] The clinical use of IT-cholinesterase inhibitors such as neostigmine is limited because of its side-effects.[189] However, low-dose spinal neostigmine may improve morphine analgesia without increasing the incidence of side effects.[190–191]

Eisenach et al.[192] performed a Phase I tolerability and safety study of the commercially available neostigmine formulation in human volunteers and found no evidence of toxicity. Studies in human volunteers have shown that intrathecal neostigmine lacks neurotoxicity and produces very low plasma concentrations,[193] by contrast to a long-lasting, measurable CSF concentration. Klamt et al.[194] reported on the successful use of bolus injection of neostigmine in two patients with cancer pain. The pain relieving effect of neostigmine was of slow onset and long duration in both patients. Gastrointestinal discomfort occurred in both cases, even with dose reduction. IT-neostigmine causes nausea and sedation in humans.[195] Intrathecal bolus injections of neostigmine (150 μg) caused mild nausea, and 500 to 750 μg caused severe nausea and vomiting. Neostigmine (150 to 750 μg) produced subjective leg weakness, decreased deep tendon reflexes, and sedation. The 750-μg dose was associated with anxiety, increased blood pressure and heart rate, and decreased end-tidal carbon dioxide.[193] To date, there are no properly conducted trials of the use of intrathecal neostigmine in cancer pain. We have no personal experience with intrathecal neostigmine and therefore cannot recommend its use in routine clinical practice for the treatment of cancer pain.

Ziconotide

The marine snail *Conus magus* produces venom that alters neuromuscular function when injected into prey. Components of this venom include ω-conopeptides that prevent voltage-gated entry of calcium within neuronal cells. A synthetically derived form of this ω-conopeptide, ziconotide (Prialt), binds to N-type voltage-sensitive calcium channels (VSCC), blocking neurotransmitter release through inhibition of calcium influx.[196]

As it is a complex protein susceptible to proteolytic enzymes, ziconotide must be administered intrathecally via continuous infusion. Adverse events can be neuropsychiatric and include depression, cognitive impairment, hallucinations, and depressed levels of consciousness. Many adverse effects are also cerebellar in origin, including nystagmus and dysmetria.[197] Elevation of serum creatine kinase levels has also been reported.

Staats et al.[198] studied the effect of IT-ziconotide on refractory pain in patients with cancer or AIDS. IT-ziconotide was titrated over 5 to 6 days, followed by a 5-day maintenance phase for responders and crossover of nonresponders to the opposite treatment group. Sixty-seven (98.5%) of 68 patients receiving ziconotide and 38 (95%) of 40 patients receiving placebo were taking opioids at baseline (median morphine equivalent dosage of 300 mg/day for the ziconotide group and 600 mg/day for the placebo group, and 36 had used IT-morphine. Because of side effects, the starting dosage of ziconotide was subsequently reduced to 0.1 μg/hour or less, with upward titrations once every 24 hours to the point of analgesic effect or to a discretionary maximum dosage of 2.4 μg/hour. Mean VAS pain intensity scores improved 53.1% (95% CI: 44.0%–62.2%) in the ziconotide group and 18.1% (95% CI: 4.8%–31.4%) in the placebo group ($P < .001$), with no loss of efficacy of ziconotide in the maintenance phase. Pain relief was moderate to complete in 52.9% of patients in the ziconotide group compared with 17.5% in the placebo group ($P < .001$). Five patients receiving ziconotide achieved complete pain relief, and 50% of patients receiving ziconotide responded to therapy, compared with 17.5% of those receiving placebo ($P = .001$). Confusion occurred much more often in patients receiving ziconotide who were older than 60 years than in those aged 60 years or younger. CNS adverse events (ie, cognitive dysfunction, vestibular symptoms, and somnolence) had a median time to resolution of 4 days (range: 0 to 58 days). Adverse events led to early discontinuation in 12 patients receiving ziconotide and in four receiving placebo. Ziconotide is extremely costly and must be titrated slowly. A significant proportion of the patients who have been trialed on this drug have experienced unacceptable and intolerable side effects to the drug. As it must be delivered intrathecally by constant infusion, its use has been restricted mainly to patients who already have an implanted pump and catheter and who have failed opioids and other drugs.

Meperidine

IT-meperidine has been used effectively for selective spinal analgesia in patients with intractable cancer pain.[199–200] Meperidine is a phenylpiperidine compound of intermediate lipid solubility. It was originally synthesized as an anticholinergic compound; however, it also has significant local anesthetic properties as well as being a μ and κ opioid receptor agonist. Phenylpiperidine opioids are known to block conduction in peripheral nerves and intrathecal administration of meperidine will provide surgical anesthesia similar to 5% hyperbaric lidocaine.[201] Although these effects may in part be explained on the basis of its cocaine-like effects,[202] meperidine has been demonstrated to block Na^+ channels with molecular pharmacologic features comparable to those of lidocaine.[203] Meperidine, unlike morphine and hydromorphone, also has activity at κ receptors, with κ activity accounting for up to 10% of its total opioid action.[204] In animal studies, κ receptor agonists have known antinociceptive effects[205] and have also been demonstrated to attenuate opioid withdrawal induced hyperalgesia.[206] Meperidine has central anticholinergic actions associated with binding to muscarinic receptors in the brain.[207]

Meperidine use is associated with the accumulation of normeperidine, a metabolite responsible for central nervous system toxicity. Since long-term use of meperidine may be associated with toxicity caused by accumulation, the safety of IT-meperidine is questionable for the treatment of cancer pain. Vranken et al.[200] studied the plasma concentrations of meperidine and normeperidine following continuous intrathecal meperidine in ten patients with neuropathic cancer pain. Plasma meperidine levels ranged from below 600 ng/mL to 1840 ng/mL and normeperidine levels from below 40 ng/mL to 423 ng/mL. Meperidine and normeperidine levels increased rapidly during the first days of intrathecal meperidine treatment in three patients. Additionally, in one patient, the plasma normeperidine concentration was higher than the meperidine concentration although the plasma concentrations remained below the level (500 ng/mL) reported to induce CNS toxicity.[208] According to Kaiko et al.,[209] who investigated the relationship between plasma concentrations of normeperidine and CNS toxicity, an increasing amount of normeperidine in plasma is responsible for increasing excitatory symptoms including nervousness, agitation, hyperreflexia, myoclonus, tremors, and seizures (median normeperidine concentrations of 303, 519, and 640 ng/mL, for no symptoms, mild symptoms and seizures, respectively). In 1979, Cousins et al.[210] described the administration of single intrathecal doses ranging from between 10 and 30 mg of meperidine to patients with severe intractable cancer pain. In these cases, pain relief for up to 48 hours was reported. Meperidine has been administered via an intrathecal pump for chronic nonmalignant pain.[211] In this case, intrathecal meperidine at doses of 10.3 mg/day provided satisfactory pain relief for 9 months with only transient dizziness being reported as a side effect. Souter et al.[199] reported on the use of intrathecal meperidine at 24 mg/day for 8 weeks with no adverse effects in a patient with cancer pain refractory to intrathecal morphine and bupivacaine. Plasma and CSF levels of meperidine and normeperidine were measured in this case. Plasma and CSF normeperidine levels were of similar magnitude (69.9 and 53.7 ng/mL, respectively); however, there was a considerable difference between the plasma and CSF meperidine levels (17.2 ng/mL and 789 ng/mL, respectively). Meperidine is very basic and it must be buffered if it is to be used with a Medtronic pump or it will corrode the pump tubing. Our experience with this drug has been exclusively with externalized delivery systems in patients with cancer.

Ketamine

Ketamine, a noncompetitive NMDA antagonist, can alter nociceptive transmission at the spinal level. Surgical anesthesia with a sensory block lasting 1 hour can be induced with 50 mg IT-ketamine.[212] In 1996, Yang et al.[213] demonstrated that IT-ketamine in combination with morphine was effective in controlling pain and improving quality of life in 20 cancer patients.

The most common commercial preparation is a recemic mixture of two enantiomers, S (+) ketamine and R (−) ketamine. In most countries, the racemic mixture is available, either preservative-free or with preservatives such as benzetholium chloride and chlorobutanol. Whereas racemic ketamine with preservatives induced mild spinal cord vacuolation as the predominant histopathologic finding,[214–215] preservative-free racemic ketamine has been shown to be devoid of neurotoxic effects after both single and repeated administration in animals.[216–218] S(+)

ketamine has four times the affinity of R (−) ketamine for the NMDA receptor and also binds to μ and κ opioid receptors. Its anesthetic potency is three times that of the racemic mixture.[219]

Vranken et al.[220] used preservative-free S (+)-ketamine intrathecally in combination with morphine, bupivacaine, and clonidine by continuous infusion in a patient with severe neuropathic cancer pain for 21 days. The patient had severe pain related to metastatic cecal carcinoma with metastatic disease to the lumbosacral plexus. Pain was inadequately controlled with an intrathecal infusion of morphine (20 mg/day), bupivacaine (60 mg/day), and clonidine 150 μg/day). Because of lower extremity weakness, the patient refused further increases in bupivacaine doses. The addition of S (+)-ketamine 20 mg/day resulted in almost complete pain relief and a reduction in both morphine and clonidine doses. Benrath et al.[221] used continuous IT-S (+)-ketamine for cancer-related neuropathic pain over a 3-month period and reported no significant side effects. S (+)-ketamine was added to morphine (120 mg/day) and clonidine (360 μg/day) at initial doses of 7.5 mg/day and increased to 50 mg/day by day 10. This resulted in a dramatic reduction in pain and allowed a reduction in morphine doses. Pain relief was deemed satisfactory over 10 weeks with a constant dose of S (+)-ketamine 22.5 mg/day, morphine 36 mg/day and clonidine 300 μg/day. Thereafter, S (+)-ketamine was increased to 30 mg/day to control a moderate increase in pain but morphine and clonidine doses were further decreased. No psychomimetic side-effects, such as sedation, dysphoria, or hallucinations, were noted at any time. The patient died 92 days after the start of S (+)-ketamine treatment with moderate pain levels at rest.

The lack of safety data on neurotoxicity, however, limits the neuraxial administration of S (+)-ketamine. Severe histopathologic abnormalities in the spinal cord and nerve roots including central chromatolysis, nerve shrinkage, neurophagia, microglial upregulation, and gliosis have been observed after intrathecal infusion of up to 50 mg/day S (+)-ketamine for 28 days in a cancer patient.[222] Kozek et al.[223] also reported on the intrathecal use of preservative-free S (+)-ketamine (22 mg/day), clonidine (540 μg/day), and morphine (58 mg/day) for 30 days in a patient with pelvic chondrosarcoma. A postmortem histological examination of the upper cervical spinal cord and the brainstem was performed after the patient died from sepsis and cardio-respiratory failure after his tumor resection. Unlike Vranken et al., they found no specific signs of neurotoxicity. Only moderate reactive gliosis in the trigeminal nuclei with activated microglia was found which was attributed to sepsis and severe illness. Stotz et al.[215] reported on the use of intrathecal ketamine in a 72-year-old woman with abdominal pain from a peritoneal malignant mesothelioma. The intrathecal catheter tip was at T7 and the patient's pain was controlled with commercially available ketamine (containing the preservative benzethonium chloride) at a mean daily dose of 67.2 mg in combination with bupivacaine 0.25%, morphine (0.12 mg/mL) and clonidine (3 μg/mL). The patient received this infusion for 7 days. At postmortem, focal lymphocytic vasculitis of the spinal cord and leptomeninges close to the catheter tip was found. The patient showed no signs of neurologic deficit before her death.

In an animal study on the histopathologic effects of IT preservative-free S (+)-ketamine, Vranken et al.[24] demonstrated mild to severe gray and white matter damage of the spinal cord. Most lesions were present around the spinal canal and consisted of small severely damaged areas resembling small infarctions. Identical subpial lesions were a frequent finding. In some spinal cords, focal white matter damage was observed. The gray matter damage ranged from central chromatolysis of motor neurons to obvious necrosis of small areas. The damage around the central canal consisted of ependymal loss and subependymal necrotic lesions. The subpial lesions showed mainly myelin loss combined with axonal swellings, necrosis, and reactive leukodiapedesis. The authors concluded that prolonged use of S (+)-ketamine had a serious toxic effect on the central nervous system in rabbits and urged appropriate caution in the use of intrathecal ketamine in humans. We do not routinely use ketamine for chronic intrathecal infusions in patients with cancer, especially if the patient is expected to survive for more than 30 days.

Midazolam

Midazolam is a $GABA_A$ receptor agonist benzodiazepine. It is a neuraxial analgesic because it reduces excitatory synaptic transmission by acting on the GABA type A/benzodiazepine receptor in interneurons, leading to a decrease in the excitability of spinal dorsal horn neurons.[225] Analgesic efficacy of IT-midazolam is demonstrated at doses below 2 mg per dose and in concentrations below 1 mg/mL. Combined intrathecal therapy with midazolam and morphine (a mixture of 2 mg midazolam and a variable dose of intrathecal morphine) also produced significant analgesia without side effects in two cancer patients resistant to large oral doses of morphine (up to 400 mg/day). Sedation and somnolence are the most commonly reported side effects. Motor dysfunction occurred only at larger doses in animals.[226]

Johansen et al.[227] reported on the histologic effects of continuous intrathecal midazolam in sheep and indicated that doses up to 15 mg/day of preservative-free midazolam were well tolerated. Single intrathecal doses of midazolam 10 mg were also reported as safe in cats.[228] However, evidence of spinal cord toxicity was found in a rabbit model after single lumbar intrathecal injections (300 μg) of midazolam.[229] Severe separation in myelin lamella of small, moderate, and large axons and honeycomb appearance, disorganization, nuclear membrane irregularity, and vacuole formation were found in the spinal medulla.

Borg and Krijnen[230] described the successful use of intrathecal midazolam and clonidine in four patients with refractory noncancer neuropathic and musculoskeletal pain. The addition of midazolam to intrathecal clonidine produced almost immediate and nearly complete pain relief that was sustained over an extensive period of time (greater than 2 years in one patient) without evidence of tolerance. Side effects were reported as minimal in these patients. Three of the four patients received intrathecal doses of midazolam of 6 mg/day and clonidine doses ranging from 450 to 600 μg/day. Aguilar et al.[122] reported on the successful addition of midazolam to a lumbar intrathecal infusion of bupivacaine and morphine over a

13-month period in a patient with severe pain associated with a sacrococcygeal chordoma. An intrathecal catheter placed at L4/5 with a subcutaneous port provided initial pain relief with a mixture of bupivacaine 3.5 mg/hour and morphine 1.35 mg/hour. For control of sudden, sharp, severe lower extremity pain, midazolam 0.15 mg/hour provided additional pain relief. Seven months later, because of progressively severe lower extremity pain, lidocaine 48.5 mg/hour was substituted for bupivacaine because of concerns of local anesthetic tachyphylaxis. At the end of treatment, the patient was receiving intrathecal morphine 3 mg/hour, midazolam 0.3 mg/hour, and lidocaine 48.5 mg/hour. The patient also self-administered hourly intrathecal boluses (up to 2 per hour) of morphine 0.5 mg, midazolam 0.05 mg, and lidocaine 8 mg. Of note, the patient remained hospitalized for the entire period after placement of the intrathecal catheter in part because of continued difficulty in controlling his pain and in part because of difficulty in continuing this system in the home setting.

SURGICAL IMPLANTATION TECHNIQUE OF EXTERNALIZED INTRATHECAL CATHETER

At the University of Washington Medical Center, we have evolved a technique for managing intractable cancer pain patients with an externalized intrathecal catheter with the intent of primarily infusing bupivacaine, not opioids. Before surgical implantation, many of these patients have had a percutaneous catheter trial of epidural bupivacaine. If adequate pain relief is obtained and after appropriate informed consent, the patient is brought to the operating room, given general anesthesia, placed in the lateral decubitus position, and the epidural catheter is removed. The desired site for the tip of the implanted catheter is marked on the skin using the fluoroscope for localization and a paper clip taped to the skin at the site of the mark. The site of catheter tip placement varies according to the site of the pain. For pain that is predominantly located in the lower extremity, catheter tips are placed under fluoroscopic guidance to approximately the L5 vertebral level. For pain that is predominantly reported in the pelvis or sacrum, catheter tips are placed in the region of T12 (conus), and for pain predominantly located in the abdomen, tips are placed at the mid-thoracic level. Before surgical draping, a site for the externalized catheter to exit the skin is marked on the upper abdomen on the nondependent side of the body.

The catheter entry site is chosen based upon the desired location of the tip so as to provide at least a four segment intrathecal course. Hence, if the tip is desired at T-12, an L4-5 or L5-S1 entry site is chosen; if the tip is planned to be at L5 or S1, a T-12 or L1 entry site is chosen with the needle angled caudally. A thoracic catheter placement is achieved via an L2-3 entry site. A midline incision of 2 inches' length is made over the spinous processes at the desired entry level and the skin margins retracted laterally with some undermining. The needle is always placed via a paramedian approach from the down side of the patient; the needle is angled steeply rostral for the lower lumbar and thoracic insertion sites and slightly caudal for the thoracolumbar insertion. The fluoroscope is used for guidance so that the dura is punctured only once, the intrathecal catheter (we have used various Medtronic [Minneapolis, MN] intrathecal catheters) threaded to the desired level using the fluoroscope and CSF flow is demonstrated. The anchoring device is placed around the catheter and sutured to the fascia and the end of the catheter is clamped.

The external segment of a DuPen catheter is then attached to a Pall rectangular filter and the system flushed with preservative-free saline. The provided DuPen trocar is placed in the end of the catheter and then is used to tunnel the catheter to the midline back incision from the abdominal site (Fig. 22.6). The antibiotic cuff is placed just below the skin. The DuPen catheter is then trimmed to a suitable length. The intrathecal catheter is trimmed to the appropriate length and the Medtronic metal connector pin inserted into it (Fig. 22.7). The connector boot is then slipped over the catheter onto the pin. The DuPen catheter is then placed over the connector pin and tied with a 2-0 silk. The connector is then sutured to the fascia with care being taken to insure that the tubing is not kinked or under tension. After antibiotic irrigation, the wound is closed in layers and a suture tied around the DuPen catheter at its exit point from the skin. Dry, sterile dressings are applied to both the back incision and the catheter egress site. When the patient reaches the PAC unit, the infusion pump, tubing and another Pall filter are bolused to fill the system and then attached to the Pall filter that was originally attached to the DuPen catheter in the operating room. A bolus of 2.6 cc is given to fill the second filter and the catheter system and an initial bolus of 1.0 cc of the drug mixture is given to the patient. The standard initial infusion rate is 0.4 cc/hour, and the customary initial infusate is a mixture of bupivacaine 0.5% (5 mg/cc) plus preservative free morphine 200 μg/cc in 100cc preservative free saline. If the patient has known intolerance to morphine, hydromorphone (1 mg/mL) is substituted.

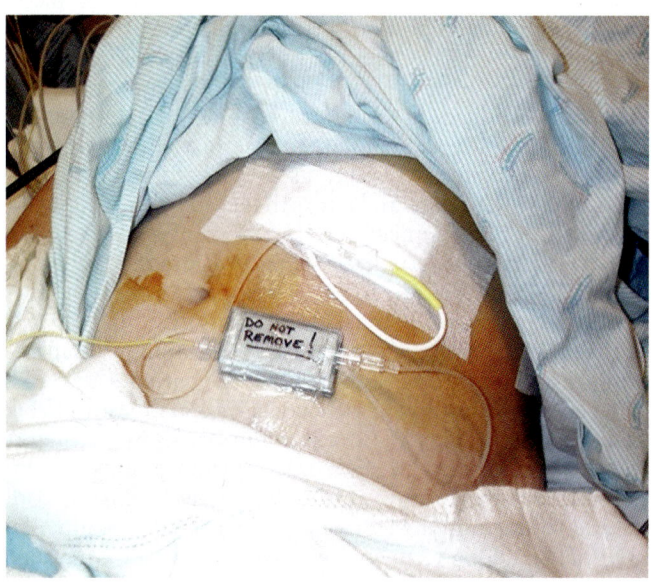

FIGURE 22.6 Externalized implanted intrathecal catheter. Two Pall rectangular filters are attached to the infusion line of the externalized pump. The catheter exit site is secured with Primapore dressing.

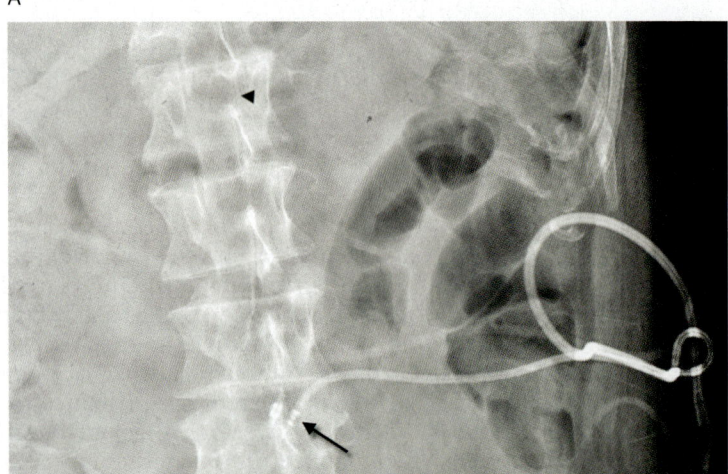 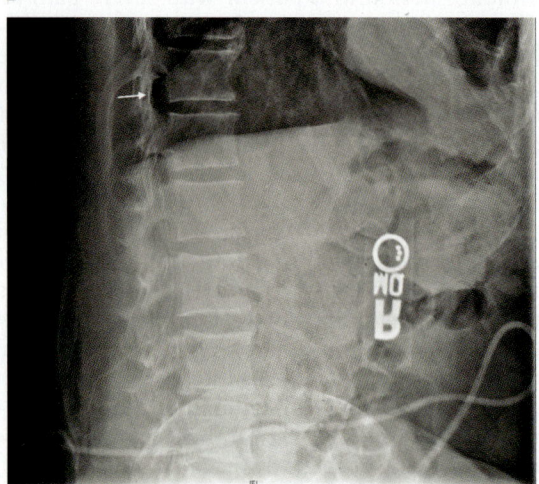

FIGURE 22.7 A 56-year-old man with recurrent left lower extremity pain and buttock pain from a recurrent pelvic chondrosarcoma involving the left buttock and encompassing the sciatic nerve at the sciatic notch. An externalized intrathecal catheter was placed for pain control. **A:** Anteroposterior view of the abdomen shows the larger tunneled system joined to the smaller intrathecal portion in the lumbar paraspinal area *(arrow)*. The catheter is directed upward in the midline *(arrow head)*. Lateral view of the spine (**B**) shows the catheter in the spinal canal with the catheter tip at approximately the T12 vertebral level *(arrow)*.

INFECTION ASSOCIATED WITH EXTERNALIZED SYSTEMS

The relative risk of CNS infections in patients with altered immune status (associated with malignancy or other causes) compared to the normal host is unknown.[231] Instrumentation of the neuraxis with placement of indwelling, externalized catheters in patients who are potentially immunocompromised would appear to be potentially risky from an infection perspective. Data comparing the use of various Hickman line and Port-a-Cath infection rates in patients with solid tumors undergoing chemotherapy suggest a threefold higher infection rate (2.54/100 catheter-days and 0.86/100 catheter-days) for Hickman lines.[232] Infections associated for these devices are usually either catheter-insertion-site related (1.4/1000 catheter-days) or catheter-related blood-stream infections (0.75/1000 catheter-days).[233] The number of manipulations, the duration of use of the device, the ability of the people performing the procedures in either the hospital or at home, the materials employed for maintenance procedures, the patients' socioeconomic conditions, and the correct functioning of the catheter are all factors that could represent a risk for catheter-related infections.[234]

The safety of externalized tunneled neuraxial catheters, particularly in relation to the development of meningitis and epidural abscess, has been questioned.[11,17,235-236] Tunneling of percutaneous catheters is mainly used in the long-term treatment of chronically ill patients. Devices used in this setting generally consist of (1) externalized, long-term intrathecal/epidural nylon or silastic catheters connected to external, electronic infusion pumps; (2) internalized, long-term intrathecal catheters (silastic) connected to implanted Medtronic Synchromed™ pumps; (c) internalized, long-term epidural nylon or silastic catheters, connected to catheter injection ports, Infusaid™ pumps; or Synchromed™ pumps.

Serious bacterial infection of the neuraxis may present as meningitis or cord compression due to abscess formation. Epidural abscess is primarily a complication of epidural catheter use; the route of infection is via the catheter entry point and the causative organism is usually Staphylococcus. Nosocomial meningitis is a complication of dural puncture (for whatever purpose) and is usually caused by streptococci of the viridians type, commonly found in the upper air passages and the vagina. Although epidural abscess most often arises in association with systemic infection,[237] it is an uncommon but devastating complication associated with continuous epidural analgesia.[238] The infectious source is either exogenous or endogenous. Exogenous sources may be contaminated equipment or medication or from the proceduralist's nasal mucosa (most commonly *Streptococcus viridans* or *Staphylcoccus aureus*). Indwelling catheters may be colonized from a superficial site and subsequently serve as a conduit for spread of infection from the skin to the epidural or intrathecal space. Endogenous causes include seeding to the site of catheter insertion from a patient source such as an open wound or decubitus ulcer.

Patients with acute bacterial meningitis may deteriorate rapidly. The initial clinical picture of meningitis is usually of headache and fever, often with backache and emetic symptoms, classical signs of meningism, drowsiness, and lethargy. Cases can be confused with dural puncture headache. If treated promptly, the condition is usually benign. In severe and untreated cases, the patient may become unrousable, with diabetes insipidus and other signs of cerebral edema. The CSF is often cloudy and shows an elevated white cell count, predominantly neutrophils, raised protein, and low glucose concentrations. Pending additional information about the responsible organism, vancomycin and a third generation cephalosporin should be given intravenously.

In the case of epidural abscess, the presenting symptom is usually backache, often extremely severe, with marked local tenderness, and, sometimes, associated radicular pain. A blood count will reveal elevated C-reactive protein and white count. Neurologic deficit may follow, in the form of leg weakness, paresthesia, bladder dysfunction, and other evidence of myelopathy or cauda equina syndrome. Diagnosis is confirmed by a contrast-enhanced MRI. Most infections are bacterial. The majority of epidural abscesses are caused by *Staphylococcus aureus*, with occasional *Streptococcus* and *Pseudomonas spp*. With catheter track infections, organisms such as *Staphylococcus epidermidis* may come from the patient's own skin flora.

Externalized Epidural Catheters

The type of catheter system may influence the development of catheter track infection. Rates of superficial and deep catheter track infections are approximately 6% with epidural systems with Dacron cuffs,[239] approximately 11% with both cuffed and noncuffed epidural catheters,[240] and 25% with noncuffed epidural catheters.[241] Overall infection rates of 23.7%[240] and 25%[242] associated with long-term epidural catheters have been reported. Severe complications, such as epidural space infections, occur at rates between 4.3% and 5.3%.

In the DuPen study, the rate of epidural and deep track catheter-related infections was one in every 1,702 days of silastic catheter use.[240] Infection of epidural catheter systems usually begins at the skin exit site. The bacteria cultured from the space are most frequently from skin flora contamination (*S. aureus* or *epidermidis*), but occasionally include *Escherichia coli*. Patients who are immunosuppressed may yield a wider variety of organisms. Catheter infections involve *S. aureus* more than 90% of the time. If organisms such as *Campylobacter* spp. appear, a contaminated infusion solution should be suspected. Track infections may also occur. Sillevis Smitt et al.[243] reported on an epidural abscess complicating long-term epidural pain relief in 11 cancer patients, 10 of whom had metastatic disease. These patients developed the abscess a median of 25 days after placement of the catheter (range: 12 to 166 days). All patients had back pain; radicular signs occurred in seven patients and spinal cord compression in two patients. MRI revealed an abscess in all 11 patients. The abscess was iso- to hypointense on T1-weighted images and hyperintense on T2-weighted images relative to spinal cord (Fig. 22.8). After I.V. gadolinium, seven lesions showed characteristic rim enhancement and three showed minimal enhancement. No signs of discitis or osteomyelitis were present, and the abscess was always localized to the posterior epidural space. Cultures were positive in all cases and revealed *S. epidermidis* in eight and *S. aureus* in three. All patients were treated with intravenous antibiotics, and four had decompressive laminectomies.

DuPen et al.[240] presented guidelines for the management of epidural catheter-related infections based upon their clinical experiences. A deep catheter/epidural infection should be suspected on clinical grounds (pain during epidural injection, soft fluctuant mass under posterior incision, decreasing epidural pain relief even with increasing dose, constant and nonspecific back pain). Thorough daily cleaning with povidone-iodine is sufficient to treat superficial track and exit site infections; topical and/or oral antibiotics should be used depending on the extent of involvement and the initial response to treatment. All deep catheter track and epidural infections require catheter removal and treatment with parenteral antibiotic therapy. The duration of treatment depends on the organism cultured. Catheters may be replaced after completion of antibiotics and an MRI scan indicates no further epidural involvement or inflammation. Deep catheter infections require in-patient management. Treat with antibiotics (usually vancomycin) for at least 10 days. The catheter should be flushed with 1 cc of saline and then aspirated. If fluid is obtained, send it for culture. Continue flushing and aspirating until the aspirate is clear. When culture results are available, shift to appropriate

A

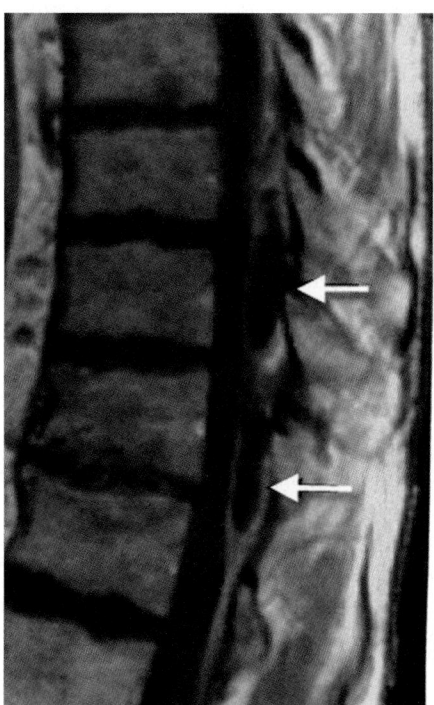

B

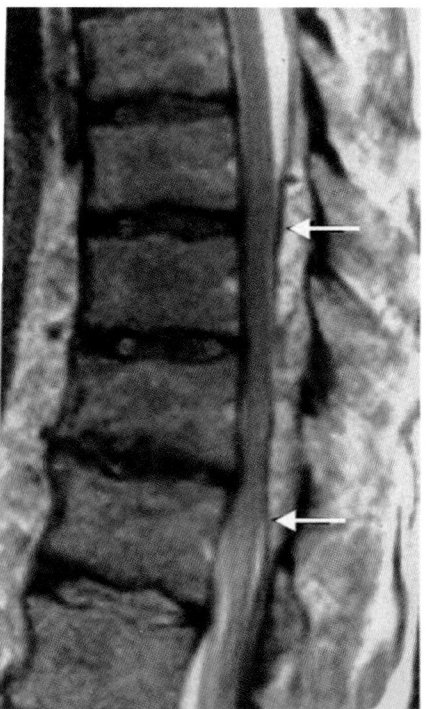

FIGURE 22.8 MRI showing spinal epidural abscess. Sagittal T1-weighted image after the administration of gadolinium (**A**) demonstrates a rim-enhancing epidural abscess (*arrows*) extending from T8 to T12. Relative to spinal cord, the lesion is iso- to hypointense on the T1-weighted image and hyperintense on the T2-weighted image (**B**). MRI, Magnetic resonance imaging. (Modified from Sillevis Smitt P, Tsafka A, van den Bent M, et al. Spinal epidural abscess complicating chronic epidural analgesia in 11 cancer patients: Clinical findings and magnetic resonance imaging. *J Neurol.* 1999; 246:815–820. Used with permission from Springer Science+Business Media.)

intravenous antibiotics as needed. The catheter should be left *in situ* until no further aspirate can be obtained (acts to decompress the epidural space) Thereafter, the catheter should be removed.

Externalized Intrathecal Catheters

Nitescu et al.[14] reviewed the risk of infectious complications associated with externalized intrathecal catheters (233 total) in 200 patients with refractory cancer pain. Patients received either intermittent injections (median: 3 per day; range: 1 to 16/day) or continuous infusions. The duration of treatment ranged from 1 to 575 days (median: 33 days), totaling 14,485 days. Catheter insertion-site infection, defined as the presence of purulent fluid at the site and signs of inflammation of the surrounding tissues, occurred in one (0.5%) patient. Tunnel exit and deep catheter track infections did not occur. Epidural abscess did not occur. Meningitis occurred in one (0.5%) patient, representing one case per 14,485 days. The authors speculated that the most important factor in preventing local infection was the secure fixation of the catheter with the externalized systems in order to prevent to-and-fro movements of the catheter and the transport of skin bacteria into the subcutaneous reactive passage formed around the catheter. The fear of meningitis has presented a major obstacle to the use of intrathecal pain treatment. However, this report and others[16,98] do not support these fears.

To minimize the risk of infection associated with externalized neuraxial systems, we recommend that the catheter be tunneled and fixed at the skin, the use of antibacterial filters (ideally, 2 rectangular Pall 0.2 micron filters in series), minimal handling of the tubing, careful exit care weekly, and education of family members on appropriate care of catheters and associated systems. We have had very few catheter-related infections in our experience with externalized intrathecal drug delivery systems.

Internalized Intrathecal Systems

Intrathecal drug delivery system (IDDS) infection occurs in approximately 1% to 2% of patients with implanted pumps.[70,244] Infections may arise from the pump, reservoir, or catheter. These infections are usually due to organisms of low virulence. The organisms most implicated in pump and catheter infections are the coagulase-negative staphylococci, such as *S. epidermidis*, which accounts for 50% to 75% of infections. The next most frequent causes of infection include *S. aureus*, Gram-negative enteric bacteria, and anaerobic diphtheroids. Meningitis is a very rare event; the reported incidence of meningitis with implanted pumps ranges from 0%[245] to less than 0.7%.[246] Frequent percutaneous refilling of implanted pumps may increase the risk for pump contamination and infection.[247] In a review of the effectiveness and complications associated with IDDS for chronic noncancer pain, one case of meningitis and six cases of wound infection in 50 patients were identified, but only a small fraction of the reviewed case series reported their complications, and the accuracy of these rates was not clear.[248]

Superficial wound infection at the site of implantation may be managed with intravenous antibiotics and local wound care. In the setting of meningitis, however, the pump probably needs to be removed although there are reports of successful treatment of intrathecal drug delivery device-associated meningitis with intravenous antibiotics and intrareservoir administration of antibiotics without removal of the pump system.[249–251] Pump pocket infection requires removal of the pump system as well as long-term intravenous antibiotic therapy. Byers et al.[252] reported on 75 cancer patients who had 87 implanted catheters. Seven infections were reported, two being meningeal. Of these, four of the patients' catheters were left in situ, and they were given antibiotics via intravenous and oral route only. They were not given intrathecal antibiotics. These four patients were not cured of infection. Schoeffler et al.[253] followed 36 consecutive patients with intrathecal systems. Six cases of meningitis were reported. Four of these intrathecal catheters were left in situ for antibiotic administration, continued pain relief, and CSF sampling. Two catheters were removed because of infection at the site of catheter entry. All six patients received intravenous antibiotics, and the four patients with in situ catheters received intrathecal aminoglycosides. In all these patients, fever and symptoms disappeared in 2 to 3 days, and CSF was sterile within 48 hours of treatment. Carputo and Philip[254] reported on a case in which meningitis secondary to an intrathecal delivery system (tunneled intrathecal catheter with Port-a-Cath, percutaneously accessed) was successfully treated with intravenous and intrathecal antibiotics while the catheter remained in situ for ongoing pain relief. Microbiologic culture of CSF grew *Klebsiella* pneumoniae, and the patient was treated with intravenous ceftriaxone (chosen because of sensitivities and ability to penetrate the CSF) for 7 days and a single dose of intrathecal dose ceftriaxone 400 mg.

We believe that the significant infection rate with implanted externalized catheters is low and should not preclude the use of this drug delivery system in appropriately selected patients when oral or systemic drug administration fails to give adequate pain relief or produces unacceptable side effects. It is clear that operator experience and attention to detail when implanting or utilizing such a system is critical. Infections with fully implanted pumps and catheters occur at a higher rate because of the large foreign object that is placed beneath the skin of the abdominal wall. Nonetheless, when this treatment strategy is indicated, it should be utilized in spite of the significant complication rate. Obtaining adequate pain relief may have some risks, but the patient is entitled to a trial if other methods of pain relief have failed.

LIMITATIONS OF NEURAXIAL THERAPY

The decision to proceed to neuraxial therapy for cancer pain management must be based upon a variety of factors. In every situation, the nociceptive process must be amenable to interruption or modulation by neuraxial medications. This is particularly true in the case of local anesthetic agents. Distribution of local anesthetics is limited in both the epidural and intrathecal spaces. Failure or inadequate delivery may occur because of anatomical (eg, lumbosacral distribution with lumbar epidural catheters), pathologic (eg, impending spinal cord occlusion from tumor growth), mechanical issues (pump, catheter failure), or choice of route (epidural vs. intrathecal). The space-occupying role of epidural metastases may reduce the efficacy of epidural pain management[255] (see "Implications of Epidural Metastasis and Spinal Canal Occlusion for Neuraxial Drug Treatment," page 296). Compared to epidural management, intrathecal administration has a lower incidence of catheter occlusion, lower malfunction rate, lower dose and volume requirements, and provides more effective pain control.[128] Life expectancy may also influence decision making. Some clinicians will preferentially consider externalized, tunneled systems if life expectancy is less than 3 months, and more sophisticated infusion devices (eg, implanted, programmable pumps) if life expectancy is greater than 3 months.[4] Financial and geographic issues limit the number of patients who can benefit from this treatment option. Although epidural externalized systems are relatively inexpensive at the outset of treatment, charges for home health care, the drug, and associated equipment including pump rental can result in a fairly rapid cost escalation. Using this particular paradigm at 15 months, a patient with an externalized system may have $100,000 or $120,000 of total charges related to the drug, the pump, home health care, and all other charges involved in his or her treatment.[256] From the perspective of cost analysis, Bedder et al.[235] suggest that implanted programmable pumps (eg, SynchroMed) become cost effective after 3 months, compared to other infusion systems. Remote geographical locations hinder access to home infusion services or limit the ability to return for specialized care in the event of pump or catheter malfunction.

Technical issues related to spinal morphine delivery (epidural or intrathecal) were reported by Crul and Delhaas in terminally ill cancer patients.[16] Technical issues included obstruction and dislocation of the catheter and infection. Treatment time varied from 10 to 366 days. During the first 20 days of treatment, the incidence of complications was different between the epidural group (8%) and the intrathecal group (25%). During the remainder of the treatment period, the complication rate rose to 55% in patients receiving epidural morphine and decreased to 5% in the intrathecal group. The most frequent complication in the epidural group was obstruction and dislocation of the catheter, presumably due to the development of epidural fibrosis. This problem became apparent in more than half of these patients during the treatment period from day 20 to 366. The prevalent complication in the intrathecal group was CSF leakage, which was observed only during the first 2 weeks of treatment. Hence, intrathecal administration is better for patients with expected survival of more than a few months.

Nitescu et al.[14] compared the rates of postinsertion complications of externalized intrathecal catheters with published rates for externalized epidural and intrathecal catheters, as well as implanted epidural and intrathecal catheters connected to subcutaneously implanted ports, reservoirs, or pumps. Standardized care after insertion in the externalized intrathecal patients included daily telephone contact with the patients, their families, or the nurse in charge, weekly dressing changes at the catheter skin outlet by the nurses, refilling of the infusion containers by nurses, exchange of the infusion systems when empty (within 1 month) and of the antibacterial filter once a month by nurses. Providers carefully avoided all contact between the connections of the syringes, cassettes, and needles with the operator's hands during filling and refilling of the infusion containers and exchange of the antibacterial filters. Table 22.5 lists the rates (as a percentage of the number of patients) of perfect function and complications of the systems in Nitescu et al. series versus the range of rates reported in the literature.[14]

Persistent CSF Leak After Dural Puncture

A CSF leak at the dural puncture site following implantation of an intrathecal catheter is typically a self-limiting complication. It is believed that CSF leakage can occur around the implanted catheter because the hole created by the needle exceeds the caliber of the catheter. A CSF leak that persists despite conservative therapy, however, may significantly increase morbidity. A persistent CSF leak may cause a post–dural puncture headache and is a cause of intracranial hypotension. Intracranial hypotension is a syndrome in which volume depletion of the CSF results in various neurologic symptoms. Most commonly, a small tear or defect in the spinal dural sac (which may occur whether spontaneously or as a result of a dural puncture) results in a CSF leakage and intracranial hypotension. Typical spinal radiographic findings include extra-arachnoid or extradural fluid collections, meningeal enhancement, engorgement of the epidural venous plexus, and tonsilar descent into the foramen magnum. MRI of the head and spine has improved the diagnosis of this syndrome, showing abnormalities including diffuse pachymeningeal enhancement, subdural fluid collections and downward displacement of the cerebral structures.

A dural cutaneous fistula may lead to meningitis; a meningocoele (hygroma) may disrupt the skin closure or contribute to the accumulation of fluid at a pump pocket site, if a pump is implanted. With persistent open leakage of CSF, complete wound debridement and surgical repair may be necessary.

Our routine treatment of CSF leak after dural puncture consists of initial conservative symptomatic treatment with progression to epidural injection of autologous blood, which can be repeated if necessary.[257] Conservative measures typically include bed rest, rehydration, the application of an abdominal binder, and liberal use of caffeine and simple analgesics. Since the epidural blood patch was introduced, it has been applied widely and safely. However, CSF leaks occasionally may persist in spite of repeated lumbar epidural blood patches. Dominguez et al.[258] described the successful application of a subdural blood patch that led to the satisfactory resolution of a persistent CSF leak after previous epidural blood patches had failed.

Fibrin glue is a preparation of pooled human plasma obtained from plasmapheresis. It has high tensile strength and tolerates highly moist environments. The fibrin clot forms a temporary biological seal of the dura until healing occurs.[259] Fibrin glue is widely applied in otology and neurosurgery as a method to achieve a watertight dural closure.[260] Crul et al.[261] described the successful use of 3 mL of lumbar epidural fibrin glue in a young patient

TABLE 22.5

RATES (PERCENTAGE OF PATIENTS) OF PERFECT FUNCTION AND COMPLICATIONS OF THE SYSTEMS IN NITESCU ET AL. SERIES VERSUS RATES REPORTED IN THE LITERATURE

System function/complication	% Rate Nitescu et al.	% Rate reported in literature
Perfect function	93	31 to 90
Accidental injury of unknown epidural tumor followed by epidural hematoma	0.5	0 to 6
Skin breakdown at insertion site	2	2 to 50
Postdural puncture headache	15.5	10
External leakage of cerebrospinal fluid	3.5	4 to 27
Cerebrospinal fluid hygroma	1.5	4 to 6.25
Hearing loss and Meniere-like syndrome	0	12
Pain on injection:		
Intermittent injection	4.5	3 to 36
Continuous infusion	0	
Catheter tip dislodgement	1.5	6 to 33
Catheter (system) occlusion	1	3 to 12
Accidental catheter withdrawal	4	3 to 22
Catheter (system) leakage	1.5	2.1 to 26.6
All mechanical complications	8.5	10 to 44
Local (catheter entry site) infection	0.5	2 to 33
Catheter track infection	0	6 to 25
Epidural abscess	0	0.6 to 25
Meningitis	0.5	1 to 25
Systemic infection	0	3
Incidence of all infections (per no. treatment days)	1/7242	1/168 to 1/2446

From Nitescu P, Sjoberg M, Appelgren L, et al. Complications of intrathecal opioids and bupivacaine in the treatment of "refractory" cancer pain *Clin J Pain*. 1995;11:45–62)

with persistent CSF leak after a lumbar puncture with a 25-gauge pencil-point needle. Gerritse et al.[262] described their experience in three cancer patients with persistent CSF leaks that had failed initial treatment with epidural blood patch. In all three patients, CSF leakage stopped within an hour of lumbar epidural injection of 3 to 4 mL of fibrin glue.

Surgical repair may be necessary in rare, persistent cases. Repair can vary from placing a purse-string suture at the site where the catheter exits through the lumbar fascia posteriorly to laminectomy and dural repair with watertight suture placement and fibrin glue. With large defects or with leakage from suture holes, a paraspinal fascial or fascia lata graft or artificial dura may be used along with fibrin glue.

NOVEL TECHNIQUES WITH INTRATHECAL THERAPY

A few reports have been published describing uncommon techniques that may have utility in properly selected patients. There are not enough published data to allow us to generate recommendations about these; they are included to make sure that the reader is aware of some of the nonstandard options.

Continuous Intracisternal and High Cervical Intrathecal Bupivacaine

Progressive tumor growth in the head and neck often leads to various types of pain localized to the distribution of both the cervical nerve roots and cranial nerves. The upper cervical components of the spinomesencephalic tract cells and cranial nerves V, VII, IX, and X are involved in mechanisms of pain from head, face, and neck structures. The pain may be limited to one side but is seldom confined to the distribution of one nerve. In patients with diffuse upper neck and head pain, the source of pain often involves multiple nerves. Cranial nerves and peripheral somatic nerves often provide overlapping nociceptive afferent input. In addition to somatic pain, burning discomfort may result from nociceptive pathways within the sympathetic chain. These circumstances restrict the usefulness of nerve blocks and peripheral neuroablative procedures.

Appelgren et al.[123] reported on 13 patients with complex, refractory pain who received continuous intracisternal or high cervical subarachnoid infusions of bupivacaine as a method to control pain in the head, face, mouth, neck, and upper extremities. Patients received bupivacaine continuously at rates of 1 to 7 (median: 1.5) mg/hour with optional bolus doses of 0.5 to 2.0 mg 2 to 4 times per hour.

They assessed efficacy utilizing VAS scores, daily dose of intracisternal bupivacaine and total opioid, amount of nocturnal sleep, and rates of adverse effects. Patients were treated from 3 to 182 days (median: 37; total: 712 days). The investigators could not evaluate one patient because of the patient's advanced senility. For most patients (11 of the remaining 12), infusions of bupivacaine provided satisfactory pain relief, decreased systemic opioid consumption, improved nocturnal sleep patterns, and improved overall function. Daily doses of intracisternal bupivacaine ranged from 20 to 118 mg (median: 37 mg). Average VAS scores decreased from 7 to 2. Total daily opioid dose decreased from median values of 53 to 36 mg parenteral morphine equivalents. Nocturnal sleep increased from median values of 2 to >6 hour. In patients with refractory pain from the shoulders and upper extremities, the intracisternal administration of bupivacaine gave less pain relief than intrathecal administration of the same bupivacaine doses at the midcervical (C4-C5) levels.

Associated side effects generally were dose related and similar to those described with more caudal sites of infusion. Signs of motor impairment of the cranial nerves occurred for the somatic fibers of the vagal nerve, expressed as hoarseness after intrathecal injection of 5.0 mg bupivacaine, in all intracisternal tests, and of the glossopharyngeal nerve (dysphagia) after a bolus dose of 7.5 mg bupivacaine. No signs of motor impairment from the other cranial nerves appeared at therapeutic doses. Paresis of the upper extremities occurred in two patients at intracisternal doses of bupivacaine of 1.5 and 5 mg/hour, respectively. No patient experienced gross impairment of phrenic nerve activity. The absence of obvious phrenic nerve paralysis is notable, and it probably reflects the greater resistance of the large motor fibers of the phrenic to the effects of local anesthetic agents.[263]

Unusual side effects included one patient experiencing severe tiredness, faintness, and malaise and one experiencing somnolence and sleep. These side effects emerged transiently with relatively high infusion rates (3 mg/hour) or large bolus doses and resolved after decreasing the infusion rate or withholding the bolus dose. They may derive from a decrease of skeletal muscle tone, inhibition of the tonic activity of the reticular substance by reduction of signals from the peripheral receptors, and loss of control of fairly specific motor tasks, such as rhythmic locomotor movements, and of eye, head, and body movements in response to optic and vestibular stimuli. No persistent neurologic deficit or death could be attributed to the intracisternal drug administration.

Appelgren et al. concluded that long-term intracisternal administration of bupivacaine might help the rare, well-selected patient with refractory pain from the head, face, and neck structures to obtain adequate pain relief when alternate methods have failed. Although the actual mechanism of pain relief is unknown, Carpenter and Rauck[264] contend that the low doses of bupivacaine used in the study suggest the possibility of a central neuronal analgesic effect. With the catheter tip being located at the height of the C1 or C2 vertebral bodies, in the lower part of the cisterna magna, local anesthetic may affect conduction on the lower seven cranial nerves, and the spinal trigeminal nucleus of the fifth nerve. Several nuclei involved in the processing of autonomic regulatory information (such as the nucleus of the tractus solitarius, and ventromedial and rostral ventrolateral medulla) may also be influenced by the infusion of bupivacaine[265] (Fig. 22.9).

Following Appelgren et al. observation that some patients reacted with increased blood pressure following intracisternal bolus doses of bupivacaine, Lambert et al.[265] studied hemodynamic changes in 16 patients with refractory pain of the head and neck associated with malignancy of the head and neck region during acute intracisternal bupivacaine administration. Intracisternal bupivacaine administration caused an almost instantaneous elevation in mean arterial blood pressure, increasing by 17 ±7 mm Hg after 10 minutes ($P < .01$). Heart rate increased in parallel (17 ±5 beats/minute), and these changes coincided with an increase in sympathetic nervous activity, peaking with an approximately 50% increase over resting level 10 min after injection ($P < .01$). By combining direct sampling of CSF, via a percutaneously placed catheter in the cisterna magna, with a noradrenaline and adrenaline isotope dilution method for examining sympathetic and adrenal medullary activity, the authors were able to quantify the release of brain neurotransmitters and examine efferent sympathetic nervous outflow in patients following intracisternal administration of bupivacaine. The observed hemodynamic changes imply that bolus doses of bupivacaine via this route of administration must be used with caution, since high con-

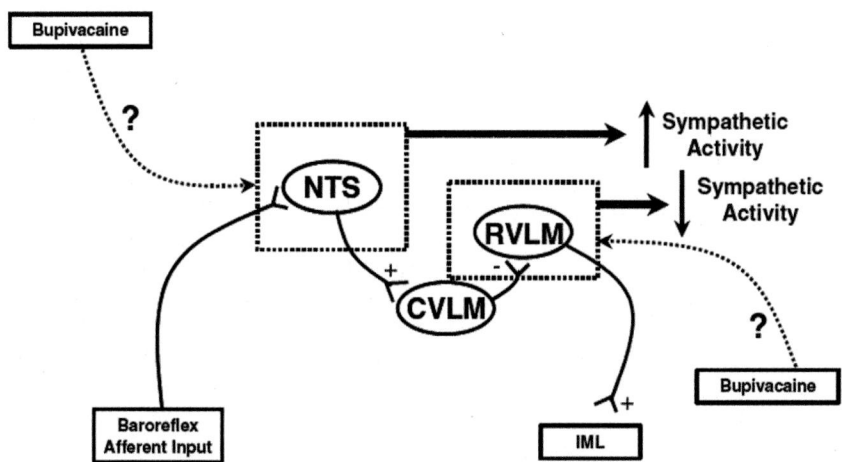

FIGURE 22.9 Hypothetical mechanism of action of intracisternal bupivacaine at the level of the medulla. Bupivacaine acts on different brainstem regions as a result of subtle variation in catheter placement, or alteration in the spread of drug. NTS, Nucleus of the tractus solitarius; RVLM, rostral ventrolateral medulla; CVLM, caudal ventrolateral medulla; IML, intermediolateral column of the spinal cord; + and −, stimulatory and inhibitory inputs, respectively. (From Lambert G, Elam M, Friberg P, et al. Acute response to intracisternal bupivacaine in patients with refractory pain of the head and neck. J Physiol. 2006;570:421–428. Used with permission of Wiley-Blackwell.)

centrations of intracisternal local anaesthetics may lead to increased risk of cardiovascular complications, including stroke and sympathetically mediated tachyarrhythmias. In an animal study assessing the neurotoxicologic effects of intracisternal liposomal bupivacaine, Malinovsky et al.[266] injected intracisternally 0.3 mL of bupivacaine 5 mg/mL. All animals had an immediate respiratory arrest and complete paralysis of the upper and lower limbs. Hypotension was observed in both the plain and liposomal bupivacaine groups and required hemodynamic support in the majority of animals. We have not utilized this route of delivery of intrathecal bupivacaine and have no personal experience upon which to base an opinion. Caution is obviously called for if this strategy is to be utilized.

Patient-Controlled Intrathecal Analgesia

A variety of medications, including morphine, bupivacaine, and clonidine, may be used both intrathecally and by PCA for the control of cancer pain. One aspect of the efficacy and high acceptance of PCA is the higher degree of satisfaction of patients who are involved in self-administration of drugs and self-monitoring of pain and side effects.[267–268] Ferrante et al.[269] demonstrated a significant reduction of the total bupivacaine requirement without any change in pain relief when comparing epidural PCA and continuous epidural infusion. Rundshagen et al. described patient-controlled intrathecal analgesia (PCIA) using bupivacaine for the control of postoperative pain[270] and Hardy et al.[271] described using PCIA morphine for cancer pain. Rauck et al.[86] evaluated the safety and efficacy of patient-activated delivery of intrathecal morphine sulfate boluses delivered by way of a novel internalized intrathecal delivery system in patients with refractory cancer pain or uncontrollable side effects. Systemic opioid use was significantly decreased throughout the study. The authors concluded that these patients achieved better pain control when managed with patient-activated intrathecal delivery via an implanted delivery system. We have utilized PCIA in carefully selected patients and believe that it can be a very useful delivery system, if the patient and support staff have received appropriate education about this technique.

IMPLICATIONS OF EPIDURAL METASTASIS AND SPINAL CANAL OCCLUSION FOR NEURAXIAL DRUG TREATMENT

The onset of back pain accompanies epidural metastasis in more than 60% of cancer patients and 80% to 95% of patients with confirmed epidural metastasis experience pain at some time during the course of the disease.[272–273] The intensity of pain and the associated neurologic deficit depends on the size of the epidural metastasis and consequently to the degree of epidural block. Patients with small epidural lesions may have no pain and no neurologic deficit.[274] The occurrence and severity of complications during insertion of epidural/intrathecal catheters may depend upon the location of the epidural tumor in relation to the puncture site, to the inserted catheter length in relation to the location of the epidural tumor,

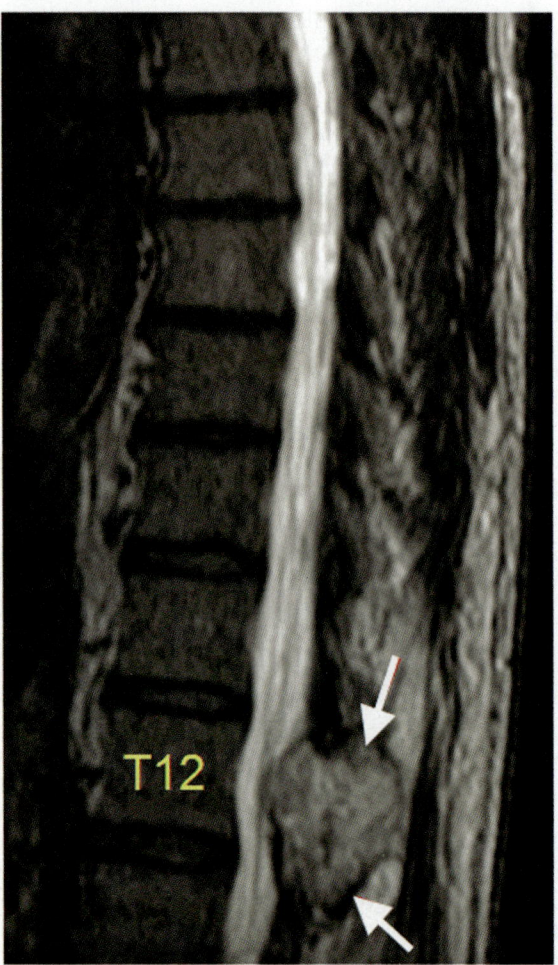

FIGURE 22.10 A 54-year-old man with metastatic melanoma to T12 vertebral body. Patient presented with severe back pain not controlled with oral opioids. MRI of spine showed extensive involvement of epidural space with canal involvement at T12 level (arrows). Patient's pain was successfully treated with placement of intrathecal catheter via a lumbar approach. The catheter tip is at the T5 vertebral level. His pain was controlled with an infusion of intrathecal morphine at 3 mg/day. MRI, Magnetic resonance imaging.

and to the degree (total or partial) of spinal canal stenosis (Fig. 22.10).

Epidural metastasis with invasion of extrathecal and intrathecal nerve roots by neoplasm, dural infiltration, and generation of reactive fibrosis in the subdural space may increase the intensity of nociceptive stimulation and hinder diffusion of drugs to the nerve roots and spinal cord, thereby reducing the effectiveness of intraspinal pain treatment (Fig. 22.11). Significant interpatient variation in daily doses of analgesics may occur for both epidural and intrathecal pain treatments. Epidural morphine doses varying from 6 to 120 mg/day at the start of treatment,[12] 16 to 600 mg/day at steady state, and 28 to 600 mg/day at the final stage of treatment have been reported.[14] Similar wide variations in epidural bupivacaine doses 96 to 2100 mg/day also occur.[109] For intrathecal treatment, morphine doses have varied from 0.8 to 200 mg/day and bupivacaine doses from 15 to 305 mg/day.[13]

Appelgren et al.[255] retrospectively reviewed 201 consecutive patients with cancer pain who received intrathecal pain treatment between 1985 and 1993. These

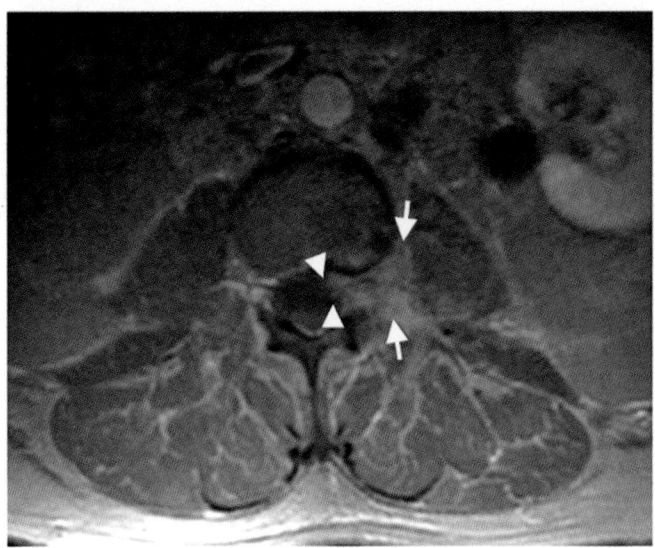

FIGURE 22.11 Axial T1 gadolinium enhanced MRI of a 57-year-old man with metastatic colorectal carcinoma involving L2 vertebral body with epidural extension indenting the spinal cord *(arrow heads)* and extending through the left foramen to the left psoas muscle *(arrow heads)*. MRI, Magnetic resonance imaging.

patients participated in a study undertaken to test the hypothesis that epidural metastasis is a common cause of "refractory" cancer pain and that its presence may affect the efficacy and the complication rates of intraspinal pain treatment. Epidural metastases occurred in 40 (70%) and spinal stenosis in 33 (58%); seven patients had total and 26 partial occlusion of the spinal canal. The presence of epidural metastasis affected catheter insertion complications, daily dosages, and complications of the intrathecal pain treatment only when it was associated with spinal canal stenosis (partial or total). During the period of intrathecal treatment, patients with confirmed epidural metastasis and complete spinal block needed significantly ($P <.05$) higher daily doses of morphine (means: 77 ±103 vs. 22±29 mg) and intrathecal bupivacaine (means: 65±44 vs. 33±20 mg) and had significantly higher rates (14% vs. 0%; $P <.05$) of radicular pain at injection and poor distribution of analgesia than those without epidural metastasis and spinal canal stenosis. Unexpected paraplegia occurred in four patients due to accidental injury during attempted dural puncture (n = 1) and collapse (due to cerebrospinal fluid leakage leading to "medullary coning" of an unknown epidural metastasis (n = 3).

Because most pathologic changes are limited to the epidural space, and the prevalence of intrathecal metastasis is 1% to 4%[275] compared to approximately 70% for epidural metastasis, epidural pain treatment is more often affected than intrathecal therapy by the presence of spinal metastasis. The risk of rapid neurologic deterioration after lumbar puncture removal of CSF below the level of a subarachnoid block has been known since 1940.[276] In such situations, it is possible that lumbar puncture may remove CSF that has acted as a critical buffer between the spinal cord and the extramedullary tumor. Hollis et al.[277] recommend avoiding lumbar puncture and intrathecal catheterization below the level of a suspected mass causing complete block, estimating the risk of neurologic deterioration at about 14% after lumbar puncture in patients with complete spinal block.

A full diagnostic evaluation, including MRI of the spine, is warranted in the patient with cancer who is being considered for spinal drug administration. We prefer the intrathecal route of delivery, as it is more reliable and is less likely to result in epidural bleeding when the catheter is placed. We have successfully placed intrathecal catheters in patients known to have epidural metastases several segments removed from the region of the dural puncture. We have obtained excellent pain relief in patients with epidural tumor deposits as well as those without disease in the spine.

References

1. Abram SE. 1992 Bonica Lecture. Advances in chronic pain management since gate control. *Reg Anesth*. 1993;18:66–81.
2. Abram SE. Continuous spinal anesthesia for cancer and chronic pain. *Reg Anesth*. 1993;18:406–413.
3. Sloan PA. Neuraxial pain relief for intractable cancer pain. *Curr Pain Headache Rep*. 2007;11:283–289.
4. Burton AW, Rajagopal A, Shah HN, et al. Epidural and intrathecal analgesia is effective in treating refractory cancer pain. *Pain Med*. 2004;5:239–247.
5. Lema MJ. Invasive analgesia techniques for advanced cancer pain. *Surg Oncol Clin N Am*. 2001;10:127–136.
6. Koulousakis A, Kuchta J, Bayarassou A, et al. Intrathecal opioids for intractable pain syndromes. *Acta Neurochir Suppl*. 2007;97:43–48.
7. Waldman SD, Coombs DW. Selection of implantable narcotic delivery systems. *Anesth Analg*. 1989;68:377–384.
8. Behar M, Magora F, Olshwang D, et al. Epidural morphine in treatment of pain. *Lancet*. 1979;1:527–529.
9. De Jong PC, Kansen PJ. A comparison of epidural catheters with or without subcutaneous injection ports for treatment of cancer pain. *Anesth Analg*. 1994;78:94–100.
10. DuPen SL, Peterson DG, Bogosian AC, et al. A new permanent exteriorized epidural catheter for narcotic self-administration to control cancer pain. *Cancer*. 1987;59:986–993.
11. Plummer JL, Cherry DA, Cousins MJ, et al. Long-term spinal administration of morphine in cancer and noncancer pain: A retrospective study. *Pain*. 1991;44:215–220.
12. Nitescu P, Appelgren L, Linder LE, et al. Epidural versus intrathecal morphine-bupivacaine: Assessment of consecutive treatments in advanced cancer pain. *J Pain Symptom Manage*. 1990;5:18–26.
13. Sjoberg M, Appelgren L, Einarsson S, et al. Long-term intrathecal morphine and bupivacaine in "refractory" cancer pain. I. Results from the first series of 52 patients. *Acta Anaesthesiol Scand*. 1991;35:30–43.
14. Nitescu P, Sjoberg M, Appelgren L, et al. Complications of intrathecal opioids and bupivacaine in the treatment of "refractory" cancer pain. *Clin J Pain*. 1995;11:45–62.
15. Brazenor GA. Long term intrathecal administration of morphine: A comparison of bolus injection via reservoir with continuous infusion by implanted pump. *Neurosurgery*. 1987;21:484–491.
16. Crul BJ, Delhaas EM. Technical complications during long-term subarachnoid or epidural administration of morphine in terminally ill cancer patients: A review of 140 cases. *Reg Anesth*. 1991;16:209–213.
17. Devulder J, Ghys L, Dhondt W, et al. Spinal analgesia in terminal care: risk versus benefit. *J Pain Symptom Manage*. 1994;9:75–81.
18. Ventafridda V, Spoldi E, Caraceni A, et al. Intraspinal morphine for cancer pain. *Acta Anaesthesiol Scand Suppl*. 1987;85:47–53.
19. Paice JA, Winkelmuller W, Burchiel K, et al. Clinical realities and economic considerations: Efficacy of intrathecal pain therapy. *J Pain Symptom Manage*. 1997;14:S14-26.
20. Smith TJ, Staats PS, Deer T, et al. Randomized clinical trial of an implantable drug delivery system compared with comprehensive medical management for refractory cancer pain: Impact on pain, drug-related toxicity, and survival. *J Clin Oncol*. 2002;20:4040–4049.
21. Stearns L, Boortz-Marx R, Du Pen S, et al. Intrathecal drug delivery for the management of cancer pain: A multidisciplinary consensus of best clinical practices. *J Support Oncol*. 2005;3:399–408.

22. Fitzgibbon D, Rapp S, Terman G, et al. Rebound hypertension and acute withdrawal associated with discontinuation of an infusion of epidural clonidine. *Anesthesiology*. 1996;84:729–731.
23. Allen JW, Horais KA, Tozier NA, et al. Opiate pharmacology of intrathecal granulomas. *Anesthesiology*. 2006;105:590–598.
24. Coffey RJ, Burchiel K. Inflammatory mass lesions associated with intrathecal drug infusion catheters: report and observations on 41 patients. *Neurosurgery*. 2002;50:78–86;discussion 86-7.
25. Max MB, Inturrisi CE, Kaiko RF, et al. Epidural and intrathecal opiates: cerebrospinal fluid and plasma profiles in patients with chronic cancer pain. *Clin Pharmacol Ther*. 1985;38:631–641.
26. Nordberg G, Hedner T, Mellstrand T, et al. Pharmacokinetic aspects of epidural morphine analgesia. *Anesthesiology*. 1983;58:545–551.
27. Onofrio BM. Treatment of chronic pain of malignant origin with intrathecal opiates. *Clin Neurosurg*. 1983;31:304–315.
28. Onofrio BM, Yaksh TL, Arnold PG. Continuous low-dose intrathecal morphine administration in the treatment of chronic pain of malignant origin. *Mayo Clin Proc*. 1981;56:516–520.
29. Rico RC, Hobika GH, Avellanosa AM, et al. Use of intrathecal and epidural morphine for pain relief in patients with malignant diseases: A preliminary report. *J Med*. 1982;13:223–231.
30. Vincenti E, Chiaranda M, Ambrosini A, et al. New trends for pain relief in gynaecologic oncology. *Eur J Gynaecol Oncol*. 1983;4:122–127.
31. Wang JK, Nauss LA, Thomas JE. Pain relief by intrathecally applied morphine in man. *Anesthesiology*. 1979;50:149–151.
32. Rawal N, Arner S, Gustafsson LL, et al. Present state of extradural and intrathecal opioid analgesia in Sweden. A nationwide follow-up survey. *Br J Anaesth*. 1987;59:791–799.
33. McQuay HJ. Opioid clinical pharmacology and routes of administration. *Br Med Bull*. 1991;47:703–717.
34. Payne R. Role of epidural and intrathecal narcotics and peptides in the management of cancer pain. *Med Clin North Am*. 1987;71:313–327.
35. Pfeifer BL, Sernaker HL, Ter Horst UM, et al. Cross-tolerance between systemic and epidural morphine in cancer patients. *Pain*. 1989;39:181–187.
36. Onofrio BM, Yaksh TL. Long-term pain relief produced by intrathecal morphine infusion in 53 patients. *J Neurosurg*. 1990;72:200–209.
37. Osenbach RK, Harvey S. Neuraxial infusion in patients with chronic intractable cancer and noncancer pain. *Curr Pain Headache Rep*. 2001;5:241–249.
38. Chrubasik J, Chrubasik S, Martin E. Patient-controlled spinal opiate analgesia in terminal cancer. Has its time really arrived? *Drugs*. 1992;43:799–804.
39. Chrubasik J, Chrubasik S, Martin E. The ideal epidural opioid—fact or fantasy? *Eur J Anaesthesiol*. 1993;10:79–100.
40. Gourlay GK, Plummer JL, Cherry DA, et al. Comparison of intermittent bolus with continuous infusion of epidural morphine in the treatment of severe cancer pain. *Pain*. 1991;47:135–140.
41. Hassenbusch SJ, Pillay PK, Magdinec M, et al. Constant infusion of morphine for intractable cancer pain using an implanted pump. *J Neurosurg*. 1990;73:405–409.
42. Mercadante S. Problems of long-term spinal opioid treatment in advanced cancer patients. *Pain*. 1999;79:1–13.
43. Bernards CM. Recent insights into the pharmacokinetics of spinal opioids and the relevance to opioid selection. *Curr Opin Anaesthesiol*. 2004;17:441–447.
44. Bernards CM, Shen DD, Sterling ES, et al. Epidural, cerebrospinal fluid, and plasma pharmacokinetics of epidural opioids (part 1): Differences among opioids. *Anesthesiology*. 2003;99:455–465.
45. Inagaki Y, Mashimo T, Yoshiya I. Time-related differential effects of epidural morphine on the neuraxis. *Anesth Analg*. 1993;76:308–315.
46. Coda BA, Brown MC, Schaffer RL, et al. A pharmacokinetic approach to resolving spinal and systemic contributions to epidural alfentanil analgesia and side-effects. *Pain*. 1995;62:329–337.
47. Ellis DJ, Millar WL, Reisner LS. A randomized double-blind comparison of epidural versus intravenous fentanyl infusion for analgesia after cesarean section. *Anesthesiology*. 1990;72:981–986.
48. Glass PS, Estok P, Ginsberg B, et al. Use of patient-controlled analgesia to compare the efficacy of epidural to intravenous fentanyl administration. *Anesth Analg*. 1992;74:345–351.
49. Loper KA, Ready LB, Downey M, et al. Epidural and intravenous fentanyl infusions are clinically equivalent after knee surgery. *Anesth Analg*. 1990;70:72–75.
50. Miguel R, Barlow I, Morrell M, et al. A prospective, randomized, double-blind comparison of epidural and intravenous sufentanil infusions. *Anesthesiology*. 1994;81:346–352.
51. Sjogren P, Banning A. Pain, sedation and reaction time during long-term treatment of cancer patients with oral and epidural opioids. *Pain*. 1989;39:5–11.
52. Hassenbusch SJ, Pillay PK, Magdinec M, et al. Constant infusion of morphine for intractable cancer pain using an implanted pump. *J Neurosurg*. 1990;73:405–409.
53. Samuelsson H, Malmberg F, Eriksson M, et al. Outcomes of epidural morphine treatment in cancer pain: nine years of clinical experience. *J Pain Symptom Manage*. 1995;10:105–112.
54. Cherry DA, Gourlay GK. CT contrast evidence of injectate encapsulation after long-term epidural administration. *Pain*. 1992;49:369–371.
55. Ummenhofer WC, Arends RH, Shen DD, et al. Comparative spinal distribution and clearance kinetics of intrathecally administered morphine, fentanyl, alfentanil, and sufentanil. *Anesthesiology*. 2000;92:739–753.
56. Cousins MJ, Mather LE. Intrathecal and epidural administration of opioids. *Anesthesiology*. 1984;61:276–310.
57. De Conno F, Caraceni A, Martini C, et al. Hyperalgesia and myoclonus with intrathecal infusion of high- dose morphine. *Pain*. 1991;47:337–339.
58. Follett KA, Hitchon PW, Piper J, et al. Response of intractable pain to continuous intrathecal morphine: A retrospective study. *Pain*. 1992;49:21–25.
59. Greenberg HS, Taren J, Ensminger WD, et al. Benefit from and tolerance to continuous intrathecal infusion of morphine for intractable cancer pain. *J Neurosurg*. 1982;57:360–364.
60. Paice JA, Penn RD, Shott S. Intraspinal morphine for chronic pain: A retrospective, multicenter study. *J Pain Symptom Manage*. 1996;11:71–80.
61. Penn RD, Paice JA. Chronic intrathecal morphine for intractable pain. *J Neurosurg*. 1987;67:182–186.
62. Schultheiss R, Schramm J, Neidhardt J. Dose changes in long- and medium-term intrathecal morphine therapy of cancer pain. *Neurosurgery*. 1992;31:664–669.
63. Wagemans MF, Bakker EN, Zuurmond WW, et al. Intrathecal administration of high-dose morphine solutions decreases the pH of cerebrospinal fluid. *Pain*. 1995;61:55–59.
64. Yaksh TL, Onofrio BM. Retrospective consideration of the doses of morphine given intrathecally by chronic infusion in 163 patients by 19 physicians. *Pain*. 1987;31:211–223.
65. Bigler D, Christensen CB, Eriksen J, et al. Morphine, morphine-6-glucuronide and morphine-3-glucuronide concentrations in plasma and cerebrospinal fluid during long-term high-dose intrathecal morphine administration. *Pain*. 1990;41:15–18.
66. Tamakawa S, Iwanami Y, Ogawa H. High-dose intrathecal morphine to control cancer pain—a case report. *J Pain Symptom Manage*. 1998;15:70–72.
67. Gestin Y, Vainio A, Pegurier AM. Long-term intrathecal infusion of morphine in the home care of patients with advanced cancer. *Acta Anaesthesiol Scand*. 1997;41:12–17.
68. Jacobson L, Chabal C, Brody MC, et al. Intrathecal methadone and morphine for postoperative analgesia: A comparison of the efficacy, duration, and side effects. *Anesthesiology*. 1989;70:742–746.
69. Chaney MA. Side effects of intrathecal and epidural opioids. *Can J Anaesth*. 1995;42:891–903.
70. Winkelmuller M, Winkelmuller W. Long-term effects of continuous intrathecal opioid treatment in chronic pain of nonmalignant etiology. *J Neurosurg*. 1996;85:458–467.
71. Abs R, Verhelst J, Maeyaert J, et al. Endocrine consequences of long-term intrathecal administration of opioids. *J Clin Endocrinol Metab*. 2000;85:2215–2222.
72. Aldrete JA, Couto da Silva JM. Leg edema from intrathecal opiate infusions. *Eur J Pain*. 2000;4:361–365.
73. North RB, Cutchis PN, Epstein JA, et al. Spinal cord compression complicating subarachnoid infusion of morphine: case report and laboratory experience. *Neurosurgery*. 1991;29:778–784.
74. Wadhwa RK, Shaya MR, Nanda A. Spinal cord compression in a patient with a pain pump for failed back syndrome: A chalk-like precipitate mimicking a spinal cord neoplasm:case report. *Neurosurgery*. 2006;58:E387.
75. Coffey RJ, Allen JW. Not all intrathecal catheter tip MRI findings are inflammatory masses. *Anesth Analg*. 2007;104:1600–1602; author reply 1602.

76. Follett KA. Intrathecal analgesia and catheter-tip inflammatory masses. *Anesthesiology.* 2003;99:5–6.
77. Allen JW, Horais KA, Tozier NA, et al. Time course and role of morphine dose and concentration in intrathecal granuloma formation in dogs: A combined magnetic resonance imaging and histopathology investigation. *Anesthesiology.* 2006;105:581–589.
78. Yaksh TL, Horais KA, Tozier NA, et al. Chronically infused intrathecal morphine in dogs. *Anesthesiology.* 2003;99:174–187.
79. Hassenbusch S, Burchiel K, Coffey RJ, et al. Management of intrathecal catheter-tip inflammatory masses: A consensus statement. *Pain Med.* 2002;3:313–323.
80. McMillan MR, Doud T, Nugent W. Catheter-associated masses in patients receiving intrathecal analgesic therapy. *Anesth Analg.* 2003;96:186–190, table of contents.
81. Mao J, Price DD, Mayer DJ. Thermal hyperalgesia in association with the development of morphine tolerance in rats: roles of excitatory amino acid receptors and protein kinase C. *J Neurosci.* 1994;14:2301–2312.
82. Mao J, Sung B, Ji RR, Lim G. Chronic morphine induces downregulation of spinal glutamate transporters: Implications in morphine tolerance and abnormal pain sensitivity. *J Neurosci.* 2002;22:8312–8323.
83. Sakurada T, Komatsu T, Sakurada S. Mechanisms of nociception evoked by intrathecal high-dose morphine. *Neurotoxicology.* 2005;26:801–809.
84. Ibuki T, Marsala M, Masuyama T, et al. Spinal amino acid release and repeated withdrawal in spinal morphine tolerant rats. *Br J Pharmacol.* 2003;138:689–697.
85. McCrory C, Diviney D, Moriarty J, et al. Comparison between repeat bolus intrathecal morphine and an epidurally delivered bupivacaine and fentanyl combination in the management of postthoracotomy pain with or without cyclooxygenase inhibition. *J Cardiothorac Vasc Anesth.* 2002;16:607–611.
86. Rauck RL, Cherry D, Boyer MF, et al. Long-term intrathecal opioid therapy with a patient-activated, implanted delivery system for the treatment of refractory cancer pain. *J Pain.* 2003;4:441–447.
87. Riba P, Ben Y, Smith AP, et al. Morphine tolerance in spinal cord is due to interaction between mu- and delta-receptors. *J Pharmacol Exp Ther.* 2002;300:265–272.
88. Stevens CW, Yaksh TL. Potency of infused spinal antinociceptive agents is inversely related to magnitude of tolerance after continuous infusion. *J Pharmacol Exp Ther.* 1989;250:1–8.
89. Yaksh TL, Kohl RL, Rudy TA. Induction of tolerance and withdrawal in rats receiving morphine in the spinal subarachnoid space. *Eur J Pharmacol.* 1977;42:275–284.
90. Dunbar S, Yaksh TL. Concurrent spinal infusion of MK801 blocks spinal tolerance and dependence induced by chronic intrathecal morphine in the rat. *Anesthesiology.* 1996;84:1177–1188.
91. Granados-Soto V, Kalcheva I, Hua X, et al. Spinal PKC activity and expression: role in tolerance produced by continuous spinal morphine infusion. *Pain.* 2000;85:395–404.
92. Sallerin-Caute B, Lazorthes Y, Deguine O, et al. Does intrathecal morphine in the treatment of cancer pain induce the development of tolerance? *Neurosurgery.* 1998;42:44–49.
93. Samuelsson H, Hedner T. Pain characterization in cancer patients and the analgetic response to epidural morphine. *Pain.* 1991;46:3–8.
94. Arner S, Arner B. Differential effects of epidural morphine in the treatment of cancer-related pain. *Acta Anaesthesiol Scand.* 1985;29:32–36.
95. Van Dongen RT, Crul BJ, van Egmond J. Intrathecal coadministration of bupivacaine diminishes morphine dose progression during long-term intrathecal infusion in cancer patients. *Clin J Pain.* 1999;15:166–172.
96. Shetter AG, Hadley MN, Wilkinson E. Administration of intraspinal morphine sulfate for the treatment of intractable cancer pain. *Neurosurgery.* 1986;18:740–747.
97. Abram SE, Mampilly GA, Milosavljevic D. Assessment of the potency and intrinsic activity of systemic versus intrathecal opioids in rats. *Anesthesiology.* 1997;87:127–134;discussion 27A–29A.
98. Van Dongen RT, Crul BJ, De Bock M. Long-term intrathecal infusion of morphine and morphine/bupivacaine mixtures in the treatment of cancer pain: A retrospective analysis of 51 cases. *Pain.* 1993;55:119–123.
99. Tseng LF, Fujimoto JM. Differential actions of intrathecal naloxone on blocking the tail-flick inhibition induced by intraventricular beta-endorphin and morphine in rats. *J Pharmacol Exp Ther.* 1985;232:74–79.
100. Lazorthes Y. Intracerebroventricular administration of morphine for control of irreducible cancer pain. *Ann N Y Acad Sci.* 1988;531:123–132.
101. Dennis GC, DeWitty RL. Long-term intraventricular infusion of morphine for intractable pain in cancer of the head and neck. *Neurosurgery.* 1990;26:404–407.
102. Ballantyne JC, Carr DB, Berkey CS, et al. Comparative efficacy of epidural, subarachnoid, and intracerebroventricular opioids in patients with pain due to cancer. *Reg Anesth.* 1996;21:542–556.
103. Ballantyne JC, Carwood CM. Comparative efficacy of epidural, subarachnoid, and intracerebroventricular opioids in patients with pain due to cancer. *Cochrane Database Syst Rev.* 2005:CD005178.
104. Yeager MP, Glass DD, Neff RK, et al. Epidural anesthesia and analgesia in high-risk surgical patients. *Anesthesiology.* 1987;66:729–736.
105. Nikolajsen L, Ilkjaer S, Christensen JH, et al. Randomised trial of epidural bupivacaine and morphine in prevention of stump and phantom pain in lower-limb amputation. *Lancet.* 1997;350:1353–1357.
106. Hjortso NC, Neumann P, Frosig F, et al. A controlled study on the effect of epidural analgesia with local anaesthetics and morphine on morbidity after abdominal surgery. *Acta Anaesthesiol Scand.* 1985;29:790–796.
107. De Leon-Casasola OA, Myers DP, Donaparthi S, et al. A comparison of postoperative epidural analgesia between patients with chronic cancer taking high doses of oral opioids versus opioid-naive patients. *Anesth Analg.* 1993;76:302–307.
108. Boudreault D, Brasseur L, Samii K, et al. Comparison of continuous epidural bupivacaine infusion plus either continuous epidural infusion or patient-controlled epidural injection of fentanyl for postoperative analgesia. *Anesth Analg.* 1991;73:132–137.
109. DuPen SL, Kharasch ED, Williams A, et al. Chronic epidural bupivacaine-opioid infusion in intractable cancer pain. *Pain.* 1992;49:293–300.
110. Akerman B, Arwestrom E, Post C. Local anesthetics potentiate spinal morphine antinociception. *Anesth Analg.* 1988;67:943–948.
111. Fink BR. Mechanisms of differential axial blockade in epidural and subarachnoid anesthesia. *Anesthesiology.* 1989;70:851–858.
112. Visser WA, Lee RA, Gielen MJ. Factors affecting the distribution of neural blockade by local anesthetics in epidural anesthesia and a comparison of lumbar versus thoracic epidural anesthesia. *Anesth Analg.* 2008;107:708–721.
113. Higuchi H, Adachi Y, Kazama T. Factors affecting the spread and duration of epidural anesthesia with ropivacaine. *Anesthesiology.* 2004;101:451–460.
114. Cousins MJ, Veering BT. Epidural neural blockade. In: Cousins MJ, Bridenbaugh PO, eds. *Neural blockade in clinical anesthesia and management of pain.* 3rd ed. Philadelphia: Lippincott, 1998:243–321.
115. Arakawa M, Aoyama Y, Ohe Y. Block of the sacral segments in lumbar epidural anaesthesia. *Br J Anaesth.* 2003;90:173–178.
116. Galindo A, Hernandez J, Benavides O, et al. Quality of spinal extradural anaesthesia: The influence of spinal nerve root diameter. *Br J Anaesth.* 1975;47:41–47.
117. Kroin JS, Ali A, York M, et al. The distribution of medication along the spinal canal after chronic intrathecal administration. *Neurosurgery.* 1993;33:226–230.
118. Van Zundert AA, Grouls RJ, Korsten HH, et al. Spinal anesthesia. Volume or concentration—what matters? *Reg Anesth.* 1996;21:112–118.
119. Kroin JS, McCarthy RJ, Penn RD, et al. The effect of chronic subarachnoid bupivacaine infusion in dogs. *Anesthesiology.* 1987;66:737–742.
120. Bernards CM. Cerebrospinal fluid and spinal cord distribution of baclofen and bupivacaine during slow intrathecal infusion in pigs. *Anesthesiology.* 2006;105:169–178.
121. Henry-Feugeas MC, Idy-Peretti I, Baledent O, et al. Origin of subarachnoid cerebrospinal fluid pulsations: A phase-contrast MR analysis. *Magn Reson Imaging.* 2000;18:387–395.
122. Aguilar JL, Espachs P, Roca G, et al. Difficult management of pain following sacrococcygeal chordoma: 13 months of subarachnoid infusion. *Pain.* 1994;59:317–320.
123. Appelgren L, Janson M, Nitescu P, et al. Continuous intracisternal and high cervical intrathecal bupivacaine analgesia in refractory head and neck pain. *Anesthesiology.* 1996;84:256–272.
124. Crul BJ, van D-RT, Snijdelaar DG, et al. Long-term continuous intrathecal administration of morphine and bupivacaine at the

125. Mercadante S. Intrathecal morphine and bupivacaine in advanced cancer pain patients implanted at home. *J Pain Symptom Manage.* 1994;9:201–207.
126. Sjoberg M, Nitescu P, Appelgren L, et al. Long-term intrathecal morphine and bupivacaine in patients with refractory cancer pain. Results from a morphine:bupivacaine dose regimen of 0.5:4.75 mg/mL. *Anesthesiology.* 1994;80:284–297.
127. Tumber PS, Fitzgibbon DR. The control of severe cancer pain by continuous intrathecal infusion and patient controlled intrathecal analgesia with morphine, bupivacaine and clonidine. *Pain.* 1998; 78:217–220.
128. Mercadante S. Neuraxial techniques for cancer pain: An opinion about unresolved therapeutic dilemmas. *Reg Anesth Pain Med.* 1999;24:74–83.
129. Mercadante S, Intravaia G, Villari P, et al. Intrathecal treatment in cancer patients unresponsive to multiple trials of systemic opioids. *Clin J Pain.* 2007;23:793–798.
130. Penn RD. Two decades of improved pain control. *J Support Oncol.* 2005;3:411–412.
131. Ready LB, Plumer MH, Haschke RH, et al. Neurotoxicity of intrathecal local anesthetics in rabbits. *Anesthesiology.* 1985;63: 364–370.
132. Hodgson PS, Neal JM, Pollock JE, et al. The neurotoxicity of drugs given intrathecally (spinal). *Anesth Analg.* 1999;88: 797–809.
133. Yamashita A, Matsumoto M, Matsumoto S, et al. A comparison of the neurotoxic effects on the spinal cord of tetracaine, lidocaine, bupivacaine, and ropivacaine administered intrathecally in rabbits. *Anesth Analg.* 2003;97:512–519.
134. Hashimoto K, Sakura S, Bollen AW, et al. Comparative toxicity of glucose and lidocaine administered intrathecally in the rat. *Reg Anesth Pain Med.* 1998;23:444–450.
135. Sakura S, Bollen AW, Ciriales R, et al. Local anesthetic neurotoxicity does not result from blockade of voltage-gated sodium channels. *Anesth Analg.* 1995;81:338–346.
136. Myers RR, Kalichman MW, Reisner LS, et al. Neurotoxicity of local anesthetics: Altered perineurial permeability, edema, and nerve fiber injury. *Anesthesiology.* 1986;64:29–35.
137. Kalichman MW, Powell HC, Myers RR. Quantitative histologic analysis of local anesthetic-induced injury to rat sciatic nerve. *J Pharmacol Exp Ther.* 1989;250:406–413.
138. Ganem EM, Vianna PT, Marques M, et al. Neurotoxicity of subarachnoid hyperbaric bupivacaine in dogs. *Reg Anesth.* 1996; 21:234–238.
139. Takenami T, Yagishita S, Murase S, et al. Neurotoxicity of intrathecally administered bupivacaine involves the posterior roots/posterior white matter and is milder than lidocaine in rats. *Reg Anesth Pain Med.* 2005;30:464–472.
140. Johnson ME. Potential neurotoxicity of spinal anesthesia with lidocaine. *Mayo Clin Proc.* 2000;75:921–932.
141. Rigler ML, Drasner K, Krejcie TC, et al. Cauda equina syndrome after continuous spinal anesthesia. *Anesth Analg.* 1991;72: 275–281.
142. Chabbouh T, Lentschener C, Zuber M, et al. Persistent cauda equina syndrome with no identifiable facilitating condition after an uneventful single spinal administration of 0.5% hyperbaric bupivacaine. *Anesth Analg.* 2005;101:1847–1848.
143. Rohm KD, Boldt J. Persisting neurologic symptoms after uncomplicated intrathecal bupivacaine. *Anesth Analg.* 2006;103:1047; author reply 1047.
144. Zeidan A, Samii K. A case of unusually prolonged hyperbaric spinal anesthesia. *Acta Anaesthesiol Scand.* 2005;49:885.
145. Johnson ME. Perineurial concentration of lidocaine is more relevant to spinal neurotoxicity than the concentration administered. *Anesth Analg.* 2000;90:766–767.
146. Li DF, Bahar M, Cole G, et al. Neurologic toxicity of the subarachnoid infusion of bupivacaine, lignocaine or 2-chloroprocaine in the rat. *Br J Anaesth.* 1985;57:424–429.
147. Sjoberg M, Karlsson PA, Nordborg C, et al. Neuropathologic findings after long-term intrathecal infusion of morphine and bupivacaine for pain treatment in cancer patients. *Anesthesiology.* 1992;76:173–186.
148. Wagemans MF, van der Valk P, Spoelder EM, et al. Neurohistopathologic findings after continuous intrathecal administration of morphine or a morphine/bupivacaine mixture in cancer pain patients. *Acta Anaesthesiol Scand.* 1997;41:1033–1038.
149. Tamsen A, Gordh T. Epidural clonidine produces analgesia. *Lancet.* 1984;2:231–232.
150. Sullivan AF, Dashwood MR, Dickenson AH. Alpha 2-adrenoceptor modulation of nociception in rat spinal cord: location, effects and interactions with morphine. *Eur J Pharm.* 1987;138:169–177.
151. Bonnet F, Boico O, Rostaing S, et al. Postoperative analgesia with extradural clonidine. *Br J Anaesth.* 1989;63:465–469.
152. Motsch J, Graber E, Ludwig K. Addition of clonidine enhances postoperative analgesia from epidural morphine: A double-blind study. *Anesthesiology.* 1990;73:1067–1073.
153. Carabine UA, Milligan KR, Mulholland D, et al. Extradural clonidine infusions for analgesia after total hip replacement. *Br J Anaesth.* 1992;68:338–343.
154. Mendez R, Eisenach JC, Kashtan K. Epidural clonidine analgesia after cesarean section. *Anesthesiology.* 1990;73:848–852.
155. Huntoon M, Eisenach JC, Boese P. Epidural clonidine after cesarean section. Appropriate dose and effect of prior local anesthetic. *Anesthesiology.* 1992;76:187–193.
156. Unnerstall JR, Kopajtic TA, Kuhar MJ. Distribution of alpha 2 agonist binding sites in the rat and human central nervous system: Analysis of some functional, anatomic correlates of the pharmacologic effects of clonidine and related adrenergic agents. *Brain Research.* 1984;319:69–101.
157. Yaksh TL. Pharmacology of spinal adrenergic systems which modulate spinal nociceptive processing. *Pharmacol Bioch Behav.* 1985;22:845–858.
158. Ono H, Mishima A, Ono S, et al. Inhibitory effects of clonidine and tizanidine on release of substance P from slices of rat spinal cord and antagonism by alpha-adrenergic receptor antagonists. *Neuropharmacology.* 1991;30:585–589.
159. Kamisaki Y, Hamada T, Maeda K, et al. Presynaptic alpha 2 adrenoceptors inhibit glutamate release from rat spinal cord synaptosomes. *J Neurochem.* 1993;60:522–526.
160. Zeng W, Chen X, Dohi S. Antinociceptive synergistic interaction between clonidine and ouabain on thermal nociceptive tests in the rat. *J Pain.* 2007;8:983–988.
161. Abelson KS, Hoglund AU. The effects of the alpha-2-adrenergic receptor agonists clonidine and rilmenidine, and antagonists yohimbine and efaroxan, on the spinal cholinergic receptor system in the rat. *Basic Clin Pharmacol Toxicol.* 2004;94:153–160.
162. Klimscha W, Tong C, Eisenach JC. Intrathecal alpha-2-adrenergic agonists stimulate acetylcholine and norepinephrine release from the spinal cord dorsal horn in sheep. An in vivo microdialysis study. *Anesthesiology.* 1997;87:110–116.
163. Honda K, Koga K, Moriyama T, et al. Intrathecal alpha-2 adrenoceptor agonist clonidine inhibits mechanical transmission in mouse spinal cord via activation of muscarinic M1 receptors. *Neurosci Lett.* 2002;322:161–164.
164. Xu Z, Chen SR, Eisenach J, et al. Role of spinal muscarinic and nicotinic receptors in clonidine-induced nitric oxide release in a rat model of neuropathic pain. *Brain Res.* 2000;861:390–398.
165. Hassenbusch SJ, Gunes S, Wachsman S, Willis KD. Intrathecal clonidine in the treatment of intractable pain: A phase I/II study. *Pain Med.* 2002;3:85–91.
166. Eisenach JC, Hood DD, Curry R. Intrathecal, but not intravenous, clonidine reduces experimental thermal or capsaicin-induced pain and hyperalgesia in normal volunteers. *Anesth Analg.* 1998; 87:591–596.
167. Boswell G, Bekersky I, Mekki Q, et al. Plasma concentrations and disposition of clonidine following a constant 14-day epidural infusion in cancer patients. *Clin Ther.* 1997;19:1024–1030.
168. Eisenach JC, Tong CY. Site of hemodynamic effects of intrathecal alpha 2-adrenergic agonists. *Anesthesiology.* 1991;74:766–771.
169. Guyenet PG, Cabot JB. Inhibition of sympathetic preganglionic neurons by catecholamines and clonidine: mediation by an alpha-adrenergic receptor. *J Neurosci.* 1981;1:908–917.
170. Jarrott B, Conway EL, Maccarrone C, et al. Clonidine: understanding its disposition, sites and mechanism of action. *Clin Exper Pharm Physiol.* 1987;14:471–479.
171. Kiowski W, Hulth'en UL, Ritz R, et al. Prejunctional alpha 2-adrenoceptors and norepinephrine release in the forearm of normal humans. *J Cardiovasc Pharm.* 1985;7(Suppl 6):S144-148.
172. Eisenach JC, Hood DD, Curry R. Relative potency of epidural to intrathecal clonidine differs between acute thermal pain and capsaicin-induced allodynia. *Pain.* 2000;84:57–64.
173. Eisenach J, Detweiler D, Hood D. Hemodynamic and analgesic actions of epidurally administered clonidine. *Anesthesiology.* 1993; 78:277–287.

174. Eisenach JC, DuPen S, Dubois M, et al. Epidural clonidine analgesia for intractable cancer pain. *Pain.* 1995;61:391–399.
175. Segal IS, Jarvis DJ, Duncan SR, et al. Clinical efficacy of oral-transdermal clonidine combinations during the perioperative period. *Anesthesiology.* 1991;74:220–225.
176. Glynn CJ, Jamous MA, Teddy PJ. Cerebrospinal fluid kinetics of epidural clonidine in man. *Pain.* 1992;49:361–367.
177. Van Essen EJ, Bovill JG, Ploeger EJ, et al. Pharmacokinetics of clonidine after epidural administration in surgical patients. Lack of correlation between plasma concentration and analgesia and blood pressure changes. *Acta Anaesthesiol Scand.* 1992;36:300–304.
178. Eisenach JC, Rauck RL, Buzzanell C, et al. Epidural clonidine analgesia for intractable cancer pain: Phase I. *Anesthesiology.* 1989;71:647–652.
179. Van Essen EJ, Bovill JG, Ploeger EJ, et al. Intrathecal morphine and clonidine for control of intractable cancer pain. A case report. *Acta Anaesthesiolog Belg.* 1988;39:109–112.
180. Coombs DW, Saunders RL, Fratkin JD, et al. Continuous intrathecal hydromorphone and clonidine for intractable cancer pain. *J Neurosurg.* 1986;64:890–894.
181. Detweiler DJ, Eisenach JC, Tong C, et al. A cholinergic interaction in alpha 2 adrenoceptor-mediated antinociception in sheep. *J Pharmacol Exp Ther.* 1993;265:536–542.
182. Filos KS, Goudas LC, Patroni O, et al. Hemodynamic and analgesic profile after intrathecal clonidine in humans. A dose-response study. *Anesthesiology.* 1994;81:591–601.
183. Ackerman LL, Follett KA, Rosenquist RW. Long-term outcomes during treatment of chronic pain with intrathecal clonidine or clonidine/opioid combinations. *J Pain Symptom Manage.* 2003;26:668–677.
184. Gillberg PG, Askmark H. Changes in cholinergic and opioid receptors in the rat spinal cord, dorsal root and sciatic nerve after ventral and dorsal root lesion. *J Neural Transm Gen Sect.* 1991;85:31–39.
185. Khan IM, Youngblood KL, Printz MP, et al. Spinal nicotinic receptor expression in spontaneously hypertensive rats. *Hypertension.* 1996;28:1093–1099.
186. Yoon MH, Choi JI, Jeong SW. Antinociception of intrathecal cholinesterase inhibitors and cholinergic receptors in rats. *Acta Anaesthesiol Scand.* 2003;47:1079–1084.
187. Hwang JH, Hwang KS, Leem JK, et al. The antiallodynic effects of intrathecal cholinesterase inhibitors in a rat model of neuropathic pain. *Anesthesiology.* 1999;90:492–499.
188. Shafer SL, Eisenach JC, Hood DD, et al. Cerebrospinal fluid pharmacokinetics and pharmacodynamics of intrathecal neostigmine methylsulfate in humans. *Anesthesiology.* 1998;89:1074–1088.
189. Chung CJ, Kim JS, Park HS, et al. The efficacy of intrathecal neostigmine, intrathecal morphine, and their combination for postcesarean section analgesia. *Anesth Analg.* 1998;87:341–346.
190. Almeida RA, Lauretti GR, Mattos AL. Antinociceptive effect of low-dose intrathecal neostigmine combined with intrathecal morphine following gynecologic surgery. *Anesthesiology.* 2003;98:495–498.
191. Tan PH, Chia YY, Lo Y, et al. Intrathecal bupivacaine with morphine or neostigmine for postoperative analgesia after total knee replacement surgery. *Can J Anaesth.* 2001;48:551–556.
192. Eisenach JC, Hood DD, Curry R. Phase I human safety assessment of intrathecal neostigmine containing methyl- and propylparabens. *Anesth Analg.* 1997;85:842–846.
193. Hood DD, Eisenach JC, Tuttle R. Phase I safety assessment of intrathecal neostigmine methylsulfate in humans. *Anesthesiology.* 1995;82:331–343.
194. Klamt JG, Dos Reis MP, Barbieri Neto J, et al. Analgesic effect of subarachnoid neostigmine in two patients with cancer pain. *Pain.* 1996;66:389–391.
195. Gurun MS, Leinbach R, Moore L, et al. Studies on the safety of glucose and paraben-containing neostigmine for intrathecal administration. *Anesth Analg.* 1997;85:317–323.
196. Kristipati R, Nadasdi L, Tarczy-Hornoch K, et al. Characterization of the binding of omega-conopeptides to different classes of non-L-type neuronal calcium channels. *Mol Cell Neurosci.* 1994;5:219–228.
197. Penn RD, Paice JA. Adverse effects associated with the intrathecal administration of ziconotide. *Pain.* 2000;85:291–296.
198. Staats PS, Yearwood T, Charapata SG, et al. Intrathecal ziconotide in the treatment of refractory pain in patients with cancer or AIDS: A randomized controlled trial. *JAMA.* 2004;291:63–70.
199. Souter KJ, Davies JM, Loeser JD, et al. Continuous Intrathecal Meperidine for Severe Refractory Cancer Pain: A Case Report. *Clin J Pain.* 2005;21:193–196.
200. Vranken JH, van der Vegt MH, van Kan HJ, et al. Plasma concentrations of meperidine and normeperidine following continuous intrathecal meperidine in patients with neuropathic cancer pain. *Acta Anaesthesiol Scand.* 2005;49:665–670.
201. Norris MC, Honet JE, Leighton BL, et al. A comparison of meperidine and lidocaine for spinal anesthesia for postpartum tubal ligation. *Reg Anesth.* 1996;21:84–88.
202. Izenwasser S, Newman AH, Cox BM, et al. The cocaine-like behavioral effects of meperidine are mediated by activity at the dopamine transporter. *Eur J Pharmacol.* 1996;297:9–17.
203. Wagner LE 2nd, Eaton M, Sabnis SS, et al. Meperidine and lidocaine block of recombinant voltage-dependent Na+ channels: Evidence that meperidine is a local anesthetic. *Anesthesiology.* 1999;91:1481–1490.
204. Magnan J, Paterson SJ, Tavani A, et al. The binding spectrum of narcotic analgesic drugs with different agonist and antagonist properties. *Naunyn Schmiedebergs Arch Pharmacol.* 1982;319:197–205.
205. Randic M, Cheng G, Kojic L. Kappa-opioid receptor agonists modulate excitatory transmission in substantia gelatinosa neurons of the rat spinal cord. *J Neurosci.* 1995;15:6809–6826.
206. Bie B, Pan ZZ. Presynaptic mechanism for anti-analgesic and anti-hyperalgesic actions of kappa-opioid receptors. *J Neurosci.* 2003;23:7262–7268.
207. Hustveit O. Binding of fentanyl and pethidine to muscarinic receptors in rat brain. *Jpn J Pharmacol.* 1994;64:57–59.
208. Hagmeyer KO, Mauro LS, Mauro VF. Meperidine-related seizures associated with patient-controlled analgesia pumps. *Ann Pharmacother.* 1993;27:29–32.
209. Kaiko RF, Foley KM, Grabinski PY, et al. Central nervous system excitatory effects of meperidine in cancer patients. *Ann Neurol.* 1983;13:180–185.
210. Cousins MJ, Mather LE, Glynn CJ, et al. Selective spinal analgesia. *Lancet.* 1979;1:1141–1142.
211. Harvey SC, O'Neil MG, Pope CA, et al. Continuous intrathecal meperidine via an implantable infusion pump for chronic, nonmalignant pain. *Ann Pharmacother.* 1997;31:1306–1308.
212. Bion JF. Intrathecal ketamine for war surgery. A preliminary study under field conditions. *Anaesthesia.* 1984;39:1023–1028.
213. Yang CY, Wong CS, Chang JY, et al. Intrathecal ketamine reduces morphine requirements in patients with terminal cancer pain. *Can J Anaesth.* 1996;43:379–383.
214. Karpinski N, Dunn J, Hansen L, et al. Subpial vacuolar myelopathy after intrathecal ketamine: report of a case. *Pain.* 1997;73:103–105.
215. Stotz M, Oehen HP, Gerber H. Histological findings after long-term infusion of intrathecal ketamine for chronic pain: A case report. *J Pain Symptom Manage.* 1999;18:223–228.
216. Brock-Utne JG, Kallichurum S, Mankowitz E, et al. Intrathecal ketamine with preservative - histological effects on spinal nerve roots of baboons. *S Afr Med J.* 1982;61:440–441.
217. Errando CL, Sifre C, Moliner S, et al. Subarachnoid ketamine in swine—pathologic findings after repeated doses: Acute toxicity study. *Reg Anesth Pain Med.* 1999;24:146–152.
218. Malinovsky JM, Lepage JY, Cozian A, et al. Is ketamine or its preservative responsible for neurotoxicity in the rabbit? *Anesthesiology.* 1993;78:109–115.
219. Meller ST. Ketamine: relief from chronic pain through actions at the NMDA receptor? *Pain.* 1996;68:435–436.
220. Vranken JH, van der Vegt MH, Kal JE, et al. Treatment of neuropathic cancer pain with continuous intrathecal administration of S+-ketamine. *Acta Anaesthesiol Scand.* 2004;48:249–252.
221. Benrath J, Scharbert G, Gustorff B, et al. Long-term intrathecal S(+)-ketamine in a patient with cancer-related neuropathic pain. *Br J Anaesth.* 2005;95:247–249.
222. Vranken JH, Troost D, Wegener JT, et al. Neuropathologic findings after continuous intrathecal administration of S(+)-ketamine for the management of neuropathic cancer pain. *Pain.* 2005;117:231–235.
223. Kozek SA, Sator-Katzenschlager S, Kress HG. Intrathecal S(+)-ketamine in refractory neuropathic cancer pain. *Pain.* 2006;121:283–284;author reply 284.
224. Vranken JH, Troost D, de Haan P, et al. Severe toxic damage to the rabbit spinal cord after intrathecal administration of preservative-free S(+)-ketamine. *Anesthesiology.* 2006;105:813–818.
225. Kohno T, Wakai A, Ataka T, et al. Actions of midazolam on excitatory transmission in dorsal horn neurons of adult rat spinal cord. *Anesthesiology.* 2006;104:338–343.

226. Nishiyama T, Hanaoka K. The synergistic interaction between midazolam and clonidine in spinally-mediated analgesia in two different pain models of rats. *Anesth Analg*. 2001;93:1025–1031.
227. Johansen MJ, Gradert TL, Satterfield WC, et al. Safety of continuous intrathecal midazolam infusion in the sheep model. *Anesth Analg*. 2004;98:1528–1535.
228. Nishiyama T, Matsukawa T, Hanaoka K. Acute phase histopathologic study of spinally administered midazolam in cats. *Anesth Analg*. 1999;89:717–720.
229. Ugur B, Basaloglu K, Yurtseven T, et al. Neurotoxicity with single dose intrathecal midazolam administration. *Eur J Anaesthesiol*. 2005;22:907–912.
230. Borg PA, Krijnen HJ. Long-term intrathecal administration of midazolam and clonidine. *Clin J Pain*. 1996;12:63–68.
231. Horlocker TT, Wedel DJ. Regional anesthesia in the immunocompromised patient. *Reg Anesth Pain Med*. 2006;31:334–345.
232. Ng F, Mastoroudes H, Paul E, et al. A comparison of Hickman line- and Port-a-Cath-associated complications in patients with solid tumours undergoing chemotherapy. *Clin Oncol (R Coll Radiol)*. 2007;19:551–556.
233. Stamou SC, Maltezou HC, Pourtsidis A, et al. Hickman-Broviac catheter-related infections in children with malignancies. *Mt Sinai J Med*. 1999;66:320–326.
234. Castagnola E, Molinari AC, Fratino G, et al. Conditions associated with infections of indwelling central venous catheters in cancer patients: A summary. *Br J Haematol*. 2003;121:233–239.
235. Bedder MD, Burchiel K, Larson A. Cost analysis of two implantable narcotic delivery systems. *J Pain Symptom Manage*. 1991;6:368–373.
236. Arner S, Rawal N, Gustafsson LL. Clinical experience of long-term treatment with epidural and intrathecal opioids—a nationwide survey. *Acta Anaesthesiol Scand*. 1988;32:253–259.
237. Martin RJ, Yuan HA. Neurosurgical care of spinal epidural, subdural, and intramedullary abscesses and arachnoiditis. *Orthop Clin North Am*. 1996;27:125–136.
238. Rathmell JP, Garahan MB, Alsofrom GF. Epidural abscess following epidural analgesia. *Reg Anesth Pain Med*. 2000;25:79–82.
239. Yue SK, St Marie B, Henrickson K. Initial clinical experience with the SKY epidural catheter. *J Pain Symptom Manage*. 1991;6:107–114.
240. DuPen SL, Peterson DG, Williams A, et al. Infection during chronic epidural catheterization: Diagnosis and treatment. *Anesthesiology*. 1990;73:905–909.
241. Hogan Q, Haddox JD, Abram S, et al. Epidural opiates and local anesthetics for the management of cancer pain. *Pain*. 1991;46:271–279.
242. Rauck RL, Eisenach JC, Jackson K, et al. Epidural clonidine treatment for refractory reflex sympathetic dystrophy. *Anesthesiology*. 1993;79:1163–1169.
243. Sillevis Smitt P, Tsafka A, van den Bent M, et al. Spinal epidural abscess complicating chronic epidural analgesia in 11 cancer patients: clinical findings and magnetic resonance imaging. *J Neurol*. 1999;246:815–820.
244. Follett KA, Naumann CP. A prospective study of catheter-related complications of intrathecal drug delivery systems. *J Pain Symptom Manage*. 2000;19:209–215.
245. Vidal J, Fenollosa P, Martin E, et al. Safety and efficacy of intrathecal baclofen infusion by implantable pump for the treatment of severe spinal spasticity: A spanish multicenter study. *Neuromodulation*. 2000;3:175–182.
246. Ochs G, Naumann C, Dimitrijevic M, et al. Intrathecal baclofen therapy for spinal origin spasticity: spinal cord injury, spinal cord disease, and multiple sclerosis. *Neuromodulation*. 1999;2:108–119.
247. Dario A, Scamoni C, Picano M, et al. The infection risk of intrathecal drug infusion pumps after multiple refill procedures. *Neuromodulation*. 2005;8:36–39.
248. Turner JA, Sears JM, Loeser JD. Programmable intrathecal opioid delivery systems for chronic noncancer pain: A systematic review of effectiveness and complications. *Clin J Pain*. 2007;23:180–195.
249. Bennett MI, Tai YM, Symonds JM. Staphylococcal meningitis following Synchromed intrathecal pump implant: A case report. *Pain*. 1994;56:243–244.
250. Boviatsis EJ, Kouyialis AT, Boutsikakis I, et al. Infected CNS infusion pumps. Is there a chance for treatment without removal? *Acta Neurochir (Wien)*. 2004;146:463–467.
251. Naveira FA, Speight KL, Rauck RL, et al. Meningitis after injection of intrathecal baclofen. *Anesth Analg*. 1996;82:1297–1299.
252. Byers K, Axelrod P, Michael S, et al. Infections complicating tunneled intraspinal catheter systems used to treat chronic pain. *Clin Infect Dis*. 1995;21:403–408.
253. Schoeffler P, Pichard E, Ramboatiana R, et al. Bacterial meningitis due to infection of a lumbar drug release system in patients with cancer pain. *Pain*. 1986;25:75–77.
254. Carputo C, Philip J. Maintenance of analgesia with an intrathecal catheter system during an episode of bacterial meningitis. *J Palliat Care*. 2004;20:59–61.
255. Appelgren L, Nordborg C, Sjoberg M, et al. Spinal epidural metastasis: Implications for spinal analgesia to treat "refractory" cancer pain. *J Pain Symptom Manage*. 1997;13:25–42.
256. Hassenbusch SJ. Cost modeling for alternate routes of administration of opioids for cancer pain. *Oncology (Williston Park)*. 1999;13:63–67.
257. Taivainen T, Pitkanen M, Tuominen M, et al. Efficacy of epidural blood patch for postdural puncture headache. *Acta Anaesthesiol Scand*. 1993;37:702–705.
258. Dominguez E, Latif O, Rozen D, et al. Subdural blood patch for the treatment of persistent CSF leak after permanent intrathecal catheter implantation: A report of two cases. *Pain Pract*. 2001;1:344–353.
259. Wiegand DA, Hartel MI, Quander T, et al. Assessment of cryoprecipitate-thrombin solution for dural repair. *Head Neck*. 1994;16:569–573.
260. Nissen AJ, Johnson AJ, Perkins RC, et al. Fibrin glue in otology and neurotology. *Am J Otol*. 1993;14:147–150.
261. Crul BJ, Gerritse BM, van Dongen RT, et al. Epidural fibrin glue injection stops persistent postdural puncture headache. *Anesthesiology*. 1999;91:576–577.
262. Gerritse BM, van Dongen RT, Crul BJ. Epidural fibrin glue injection stops persistent cerebrospinal fluid leak during long-term intrathecal catheterization. *Anesth Analg*. 1997;84:1140–1141.
263. Greene NM. *Physiology of spinal anesthesia*. 3rd ed. Baltimore, Williams & Wilkins, 1983:149.
264. Carpenter RL, Rauck RL. Refractory head and neck pain. A difficult problem and a new alternative therapy [editorial]. *Anesthesiology*. 1996;84:249–252.
265. Lambert G, Elam M, Friberg P, et al. Acute response to intracisternal bupivacaine in patients with refractory pain of the head and neck. *J Physiol*. 2006;570:421–428.
266. Malinovsky JM, Benhamou D, Alafandy M, et al. Neurotoxicological assessment after intracisternal injection of liposomal bupivacaine in rabbits. *Anesth Analg*. 1997;85:1331–1336.
267. Jamison RN, Taft K, Oh JP, et al. Psychosocial and pharmacologic predictors of satisfaction with intravenous patient-controlled analgesia. *Anesth Analg*. 1993;77:121–125.
268. Chapman CR. Psychological aspects of postoperative pain control. *Acta Anaesthesiol Belg*. 1992;43:41–52.
269. Ferrante FM, Lu L, Jamison SB, et al. Patient-controlled epidural analgesia: Demand dosing. *Anesth Analg*. 1991;73:547–552.
270. Rundshagen I, Standl T, Kochs E, et al. Continuous spinal analgesia. Comparison between patient-controlled and bolus administration of plain bupivacaine for postoperative pain relief. *Reg Anesth*. 1997;22:150–156.
271. Hardy PA, Wells JC. Patient-controlled intrathecal morphine for cancer pain. A method used to assess morphine requirements and bolus doses. *Clin J Pain*. 1990;6:57–59.
272. Mullins GM, Flynn JP, el-Mahdi AM, et al. Malignant lymphoma of the spinal epidural space. *Ann Intern Med*. 1971;74:416–423.
273. Lewis DW, Packer RJ, Raney B, et al. Incidence, presentation, and outcome of spinal cord disease in children with systemic cancer. *Pediatrics*. 1986;78:438–443.
274. Portenoy RK, Galer BS, Salamon O, et al. Identification of epidural neoplasm. Radiography and bone scintigraphy in the symptomatic and asymptomatic spine. *Cancer*. 1989;64:2207–2213.
275. Barron KD, Hirano A, Araki S, et al. Experiences with metastatic neoplasms involving the spinal cord. *Neurology*. 1959;9:91–106.
276. Eaton LM, Craig WM. Tumor of the spinal cord: sudden paralysis following lumbar puncture. *Proc Staff Meet Mayo Clin*. 1940;15:170–172.
277. Hollis PH, Malis LI, Zappulla RA. Neurologic deterioration after lumbar puncture below complete spinal subarachnoid block. *J Neurosurg*. 1986;64:253–256.

CHAPTER 23 ■ SPINE AND BONE PAIN

METASTATIC SPINAL DISEASE

Metastases of the spine may occur in the spinal cord (intramedullary), in the subarachnoid space (extramedullary), epidural space, and vertebral bodies. Intramedullary metastases are relatively rare (1% to 3% of cancer patients), and originate from the tumors outside the central nervous system (CNS; most commonly breast and lung cancers) as well as from CNS tumors such as glioblastoma, medulloblastoma, and ependymoma. Tumor spread occurs via blood or due to the cord penetration from leptomeningeal tumors. Intramedullary metastases may be single or multiple. Intramedullary metastases show low signal intensity on T1-weighted (T1W) magnetic resonance imaging (MRI) and high signal intensity on T2-weighted (T2W) images, with heterogeneous contrast enhancement.

Leptomeningeal metastases have the same origin as the intramedullary ones, with the exception of acute leukemia, which occurs frequently in the dura. The intradural involvement (carcinomatous meningitis) results in thickened leptomeninges. As the tumor increases, nodules and/or plaques appear in the subarachnoid spaces. Myelography and intrathecal contrast-enhanced computed tomography (CT) reveal nodular filling defects suggesting leptomeningeal disease, which should be confirmed by positive findings on cerebrospinal fluid (CSF) study. Contrast-enhanced MRI will also identify the nodules and the dura involvement as area of contrast enhancement. Leptomeningeal involvement is most commonly seen in melanoma, breast, and lung cancer. Tumor reaches the leptomeninges by hematogenous spread or by direct extension from preexisting parenchymal tumor deposits. Tumor cells are then disseminated throughout the neuraxis by CSF flow. Patients may present with signs and symptoms suggestive of local injury to nerves (cranial nerve palsies, radicular weakness, paresthesias, or pain); direct invasion into the brain or spinal tissues or interruption of blood supply to those tissues (focal findings or seizures); obstruction of normal CSF flow pathways (headache and increased intracranial pressure); interference of normal brain function (encephalopathy); or perivascular infiltration by tumor cells, leading to local ischemia and hence stroke-like symptoms. Without treatment, the median survival is 4 to 6 weeks, and death usually occurs as a result of progressive neurologic dysfunction. Often, leptomeningeal metastases are a manifestation of end-stage disease, and symptom management may be the most appropriate care.

Epidural and paraspinal lesions are closely related to those of vertebral bodies. On MRI, the tumor cells infiltrate and replace the fatty epidural spaces, with isohypointensity on T1W imaging, and high signal on T2W imaging, with homogeneous enhancement on postcontrast studies. Metastases of the vertebral bodies are the most frequent pathology of the spine. MRI is the method of choice in symptomatic patients for detecting and defining vertebral body metastases. Daldrup-Link et al.[1] noted that positron-emission tomography (PET) scanning had a higher sensitivity (90%) for detection of bone metastases in young adults than whole-body MRI (82%) and skeletal scintigraphy (71%). Foraminal and intracanalar epidural extension of lesions is well defined on postcontrast MRI images. On T1W images the osteolytic metastasis by tumoral infiltration of the bone marrow shows hypointense signal related to isointense signal of the bone, whereas on T2W imaging, metastases show a high signal, easily depicted on Short T1 Inversion Recovery (STIR) and Spectral Presaturation by Inversion Recovery (SPIR) sequences.

The most frequent presentation of spinal tumors is axial pain. A thorough spinal examination includes assessment of local tenderness, deformity, limitation of motion, and signs of nerve root or cord compression. Management is guided by three key issues: neurologic compromise, spinal instability, and individual patient factors. Standard treatment options for spinal tumors include radiation therapy alone, radionuclide therapy, radiation plus systemic chemotherapy, hormonal therapy, or surgical decompression and/or stabilization followed by radiation.

The role of radiation therapy in the treatment of metastatic tumors of the spine is well established and is often the initial treatment modality.[2] The goals of local radiation therapy in the treatment of spinal tumors are palliation of pain, prevention of pathologic fractures, and halting progression of or reversing neurologic compromise. A primary factor that limits radiation dose for local vertebral tumor control with conventional radiation therapy is the relatively low tolerance of the spinal cord to radiation.[3] Conventional external beam radiation lacks the accuracy to deliver large single-fraction doses of radiation to the spine near radiosensitive structures such as the spinal cord. Consequently, the low tolerance of the spinal cord to radiation often limits the treatment dose to a level that is far below the optimal therapeutic dose thus limiting the optimal clinical response.

Radiosurgery is defined as the delivery of a highly conformal, large single-fraction radiation dose by a stereotactic approach to a localized intracranial or extracranial tumor. The goal of radiosurgery is cessation of tumor growth and preservation of neurologic function. Precise confinement of the radiation dose should increase the likelihood of successful tumor control while minimizing the risk of spinal cord injury. Radiosurgery has been shown to be very effective for controlling intracranial malignancies.[4] Stereotactic radiosurgery for tumors of the spine has also been demonstrated to be accurate, safe, and efficacious.[5]

The emerging technique of spinal radiosurgery represents a logical extension of the current state-of-the-art radiation therapy. Technological developments include imaging technology for three-dimensional localization and pretreatment planning, the advent of intensity-modulated radiated therapy, and a higher degree of accuracy in achieving target dose conformation while sparing normal surrounding tissue. Unlike conventional radiation therapy that delivers a full dose to both the vertebral body and the spinal cord, the CyberKnife Image-Guided Radiosurgery System (Accuray, Sunnyvale, CA) can deliver a single high-dose fraction of radiation that conforms to the target tissue while sparing most of the adjacent spinal cord. Fiducials are placed using fluoroscopic guidance using a percutaneous technique. Fiducial placement procedure is performed in the operating room in an outpatient setting. A limit of 8 Gy is set as the maximum spinal cord dose for treatment planning calculations. A limit of 2 Gy is set as the maximum dose to each of the kidneys. A limit of 4 Gy is set as the maximum dose to the bowel. This especially becomes important in the treatment of lower thoracic and lumbar vertebrae, even more so if the patient has undergone a nephrectomy or received nephrotoxic chemotherapy. Potential lesions for spinal radiosurgery are listed in Table 23.1.

Gerszten et al.[6] reported that spinal radiosurgery was highly effective in decreasing pain in patients with spinal tumors. Long-term pain improvement occurred in 96% of women with breast cancer, 96% of patients with melanoma, 94% of patients with renal cell carcinoma, and 92% of patients with neurofibromatosis Type 1. Pain usually decreased within weeks after treatment, and occasionally within days. Spinal radiosurgery was also effective at alleviating radicular pain caused by tumor compression of adjacent nerve roots.

MANAGEMENT OF EPIDURAL SPINAL CORD COMPRESSION

Epidural spinal cord compression (ESCC) is a neurologic emergency requiring immediate attention. ESCC usually occurs in patients with disseminated disease. The patterns of compression, as identified by magnetic resonance imaging (MRI) scan, appear to be predominantly soft tissue epidural disease.[7] Figure 23.1 outlines a treatment algorithm of patients with symptomatic epidural spinal metastasis. Treatment of patients with coexisting pain and neurologic deficits should be prioritized according to neurologic deficit.

The therapy instituted depends on several factors, including the patient's condition at the time of presentation, the nature of the underlying malignancy, the extent of systemic disease burden, and patient prognosis.[8] The goals of treatment are pain relief, preservation or recovery of neurologic function, and preservation of spinal stability. Prompt administration of corticosteroids is standard if symptomatic spinal cord compression is confirmed or strongly suspected on clinical grounds. However, there is no general agreement concerning the dosage and the schedule. Dexamethasone is the most commonly used corticosteroid, in doses of 10 to 100 mg I.V. bolus (according to clinical decision based on the course of neurologic deficit, prognosis, and clinical experience) followed by 16 to 96 mg daily orally. Commonly, the regimen is 96 mg I.V. bolus of dexamethasone followed by 96 mg per day orally for 3 days and a 10-day taper. The indications for chemotherapy in the treatment of spinal cord compression are very limited and in general should be considered as the sole therapy for adults with chemosensitive tumors (lymphoma, myeloma, breast, or germ cell tumors) who are not candidates for surgery or radiation.

The best treatment for ESCC is not well defined, and the choice between surgery with radiation or radiation alone is debatable. Management by radiation must balance the need to deliver a sufficient dose of radiation to kill the tumor and the need to avoid further injuring the spinal cord. Radiation volume is usually defined by myelography, computed tomography (CT), or MRI. The standard radiation volume should include the site of cord compression and should extend two vertebral bodies above and below.[9] For patients with ESCC from solid tumors, 30 Gy in 10 fractions is considered the standard of care.[10] Special techniques such as image-guided intensity modulated radiation therapy (IG-IMRT) or stereotactic body radiation therapy (SBRT) should be considered. However, the routine use of IG-IMRT or SBRT are currently not recommended, because the technology is expensive, and it has yet to show definite benefit over conventional delivery of radiation in a patient population that has a median survival of 6 months or less.[10] The restrictions imposed by the radiation tolerance of the cord can limit the success of therapy. The ceiling of response, defined as maintaining pretherapeutic level of ambulation/motor function, is 80% with radiation therapy alone.[5] This is particularly true with extensive tumor burdens, like spinal cord compression associated with a paravertebral mass, which require high doses of radiation to achieve local control. Lung cancers, specifically apical tumors, account for 60% of the presentations of epidural spinal cord compression associated with a paravertebral mass. Complete response to radiation therapy is achieved in 30% of all tumor types, including breast cancer and malignant melanoma.[11] Radiosensitive tumors, like lymphoproliferative malignancies, multiple myeloma, and germ cell tumors, have a better outcome, with 77% of these tumors achieving a complete response to radiation alone.

TABLE 23.1

POTENTIAL LESIONS FOR SPINAL RADIOSURGERY

Well-circumscribed lesion
Minimal spinal cord compromise
Radioresistant lesions that would benefit from a radiosurgical boost
Residual tumor after surgery
Previously irradiated lesions precluding further external bean radiation
Recurrent surgical lesions
Relatively short life expectancy as an exclusion for open surgical intervention

(Modified from Gerszten PC, Burton SA. Clinical assessment of stereotactic IGRT: Spinal radiosurgery. *Med Dosim.* 2008;33:107–116. Copyright 2008 American Association of Medical Dosimetrists; published by Elsevier, Inc.)

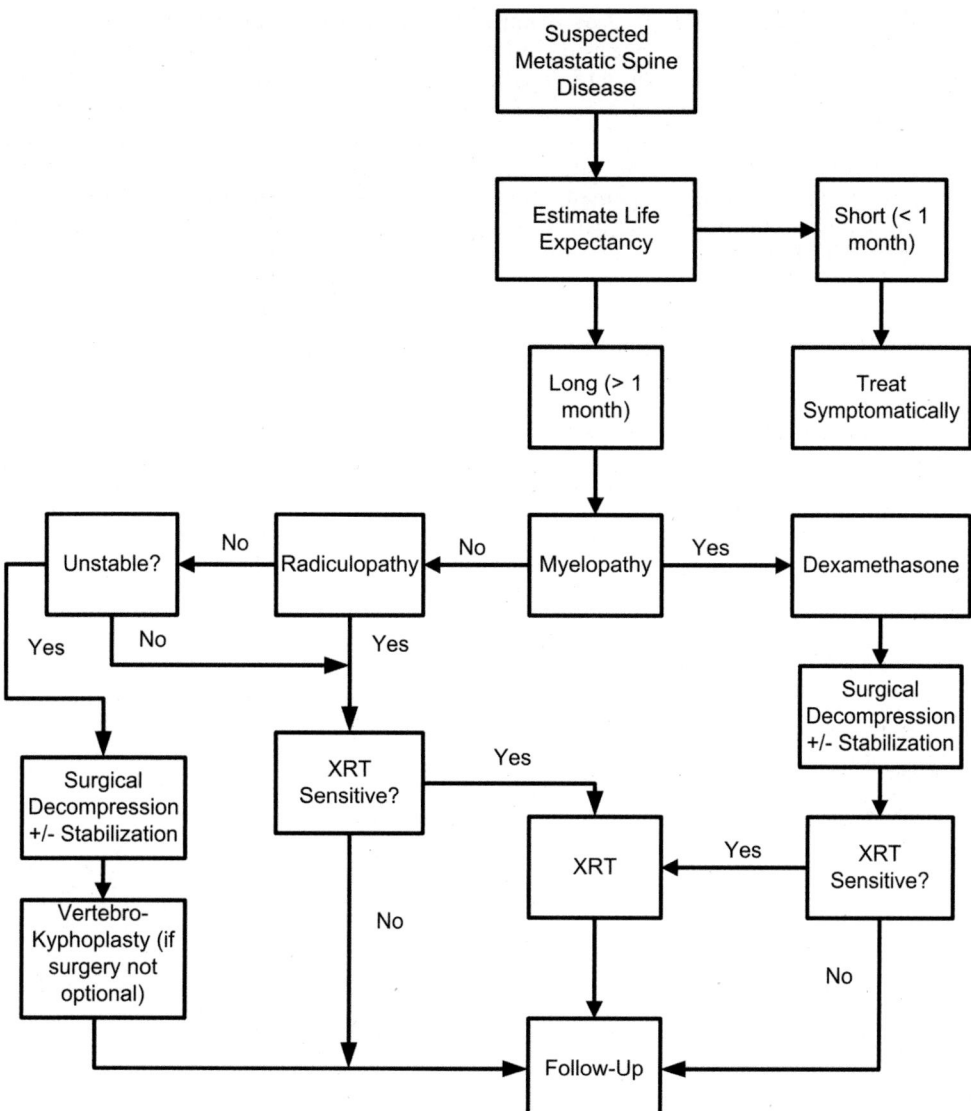

FIGURE 23.1 Treatment algorithm of patients with symptomatic epidural spinal metastasis. XRT, Radiation therapy.

Combining surgery with radiation therapy may help improve therapeutic outcome. In some cases, surgical decompression by vertebrectomy or laminectomy can promptly reduce pain and improve neurologic status. These clinical improvements follow promptly relieving the mechanical compression produced by collapse of a vertebral body, and improving spinal stability. Surgical intervention is an alternative for patients presenting with a high-grade epidural lesion, particularly a lesion because of a radiation insensitive tumor. Surgery often is the only available option for therapy, because previously administered radiation may preclude further radiation in the area of compression. This is often the case in lung cancer because over 70% of spinal cord involvement in lung cancer is located in the thoracic spine, and many of these patients have received mediastinal radiation. Surgical intervention may provide significant benefit in specific groups with spinal cord or cauda equina compression. Patient selection should depend upon prognostic factors, so far as possible. For example, median survival in breast cancer patients with epidural metastases is significantly less if visceral metastases are evident.[12] Even patients with advanced malignancies may benefit from surgical intervention if it is possible to maintain neurologic integrity.[13] Decompressive laminectomy is suitable for posterior tumors in order to relieve spinal cord compression and to remove the lesion but is not considered helpful for the majority of compressions (which occur in the anterior epidural space) as laminectomy has been associated with a high rate of spinal instability[14] and poor neurologic outcome.[15] Anterior decompression (vertebral body resection) and stabilization is suitable in carefully selected patients (in good medical condition, with focal anterior ESCC and paraparesis), when performed in highly specialized centers. Many now advocate direct decompressive and maximal-debulking surgery with intraoperative stabilization of the spine (in appropriate cases) followed by postoperative radiation therapy.[10]

Measures of response involve pain and functional status. With radiation therapy alone, back pain resolves in 60% to 80% of patients.[16–19] Improvement in motor and autonomic dysfunction occurs in 40% to 60% of cases.[16–17] Pretreatment functional status is maintained at 3 years in follow-up after radiation therapy in over 90% of surviving patients.

FOCUSED MANAGEMENT STRATEGIES FOR PAINFUL BONE METASTASES

Metastasis to bone is a significant problem for a large number of cancer patients; up to 85% of patients dying from breast, prostate, or lung cancer primary tumors demonstrate bone involvement at autopsy.[20] The morbidity of bone metastases can become significant due to pain and pathologic fracture. Pharmacologic management of pain associated with bone metastases is the mainstay of treatment and should follow the principles outlined in Chapter 16. Delaney et al.[21] suggest an algorithmic approach to this problem based on well-designed randomized controlled trials, systematic reviews, or mega-analysis of published therapies (Fig. 23.2).

Not all patients with bone metastases exhibit symptoms, but as many as two thirds of patients with metastatic bone disease experience severe pain, particularly those who are in advanced stages of their diseases.[22] Therapeutic strategies for painful bone metastases are listed in Table 23.2. The site of bone metastases significantly influences management strategies. In breast cancer patients, solitary bone metastases have different management implications than multiple skeletal metastases. Koizumi et al.[23] showed in a multivariate analysis that a solitary metastatic bone lesion ($P = .002$) is an independent favorable prognostic factor in patients with skeletal metastasis and patients with solitary lesions live longer than patients with multiple metastases. Furthermore, although external beam radiation therapy remains the mainstay of pain palliation of solitary lesions, bone-seeking radiopharmaceuticals may be used in preference for the treatment of multiple painful osseous lesions.[24]

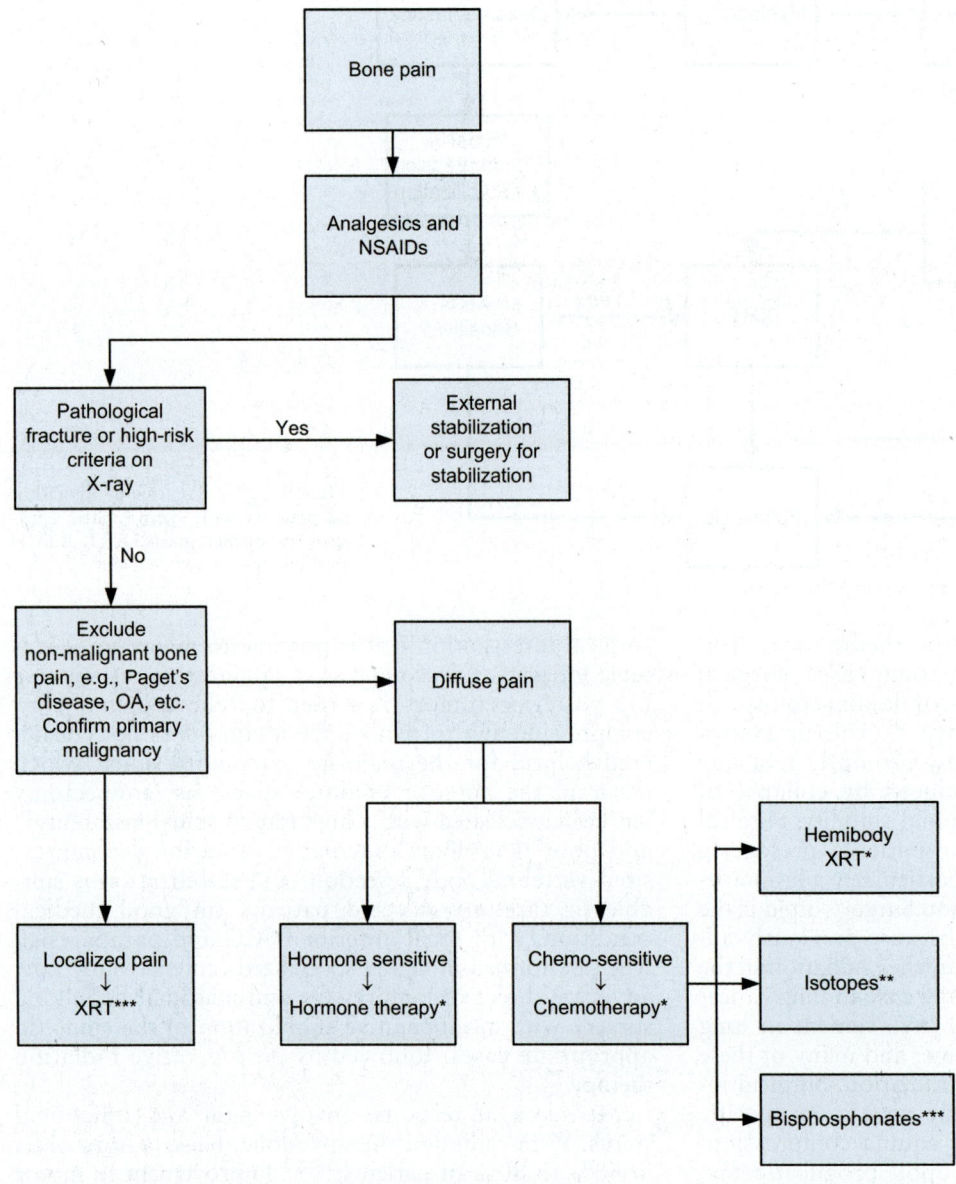

FIGURE 23.2 Overview of the management of metastatic bone pain.

*Nonrandomized controlled trials, cohort study, and so on.
**One or more well-designed randomized controlled trials.
***Systematic review or meta-analysis.
(Modified from Delaney A, Fleetwood-Walker SM, Colvin LA, et al. Translational medicine: Cancer pain mechanisms and management. *Br J Anaesth*. 2008;101:87–94. By permission of Oxford University Press.)

TABLE 23.2
STRATEGIES FOR MANAGING PAINFUL BONE METASTASES

- Base treatments or treatments directed towards oncologic illness
- Conventional analgesics, eg, acetaminophen and nonsteroidal anti-inflammatory drugs, with or without opioid
- Radiation therapy for localized bone metastases
- Specific drugs for bone pain that work on the bone tumor-induced alteration, eg, bisphosphonates (which inhibit osteoclastic activity and reduce bone resorption), radiopharmaceuticals, or calcitonin
- Surgery (stabilization of bones at risk for fracture)
- Vertebroplasty/kyphoplasty
- Radiofrequency/cryoablation

Chemotherapy

Bone metastasis represents systemic spread of disease, and oncologists often treat bone metastases with systemic therapies, such as chemotherapy and hormonal therapy.[25,26] The analgesic effect of systemic chemotherapy depends mainly on the chemosensitivity of the specific primary tumor. Chemotherapeutic options can provide excellent pain relief, especially in breast or prostate cancer patients. Hormone therapy is mainly used in hormone-sensitive breast cancer (tamoxifen, letrozole, anastrozole)[27] and prostate cancer (antiandrogens and gonadotrophin-releasing hormone analogues).[28]

Bisphosphonates

Physiologic bone turnover maintains normal skeletal integrity through a coupled process of bone resorption, mediated by osteoclasts, followed by new bone formation. Major features of the pathogenesis of tumor-associated skeletal destruction are enhanced osteoclast-mediated bone resorption and disruption of normal bone formation. Bisphosphonates, by inhibiting bone turnover and decreasing the resorption of bone, are useful in the management of bone metastases. The effects of these agents are complex and include antiosteoclastic activity, suppression of progression of bone metastases, alteration of cell activity and apoptosis, antiangiogenic properties, and immunomodulator effects. Their role is most clearly defined in breast cancer and multiple myeloma but clinical benefit may extend the entire spectrum of metastatic bone disease.[29,30] Of interest, some authors suggest that the use of third-generation bisphosphonates such as zoledronic acid may have changed the computed tomography (CT) appearance of osteolytic bone metastases from breast cancer to an osteosclerotic appearance.[31] Zoledronic acid is the only bisphosphonate that has demonstrated statistically significant, long-term clinical benefits through the prevention and delay of skeletal-related events in patients with metastatic prostate cancer or renal cell carcinoma[32] and is the only bisphosphonate to show efficacy in prostate cancer, lung cancer, and other solid tumors.[33]

Radiopharmaceuticals

The clinical development of bone-seeking radiopharmaceuticals is based on the rationale that medium- to high-energy β particle radiation, targeted and delivered to skeletal sites involved with tumor, can result in more effective antitumor activity while sparing normal tissues the damaging effects of radiation. Metastatic lesions that produce a significant osteoblastic response in bone will concentrate bone precursors such as the radiopharmaceuticals.

Radiopharmaceuticals bind to the bone matrix in areas of increased bone turnover due to metastatic response. β rays from the specific radionuclide, bound to its carrier ligand, result in the therapeutic effect. These agents bind to hydroxyapatite, most actively at the tumor-bone interface of osteoblastic lesions, where they deliver therapeutic doses of radiation with tissue penetration limited to a few millimeters. This limited penetration allows multiple sites and diffuse disease to be treated while sparing most of the surrounding healthy tissue. The sole significant toxicity is due to the effect of β particle radiation on rapidly dividing cells in the adjacent bone marrow. By calculating the percentage of the skeleton involved with metastases, combined with the dosage and the patients' bone marrow reserve, hematologic toxicity can be predicted. Contraindications for the use of bone-seeking radiopharmaceuticals are thrombocytopenia (<100,000/mL) or leukopenia (<3000/mL), acute renal insufficiency, and pregnancy. The aim of the treatment is palliation of pain, improvement of the patients' quality of life, reduced intake of analgesics, reduced use of chemotherapy and external beam radiotherapy, and improvement of disease-free survival.

Onset of pain relief may occur as early as 3 to 6 days, but more typically begins within 1 to 2 weeks of administration, with occasional responses seen after a latency of up to 4 weeks. The duration of pain relief is typically on the order of 1 to 6 months, after which treatment may be repeated multiple times, if necessary.[34,35]

Various radiopharmaceuticals have been developed for this purpose. Each has its own characteristics. These radiopharmaceuticals include samarium-153-ethylenediaminetetramethylene phosphonic acid (Sm-153 EDTMP) and strontium-89-chloride, which are approved in the United States and Europe, as well as the not universally approved rhenium-186-hydroxyethane diphosphonic acid (Re-186 HEDP). Depending on the half-life and radiation energy of the specific radionuclide, they exert a different effect and toxicity profile. In most cases, bone marrow toxicity is limited and reversible, which makes repetitive treatment relatively safe.

Evidence supporting the use of radiopharmaceuticals is greatest for prostate (nearly always osteoblastic) and breast (usually mixed osteoblastic/osteoclastic) malignancies.[34] Data are limited for solid tumors with bone tropisms such as lung, renal, and thyroid cancer. The most significant toxicity of these agents is reversible, moderate myelosuppression. Drops in leukocyte and platelet counts are generally in the range of 30% to 70% and correlate with existing marrow reserve. Myelosuppression generally begins between weeks 2 and 4, reaches a nadir between 4 to 6 weeks, and resolves by 8 to 12 weeks. Complete blood counts should be monitored biweekly until acceptable marrow recovery is observed.

Surgery

Structural weakness secondary to extensive bone loss is not acutely reversed with medical or radiation therapy. The local effects of chemotherapy and radiation depress the rate of bone regeneration in compromised areas. In such cases, an approach that supports the bone during recovery is often necessary. Long-bone fractures most commonly occur in the femur and humerus and are typically internally fixed by intramedullary devices that control impaction, distraction, and torquing stresses by the use of proximal and distal interlocking fixation. Orthotic devices can often protect upper-extremity lesions. The lower extremity is less tolerant, largely because of the high stress experienced during ambulation. Impending fractures of the lower extremity generally require surgical stabilization with fracture fixation devices or prosthetic reconstruction. In general, the only indication for endoprosthesis is an intracapsular or very proximal lesion. In almost all other cases, intramedullary nailing is preferred.[36] The humerus is the second most common long-bone site of metastatic disease, and the proximal third and diaphysis are frequent sites. Purely lytic disease and cortical bone destruction increase the risk of fracture more than 50% (Fig. 23.3). For most patients, external beam irradiation is effective as a means of pain control and halting bone destruction. Fractures of the head or surgical neck of the humerus can be treated with standard endoprostheses, whereas extensive proximal bone destruction is treated with custom proximal humeral replacements. Impending and complete diaphyseal fractures can be treated effectively with either intramedullary nail fixation or plate fixation.[37] Rigid fixation, which can be achieved with dual plate fixation, is optimal because patients can begin immediate unrestricted activities using the upper extremity. The indications for prophylactic fixation of impending fractures remain poorly defined. Table 23.3 lists guidelines for indications for prophylactic fixation of impending long bone fractures.

One of the problems with plain x-rays is that bone loss must approach 30% to 50% before it becomes apparent. In addition, in metastatic lesions characterized by bone production (eg, prostate), clear evidence of bone destruction can be difficult to assess by plain radiography. Once a pathological fracture has occurred, aggressive surgical treatment is normally in order. Patients who are medically unstable or who have a life expectancy of less than 4 weeks are not surgical candidates. Habermann[38] found that 97% of patients had good to excellent pain relief after internal fixation or prosthetic replacement. Harrington[39] reported a success rate of 95% in returning patients to prefracture ambulatory status with surgical intervention. Current fracture fixation methods have led to improved patient survival, from 24.6 months to 11.6 months, after pathologic fracture.[39]

The spine is the most common site for skeletal metastasis. Oncologists can manage most spinal metastases conservatively. CT and MRI of the spine are reserved for patients who present with radiologic evidence of vertebral body compression >50% or who present with neurological involvement suggestive of nerve root or spinal cord compression. Once the workup is complete, patients fall into five categories, depending on the extent of neurological involvement or bone destruction (Table 23.4). Patients with spinal metastases that symptomatically compress spinal cord of nerve roots are discussed in Chapter 21.

The majority of patients fall into categories I, II, or III and they are candidates for nonoperative treatment with

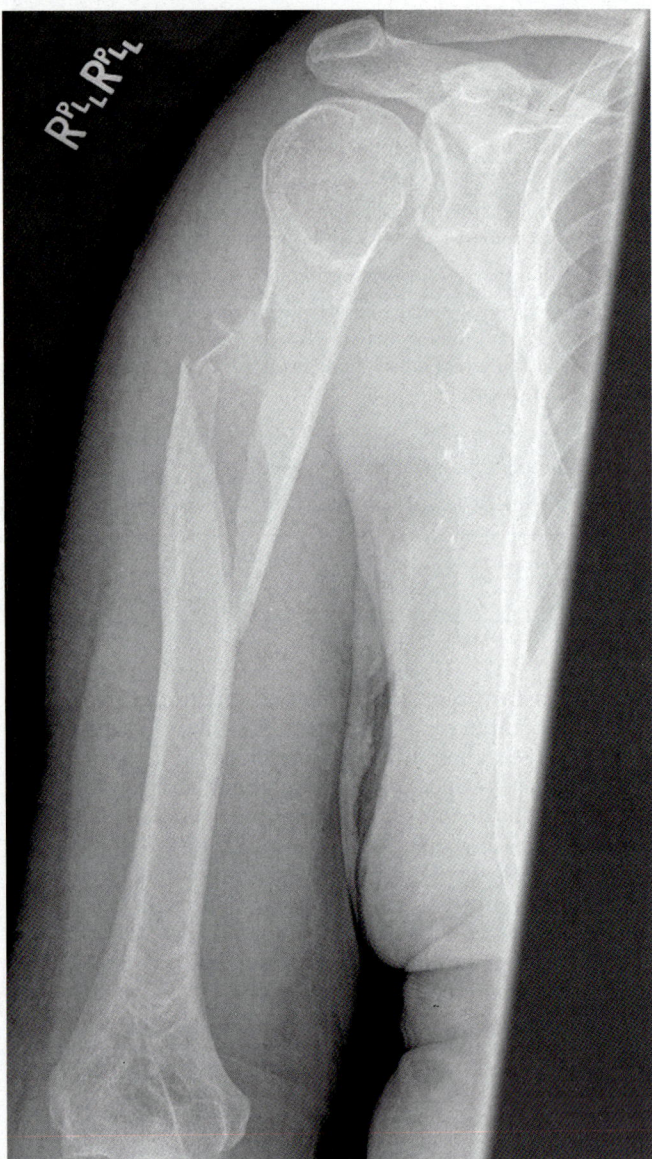

FIGURE 23.3 A 56-year-old man with metastatic melanoma presented with sudden onset right upper extremity pain. Plain x-ray of the upper extremity showed a spiral displaced fracture of the humerus secondary to metastases.

TABLE 23.3

INDICATIONS FOR PROPHYLACTIC FIXATION OF IMPENDING LONG-BONE FRACTURES

Cortical bone destruction of >50%
Lesion of >2.5 cm in the proximal femur
Pathological avulsion fracture of the lesser trochanter
Persisting stress pain despite irradiation

(With permission from Harrington KD. *Orthopaedic management of metastatic bone disease*. St. Louis, Mo.: CV Mosby, 1988.)

TABLE 23.4
CATEGORIES OF SKELETAL SPINAL METASTASIS

Class	Degree of Involvement
I	No major neurological involvement
II	Involvement of bone without collapse and instability
III	Major neurological involvement (sensory or motor) without significant bone involvement
IV	Vertebral collapse with pain due to mechanical causes or instability but without significant neurological impairment
V	Vertebral collapse or instability combined with major neurological impairment

(Data from Harrington KD. Metastatic disease of the spine. *J Bone Joint Surg (Am)*. 1986;68:1110–1115. Reprinted with permission from The Journal of Bone and Joint Surgery Inc.)

chemotherapy, hormonal manipulation, radiation therapy, or a combination of these. Operative intervention is reserved for patients in categories IV or V. The treatment of choice is anterior resection of the diseased vertebral body and reconstruction with bone graft or methylmethacrylate and anterior or posterior spinal instrumentation as needed. Advances in spinal instrumentation have resulted in better methods for the stabilization of vertebral body collapse secondary to metastatic disease[40] (Fig 23.4).

Radiation

Radiation remains the treatment of choice, and radiation therapy given in a single fraction has proven to be an efficient and cost-effective alternative to traditional multifraction radiation courses.[41] However, surveys in the United States indicated that 30 Gy over 10 sessions was most commonly used in the treatment of bone metastases, and 90% to 100% of these oncologists preferred multiple- over single-fraction radiation therapy.[42] Radiation therapy is usually effective at reducing pain from painful bone metastases. There is no evidence of any difference in efficacy between different fractionation schedules, or of a dose-response with total dose of radiation.[43] For treatment of generalized bone pain from multiple bone metastases, both hemibody irradiation and radioisotopes can reduce the number of painful new sites. A pain flare is common after palliative radiation for osseous metastases and patients receiving single-fraction radiotherapy may be at higher risk.[44] The use of prophylactic dexamethasone in doses of 8 mg may be helpful in attenuating this flare.[45]

Vertebroplasty/Kyphoplasty

Percutaneous vertebroplasty (PVP) involves the injection of polymethyl methacrylate (PMMA), or other nonacrylic cements, through a large needle within the vertebral body under radiologic guidance. A transpedicular approach is used typically in the lower lumbar spine, but in the upper lumbar spine because of the smaller diameter and more sagitally oriented pedicles, an extrapedicular approach may be preferred. Biplanar fluoroscopy is used to ensure adequate visualization to minimize the risk of spread of PMMA outside of the vertebral body into the retroperitoneum, the spinal canal, or the paraspinal tissues.

Kyphoplasty involves the use of a balloon tamp to both create a void in the vertebral body and to elevate the depressed endplates to reduce the deformity of the vertebral body. It involves the percutaneous placement of balloon tamps into the vertebral body, followed by an inflation/deflation sequence to create a cavity before PMMA injection. After removal of the tamp, the PMMA fixes and stabilizes the fracture. The balloon tamp is a high-pressure balloon designed to force the vertebral body back to its original height. The technique is illustrated in Figure 23.5. The goals of treatment include pain relief, fracture stabilization, restoration of vertebral height, and strengthening of the vertebral body to reduce the risk of a future fracture at the same level.

The main indication for vertebroplasty is back pain associated with osteoporotic vertebral fractures refractory to medical treatment (Fig. 23.6). Other indications for PVP are painful vertebral fractures related to malignant or benign tumors, including multiple myeloma or, less frequently, fractures associated with osteonecrosis. Absolute and relative indications for vertebroplasty are listed in Table 23.5. Because medical therapy is considered to have failed only after a period of at least 4 weeks, the fractures that are considered for vertebroplasty almost always are subacute: typically between 4 and 12 weeks old. Vertebroplasty has been performed in the acute phase (<4 weeks) for several indications, including osteoporosis, multiple myeloma, and trauma-induced fractures, including burst fractures; however, this may lead to a higher risk for complications such as cement leakage. Although most fractures treated with PVP are subacute and less than 1 year old, there may also be benefit in treating fractures more than 1 year old.[46]

Vertebroplasty is useful for alleviating pain, for providing mechanical stabilization, and improving posture, especially in osteolytic neoplasms.[47] Although spinal canal compromise due to retropulsed bony fragments

TABLE 23.5
INDICATIONS FOR VERTEBROPLASTY

Absolute	Relative
Painful metastatic lesion with intact posterior vertebral cortex	Chronic painful vertebral compression fracture without nonunion
Subacute (<3 months) painful fracture refractory to best medical therapy	Acute fracture with associated kyphosis ≥20 degrees
Progressive kyphosis to ≥20 degrees in subacute fracture	Acute fracture with collapse ≥40 degrees
Chronic (>3 months) painful fracture with nonunion	Acute-on-subacute chronic fracture
	Recurrent discomfort at level of previous vertebroplasty refractory to medical therapy

(From Heran, MK, Legrehn GM and Munk PL. Current concepts and techniques in percutaneous vertebroplasty. *Orthop Clin North Am*. 2006; 37:409–434. With permission from Elsevier, Inc.)

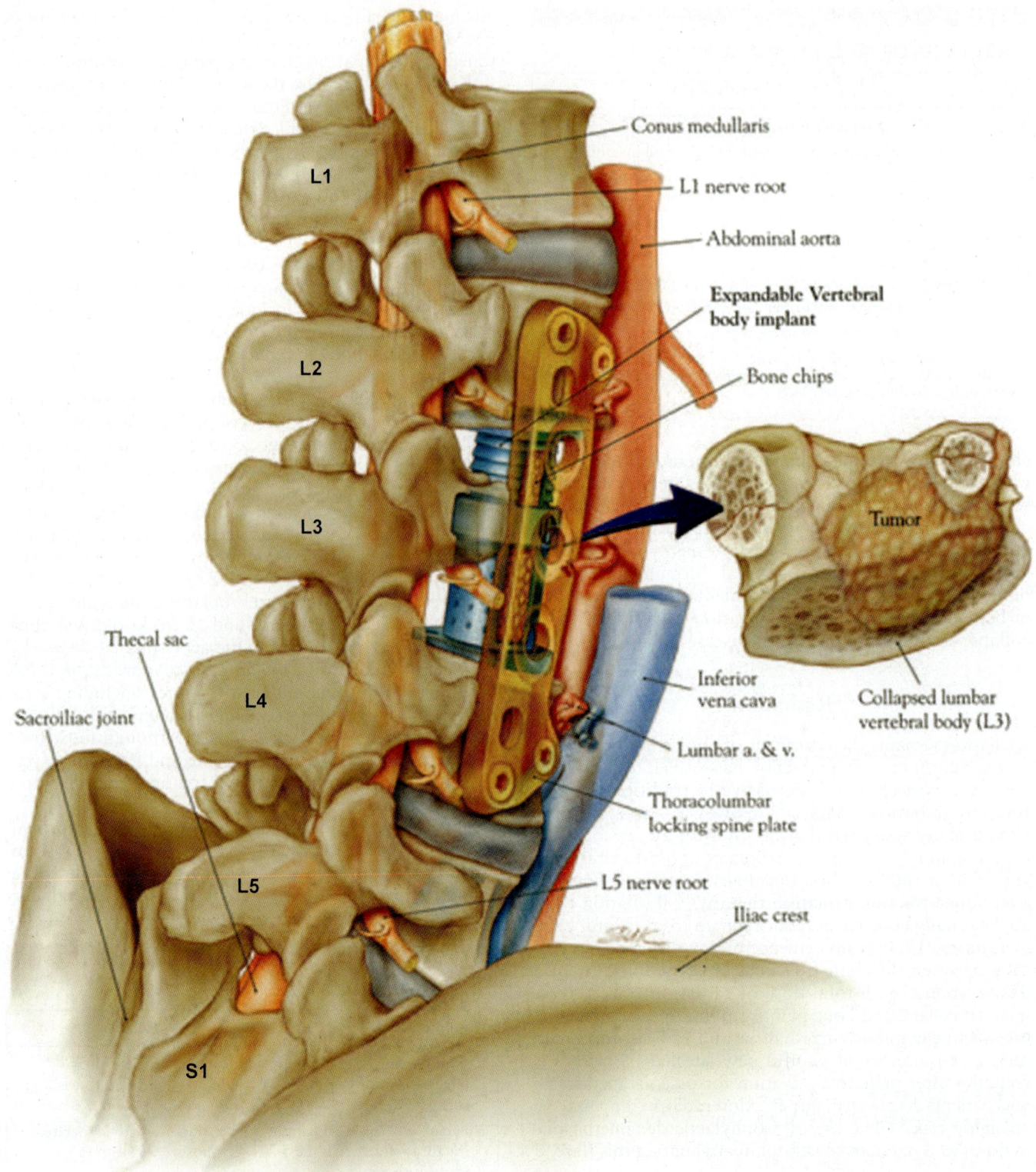

FIGURE 23.4 Surgical instrumentation of the lumbar spine. (From Holman PJ, et al. Surgical management of metastatic disease of the lumbar spine: Experience with 139 patients. *J Neurosurg Spine*. 2005;2:550–563. Figure reprinted by permission of *Journal of Neurosurgery Spine* and Ian Suk, illustrator.)

or epidural neoplastic extension presents a significant risk, vertebroplasty has been performed safely in this setting.[48,49]

Cheung et al.[50] reported on the effects of PPV in 30 patients with intractable pain from vertebral metastases (13 patients, many of whom were resistant to palliative radiation therapy) and patients with intractable painful osteoporotic fractures (17 patients) who were treated with parapedicular or transpedicular injection of PMMA. PVP in osteoporotic and metastatic fractures signifi-

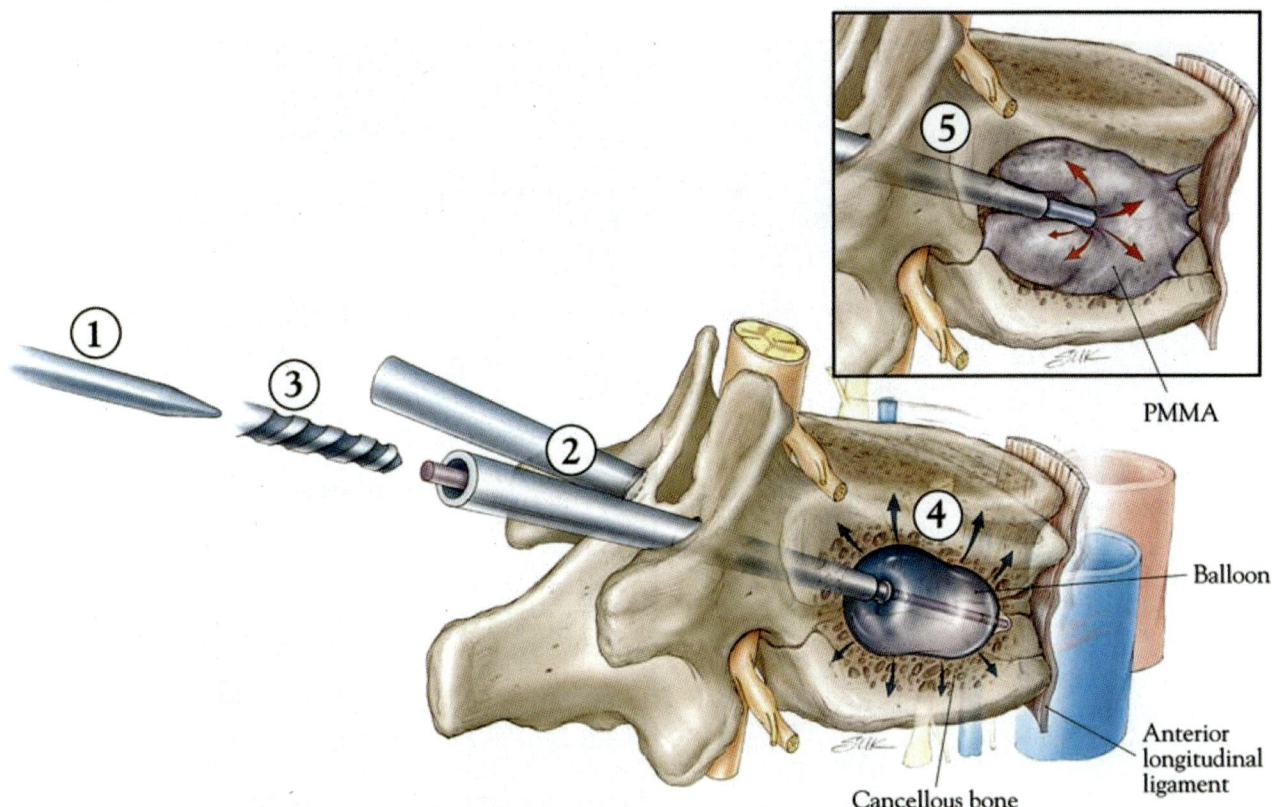

FIGURE 23.5 Technique for kyphoplasty. Using a bilateral transpedicular approach, bone biopsy needles are directed into the posterior third of the VB. Guide pins *(K-wires)* are used to exchange the biopsy needles for blunt cannulated obturators (1). Working cannulas (2) are then advanced, and the obturators and K-wires are removed. A hand mounted drill (3) creates bilateral channels within the anterior aspect of the VB for placement of the inflatable bone tamps (4). Balloon inflation allows restoration of VB height. *Inset:* The tamps are removed and the osseous void is filled with polymethyl methacrylate displaced from bone cement cannulae. (5) VB, Vertebral body.
(From Fourney DR, Schomer DF, Nader R, et al. Percutaneous vertebroplasty and kyphoplasty for painful vertebral body fractures in cancer patients. *J Neurosurg.* 2003;98:21–30.)

cantly improved many patients' global quality of life scores and function by markedly decreasing their back pain and reducing their intake of pain medications. The procedure was deemed safe with no serious complications noted. Weill et al.[47] reported on 33 patients who had cancer with spinal metastases and were treated with vertebroplasty and then followed for 6 months. Seventy-three percent showed marked improvement, 21% had moderate improvement, and 6% experienced no improvement. The improvement was durable in 73% of patients at 6 months. Fourney et al.[51] described 84% of their oncologic patient group as having marked or complete pain relief following vertebroplasty, with an absence of symptomatic cement leakage–mediated complications. In this study, 97 (65 vertebroplasty and 32 kyphoplasty) procedures were performed in 56 patients during 58 treatment sessions.

Percutaneous Radio-frequency/Cryoablation

Radiofrequency (RF) ablation is a technique whereby an alternating electrical current operating in the frequency of radiowaves (460 to 480 kHz) is emitted from the tip of an electrode or needle placed directly into the tissue. The alternating current causes the local ions to oscillate, producing heat and inducing cell death by coagulative necrosis. Newly developed percutaneous cryoprobes are based on delivery of argon gas through a segmentally insulated probe, with rapid expansion of the gas resulting in rapid cooling, reaching −100°C within a few seconds.

Percutaneous ablation may be useful for managing pain from bony metastatic disease. These image-guided treatments can be performed precisely, allowing safe treatment of complex metastatic tumors. A single ablation treatment may be effective, is well tolerated, and often provides a long duration of pain relief.[52,53] Callstrom et al.[52] published a single-arm, paired-comparison, observational study involving 12 patients with a single painful osteolytic metastasis; each patient served as his or her own control. Radiation therapy or chemotherapy had failed to provide pain relief. All treated lesions were osteolytic, with a combination of bone destruction and soft tissue mass. A single lesion was treated in all 12 patients. The size of the treated lesion ranged from 1 to 11 cm. One patient with a large lesion was treated in two separate sessions 6 weeks apart, and the remaining 11 patients were treated in a single RF session. Before RF ablation, the mean worst pain score in a 24-hour period in the 12 patients was 8.0 (range: 6 to 10). At 4 weeks post-RF treatment, the recorded mean worst pain had decreased to 3.1 ($P < .001$). No major complications from RF ablation were observed in these 12 patients. Most experience currently with percutaneous RF ablation for the treatment of bone tumors is with osteoid osteomas.[54] Thanos et al.[55] used CT-guided RF ablation in the

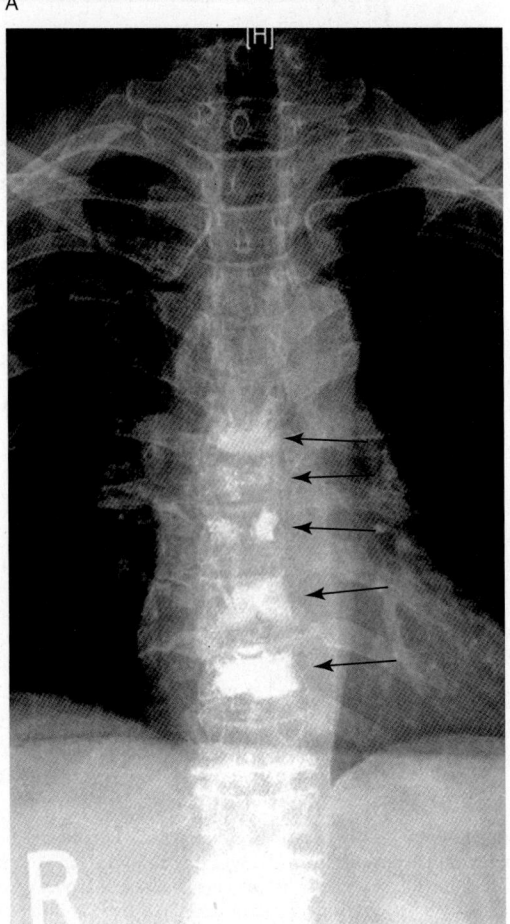
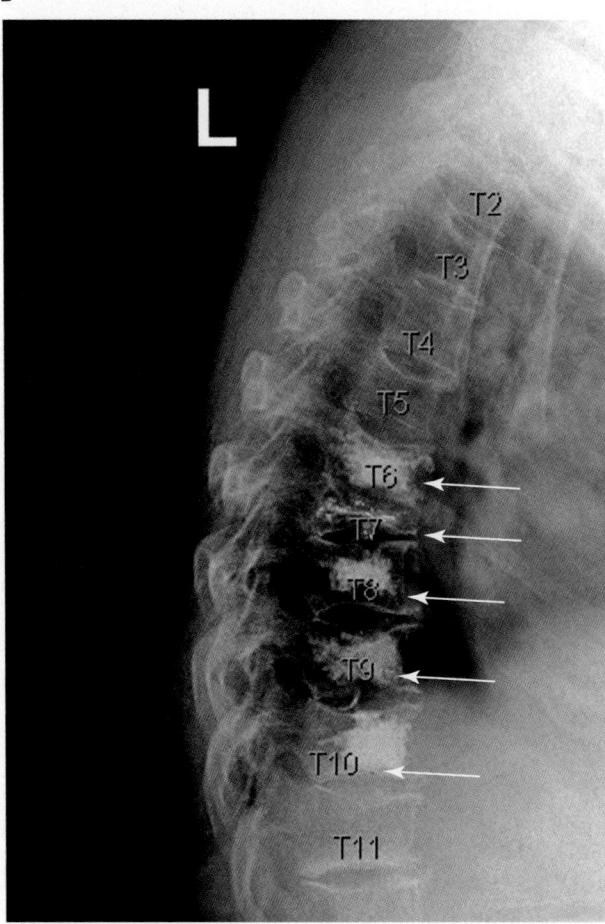

FIGURE 23.6 A 65-year-old woman with multiple thoracolumbar compression fractures secondary to chronic steroid therapy. The patient was treated with multilevel vertebroplasties *(arrows)* (**A**). She also has evidence of severe kyphosis (**B**).

treatment of 30 patients (34 lesions) with painful bone metastases. There was a significant decrease in the mean past-24-h Brief Pain Inventory (BPI) score for worst pain, for average pain, and for pain interference during daily life (4.7, 4.8, and 5.3 units, respectively) 4 and 8 weeks after treatment.

Callstrom et al.[56] also investigated the safety and effectiveness of percutaneous cryoablation for the reduction of pain, improvement in the activities of daily life, and reduction in the use of analgesic medications for 14 patients with painful bone metastases. Treated lesions were 1 to 11 cm in diameter. Before cryoablation, the mean score for worst pain in a 24-hour period was 6.7 of 10; the score decreased to 3.8 ($P = .003$) 4 weeks after treatment. Mean pain interference with activities of daily living was 5.5 of 10 before treatment and decreased to 3.2 ($P = .004$) 4 weeks after treatment. All eight patients for whom opioids were prescribed before the procedure reported a reduction in these medications after cryoablation. No serious complications were observed.

References

1. Daldrup-Link HE, Franzius C, Link TM, et al. Whole-body MR imaging for detection of bone metastases in children and young adults: Comparison with skeletal scintigraphy and FDG PET. *AJR Am J Roentgenol.* 2001;177:229–236.
2. Faul CM, Flickinger JC. The use of radiation in the management of spinal metastases. *J Neurooncol.* 1995;23:149–161.
3. Schultheiss TE. The radiation dose-response of the human spinal cord. *Int J Radiat Oncol Biol Phys.* 2008;71:1455–1459.
4. Kondziolka D, Levy EI, Niranjan A, et al. Long-term outcomes after meningioma radiosurgery: Physician and patient perspectives. *J Neurosurg.* 1999;91:44–50.
5. Gerszten PC, Ozhasoglu C, Burton SA, et al. CyberKnife frameless stereotactic radiosurgery for spinal lesions: Cexperience in 125 cases. *Neurosurgery.* 2004;55:89–98; discussion 98–99.
6. Gerszten PC, Burton SA. Clinical assessment of stereotactic IGRT: Spinal radiosurgery. *Med Dosim.* 2008;33:107–116.
7. Pigott KH, Baddeley H, Maher EJ. Pattern of disease in spinal cord compression on MRI scan and implications for treatment. *Clin Oncol (R Coll Radiol).* 1994;6:7–10.
8. Cavaliere R, Schiff D. Epidural spinal cord compression. *Curr Treat Options Neurol.* 2004;6:285–295.
9. Quinn JA, DeAngelis LM. Neurologic emergencies in the cancer patient. *Semin Oncol.* 2000;27:311–321.
10. Kwok Y, Tibbs PA, Patchell RA. Clinical approach to metastatic epidural spinal cord compression. *Hematol Oncol Clin North Am.* 2006;20:1297–1305.
11. Leviov M, Dale J, Stein M, et al. The management of metastatic spinal cord compression: A radiotherapeutic success ceiling. *Int J Radiat Oncol Biol Phys.* 1993;27:231–234.
12. Boogerd W, van der Sande JJ, Kroger R. Early diagnosis and treatment of spinal epidural metastasis in breast cancer: A prospective study. *J Neurol Neurosurg Psychiatry.* 1992;55:1188–1193.
13. Ingham J, Beveridge A, Cooney NJ. The management of spinal cord compression in patients with advanced malignancy. *J Pain Symptom Manage.* 1993;8:1–6.
14. Loblaw DA, Laperriere NJ. Emergency treatment of malignant extradural spinal cord compression: An evidence-based guideline. *J Clin Oncol.* 1998;16:1613–1624.

15. Schoeggl A, Reddy M, Matula C. Neurological outcome following laminectomy in spinal metastases. *Spinal Cord.* 2002;40:363–366.
16. Maranzano E, Latini P, Checcaglini F, et al. Radiation therapy in metastatic spinal cord compression. A prospective analysis of 105 consecutive patients. *Cancer.* 1991;67:1311–1317.
17. Maranzano E, Latini P, Checcaglini F, et al. Radiation therapy of spinal cord compression caused by breast cancer: Report of a prospective trial. *Int J Radiat Oncol Biol Phys.* 1992;24:301–306.
18. Russi EG, Pergolizzi S, Gaeta M, et al. Palliative-radiotherapy in lumbosacral carcinomatous neuropathy. *Radiother Oncol.* 1993;26:172–173.
19. Turner S, Marosszeky B, Timms I, et al. Malignant spinal cord compression: A prospective evaluation. *Int J Radiat Oncol Biol Phys.* 1993;26:141–146.
20. Nielsen OS, Munro AJ, Tannock IF. Bone metastases: Pathophysiology and management policy. *J Clin Oncol.* 1991;9:509–524.
21. Delaney A, Fleetwood-Walker SM, Colvin LA, et al. Translational medicine: Cancer pain mechanisms and management. *Br J Anaesth.* 2008;101:87–94.
22. Coleman RE. Clinical features of metastatic bone disease and risk of skeletal morbidity. *Clin Cancer Res.* 2006;12:6243s–6249s.
23. Koizumi M, Yoshimoto M, Kasumi F, et al. Comparison between solitary and multiple skeletal metastatic lesions of breast cancer patients. *Ann Oncol.* 2003;14:1234–1240.
24. Pandit-Taskar N, Batraki M, et al. Radiopharmaceutical therapy for palliation of bone pain from osseous metastases. *J Nucl Med.* 2004;45:1358–1365.
25. Scheid V, Buzdar AU, Smith TL, et al. Clinical course of breast cancer patients with osseous metastasis treated with combination chemotherapy. *Cancer.* 1986;58:2589–2593.
26. Wood BC. Hormone treatments in the common "hormone-dependent" carcinomas. *Palliat Med.* 1993;7:257–272.
27. Rastelli F, Crispino S. Factors predictive of response to hormone therapy in breast cancer. *Tumori.* 2008;94:370–383.
28. Ramirez ML, Keane TE, Evans CP. Managing prostate cancer: The role of hormone therapy. *Can J Urol.* 2007;14(Suppl 1):10–18.
29. Coleman RE, Purohit OP, Vinholes JJ. The future of bisphosphonates in cancer. *Acta Oncol.* 1996;35 Suppl 5:23–29.
30. Coleman RE, Purohit OP, Vinholes JJ, et al. High dose pamidronate: Clinical and biochemical effects in metastatic bone disease. *Cancer.* 1997;80:1686–1690.
31. Quattrocchi CC, Piciucchi S, Sammarra M, et al. Bone metastases in breast cancer: Higher prevalence of osteosclerotic lesions. *Radiol Med (Torino).* 2007;112:1049–1059.
32. Saad F. New research findings on zoledronic acid: Survival, pain, and anti-tumour effects. *Cancer Treat Rev.* 2008;34:183–192.
33. Major P. Optimal management of metastatic bone disease. *Eur J Oncol Nurs.* 2007;11(Suppl 2):S32–S37.
34. Lewington VJ. A practical guide to targeted therapy for bone pain palliation. *Nucl Med Commun.* 2002;23:833–836.
35. Pons F, Herranz R, Garcia A, et al. Strontium-89 for palliation of pain from bone metastases in patients with prostate and breast cancer. *Eur J Nucl Med.* 1997;24:1210–1214.
36. Fourneau I, Broos P. Pathologic fractures due to metastatic disease. A retrospective study of 160 surgically treated fractures. *Acta Chir Belg.* 1998;98:255–260.
37. Frassica FJ, Frassica DA. Evaluation and treatment of metastases to the humerus. *Clin Orthop Relat Res.* 2003:S212–S218.
38. Habermann ET, Sachs R, Stern RE, et al. The pathology and treatment of metastatic disease of the femur. *Clin Orthop.* 1982:70–82.
39. Harrington KD. *Orthopaedic management of metastatic bone disease.* St. Louis, Miss: CV Mosby, 1988.
40. Taneichi H, Kaneda K, Takeda N, et al. Risk factors and probability of vertebral body collapse in metastases of the thoracic and lumbar spine. *Spine.* 1997;22:239–245.
41. Janjan N. Bone metastases: Approaches to management. *Semin Oncol.* 2001;28:28–34.
42. Bradley NM, Husted J, Sey MS, et al. Review of patterns of practice and patients' preferences in the treatment of bone metastases with palliative radiotherapy. *Support Care Cancer.* 2007;15:373–385.
43. McQuay HJ, Collins SL, Carroll D, et al. Radiotherapy for the palliation of painful bone metastases. *Cochrane Database Syst Rev.* 2000:CD001793.
44. Loblaw DA, Wu JS, Kirkbride P, et al. Pain flare in patients with bone metastases after palliative radiotherapy—a nested randomized control trial. *Support Care Cancer.* 2007;15:451–455.
45. Chow E, Loblaw A, Harris K, et al. Dexamethasone for the prophylaxis of radiation-induced pain flare after palliative radiotherapy for bone metastases: A pilot study. *Support Care Cancer.* 2007;15:643–647.
46. Brown DB, Gilula LA, Sehgal M, et al. Treatment of chronic symptomatic vertebral compression fractures with percutaneous vertebroplasty. *AJR Am J Roentgenol.* 2004;182:319–322.
47. Weill A, Chiras J, Simon JM, et al. Spinal metastases: Indications for and results of percutaneous injection of acrylic surgical cement. *Radiology.* 1996;199:241–247.
48. Appel NB, Gilula LA. Percutaneous vertebroplasty in patients with spinal canal compromise. *AJR Am J Roentgeno.* 2004;182:947–951.
49. Shimony JS, Gilula LA, Zeller AJ, et al. Percutaneous vertebroplasty for malignant compression fractures with epidural involvement. *Radiology.* 2004;232:846–853.
50. Cheung G, Chow E, Holden L, et al. Percutaneous vertebroplasty in patients with intractable pain from osteoporotic or metastatic fractures: A prospective study using quality-of-life assessment. *Can Assoc Radiol J.* 2006;57:13–21.
51. Fourney DR, Schomer DF, Nader R, et al. Percutaneous vertebroplasty and kyphoplasty for painful vertebral body fractures in cancer patients. *J Neurosurg.* 2003;98:21–30.
52. Callstrom MR, Charboneau JW, Goetz MP, et al. Painful metastases involving bone: Feasibility of percutaneous CT- and US-guided radio-frequency ablation. *Radiology.* 2002;224:87–97.
53. Camann WR, Denney RA, Holby ED, et al. A comparison of intrathecal, epidural, and intravenous sufentanil for labor analgesia. *Anesthesiology.* 1992;77:884–887.
54. Ghanem I. The management of osteoid osteoma: Updates and controversies. *Curr Opin Pediatr.* 2006;18:36–41.
55. Thanos L, Mylona S, Galani P, et al. Radiofrequency ablation of osseous metastases for the palliation of pain. *Skeletal Radiol.* 2008;37:189–194.
56. Callstrom MR, Atwell TD, Charboneau JW, et al. Painful metastases involving bone: Percutaneous image-guided cryoablation—prospective trial interim analysis. *Radiology.* 2006;241:572–580.

CHAPTER 24 ■ DEPRESSION, ANXIETY, AND SLEEP

Desire for hastened death among terminally ill cancer patients is not uncommon.[1,2] Depression and hopelessness are predictors of desire for hastened death in this population and provide independent and unique contributions. Interventions addressing depression, hopelessness, and social support are important aspects of adequate palliative care, particularly as it relates to desire for hastened death. Miovic and Block[3] reported that approximately 50% of patients with advanced cancer meet criteria for a psychiatric disorder, the most common being adjustment disorders (11% to 35%) and major depression (5% to 26%).

Treatment decisions for depression in the cancer patient presume that a thorough medical and psychiatric assessment has led to an accurate diagnosis that will allow specific and effective intervention. Tumor involvement of the CNS, hyperparathyroidism, and adrenal insufficiency may contribute to mood disorders. Patients with severe depression and/or suicidal ideation or intent require psychiatric consultation. Before planning an intervention, the physician should consider a history of previous depressive episodes and substance (including alcohol) abuse, family history of depression and suicide, concurrent life stresses, losses secondary to cancer (eg, financial, social, and occupation) in addition to loss of good health, and the availability of social support. Once it becomes clear that the patient is depressed, one must consider coexisting organic factors before starting treatment.

Standard therapeutic approaches such as the use of corticosteroids,[4] chemotherapeutic agents (tamoxifen,[5] asparaginase,[6] interferon,[7] and interleukin),[8] whole brain radiation,[9] and amphotericin[10] can cause or exacerbate depressive symptoms in cancer patients (Table 24.1). Likewise the presence of brain metastases or tumors,[11] metabolic and endocrine complications,[12] and paraneoplastic syndromes[13] often contribute to the presence of depressive symptoms.

Depressed patients with cancer should be treated with a combination of psychological treatments (cognitive behavioral and supportive psychotherapy) and psychopharmacological interventions (antidepressants and psychostimulants). For patients with cancer pain, interventions that help diminish mood disturbance also help reduce pain.[14] Reducing severe pain may help relieve depression. In cancer patients with depressive disorders or with significant depressive symptoms, studies thus far provided only modest evidence for the benefit of pharmacological and psychosocial interventions.[2]

TABLE 24.1

CHEMOTHERAPEUTIC DRUGS ASSOCIATED WITH DEPRESSION

Corticosteroids
Vinblastine
Vincristine
Vinorelbine
Interferon
Procarbazine
Asparaginase
Tamoxifen

PSYCHOTHERAPY

The goals of psychotherapy are to reduce emotional distress and to improve morale, coping ability, self-esteem, sense of control, and resolution of problems. It consists of four basic components—social support, emotional expression, cognitive restructuring, and coping skills training. Different formats for psychosocial support and therapy exist, including psychoeducation, cognitive-behavioral therapy, supportive therapy, and individual therapy, each of which may be more useful depending on the stage of illness and the individual's attributes and circumstances. Although psychotherapy can be an effective treatment for depression in cancer patients, pharmacotherapy is frequently needed, because terminally ill patients often cannot participate fully in psychotherapy.

ANTIDEPRESSANT MEDICATIONS

Antidepressant medications should be considered for the treatment of moderate to severe major depression in cancer patients. Current evidence does not support the relative superiority of one pharmacologic treatment over another, nor the superiority of pharmacologic treatment over psychosocial interventions.[2] The choice of an antidepressant should be based on individual medication and patient factors: the side effect profiles of the medication, tolerability of treatment (including the potential for interaction with other current medications), response to previous treatment, and patient preference. Antidepressants commonly used in cancer patients are listed in Table 24.2.

The side effect profile with the newer antidepressants, including the selective serotonin reuptake inhibitors (SSRIs) and the mixed-action antidepressants appear to show fewer side effects than the tricyclic antidepressants (TCAs) and monoamine oxidase inhibitors (MAOIs). The SSRIs and mixed-action antidepressants should be considered first-line treatments for depression in cancer patients. Commonly used SSRIs include fluoxetine, sertaline, paroxetine, fluvoxamine, citalopram, and escitalopram. The most common side effects associated with the SSRIs

TABLE 24.2

ANTIDEPRESSANTS IN CANCER PATIENTS

	Agent	Oral Starting Dose (mg)	Therapeutic Dose (mg)	Remarks
SSRIs	Sertaline (Zoloft)	25	50–200	Few drug interactions. Useful in OCD. $T_{1/2}$ = 24 hr
	Paroxetine (Paxil)	5–10	10–60	More anticholinergic; weight gain; CR available. $T_{1/2}$ = 21 hr
	Escitalopram (Lexapro)	5–10	10–20	Few drug interactions; $T_{1/2}$ = 30 hr
	Citalopram (Celexa)	10	10–60	Few drug interactions; $T_{1/2}$ = 35 hr
	Fluoxetine (Prozac)	5–10	20–60	Stimulating; $T_{1/2}$ = 1–3 d
	Fluvoxamine (Luvox)	25	50–300	Sedating; indicated OCD; off-label use for depression. $T_{1/2}$ = 14 hr
TCAs	Amitriptyline (Elavil)	10–25	50–150	Sedating
	Nortriptyline (Pamelor)	10–25	50–150	Blood levels can be checked.
	Desipramine (Norpramin)	10–25	50–150	Least sedating
Others	Trazodone (Desyrel)	25–50	150–300	Sedating; risk of priapism
	Buproprion (Wellbutrin, Wellbutrin SR, Wellbutrin XL)	75–100	150–450	Minimal effect on weight and sexual dysfunction; seizure risk at higher dose; IR max dose = 150 mg tid; SR max dose = 200 mg bid; XL max dose = 450 mg once daily
	Duloxetine (Cymbalta)	20	40–60	Approved for PDN and PHN pain
	Mirtazapine (Remeron)	15	15–45	Sedating
	Venlafaxine (Effexor, Effexor XR)	18.75–37.5	75–300	May elevate BP; ER available (max 225 mg/day)

SSRIs, selective serotonin reuptake inhibitors; TCAs, tricyclic antidepressants; OCD, obsessive-compulsive disorder; CR, controlled release; ER, XL, extended release; SR, slow release; IR, immediate release; $T_{1/2}$, half-life; PD, painful diabetic neuropathy; PHN, postherpetic neuralgia.

are nausea, headache, sleep disturbance, sexual dysfunction, appetite suppression, and anxiety with the first few days of use. There are important differences in these agents including half-life, drug interactions, and individual side effect profiles. Fluoxetine, for example, has the longest half-life resulting in little if any risk of SSRI discontinuation syndrome with abrupt withdrawal. Because of the relatively short half-life (< 24 hours) of the other SSRIs, patients are at risk for developing significant psychiatric, neurologic, gastrointestinal, or flulike symptoms after abrupt withdrawal. All SSRIs are equally efficacious, with depressive symptoms improving 2 to 4 weeks after a therapeutic dose. Paroxetine causes the most anticholinergic side effects of the SSRIs and causes the most weight gain. Fluvoxamine and paroxetine are the more sedating, whereas fluoxetine is the most stimulating. Sertraline, citalopram, and escitalopram have fewer drug interactions, whereas fluvoxamine has the most, and this feature often limits its use.

TCAs act on multiple receptors (including muscarinic, cholinergic, histaminic, and adrenergic receptors) and side effects include dry mouth, constipation, confusion, urinary retention, sedation, weight gain, and orthostatic hypotension. These agents are potentially helpful for cancer patients with insomnia, pain, and depression and can be effective in relatively low doses. Dosing may be initiated at 10 to 25 mg at bedtime and the dose increased every 2 to 3 days until benefit is achieved. The effects on appetite and sleep are frequently very rapid; the effects on mood may be delayed or not clinically apparent. The choice of TCA depends on the nature of the depressive symptoms, coexistent medical problems, and side effects of the particular drug. The depressed patient who has insomnia may benefit from the use of a TCA that has sedating properties, such as amitriptyline or doxepin. Patients with psychomotor slowing will benefit from agents with the least sedating properties, such as desipramine. Patients with stomatitis secondary to chemotherapy or radiation therapy, or who have slow intestinal motility should receive agents with the least anticholinergic effects such as desipramine or nortriptyline. Imipramine, doxepin, amitriptyline, desipramine, and nortriptyline have been used in the management of neuropathic pain in cancer patients.[15] Dosing is similar to the treatment of depression, and analgesic efficacy, if it occurs, is usually observed at a dose of 50 to 150 mg daily; higher doses are sometimes necessary.

The novel and mixed-action antidepressants (venlafaxine, duloxetine, bupropion, trazodone, and mirtazapine) differ from the SSRIs in their mechanism of action, resulting in their different side effect profiles. Venlafaxine and duloxetine are serotonin/norepinephrine uptake inhibitors, with venlafaxine inhibiting serotonin reuptake at lower doses, thereby sharing some of the side effects of the SSRIs while inhibiting norepinephrine reuptake at higher doses. At higher doses (>225 mg/day) venlafaxine may contribute to hypertension. Both duloxetine and venlafaxine have been shown to improve neuropathic pain and peripheral neuropathy in cancer patients. Bupropion is primarily a noradrenergic agent that increases dopamine reuptake at higher doses. Its stimulating effects may be beneficial to the depressed cancer patient with fatigue. Bupropion has fewer gastrointestinal side effects than the SSRIs and tends to cause constipation more frequently than nausea, vomiting, or diarrhea. It increases the rise for seizures at higher doses and should be avoided or used with caution in patients with seizure disorders or organic brain pathology. Venlafaxine, trazodone, mirtazapine, and SSRIs are useful in managing hot flashes.[16,17] Mirtazapine is a noradrenergic and specific serotonergic antidepressant.[18] It has low affinity for muscarinic, cholinergic, and dopaminergic receptors, but a high affinity for H1 histaminic receptors. It antagonizes serotonin (5-HT) 5-HT$_2$ and 5-HT$_3$ receptors, resulting in increased serotonin release through 5-HT^1. The drug's activity at these receptors may result in a variety of features, including sedation, anxiolysis, appetite stimulation, and antiemesis. These clearly have potential advantages in the oncology population.

PSYCHOSTIMULANTS

Psychostimulants such as dextroamphetamine (Dexedrine), methylphenidate (Ritalin), dexmethylphenidate (Focalin), pemoline (Cylert), and modafinil (Provigil) help diminish sedation related to opioids and are useful antidepressants in the medically ill. Concerns about hepatotoxicity and liver failure[19] led to the discontinuation of pemoline in May 2005 in the United States. Advantages in the use of psychostimulants in the cancer patient include a decrease in fatigue, improved concentration and attention, and appetite stimulation. Potential issues with the use of psychostimulants include nightmares, agitation, insomnia, and lower seizure threshold. The primary role of psychostimulants in advanced cancer is the treatment of symptoms such as cancer-related fatigue, opioid-induced sedation, depression, and cognitive dysfunction.

Methylphenidate is a piperidine-derived CNS stimulant structurally related to amphetamines. Dexmethylphenidate (Focalin), the d-enantiomer of methylphenidate, may have a role in the treatment of cancer-related fatigue. Dexmethylphenidate has approximately 6-hour duration of effect (the XR version spans 12 hours, covering a full day). Methylphenidate has binding affinity for both the dopamine transporter and norepinephrine transporter, with the D-isomer displaying a prominent affinity for the latter. After standard oral doses, peak plasma levels occur in 1 to 3 hours with a plasma half-life of 1.5 to 2.5 hours. Side effects include difficulty sleeping, stomachaches, headaches, lack of hunger (leading to weight loss), and dry mouth. Methylphenidate is available in 5-, 10-, and 20-mg tablets, as well as a 20-mg sustained-release tablet in which the drug is embedded in a wax matrix. Sustained-release methylphenidate has a longer T_{max} (3 to 4 hours) and $T_{1/2}$ (4 hours). Methylphenidate is also available as a transdermal patch. Approved uses for methylphenidate include attention deficit hyperactivity disorder and narcolepsy. Hypoactive delirium unexplained by an underlying cause (metabolic or drug-induced) and depression in patients with advanced cancer can be improved by the administration of methylphenidate.[20,21] In 30 patients with malignant gliomas treated with methylphenidate, improvements in cognitive functioning and performance status were demonstrated despite ongoing neurologic injury due to disease progression or radiation therapy in half of these patients.[22] In a randomized, double-blind, placebo-controlled crossover trial of 32 patients with advanced cancer receiving chronic opioid therapy, statistically significant reductions in pain intensity and sedation were seen with the use of methylphenidate.[23] Further benefits on opioid sedation were also observed but tolerance to this effect was seen over a period of one month.[24]

Dextroamphetamine is a dextrorotatory stereoisomer of amphetamine and is also called dexamphetamine. The mechanism of action is unknown. In animals, it blocks dopamine and norepinephrine reuptake from central presynaptic neurons, inhibits MAOI activity, and facilitates catecholamine release. Dextroamphetamine also has peripheral α and β sympathomimetic actions, including elevation of both diastolic and systolic blood pressure. Dextroamphetamine (0.215 mg/kg) antagonized respiratory depression caused by low-dose morphine (0.15 mg/kg) over a 5-hour period as measured by CO_2 response curves and isohypercapnic minute ventilationin healthy volunteers, but did not reverse respiratory depression at higher doses of morphine (0.3 mg/kg).[25] Mitler et al.[26] suggested that both dextroamphetamine and methylphenidate were effective in treating somnolence in narcolepsy patients. Methamphetamine is subject to abuse and concerns have been expressed on the misuse of methamphetamine particularly in youths and young adults.[27] Treatment with dextroamphetamine or methylphenidate usually begins with a dose of 2.5 mg on awakening and at noon. The dosage is slowly increased over several days until a desired effect is achieved or side effects (overstimulation, anxiety, insomnia, paranoia, and confusion) become apparent. Occasional doses of 60 mg per day are required, but doses of not more than 30 mg per day are more typical.

Modafinil improves wakefulness and has been approved by the Food and Drug Administration (FDA) for the treatment of narcolepsy,[28] obstructive sleep apnea,[29] and shift-work sleep disorder.[30] Short-term clinical studies have shown improved wakefulness in patients with other conditions such as multiple sclerosis,[31] major depression,[32] and Parkinson disease.[33] The most commonly reported adverse effects of modafinil treatment were headache, infection, nausea, nervousness, anxiety, and insomnia, all of which were generally mild.

ANXIOLYTICS

Several types of anxiety syndromes can appear in cancer patients with and without pain. These include reactive anxiety related to the stress of cancer and its treatment, anxiety that is a manifestation of a medical or physiologic problem related to cancer such as uncontrolled pain, and chronic anxiety disorders that predate the cancer diagnosis but are exacerbated during illness. The most effective management of anxiety in cancer patients is multimodal, including psychotherapy, behavioral therapy, and pharmacologic management. The severity of symptoms is the most useful guide in deciding whether a pharmacologic approach should be tried. Oftentimes, the first-line drugs for the treatment of anxiety in cancer patients are benzodiazepines. In addition, short- to medium-acting benzodiazepines as well as the nonbenzodiazepine hypnotics (zolpidem, zaleplon, or eszopiclone) may be effective for insomnia, but only on a short-term basis. In general, benzodiazepines should be used in conjunction with other interventions (psychological treatments, antidepressants, other drugs), although such interventions have a slower onset of action.

The major clinical advantages of benzodiazepines are high efficacy and rapid onset of action. The main actions of benzodiazepines (hypnotic, anxiolytic, anticonvulsant, myorelaxant, and amnesic) confer a therapeutic advantage in a wide range of conditions. Adverse effects include psychomotor impairment, mental status changes especially in the elderly, drowsiness and sedation, and occasionally paradoxical excitement.

Indications for benzodiazepines include acute stress reactions, episodic anxiety, fluctuations in generalized anxiety, and as initial treatment for severe panic and agoraphobia. For the treatment of panic disorder and agoraphobia, the benzodiazepine, alprazolam, and antidepressant medications (TCAs, SSRIs, and MAOIs) are useful. The apparent efficacy of benzodiazepines in patients with major depressive disorder may depend on the patient's level of anxiety.

Because drug interactions and decreased clearance are often factors in treating cancer pain patients, benzodiazepines with shorter half-lives may be more desirable. Compared with other benzodiazepines, alprazolam has particular efficacy in the treatment of panic disorders and may have antidepressant effects. It may help cancer patients who have mixed symptoms of anxiety and depression. Alprazolam is associated with a low incidence of side effects but may cause physical dependence, withdrawal, and sedation. Alprazolam should not be considered as a first-line treatment option, but may be considered when agents such as SSRIs are not effective or well tolerated.[34] A typical starting dose is 0.25 mg tid. Clonazepam, a benzodiazepine with anticonvulsant and anxiolytic properties, is increasingly used in various psychiatric disorders.[35] In addition to activation of the benzodiazepine-GABA receptor complex, unlike many other benzodiazepines, clonazepam appears to have serotonergic effects, which may contribute to its psychotropic and antimyoclonic effects.[36] Clonazepam is a high-potency benzodiazepine with greater receptor affinity than, for example, alprazolam; it is approximately twice as potent as alprazolam on a mg-per-mg basis and may potentially achieve a therapeutic effect at lower doses. Clonazepam also has a long elimination half-life (typically 30 to 40 hours), high bioavailability, and a rapid onset of action. Maximum plasma concentrations occur 1 to 4 hours after oral administration and responses can be seen as quickly as 1 to 2 hours postdose. The long half-life and higher potency of clonazepam may allow easier tapering of dosage and potentially fewer withdrawal symptoms compared to other benzodiazepines when tapered. Somnolence is the most frequent adverse event associated with clonazepam therapy in clinical studies.[35] Although withdrawal symptoms can occur with abrupt discontinuation, the longer half-life of clonazepam (allowing administration twice daily, as opposed to four times daily for alprazolam) minimizes the risk of interdose rebound anxiety.

Although benzodiazepines relieve acute anxiety, they are relatively ineffective for chronic anxiety disorders.[37] Drugs such as antidepressants and anxiolytics like buspirone, which combine anxiolytic and antidepressant actions, are more effective for the management of chronic anxiety. The role of 5-HT in the treatment of depressive and anxiety disorders is underscored by the therapeutic action of selective 5-HT reuptake inhibitors acting to enhance the degree of activation of various 5-HT receptor subtypes. The 5-HT^{1A} receptors are particularly relevant to the antidepressant and anxiolytic responses in human beings. They are located presynaptically in the raphe nuclei, where they act as cell body autoreceptors to inhibit the firing rate of 5-HT neurons, and are located postsynaptically in limbic and cortical regions, where they also attenuate firing activity.[38] Buspirone is a 5-HT^{1A} agonist. The starting dose of buspirone is 5 mg tid. Dosage may be increased by 5 mg/day until the desired effect is achieved. The usual daily maximum dose is 60 mg with a usual dose of 20 to 30 mg/day. Onset of anxiolysis is delayed relative to benzodiazepine and it is not uncommon for onset of effect to occur after 5 to 10 days.

PSYCHIATRIC DRUG INTERACTION ISSUES IN CANCER THERAPY

Potential drug interactions are not uncommon among cancer patients and most often involve medications to treat comorbid conditions.[39] Tamoxifen, a selective estrogen receptor modulator, is converted to 4-hydroxy-tamoxifen and other active metabolites by cytochrome P450 (CYP) enzymes. Tamoxifen is metabolized to an extremely potent antiestrogen by CYP P450 2D6, 2C9, and 3A isoforms. Endoxifen is an active tamoxifen metabolite that is generated via CYP3A4-mediated N-demethylation and CYP2D6-mediated hydroxylation. SSRIs, which are often prescribed to alleviate tamoxifen-associated hot flashes, can inhibit CYPs. Stearns et al.[40] tested the effects of coadministration of tamoxifen and the SSRI paroxetine, an inhibitor of CYP2D6, on tamoxifen metabolism. Coadministration of paroxetine decreased the plasma concentration of endoxifen potentially reducing the effectiveness of tamoxifen in this patient population. Jin et al.[41] also examined the effects of concomitant use of SSRIs in women taking tamoxifen and similarly concluded that interactions between CYP2D6 polymorphisms and coadministered antidepressants and other drugs that are CYP2D6 inhibitors may be associated with altered tamoxifen activity. Since the prevalence of depression in breast cancer patients is nearly triple that of the general population, it is likely that a subgroup of breast cancer patients will receive long-term treatment with both an SSRI and tamoxifen.[42] Although the interactions of SSRIs with tamoxifen therapy are somewhat controversial, these agents should be used with caution in this setting, particularly if alternative treatment options are available.

MANAGEMENT OF SLEEP DISTURBANCES IN CANCER PATIENTS

Sleep disorders, such as difficulty falling asleep, problems maintaining sleep, poor sleep efficiency, early awakening, and excessive daytime sleepiness, are prevalent in patients with cancer, and particularly so in those who have chronic pain. Insomnia is defined as difficulty with the initiation, maintenance, duration, or quality of sleep that results in the impairment of daytime functioning, despite adequate opportunity and circumstances for sleep. Adult insomnia may be classified as primary or secondary (Table 24.3). Some studies estimate that approximately one half of

TABLE 24.3

CLASSIFICATION OF ADULT INSOMNIA

Primary insomnia
- Idiopathic insomnia—insomnia arising in infancy or childhood with a persistent, unremitting course.
- Psychophysiologic insomnia—insomnia due to a maladaptive conditioned response in which the patient learns to associate the bed environment with heightened arousal rather than sleep; onset often associated with an event causing acute insomnia, with the sleep disturbance persisting despite resolution of the precipitating factor.
- Paradoxical insomnia (sleep-state misperception)—insomnia characterized by a marked mismatch between the patient's description of sleep duration and objective polysomnographic findings.

Secondary insomnia
- Adjustment insomnia—insomnia associated with active psychosocial stressors.
- Inadequate sleep hygiene—insomnia associated with lifestyle habits that impair sleep.
- Insomnia due to a psychiatric disorder—Insomnia due to an active psychiatric disorder, such as anxiety or depression.
- Insomnia due to a medical condition—insomnia due to a condition such as restless legs syndrome, chronic pain, nocturnal cough or dyspnea, or hot flashes.
- Insomnia due to a drug or substance—insomnia due to consumption or discontinuation of medication, drugs of abuse, alcohol, or caffeine.

(From Silber MH. Clinical practice, chronic insomnia. *N Eng J Med.* 2005; 353:803–810.) Copyright 2005, Massachusetts Medical Society. All rights reserved.

patients with cancer suffer from insomnia, with 23% to 44% reporting insomnia-related issues up to several years after diagnosis and treatment.[43,44] The critical role of sleep in health and disease has been underscored by research that further defines the relationship between sleep and myriad physiologic and psychological functions as well as quality of life. In a study of 954 cancer patients, Lis et al. reported that insomnia strongly correlated with patient satisfaction with quality of life.[45] Patients with cancer report insomnia, poor sleep quality, and short sleep duration. Insomnia is commonly defined by its duration as transient (less than 2 weeks), short-term (lasting 2 to 4 weeks), and chronic (lasting more than 4 weeks).[46] Several tools have been used to assess for sleep disturbance. One such tool is the Pittsburgh Sleep Quality Index (Appendix I).

Precipitating factors for insomnia in patients with cancer include the diagnosis of cancer, the type and stage of cancer, pain, side effects of treatment (eg, nausea, vomiting, and so on) or the direct iatrogenic effects of treatment on sleep (Fig. 24.1). Hopelessness, pain treatment, and "interference of pain with mood" may influence the quality of sleep in advanced stages of cancer.[47] A significant proportion of prescriptions written for cancer patients are for hypnotics.[48]

Sleep disturbances can persist for many years in cancer survivors. In a study of 982 patients (mean age: 65 years) with six different types of cancer, a "sleep survey" questionnaire was used to evaluate the presence of various sleep problems (eg, insomnia due to difficulty falling asleep, waking up several times a night, waking up for a long time, or waking up too early).[49] The most prevalent problems reported by this patient sample were: fatigue (44%), insomnia (31%), and excessive sleepiness (28%). The authors noted that patients who reported being overly fatigued were 2.5 times more likely to have insomnia than others. Of the 300 patients reporting insomnia, 76% noted waking several times a night, 44% had difficulty falling asleep, 35% reported waking for a long time, and 33% woke up too early. The duration of insomnia was 6 months or longer in 75% of cases. Correlations between fatigue and sleep problems are evident in some cancer patients more than a year after completion of their treatment.[50] Servaes et al.[51] reported in disease-free breast cancer survivors at a mean of 29 months after completion of treatment that women who were severely fatigued experienced significantly greater sleep disturbance than women with less fatigue. Other correlates with fatigue and insomnia include feelings of drowsiness, daytime sleepiness, and napping.[52]

Effective management of insomnia begins with its recognition and adequate assessment.[53] To achieve optimal patient outcomes, clinicians should differentiate acute from chronic insomnia and distinguish primary insomnia from sleep disorders that occur with comorbid conditions, most notably psychiatric illnesses such as circadian rhythm disturbances, and pain. In the cancer patient with pain and insomnia, it is essential to address the pain complaint concomitantly with sleep disturbance. Nonpharmacologic interventions for insomnia include sleep-hygiene education, stimulus-control therapy, relaxation therapy, and sleep-restriction therapy. The most common pharmacologic therapies for insomnia are benzodiazepines, benzodiazepine-receptor agonists, melatonin-receptor agonists, and antidepressants. Choice of a specific agent should be based on patient-specific factors, including age, proposed length of treatment, primary sleep complaint, history of drug or alcohol abuse, and cost.

Good sleep hygiene behaviors may help improve sleep disorders in cancer patients (Table 24.4). Cognitive-behavioral therapy for insomnia appears promising for individuals with major depression and comorbid insom-

TABLE 24.4

GOOD SLEEP HYGIENE BEHAVIORS FOR CANCER PATIENTS

Keep a regular time for sleeping and waking up
Before sleeping, keep activities calm.
Avoid going to bed unless sleepy.
If there is difficulty falling asleep, get out of bed and engage in a calm activity until sleepy.
Don't sleep excessively.
Exercise regularly, preferably 6 hours before sleeping.
Avoid heavy food intake in the evening.
Avoid stimulants (particularly caffeine).
Avoid alcohol.
Limit daytime napping.

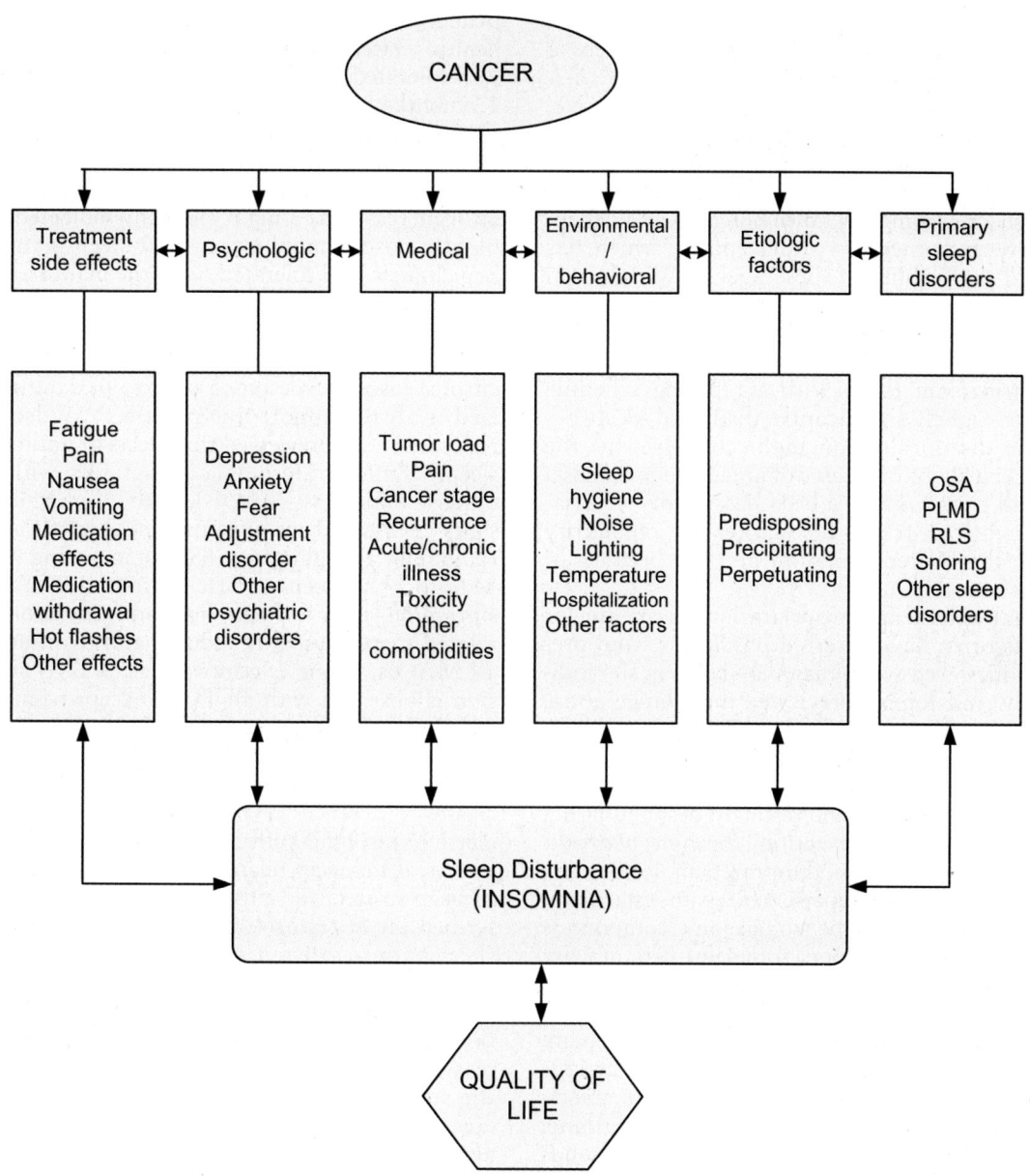

FIGURE 24.1 Potential factors contributing to the pathogenesis of cancer-related insomnia. OSA, Obstructive sleep apnea; PLMD, periodic limb movement disorder; RLS, restless leg syndrome. (Modified from Graci G, Pathogenesis and mangement of cancer-related incomnia, *Oncol*, 2005;3:349–359.).

nia for alleviating both depression and insomnia.[54] Hypnotics have a role in the management of acute insomnia; however, the efficacy and safety of pharmacologic interventions in the management of chronic insomnia are unclear. Pharmacotherapy is generally not recommended in the treatment of chronic insomnia, except on a short-term basis (usually accepted as 7 to 10 days). Many of the hypnotics are approved by the FDA only for short-term management of insomnia. Over-the-counter hypnotic medications, including antihistamines, are not generally recommended because of the potential for abuse, tolerance, and unsupervised dose escalation. Hypnotic agents, both benzodiazepines (Temazepam [Restoril], Estazolam [ProSom], Triazolam [Halcion]), and nonbenzodiazepines (Zolpidem [Ambien], Zaleplon [Sonata], Eszopiclone [Lunesta]), are commonly prescribed for sleep problems. Medications with longer half-lives are associated with residual effects such as daytime sedation and cognitive impairment. If used chronically, these agents may also result in rebound insomnia. Nonbenzodiazepine hypnotics such as zolpidem (Ambien) and zaleplon (Sonata) have shorter half-lives and are less frequently associated with daytime residual effects.[55]

Pharmacologic manipulation of gamma-aminobutyric acid (GABA) and GABA-A receptors has differential effects on sleep onset and sleep maintenance insomnia.[56] GABA-A receptors are the target for the most widely prescribed sleep medicines (benzodiazepines and benzodiazepine-receptor agonists). Benzodiazepines act through the GABA-receptor complex by affecting chloride flux. Benzodiazepine-receptor agonists bind to the same receptor complex but have different affinities for various receptor subclasses. The receptor is a ligand-gated ion channel, activated by the amino acid neurotransmitter GABA, which normally results in hyperpolarization of neurons leading to reduced action potential firing, and thereby a reduction in neuronal activity.[57] Modulation of GABA-A receptor activity by benzodiazepines produces sedative, hypnotic, anxiolytic, and anticonvulsant activities.

Short half-life benzodiazepines, such as triazolam, have been particularly useful in treating insomnia, but concerns have been raised regarding tolerance potential and dependence liability of classical benzodiazepines, which has led to reduced prescribing of these agents. Withdrawal effects, especially insomnia, can occur after discontinuation of triazolam even after very short-term use. Roehrs et al.[58] noted that after abrupt discontinuation of 6 nights of 0.50 mg triazolam (even with a tapering schedule during the six nights) significantly disturbed sleep occurred on the discontinuation night compared to the baseline night. Furthermore, cases of anterograde amnesia associated with triazolam have been described.[59,60] Triazolam was removed from the market by regulatory authorities in the United Kingdom in 1991 because of abuse liability issues.[61]

Recreational abuse, inappropriate long-term use, or adverse effects often have deterred physicians from prescribing hypnotics even when they may be clinically indicated. Griffiths and Johnson reviewed the relative abuse liability of different hypnotic drugs.[62] The relative likelihood of abuse scores of 19 hypnotic compounds range from 100 (most likely) for pentobarbital to 0 (least likely) for trazodone and ramelteon. Interestingly, despite sharing a common molecular site of action, the nine benzodiazepine compounds (diazepam, flunitrazepam, lorazepam, temazepam, triazolam, flurazepam, oxazepam, estazolam, quazepam) and the four nonbenzodiazepine compounds (zaleplon, eszopiclone, zopiclone, zolpidem) with activity at the benzodiazepine receptor binding site show a wide range of abuse liability scores, ranging from highs of 67 for diazepam and flunitrazepam to 13 for quazepam. Also of interest is that the three compounds with actions not mediated through a GABA receptor site were associated with a low likelihood of abuse (diphenhydramine, trazodone, and ramelteon). All three of these compounds produce an atypical profile of subjective effects, with diphenhydramine and trazodone producing greater adverse side effects than the classic hypnotics and ramelteon producing no detectable subjective effects at up to 20 times the recommended therapeutic dose.

Hair et al.[63] reviewed *Eszopiclone* (Lunesta), a nonbenzodiazepine hypnotic agent that is approved in the United States as an oral, once-nightly therapy for insomnia in adults. Eszopiclone is rapidly absorbed after oral administration without any next-day clinical residual effects being detected. Trials of up to 6 months' duration have shown that eszopiclone significantly improves both sleep onset and sleep maintenance compared with placebo in adult and elderly patients with primary insomnia. Eszopiclone for 4 to 8 weeks also significantly improved sleep parameters compared with placebo in patients with insomnia coexisting with other conditions that also disturb sleep (comorbid insomnia), and improved certain measures of the comorbid conditions to a greater extent than the standard therapies alone. Short-term eszopiclone produced improvements in daytime functioning in patients with comorbid insomnia. Six months' therapy in adults with primary insomnia improved daytime functioning and health-related quality of life. Eszopiclone was generally well tolerated. There was no evidence of tolerance during 12 months of treatment with this agent. On discontinuation of eszopiclone, there was no rebound insomnia or serious withdrawal effects. Dosing of eszopiclone should begin at 2 mg for nonelderly patients and may be initiated at or increased to 3 mg if clinically indicated.[64] The 3-mg nightly dose is more effective at sleep maintenance. Eszopiclone is well tolerated, with the main treatment-emergent side effects being unpleasant taste, headache, and dizziness.

Sedating antidepressants have also been prescribed for chronic insomnia despite a paucity of data from randomized trials to support this practice.[65] Wilson and Argyropoulos[66] have reviewed the effects of antidepressants on sleep. Of interest, insomnia is often seen with monoamine oxidase inhibitors (MAOIs), with all tricyclic antidepressants (TCAs) except amitriptyline, and all selective serotonin reuptake inhibitors (SSRIs), including venlafaxine.[25] Sedation has been reported with all TCAs except desipramine, with mirtazapine and nefazodone, the TCA-related maprotiline, trazodone, and mianserin, and with all MAOIs. Rapid eye movement (REM) sleep suppression is observed with all TCAs except trimipramine, but especially clomipramine, with all MAOIs and SSRIs and with venlafaxine, trazodone, and bupropion. The effect on sleep varies between compounds within antidepressant classes, differences relating to the amount of sedative or alerting (insomnia) effects, changes to baseline sleep parameters, differences relating to REM sleep, and the degree of sleep-related side effects.[67] In 1988, Mouret et al.[68] described the effect of 400 to 600 mg of trazodone on the sleep patterns of ten depressed in-patients treated for 5 weeks. From the beginning of treatment, there was a hypnotic-like effect from the drug (increase in total duration of sleep and stage II, decrease in sleep latency and intrasleep awakenings). In addition, records at the end of the study showed an increase in delta sleep and an increase in REM latency, an effect classically associated with an antidepressant action. Prescription of adjunctive trazodone 50 to 150 mg is a common clinical practice to treat comorbid insomnia during antidepressant therapy.[69] However, the efficacy of trazodone for sleep maintenance is questionable.[70] Mirtazapine is a noradrenergic and specific serotonergic antidepressant which has predominantly been evaluated in the treatment of major depression. The drug had equivalent efficacy to tricyclic antidepressants and it was at least as effective as trazodone in the majority of available short-term trials in patients with moderate or severe depression, including those with baseline anxiety symptoms or sleep disturbance and the elderly.[71] There is also a potential beneficial effect of mirtazapine in the treatment of patients with pain and concomitant depression at mean daily dose of 34.5 (10.4 mg).[72] This implies that patients may benefit with average nightly doses of mirtazapine 30 mg.

Melatonin is a hormone that has been associated with soporific effects. Ramelteon (Rozerem), a MT1 and MT2 melatonin receptor selective agonist, was approved by the Food and Drug Administration (FDA) in 2005 and is the only medication indicated for the long-term treatment of insomnia that is not a controlled substance. The MT1 and

MT2 receptors are believed to mediate the circadian rhythm in mammals.[73] Ramelteon does not have a direct sedating effect, but rather enhances sleep through effects on sleep regulatory mechanisms within the suprachiasmatic nucleus of the hypothalamus.[74] Simpson and Curran[75] reviewed its use in insomnia. In patients with chronic insomnia, objectively assessed latency to persistent sleep at week 1 was improved with oral ramelteon 8 mg administered 30 minutes before bedtime, compared with placebo, and this effect was maintained throughout the duration of 5-week and 6-month clinical studies. Subjectively-assessed sleep latency improved in some, but not all, studies. When a statistically significant improvement in sleep latency occurred at week 1, the effect was maintained throughout the duration of the 5-week studies, but not at all timepoints throughout a 6-month study. Improvements in objectively assessed total sleep time and sleep efficiency were only reported during the first week of treatment. Improvements in other objective or subjective measures of sleep were not consistent. Ramelteon was generally well tolerated and did not impair next-day cognitive or motor performance. Safety data from short-term studies showed advantages of ramelteon over other sleep agents including no potential for abuse, no rebound insomnia, and lack of effect on motor and cognitive function. Adverse effects seen most frequently in ramelteon clinical trials were headache, somnolence, fatigue, nausea, dizziness, and insomnia with the overall incidence similar to that of placebo.[76]

In patients who complain of persistent insomnia, we recommend the use of Pittsburgh Sleep Quality Index for insomnia assessment. We always try to make use of cognitive behavioral therapy management strategies for all patients. When these are not adequate, and pharmacologic therapy is deemed necessary, we initiate therapy with low doses of trazodone (50 to 100 mg qhs). If this proves ineffective, and we anticipate pharmacologic therapy continuing for 3 to 6 months, we use eszopiclone. For therapy anticipated to continue beyond 6 months, we switch to ramelteon. Doses and drugs must be tailored to individual patient's response.

References

1. Breitbart W, Rosenfeld B, Pessin H, et al. Depression, hopelessness, and desire for hastened death in terminally ill patients with cancer. *JAMA*. 2000;284:2907–2911.
2. Rodin G, Zimmermann C, Rydall A, et al. The desire for hastened death in patients with metastatic cancer. *J Pain Symptom Manage*. 2007;33:661–675.
3. Miovic M, Block S. Psychiatric disorders in advanced cancer. *Cancer*. 2007;110:1665–1676.
4. Drigan R, Spirito A, Gelber RD. Behavioral effects of corticosteroids in children with acute lymphoblastic leukemia. *Med Pediatr Oncol*. 1992;20:13–21.
5. Shariff S, Cumming CE, Lees A, et al. Mood disorder in women with early breast cancer taking tamoxifen, an estradiol receptor antagonist. An expected or unexpected effect? *Ann N Y Acad Sci*. 1995;761:365–368.
6. Cetin M, Yetgin S, Kara A, et al. Hyperglycemia, ketoacidosis and other complications of L-asparaginase in children with acute lymphoblastic leukemia. *J Med*. 1994;25:219–229.
7. Adams F, Quesada JR, Gutterman JU. Neuropsychiatric manifestations of human leukocyte interferon therapy in patients with cancer. *JAMA*. 1984;252:938–941.
8. Denicoff KD, Rubinow DR, Papa MZ, et al. The neuropsychiatric effects of treatment with interleukin-2 and lymphokine-activated killer cells. *Ann Intern Med*. 1987;107:293–300.
9. DeAngelis LM, Delattre JY, Posner JB. Radiation-induced dementia in patients cured of brain metastases. *Neurology*. 1989;39:789–796.
10. Weddington WW, Jr. Delirium and depression associated with amphotericin B. *Psychosomatics*. 1982;23:1076–1078.
11. Filley CM, Kleinschmidt-DeMasters BK. Neurobehavioral presentations of brain neoplasms. *West J Med*. 1995;163:19–25.
12. Patchell RA, Posner JB. Neurologic complications of systemic cancer. *Neurol Clin*. 1985;3:729–750.
13. Dalmau JO, Posner JB. Paraneoplastic syndromes affecting the nervous system. *Semin Oncol*. 1997;24:318–328.
14. Spiegel D, Bloom JR. Pain in metastatic breast cancer. *Cancer*. 1983;52:341–345.
15. Berger A, Dukes E, Mercadante S, et al. Use of antiepileptics and tricyclic antidepressants in cancer patients with neuropathic pain. *Eur J Cancer Care (Engl)*. 2006;15:138–145.
16. Hoda D, Perez DG, Loprinzi CL. Hot flashes in breast cancer survivors. *Breast J*. 2003;9:431–438.
17. Pansini F, Albertazzi P, Bonaccorsi G, et al. Trazodone: A non-hormonal alternative for neurovegetative climacteric symptoms. *Clin Exp Obstet Gynecol*. 1995;22:341–344.
18. Gillman PK. A systematic review of the serotonergic effects of mirtazapine in humans: Implications for its dual action status. *Hum Psychopharmacol*. 2006;21:117–125.
19. Shevell M, Schreiber R. Pemoline-associated hepatic failure: A critical analysis of the literature. *Pediatr Neurol*. 1997;16:14–16.
20. Gagnon B, Low G, Schreier G. Methylphenidate hydrochloride improves cognitive function in patients with advanced cancer and hypoactive delirium: A prospective clinical study. *J Psychiatry Neurosci*. 2005;30:100–107.
21. Homsi J, Walsh D, Nelson KA, et al. Methylphenidate for depression in hospice practice: A case series. *Am J Hosp Palliat Care*. 2000;17:393–398.
22. Meyers CA, Weitzner MA, Valentine AD, et al. Methylphenidate therapy improves cognition, mood, and function of brain tumor patients. *J Clin Oncol*. 1998;16:2522–2527.
23. Bruera E, Chadwick S, Brenneis C, et al. Methylphenidate associated with narcotics for the treatment of cancer pain. *Cancer Treat Rep*. 1987;71:67–70.
24. Bruera E, Brenneis C, Paterson AH, et al. Use of methylphenidate as an adjuvant to narcotic analgesics in patients with advanced cancer. *J Pain Symptom Manage*. 1989;4:3–6.
25. Bourke DL, Allen PD, Rosenberg M, et al. Dextroamphetamine with morphine: Respiratory effects. *J Clin Pharmacol*. 1983;23:65–70.
26. Mitler MM, Hajdukovic R, Erman M, et al. Narcolepsy. *J Clin Neurophysiol*. 1990;7:93–118.
27. Wu LT, Pilowsky DJ, Schlenger WE, et al. Misuse of methamphetamine and prescription stimulants among youths and young adults in the community. *Drug Alcohol Depend*. 2007;89:195–205.
28. Randomized trial of modafinil as a treatment for the excessive daytime somnolence of narcolepsy: US Modafinil in Narcolepsy Multicenter Study Group. *Neurology*. 2000;54:1166–1175.
29. Pack AI, Black JE, Schwartz JR, et al. Modafinil as adjunct therapy for daytime sleepiness in obstructive sleep apnea. *Am J Respir Crit Care Med*. 2001;164:1675–1681.
30. Czeisler CA, Walsh JK, Roth T, et al. Modafinil for excessive sleepiness associated with shift-work sleep disorder. *N Engl J Med*. 2005;353:476–486.
31. Zifko UA, Rupp M, Schwarz S, et al. Modafinil in treatment of fatigue in multiple sclerosis. Results of an open-label study. *J Neurol*. 2002;249:983–987.
32. DeBattista C, Lembke A, Solvason HB, et al. A prospective trial of modafinil as an adjunctive treatment of major depression. *J Clin Psychopharmacol*. 2004;24:87–90.
33. Adler CH, Caviness JN, Hentz JG, et al. Randomized trial of modafinil for treating subjective daytime sleepiness in patients with Parkinson's disease. *Mov Disord*. 2003;18:287–293.
34. Verster JC, Volkerts ER. Clinical pharmacology, clinical efficacy, and behavioral toxicity of alprazolam: A review of the literature. *CNS Drug Rev*. 2004;10:45–76.
35. Nardi AE, Perna G. Clonazepam in the treatment of psychiatric disorders: An update. *Int Clin Psychopharmacol*. 2006;21:131–142.
36. Moroz G. High-potency benzodiazepines: Recent clinical results. *J Clin Psychiatry*. 2004;65 Suppl 5:13–18.
37. Dellemijn PL, Fields HL. Do benzodiazepines have a role in chronic pain management? *Pain*. 1994;57:137–152.

38. Blier P, Ward NM. Is there a role for 5-HT1A agonists in the treatment of depression? *Biol Psychiatry.* 2003;53:193–203.
39. Riechelmann RP, Tannock IF, Wang L, et al. Potential drug interactions and duplicate prescriptions among cancer patients. *J Natl Cancer Inst.* 2007;99:592–600.
40. Stearns V, Johnson MD, Rae JM, et al. Active tamoxifen metabolite plasma concentrations after coadministration of tamoxifen and the selective serotonin reuptake inhibitor paroxetine. *J Natl Cancer Inst.* 2003;95:1758–1764.
41. Jin Y, Desta Z, Stearns V, et al. CYP2D6 genotype, antidepressant use, and tamoxifen metabolism during adjuvant breast cancer treatment. *J Natl Cancer Inst.* 2005;97:30–39.
42. Lehmann D, Nelsen J, Ramanath V, et al. Lack of attenuation in the antitumor effect of tamoxifen by chronic CYP isoform inhibition. *J Clin Pharmacol.* 2004;44:861–865.
43. Lindley C, Vasa S, Sawyer WT, et al. Quality of life and preferences for treatment following systemic adjuvant therapy for early-stage breast cancer. *J Clin Oncol.* 1998;16:1380–1387.
44. Savard J, Morin CM. Insomnia in the context of cancer: A review of a neglected problem. *J Clin Oncol.* 2001;19:895–908.
45. Lis CG, Gupta D, Grutsch JF. The relationship between insomnia and patient satisfaction with quality of life in cancer. *Support Care Cancer.* 2008;16:261–266.
46. Maczaj M. Pharmacologic treatment of insomnia. *Drugs.* 1993;45:44–55.
47. Mystakidou K, Parpa E, Tsilika E, et al. Sleep quality in advanced cancer patients. *J Psychosom Res.* 2007;62:527–533.
48. Stiefel FC, Kornblith AB, Holland JC. Changes in the prescription patterns of psychotropic drugs for cancer patients during a 10-year period. *Cancer.* 1990;65:1048–1053.
49. Davidson JR, MacLean AW, Brundage MD, et al. Sleep disturbance in cancer patients. *Soc Sci Med.* 2002;54:1309–1321.
50. Bower JE, Ganz PA, Desmond KA, et al. Fatigue in breast cancer survivors: Occurrence, correlates, and impact on quality of life. *J Clin Oncol.* 2000;18:743–753.
51. Servaes P, Verhagen CA, Bleijenberg G. Relations between fatigue, neuropsychological functioning, and physical activity after treatment for breast carcinoma: Daily self-report and objective behavior. *Cancer.* 2002;95:2017–2026.
52. Le Guen Y, Gagnadoux F, Hureaux J, et al. Sleep disturbances and impaired daytime functioning in outpatients with newly diagnosed lung cancer. *Lung Cancer.* 2007;58:139–143.
53. Sateia MJ, Pigeon WR. Identification and management of insomnia. *Med Clin North Am.* 2004;88:567–596.
54. Manber R, Edinger JD, Gress JL, et al. Cognitive behavioral therapy for insomnia enhances depression outcome in patients with comorbid major depressive disorder and insomnia. *Sleep.* 2008;31:489–495.
55. Dooley M, Plosker GL. Zaleplon: A review of its use in the treatment of insomnia. *Drugs.* 2000;60:413–445.
56. Agosto J, Choi JC, Parisky KM, et al. Modulation of GABAA receptor desensitization uncouples sleep onset and maintenance in Drosophila. *Nat Neurosci.* 2008;11:354–359.
57. Bateson AN. The benzodiazepine site of the GABAA receptor: An old target with new potential? *Sleep Med.* 2004;5 Suppl 1:S9-15.
58. Roehrs T, Merlotti L, Zorick F, et al. Rebound insomnia in normals and patients with insomnia after abrupt and tapered discontinuation. *Psychopharmacology (Berl).* 1992;108:67–71.
59. Ansseau M, Poncelet PF, Schmitz D. High dose triazolam and anterograde amnesia. *BMJ.* 1992;304:1178.
60. Hung DZ, Tsai WJ, Deng JF. Anterograde amnesia in triazolam overdose despite flumazenil treatment: A case report. *Hum Exp Toxicol.* 1992;11:289–290.
61. Nazareth I, Ashworth M, Hammond J, et al. Withdrawal of triazolam's product license: Effect on patients 18 months later. *Addiction.* 1995;90:927–934.
62. Griffiths RR, Johnson MW. Relative abuse liability of hypnotic drugs: A conceptual framework and algorithm for differentiating among compounds. *J Clin Psychiatry.* 2005;66 Suppl 9:31–41.
63. Hair PI, McCormack PL, Curran MP. Eszopiclone: A review of its use in the treatment of insomnia. *Drugs.* 2008;68:1415–1434.
64. Brielmaier BD. Eszopiclone (Lunesta): A new nonbenzodiazepine hypnotic agent. *Proc (Bayl Univ Med Cent).* 2006;19:54–59.
65. Curry DT, Eisenstein RD, Walsh JK. Pharmacologic management of insomnia: Past, present, and future. *Psychiatr Clin North Am.* 2006;29:871–893.
66. Wilson S, Argyropoulos S. Antidepressants and sleep: A qualitative review of the literature. *Drugs.* 2005;65:927–947.
67. Mayers AG, Baldwin DS. Antidepressants and their effect on sleep. *Hum Psychopharmacol.* 2005;20:533–559.
68. Mouret J, Lemoine P, Minuit MP, et al. Effects of trazodone on the sleep of depressed subjects—a polygraphic study. *Psychopharmacology (Berl).* 1988;95 Suppl:S37-43.
69. Becker PM. Treatment of sleep dysfunction and psychiatric disorders. *Curr Treat Options Neurol.* 2006;8:367–375.
70. Rosenberg RP. Sleep maintenance insomnia: Strengths and weaknesses of current pharmacologic therapies. *Ann Clin Psychiatry.* 2006;18:49–56.
71. Holm KJ, Markham A. Mirtazapine: A review of its use in major depression. *Drugs.* 1999;57:607–631.
72. Freynhagen R, Muth-Selbach U, Lipfert P, et al. The effect of mirtazapine in patients with chronic pain and concomitant depression. *Curr Med Res Opin.* 2006;22:257–264.
73. Zlotos DP. Recent advances in melatonin receptor ligands. *Arch Pharm (Weinheim).* 2005;338:229–247.
74. Neubauer DN. A review of ramelteon in the treatment of sleep disorders. *Neuropsychiatr Dis Treat.* 2008;4:69–79.
75. Simpson D, Curran MP. Ramelteon: A review of its use in insomnia. *Drugs.* 2008;68:1901–1919.
76. Reynoldson JN, Elliott E, Sr., Nelson LA. Ramelteon: A novel approach in the treatment of insomnia. *Ann Pharmacother.* 2008;42:1262–1271.

CHAPTER 25 ■ RELATED ISSUES

HOME CARE

Home care is a dynamic component of the health care system. In the United States, several factors have contributed towards change as well as growth in the home care industry. Over the last two decades, the use of home care and home infusion therapy continues to expand and grow. Several areas may account for this growth. Prospective payment for hospital services and diagnosis-related groups for Medicare patients, implemented in the mid-1980s, resulted in earlier discharge from hospital. An aging population and improved survival rates for chronic illnesses, including cancer, have led to an increased use of home care. In addition, marketplace regulation has forced the delivery of health care from its traditionally hospital-based center of services into alternative settings. For individuals requiring long-term therapy (such as those requiring lifelong intravenous nutrition support) inpatient care is not only expensive, but also prevents the individual from resuming normal lifestyle and work activities. Advances in pain management technology, such as ambulatory patient-controlled analgesias (PCA)s and the use of silicone subcutaneously tunneled neuraxial catheters have expanded the scope and success of interventional pain management beyond the hospital to the home. Potential benefits of home infusion therapy include decreased health care costs, patient/caregiver convenience, less time spent in hospital with the ability to extend interventional pain management strategies into the patient's home. A possible disadvantage to home infusion therapy may include the additional burden placed on the patient/caregiver in terms of role responsibilities and schedules. Home care agencies must have explicitly defined policies and procedures consistent with regulatory bodies and national and regional standards of practice.

A provider of infusion therapy must be a licensed pharmacy or work in conjunction with a licensed pharmacy. Pharmacies are licensed by the board of pharmacy of the state in which they are located. State boards of pharmacies maintain requirements. For many patients, home nursing services are also provided to educate patients and their caregivers regarding administering the drug therapy, complying with the prescribed dosing schedule, understanding the drug delivery device being used (an infusion pump or other device), and other important information regarding the treatment regimen. Drug therapies commonly administered via infusion at home include antibiotics, chemotherapy, pain management, parenteral nutrition, and immune globulin. Diagnoses commonly requiring infusion therapy include infections that are unresponsive to oral antibiotics, cancer and cancer-related pain, gastrointestinal (GI) diseases or disorders which prevent normal functioning of the GI system, congestive heart failure, immune disorders, growth hormone deficiencies, and more.

Ambulatory infusion pumps are either designed to be therapy-specific, or are multipurpose, enabling treatments such as chemotherapy, systemic antibiotics, total parenteral nutrition, hydration therapy, and opioid pain control. Recent developments in pump design include remote access capability by modem with the ability to change pump settings and download data.

Home-based PCA therapy provides select patients with the ability to deliver analgesia based on their own perception of need. PCA therapy may be superior to oral analgesia, especially in the treatment of severe, fluctuating pain. Patient selection criteria include intact cognition and proper supervision from a family member or health professional. A collaborative interdisciplinary approach is necessary for effective pain control for the cancer patient receiving interventional pain management at home. Collaboration among the patient, the patient's family, the home care nurse and home care agency, and the patient's physician is necessary. The physician remains responsible for determining the appropriate drug, bolus dose, background infusion rate, and lockout interval.

PCA is increasingly more commonly used in the home setting as an effective option in pain management. As discussed above, the subcutaneous and intravenous routes are the primary methods of administration. The availability of a central vascular access device such as a tunneled or peripherally inserted central catheter (PICC) offers advantages over peripheral access to ensure safe and consistent administration of intravenous analgesia.

The safety and efficacy of home-based PCA opioid therapy has not been extensively reported as in-hospital use. One study,[1] however, reported on the use of morphine PCA in the home environment of 143 preterminally and terminally ill tumor patients suffering either from excruciating chronic pain or severe chronic/acute complex pain that could not be relieved adequately by oral analgesia. After initial dose adjustment, which lasted 2 to 3 days, the median morphine was 93 mg/day (range: 12 to 464 mg/day). This median was 28% lower than the median dose administered orally prior to PCA therapy. During the course of treatment, morphine requirements increased by a median of 2.3 mg/day (range: −29 to 52 mg/day). Most patients were treated continuously in the home care setting until death, the median duration of treatment was 27 days (range: 1 to 437 days). Terminal morphine demands reached a median of 188 mg/day (range: 15 to 1008 mg/day). The authors concluded that PCA was both safe and effective in the home environment, attaining excellent results in 95 (66%) patients and satisfactory pain relief in 43 (30%). PCA was considered insufficient in five (4%) cases. Side effects, in general, were considered mild, the most common being constipation, fatigue, and nausea.

Although further study is warranted, safe provision of domiciliary interventional pain management probably requires selection of appropriate patients, effective patient and caregiver education, well-defined policies, and use of experienced and knowledgeable home care agencies. We work very hard to establish domiciliary pain management whenever this is a feasible option for a cancer patient. It is our belief that it is both better and more effective for the patient and his or her family.

COMPLEMENTARY AND ALTERNATIVE MEDICINE

Complementary and alternative medicine (CAM) should be considered a group of diverse medical and health care systems, practices, and products that are not presently considered to be part of conventional medicine. The National Center for Complementary and Alternative Medicine (NCCAM) is a federally funded agency within the National Institutes of Health (NIH) and Department of Health and Human Services. NCCAM groups CAM practices into whole medical systems (eg, homeopathic and naturopathic medicine, systems that have developed in non Western cultures), mind-body medicine (eg, meditation, prayer, mental healing), biologically-based practices (eg, dietary supplements, herbal products), manipulative and body-based practices (eg, manipulation, massage), and energy medicine (eg, reiki, therapeutic touch, magnetic fields). CAM therapies are used widely among cancer patients.[2]

These therapies have been used as an alternative to conventional medicine (alternative medicine) and complementary to conventional medicine (complementary medicine). Most cancer patients use CAM with the hope of boosting the immune system, relieving pain, and controlling side effects related to disease or treatment. Only a minority of patients include CAM in the treatment plan with curative intent. Frequently, patients do not discuss CAM therapies with physicians.[3] Mansky and Wallerstedt[4] reported that the CAM domains of mind-body medicine, CAM botanicals, manipulative practices, and energy medicine were widely used as complementary approaches to palliative cancer care and cancer symptom management. In the area of cancer symptom management, auricular acupuncture, therapeutic touch, and hypnosis may help to manage cancer pain. Music therapy, massage, and hypnosis may have an effect on anxiety, and both acupuncture and massage may have a therapeutic role in cancer fatigue.

Acupuncture and selected botanicals may reduce chemotherapy-induced nausea and emesis, and hypnosis and guided imagery may be beneficial in anticipatory nausea and vomiting. Transcendental meditation and the mindfulness-based stress reduction can play a role in the management of depressed mood and anxiety. Black cohosh and phytoestrogen-rich foods may reduce vasomotor symptoms in postmenopausal women. Although there have been many trials of CAM therapies for cancer pain and a few expert reviews, there is a lack of rigorous systematic review.[5] Furthermore, studies have found that there is considerable variation in the search for CAM studies, making systematic reviews prone to bias.[6] Bardia et al.,[5] in a systematic review of CAM therapies for cancer-related pain, demonstrated the paucity of well-designed, multi-institutional trials. Most trials were of short duration, had small numbers without sample size justification, and did not report the adverse effects of CAM intervention.

However, some data existed suggesting that mind-body medicine (hypnosis, imagery, and relaxation) may have some efficacy in decreasing cancer pain. Pan et al.[7] had similar conclusions regarding the role of CAM therapies in the management of pain, dyspnea, and nausea and vomiting in patients near the end of life. The heterogeneity of pain syndromes has made broad, sweeping conclusions about the efficacy of acupuncture difficult. An NIH consensus conference[8] on the use of acupuncture for pain concluded that while there have been many studies of its potential usefulness, many of these studies provide equivocal results because of design, sample size, and other factors. However, promising results have emerged, for example, showing efficacy of acupuncture in adult postoperative and chemotherapy nausea and vomiting and in postoperative dental pain. There are other situations such as addiction, stroke rehabilitation, headache, menstrual cramps, tennis elbow, fibromyalgia, myofascial pain, osteoarthritis, low back pain, carpal tunnel syndrome, and asthma, in which acupuncture may be useful as an adjunct treatment or an acceptable alternative or be included in a comprehensive management program.

NANOTECHNOLOGY AND CANCER

Nanotechnology is a broad term covering the building of structures and "machines" on an atomic or molecular scale—in the range from 1 to 100 nm. Nanoscience is the study of the fundamental principles of molecules and structures with at least one dimension between 1 and 100 nm. Nanotechnology offers the unprecedented and paradigm-changing opportunity to study and interact with normal and cancer cells in real time at the molecular and cellular scales during the earliest stages of the cancer process (Fig. 25.1). It has the potential to radically increase options for prevention, diagnosis, and treatment of cancer. Liposomes, the "first generation" of nanoscale drug delivery devices, were developed to deliver anticancer therapeutics directly at tumors. Specifically, liposomal doxorubicin is being used to treat certain forms of cancer, whereas liposomal amphotericin B treats fungal infections often associated with aggressive anticancer treatments. Abraxane is the albumin-bound, 130-nm particle form of paclitaxel, approved by the Food and Drug Administration (FDA) for the treatment of metastatic breast cancer, may also be considered a first generation nano delivered drug. It was developed to avoid solvent-related toxicities in free paclitaxel and to exploit the albumin receptor-mediated endothelial transport. Other clinical applications of nanotechnology have focused on identifying cancer in its earliest stages, visualizing development of the disease, delivering improved therapy to increase the effectiveness and reduce side effects of drugs, and capturing early signals of drug efficacy.

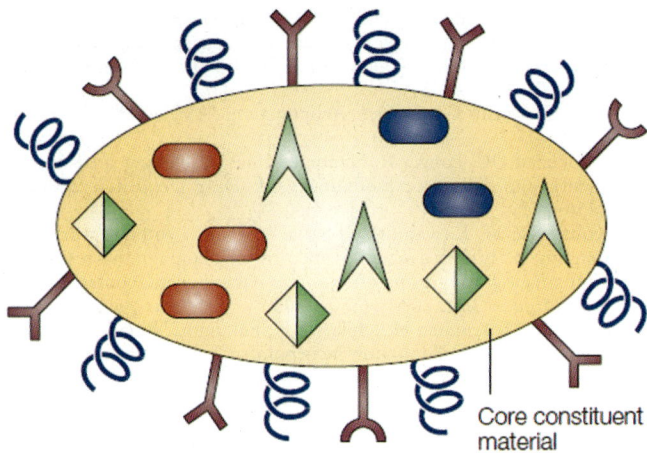

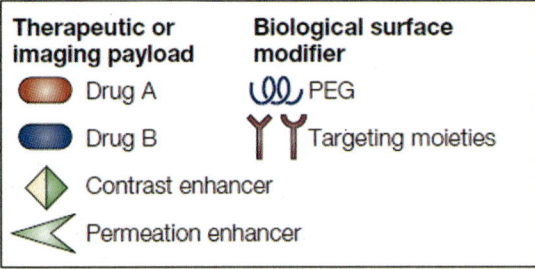

FIGURE 25.1 Multifunctional nanoparticle. Illustrated are (1) the ability to carry one or more therapeutic agents, (2) biomolecular targeting through one or more conjugated antibodies, (3) imaging signal amplification by way of coencapsulated contrast agents, (4) biobarrier avoidance as illustrated by an endothelial tight-junction opening permeation enhancer and by polyethylene glycol (PEG) for the avoidance of macrophage uptake by macrophages (From Ferrari M. Cancer nanotechnology: opportunities and challenges. *Nat Rev Cancer*. 2005; 5:(3):161-171.) Reprinted by permission from Macmillan Publishers Ltd: Copyright 2005.

Nanotechnology involves the application of nanostructures into useful nanoscale devices. Nanomedical developments range from nanoparticles for molecular diagnostics, imaging, and therapy to integrated medical nanosystems, which may in the future perform complex repair actions at the cellular level inside the body. The areas where micro- and nanotechnology may be applied in biomedicine include detection of molecular changes responsible for disease pathogenesis, disease diagnosis and imaging, drug delivery and therapy, multifunctional systems for combined therapeutic and diagnostic applications, vehicles to report the in vivo efficacy of a therapeutic agent, and nanoscale-enabling technologies which will accelerate scientific discovery and basic research.[9]

Nanotechnology and biology share many similarities. The most complicated organisms are made up of tiny cells constructed from nanoscale building blocks: proteins, lipids, nucleic acids, and other complex biological molecules. Nanotechnology utilizes nanostructures made from semiconductors, metals, plastic, or glass. The major requirement for implantable drug delivery devices is controlled release of therapeutic agents as a continuous process over an extended period of time. The goal is to achieve a continuous drug release profile consistent with zero-order kinetics where the concentration of the drug remains constant throughout the delivery period. Drug delivery systems with a zero-order release rate have several potential therapeutic advantages, including in vivo predictability of release rate on the basis of in vitro data, minimized peak plasma levels and reduced risk of adverse reactions, predictable and extended duration of action, reduced inconvenience of frequent redosing, and improved patient compliance.

Nanomaterials have the inherent advantage of possessing unique functional properties for cancer detection and treatment. Kobayashi et al.[10] used nanosized formulation of G6 contrast agents for studying lymphatic drainage by magnetic resonance imaging (MRI) for understanding the metastases of breast cancer. Similarly, Shikata et al.[11] encapsulated gadolinium in chitosan nanoparticles for neuron capture therapy of cancer. Veiseh et al.[12] developed a "nanoprobe" consisting of PEG (polyethylene glycol)-coated iron oxide nanoparticles. These nanoprobes had preferential uptake in glioma cells and were used for real-time imaging and correlation of preoperative images with intraoperative pathology of gliomas at cellular-level resolution.

The advent of novel cancer therapeutics from nanotechnology has slowly evolved from nanoencapsulated drug formulations to nanosized functional nanoparticles. Such functional nanoparticles are engineered to ensure delivery of ionizing radiation, chemotherapeutic agents, or thermal dose specifically to malignant tissues. Sengupta et al.[13] developed nanocells targeted to malignant tissues. The nanocell comprises a nuclear nanoparticle within an extranuclear pegylated-lipid envelope and is preferentially taken up by the tumor. The nanocell enables a temporal release of two drugs: the outer envelope first releases an antiangiogenesis agent, causing a vascular shutdown; the inner nanoparticle, which is trapped inside the tumor, then releases a chemotherapy agent. This focal release within a tumor results in improved therapeutic index with reduced toxicity.

The most common nanotech platforms today include polymeric nanoparticles, nanoshells, micelles, liposomes, dendrimers, nucleic acid–based nanoconstructs, engineered viral nanoparticles, magnetic nanoparticles, silicon oxide nanoparticles, and quantum dots. Implanted controlled drug delivery systems based on degradable biomaterials have great potential in pain management. Various materials such as viscous liquids, gel or semisolids, rods or fibers, pellets and minipellets, pastes, fills, discs, wafers, matrices, and squares have been studied.

There has been steady progress in the development of nanosized hybrid therapeutics and drug delivery systems. Many of the approved products in clinical use are anticancer therapies. These include liposomes (eg, DaunoXome), polymer-coated liposomes (Doxil), polymeric drugs (Copaxone), antibodies (Herceptin, Avastin) and antibody conjugates (Mylotarg), polymer-protein conjugates (Neulasta), and a nanoparticle-containing paclitaxel (Abraxane). The first preliminary data on the application of the local anesthetics loaded into implantable biodegradable polymers in humans for intercostal nerve block was reported in 2003.[14] Holte et al.[15] also examined the effect of bupivacaine-loaded polylactide-co-glycolide (PLGA) microcapsules implanted subcutaneously in an experimental pain model in humans, in the presence or absence of dexamethasone. They found that the examined system provided a longer period of pain relief in the presence of dexamethasone. Nanotechnology is a promising new scientific endeavor that will have significant impact upon the treatment of cancer itself as well as pain ascribed to malignant diseases. Betbeder et al.[16] studied the antinociceptive activity and blood and brain delivery of nasal morphine with Biovector nanoparticles in mice and reported that the presence of nanoparticles only at a very specific dose increased the antinociceptive activity of morphine. As these nanoparticles appear to be well tolerated in humans after nasal administration, there is potential for use of this system in humans.

References

1. Meuret G, Jocham H. Patient-controlled analgesia (PCA) in the domiciliary care of tumour patients. *Cancer Treat Rev.* 1996; 22(Suppl A):137–140.
2. Cassileth B, Trevisan C, Gubili J. Complementary therapies for cancer pain. *Curr Pain Headache Rep.* 2007;11:265–269.
3. Adler SR, Fosket JR. Disclosing complementary and alternative medicine use in the medical encounter: A qualitative study in women with breast cancer. *J Fam Pract.* 1999;48:453–458.
4. Mansky PJ, Wallerstedt DB. Complementary medicine in palliative care and cancer symptom management. *Cancer J.* 2006;12:425–431.
5. Bardia A, Barton DL, Prokop LJ, et al: Efficacy of complementary and alternative medicine therapies in relieving cancer pain: A systematic review. *J Clin Oncol.* 2006;24:5457–5464.
6. Sood A, Sood R, Bauer BA, et al: Cochrane systematic reviews in acupuncture: Methodological diversity in database searching. *J Altern Complement Med.* 2005;11:719–722.
7. Pan CX, Morrison RS, Ness J, et al. Complementary and alternative medicine in the management of pain, dyspnea, and nausea and vomiting near the end of life. A systematic review. *J Pain Symptom Manage.* 2000;20:374–387.
8. NIH Consensus Conference. Acupuncture. *JAMA.* 1998;280:1518–1524.
9. Farokhzad OC, Langer R. Nanomedicine: Developing smarter therapeutic and diagnostic modalities. *Adv Drug Deliv Rev.* 2006;58:1456–1459.
10. Kobayashi H, Kawamoto S, Sakai Y, et al. Lymphatic drainage imaging of breast cancer in mice by micro-magnetic resonance lymphangiography using a nano-size paramagnetic contrast agent. *J Natl Cancer Inst.* 2004;96:703–708.
11. Shikata F, Tokumitsu H, Ichikawa H, Fukumori Y. In vitro cellular accumulation of gadolinium incorporated into chitosan nanoparticles designed for neutron-capture therapy of cancer. *Eur J Pharm Biopharm.* 2002;53:157–163.
12. Veiseh O, Sun C, Gunn J, et al. Optical and MRI multifunctional nanoprobe for targeting gliomas. *Nano Lett.* 2005;5:1003–1008.
13. Sengupta S, Eavarone D, Capila I, et al. Temporal targeting of tumour cells and neovasculature with a nanoscale delivery system. *Nature.* 2005;436:568–572.
14. Kopacz DJ, Lacouture PG, Wu D, et al. The dose response and effects of dexamethasone on bupivacaine microcapsules for intercostal blockade (T9 to T11) in healthy volunteers. *Anesth Analg.* 2003;96:2576–2582.
15. Holte K, Werner MU, Lacouture PG, Kehlet H. Dexamethasone prolongs local analgesia after subcutaneous infiltration of bupivacaine microcapsules in human volunteers. *Anesthesiology.* 2002;96:1131–1135.
16. Betbeder D, Sperandio S, Latapie JP, et al. Biovector nanoparticles improve antinociceptive efficacy of nasal morphine. *Pharm Res.* 2000;17:743–748.

CHAPTER 26 ■ SPECIALIZED PAIN MANAGEMENT

Advances in cancer detection and early diagnosis, more effective treatments, and the adoption of healthier lifestyles by those at risk for cancer have resulted in a dramatic increase in the number of individuals living longer with their cancer. In many instances, cancer has become a survivable illness. Cancer survivors constitute 3.5% of the United States population, but second primary malignancies among this high-risk group now account for 16% of all cancer incidence.[1] The 5-year survival for many cancer sites exceeds 50%, suggesting that these patients are living longer and may be considered to have a chronic illness.[2] Cancer survivors are high health care utilizers affecting distinct health care domains owing to therapeutic exposures, genetic predisposition, and/or lifestyle risk factors.

Improved quality of life (QoL) is the goal of survivorship. Survivors should understand the importance of pain control as a vital component of this process. Patient, professional, and system-related barriers that are seen during active treatment may continue to hinder optimal pain relief during survivorship.[3] For clinicians to be understanding of the very complex needs of patients with cancer, it is requisite that they be aware of often unspoken expressions of a patient's anxieties about pain and suffering, loss of control over personal destiny, dread of dying and of the end of cherished relationships.[4]

New pain complaints or side effects from treatment (ie, pharmacotherapeutic or cancer treatment) require careful evaluation and management. Survivors and families need to understand their fundamental role as part of the treatment team and that successful survivorship may be dependent on their sharing any concerns or fears related to pain management. Educational tools that are easy to read and understand should be available for all patient populations. Health care providers should work to educate not only survivors and families who are currently in treatment, but also the entire community of the availability and importance of pain management in successful cancer survivorship.

The issues of pain management in these patients are often very similar to those of any chronic nonmalignant pain patient, although there are some exceptions. The potential for disease recurrence is always possible. Any new pain may imply the possibility of either a new disease process or recurrence, thus making patient interpretation of painful symptoms more difficult. Some studies suggest that fear of recurrence is negatively correlated with QoL.[5] Successful pain management for cancer survivors begins with detailed assessment, includes good health care team communication, the initiation of appropriate interventions, and ongoing reassessment of any interventions.

The natural history of chronic pain in cancer patients differs in that the initial pain complaint is often of significant intensity during the initial treatment phase, followed by chronic, less intense pain during remission.[6] Thus, cancer patients often start on opioid therapy during curative treatment and then develop chronic pain. Opioid treatment may often be continued without recognition of its potential hazards in a patient who no longer has pain from cancer. There may not be an obvious point at which the necessity for continued opioid therapy has been questioned. Uncontrolled and frequently escalating opioid therapy may not be the optimal therapy for chronic pain conditions such as myofascial pain associated with deactivation, particularly if opioid use is the primary focus of care. Problematic opioid use may be recognized in these circumstances by unchanged or decreasing functional status with escalating opioid use. Deciding when opioid therapy is more harmful than beneficial can be difficult. The prescribing clinician must determine if opioid treatment should be continued, stabilized, or discontinued. A tapering schedule is the wisest way to discontinue opioids.

Long-term survivors may have other issues, which can include functional deficits, pain, fatigue, lymphedema, and altered bowel and bladder function. Simple activities such as mobility and the ability to perform self-care can be limited. In addition, reintegration into society with activities such as driving, social interaction, and return to work can be problematic. Cancer rehabilitation may improve QoL by minimizing disability and handicap caused by cancer and its treatment.[7]

Several different factors potentiate the risk for chronic comorbid conditions among cancer survivors. These include metabolic syndrome associated disease (obesity, diabetes, and cardiovascular disease), osteoporosis, and decreased functional status. Obesity is a well-established risk factor for cancers of the breast (postmenopausal), colon, kidney (renal cell), esophagus (adenocarcinoma), and endometrium; thus, a large proportion of cancer patients tend to be overweight or obese at the time of diagnosis.[8] Additional weight gain can also occur during and after cancer treatment in breast cancer, testicular, and gastrointestinal cancer patients. Because obesity is associated with cancer recurrence in both breast and prostate cancer, and reduced QoL among survivors, there is compelling evidence to support weight control efforts in this population.[9] Obesity is a common manifestation of several metabolic disorders that are frequently observed among cancer survivors. These disorders are grouped under the umbrella term, "the metabolic syndrome," and also include diabetes and cardiovascular disease (CVD). Insulin resistance is the underlying event associated with the metabolic syndrome and co-occurs with hyperinsulinemia and/or diabetes.[10] CVD is a major health issue among survivors, evidenced by mortality data which show that half of noncancer-related deaths are attributed to CVD.[11] Risk is especially high among men with prostate cancer who receive hormone ablation therapy, as well as patients who receive adriamycin, and radiation therapy to fields surrounding the heart.[12] Clinical studies suggest that osteoporosis remains an important health concern among survivors.[13] Functional status is often lowest immediately after treatment and tends to improve over time; however, the presence of pain and co-occurring diseases may affect this relationship.[14] Cancer survivors demonstrate almost a twofold increase in having at least one functional limitation, and, in the presence of another comorbid condition, the odds ratio increases to 5.06 (95% confidence interval [CI]: 4.47–5.72).[15]

Possible late effects of cancer and its treatment are listed in Table 26.1.

The constantly evolving effect of a philosophical shift in cancer treatment from a primarily seek-and-destroy mindset toward one reflecting the importance of both curing the disease and controlling its attendant adverse sequelae significantly affects the cancer survivorship research paradigm. Cancer treatments today are increasingly used in the context of the survivor's life, striving toward minimal toxicity yet optimal effectiveness and with recognition of the importance of interdisciplinary care and management. This philosophy must be communicated to researchers and care providers across diverse settings to promote its incorporation into the design of the next generation of cancer survivorship investigations. Aziz[16] summarizes the paradigm of cancer survivorship research as one that:

1. Seeks to identify, examine, prevent and control adverse sequelae of cancer and its treatment;
2. Manages, treats, and prevents comorbidities;
3. Incorporates health promotion and lifestyle interventions to optimize health after cancer treatment;
4. Defines optimal follow-up care and surveillance strategies and guidelines for all survivors;
5. Pays special attention to disparities in survivorship outcomes by age, income, ethnicity, geography, or cancer site; and
6. Explores the impact of the survivorship experience on the family (and vice versa).

TABLE 26.1

LATE SEQUELAE OF CANCER AND ITS TREATMENT

Organ System	Late Effect/Sequelae of Radiation Therapy	Late Effect/Sequelae of Chemotherapy	Chemotherapeutic Drugs Responsible
Bone and soft tissues	Short stature; atrophy, fibrosis, osteonecrosis	Avascular necrosis	Steroids
Cardiovascular	Pericardial effusion; pericarditis; CAD	Cardiomyopathy; CHF	Anthracyclines, cyclophosphamide
Pulmonary	Pulmonary fibrosis; decreased lung volumes	Pulmonary fibrosis, interstitial pneumonitis	Bleomycin, carmustine, methotrexate, anthracyclines
CNS	Neuropsychological deficits, structural changes, hemorrhage	Neuropsychological deficits, structural changes; hemiplegia; seizure	Methotrexate
Peripheral nervous system	—	Peripheral neuropathy; hearing loss	Platinum analogs, vinca alkaloids
Hematologic	Cytopenia, myelodysplasia	Myelodysplastic syndromes	Alkylating agents
Renal	Decreased creatinine clearance; hypertension	Decreased creatinine clearance; increased creatinine clearance; renal failure; delayed renal failure	Platinum analogs, methotrexate, nitrosoureas
Genitourinary	Bladder fibrosis, contractures	Bladder fibrosis; hemorrhagic cystitis	Cyclophosphamide
Gastrointestinal	Malabsorption; stricture; abnormal LFT	Abnormal LFT; hepatic fibrosis; cirrhosis	Methotrexate, carmustine
Pituitary	Growth hormone deficiency; pituitary deficiency	—	—
Thyroid	Hypothyroidism; nodules	—	—
Gonadal	Men: risk of sterility, Leydig cell dysfunction. Women: ovarian failure, early menopause	Men: sterility. Women: sterility, premature menopause	Alkylating agents, Procarbazine
Dental/oral health	Poor enamel and root formation; dry mouth	Tooth decay	Multiple
Opthalmologic	Cataracts; retinopathy	Cataracts	Steroids

CAD, coronary artery disease; CHF, congestive heart failure; CNS, central nervous system; LFT, liver function test. (Reused with permission from Aziz NM. Cancer survivorship research: State of knowledge, challenges and opportunities. *Acta Oncol*. 2007;46:417–432. Copyright Informa Healthcare, with permission of Taylor & Francis Group, http://www.informaworld.com)

Psychological interventions designed to assist patients with chronic pain and associated disability and emotional distress may be suitable alternatives to more traditional medical and rehabilitative approaches. These interventions, commonly labeled cognitive-behavioral therapy, typically emphasize the development of personal control and self-management by means of active, structured techniques. Treatment focuses on modifying negative thinking, particularly thoughts of helplessness and hopelessness, and promoting increased activity and productive functioning. However, a subset of patients frequently does not successfully engage in such activities.[17] Ultimately, if a patient with a stable, chronic pain complaint is not motivated to change behaviors that influence functional status, it is highly unlikely that treatment will succeed. Kerns et al.[18] investigated the validity of a self-reported questionnaire, Pain Stages of Change Questionnaire (PSOCQ), to predict a patient's readiness to adopt a self-management approach to their chronic pain condition. Four factors—precontemplation, contemplation, action, and maintenance—were found to influence readiness to change. Using PSOCQ, Burns et al.[19] suggest that any advantage enjoyed by patients with predominant action attitudes at pretreatment may be enhanced by consolidating a pain self-management approach during treatment. By contrast, late-treatment gains of patients initially taking a predominant precontemplation stance were unaffected by their degree of early-treatment attitude changes. Because none of the most commonly prescribed treatment regimens are sufficient to eliminate many chronic pain complaints, Turk et al.[20] believe a more realistic approach will likely combine pharmacologic, physical, and psychological components tailored to each patient's needs and that cognitive-behavioral therapy alone or within the context of an interdisciplinary pain rehabilitation program has the greatest empirical evidence for success. Goal achievement is considered an important measure of outcome by clinicians working with patients in physical and neurologic rehabilitation settings.[21] Zaza et al.[22] believes the use of goal attainment scaling (GAS) is an appropriate technique for guiding and monitoring the treatment of individual chronic pain patients, and may provide a useful tool for evaluating chronic pain programs. The use of GAS scores as an independent criterion of patient-relevant improvement also proved useful in a study of 73 patients with chronic musculoskeletal pain as those patients who achieved highly successful goal achievement have also shown clinically meaningful improvements on other measures.[23]

THE SPECIALTY OF PAIN MEDICINE

The diagnosis and treatment of patients with pain has long been part of the physician's responsibilities, but it is only in the past 30 years that pain medicine has attracted enough attention to begin to develop into a specialty of medicine. The provision of health care has become much more complex in this era, and pain management is practiced both by physicians and other health care providers such as psychologists, nurses, mid-level practitioners, and physical therapists. Medical knowledge about pain and interest in the sciences basic to pain relief has accelerated markedly over the past several decades. Over the years, pain medicine has utilized many strategies beyond the biomedical framework of traditional medicine. Certainly, the biopsychosocial approach, as first elucidated by Engel, has fueled the development of both research and treatments for pain.[24] In the late 1990s and early 2000s, the practice of interventional pain management expanded, leading to a schism in pain medicine and vigorous arguments as to what should characterize pain medicine.

The American Academy of Pain Medicine (AAPM) has defined *pain medicine* and the *pain specialist*. "Pain Medicine is a primary medical specialty based on a distinct body of knowledge and a well-defined scope of clinical practice that is founded on science, research and education. It is concerned with the study of pain, the prevention of pain and the evaluation, treatment and rehabilitation of persons in pain. A comprehensive evaluation incorporates the physical, psychological, cognitive and sociocultural contributions to pain. The treatment protocol may include pharmacological, invasive, behavioral, cognitive, rehabilitative and complementary strategies provided in a concurrent focused and patient specific manner. The Pain Medicine physician often serves the patient as a frontline physician regarding their pain, but also may serve as a consultant to other physicians, direct an interdisciplinary/multidisciplinary treatment team, conduct research or advocate for the patient's pain care with public and private agencies. The Pain Medicine physician may work in a variety of settings including office, clinic, hospital, university, or governmental/ public agencies." The American Board of Medical Specialties (ABMS) describes a medical specialty as "a defined area of medical practice, which connotes special knowledge and ability resulting from specialized effort and training in the special field."

Because the diagnosis and treatment of pain is in the purview of all clinical disciplines, pain medicine encompasses many specialties, but its identity is still evolving. Various disciplines in medicine practice pain medicine (Table 26.2). Within any medical specialty, there is a process of training and certification appropriate for that specialty. Unfortunately, there are no universally-recognized certifying, accrediting, or training organizations in pain medicine. Consequently, it is difficult to determine whether a physician is expert in the management of pain in general, or of cancer pain in specific. Standards differ in countries in the developed world; in the developing world,

TABLE 26.2

MEDICAL DISCIPLINES PRACTICING PAIN MEDICINE

Anesthesiology
Physical Medicine and Rehabilitation
Neurology
Psychiatry
Neurosurgery
Radiology
Rheumatology
Emergency Medicine
Family Practice
Internal Medicine
General Surgery
Orthopedic Surgery

the shortage of health care providers limits access to pain management specialists. There are both national and international organizations that offer aspects of certification, accreditation and training; it is possible to acquire many wall decorations that do not really attest to an individual's competence, or a treatment program's expertise.

Historically, the International Association for the Study of Pain (IASP) was the first formally organized group to address research, education and clinical care in pain. Founded in 1975 at its First World Congress on Pain in Florence, this group immediately set about developing educational materials and curricula for health care professionals. However, due to the multinational and multiprofessional nature of this organization, its leadership decided that no programs for certification of individuals or accreditation of treatment or educational programs would be established. The American Pain Society (APS), a national chapter of IASP, held its first meeting in 1978 and was strongly modeled upon IASP for its mission and goals. It, too, was multiprofessional and included both basic scientists and clinicians of different types. The issues of establishing certification and accreditation were fiercely debated; lack of resources in this new and small organization as well as the desire to represent all professionals interested in pain led to a policy of not developing physician certification or accreditation of treatment programs. APS did establish, in conjunction with the Commission on Accreditation of Rehabilitation Facilities (CARF), a program to accredit treatment facilities that were established using a cognitive/behavioral, multidisciplinary model; CARF had the resources to add this program to its existing accreditation activities and CARF accreditation has been available since the early 1980s for American treatment programs.

Some members of APS thought that physicians should establish an organization that would obtain recognition from the American Medical Association (AMA) and ABMS for the development of a specialty in pain medicine, board certification, and the accreditation of training programs. On this basis, the American Academy of Algology was founded in 1983. This name was subsequently changed to the American Academy of Pain Medicine (AAPM). The physicians who belong to this organization have worked diligently to obtain recognition from the AMA and to establish a certification system for physicians. Neither the AMA nor the ABMS have fully recognized the AAPM at the time of this writing. Within AAPM, there is no recognition of subspecialties such as acute pain or cancer pain management. They do offer a board certification in pain medicine (ABPM) to physicians who have completed an ABMS approved residency, undergone appropriate training in pain management, have practical experience in pain management, and have successfully completed a written examination. They do not accredit training programs in pain management at this time. Because there is no accreditation of individual training programs, the education of pain specialists is not standardized. There is no bias towards interventional pain practice in AAPM certification.

The American Board of Anesthesiology (ABA) approved a certificate of added qualification in pain management in 1991. Initially, the process was entirely within anesthesiology and only ABA-eligible or certified physicians were allowed to enter into ABA-sponsored training programs or sit for their examination. This certificate was followed by applications for subspecialty certificates in pain management from the American Board of Psychiatry and Neurology (ABPN) and the American Board of Physical Medicine and Rehabilitation (ABPMR) in 2000. An institution can only have one pain training program, subsequent to this agreement. Physicians holding ABMS-approved certification in any clinical specialty can now enroll in a pain management training program and sit for the examination. The eligibility to sit for the examination is determined by completion of an ABMS-approved residency and successful completion of an accredited pain management training program. Although broad curricular content is specified in the accreditation process, training programs are highly variable in the aspects of pain management that they include. However, these training programs tend to have a bias towards interventional pain management.

Another organization that offers certification and accreditation of training programs is the American Academy of Pain Management (AAPMan). Since 1988, this group has offered certification to individuals from a wide array of health care professions on the basis of training and experience and personal recommendation. It also accredits clinical programs. It does not have standing within organized medicine, except within the State of California.

The American Society of Interventional Pain Practice offers certification via the American Board of Interventional Pain Practice (ABIPP) to those physicians who have pain practice experience and training and who pass a written and oral examination that is based mainly upon the World Institute of Pain's examination to be a fellow in interventional pain practice (FIPP). This certification is primarily focused upon interventional procedures and is unique in that the examination includes demonstrating the ability to perform a variety of procedures on cadavers.

There are also certification processes within the palliative care community that are relevant to the management of pain associated with cancer. They are, however, not focused upon pain management, but have a much broader agenda.

None of the available certifications attest to one's abilities to diagnose or manage pain in cancer patients. It seems likely that those organizations that address multidisciplinary and multimodal care for the patient will provide better training for the diagnosis and management of cancer-related pain. At this time, it is primarily the practitioner's experience and attitudes that will lead to optimal services for the cancer patient with pain; one cannot rely on the certification process to identify qualified cancer pain management specialists. Training within a recognized cancer center is probably the best single factor that identifies a potential cancer pain specialist.

THE ROLE OF THE CANCER PAIN SPECIALIST IN PALLIATIVE CARE

The practice of oncology is characterized by challenging communication tasks that make it difficult to ensure optimal physician–patient information sharing and care planning. Discussions of diagnosis, prognosis, and patient goals are essential processes that inform decisions. Domains of information and care planning that are important for high-quality cancer care include integration of palliation into cancer care, advance care planning, sentinel events as markers for the need to readdress a patient's goals of care, and continuity of care planning. Palliative care is a person-centered approach concerned with physical, psychosocial, and spiritual care in progressive disease. It focuses on both the quality of life remaining to patients and supporting their families and those close to them. Primary palliative care refers to the basic skills and competencies required of all physicians and other health care professionals. Secondary palliative care refers to the specialist clinicians and organizations that provide consultation and specialty care. Tertiary palliative care refers to the academic medical centers where specialist knowledge for the most complex cases is practiced, researched, and taught. Compared to conventional care, specialist teams in palliative care improve satisfaction and identify and deal with more patient and family needs. Moreover, multiprofessional approaches to palliative care reduce the overall cost of care by reducing the amount of time patients spend in acute hospital settings.[25]

Palliative services may need to provide pain control for 2,800 patients per 1 million population dying from cancer each year and 3,400 patients per 1 million with noncancer terminal illness.[26] Effective pain management is one of the integral aims of palliative care. Although pharmacologic approaches (enteral or systemically administered) to tumor-associated pain management are effective in >90% of cases,[27] it may be argued that the highly selected cohort of patients seen by specialist palliative care teams with a preponderance of difficult pain syndromes may require a greater frequency of interventions, such as neuraxial drug infusion or neurolysis, peripheral nerve block, celiac plexus, and cordotomy.[28] Some studies suggest that palliative care units with access to pain specialists may, in fact, underutilize these services.[28–29] Factors that may improve utilization of services include increased interprofessional understanding of skills and a thorough exploration of roles and function within the multidisciplinary team at a local level.[29]

Patients with cancer pain who may require advanced pain management techniques have complex needs which require an interdisciplinary approach which should include holistic assessment and exploration of needs from a variety of professionals, including pain specialists. There has been a shift of practice from neurodestructive techniques to neuraxial infusions over the years. Neuraxial infusions are reported to be available to inpatients in most institutions, although this procedure may not be universally available to cancer patients, particularly in a home setting. Maintaining supplies and troubleshooting outside hospital is problematic. Finally, the availability of neurodestructive interventions is limited, for there are few practitioners trained to perform percutaneous cordotomy and similar ablative procedures.

References

1. Travis LB, Rabkin CS, Brown LM, et al. Cancer survivorship—genetic susceptibility and second primary cancers: Research strategies and recommendations. *J Natl Cancer Inst.* 2006;98:15–25.
2. Gerber LH. Cancer rehabilitation into the future. *Cancer.* 2001;92:975–979.
3. Sun V, Borneman T, Piper B, et al. Barriers to pain assessment and management in cancer survivorship. *J Cancer Surviv.* 2008;2:65–71.
4. Zebrack B. Reflections of a cancer survivor/research scientist. *Cancer.* 2003;97:2707–2709.
5. Van den Beuken-Van Everdingen MH, Peters ML, et al. Concerns of former breast cancer patients about disease recurrence: A validation and prevalence study. *Psychooncology.* 2008;17:1137–1145.
6. Ballantyne JC. Opioid misuse in oncology pain patients. *Curr Pain Headache Rep.* 2007;11:276–282.
7. Yadav R. Rehabilitation of surgical cancer patients at University of Texas M.D. Anderson Cancer Center. *J Surg Oncol.* 2007;95:361–369.
8. Bergstrom A, Pisani P, Tenet V, et al. Overweight as an avoidable cause of cancer in Europe. *Int J Cancer.* 2001;91:421–430.
9. Nuver J, Smit AJ, Postma A, et al. The metabolic syndrome in long-term cancer survivors, an important target for secondary preventive measures. *Cancer Treat Rev* 2002;28:195–214.
10. Yoshikawa T, Noguchi Y, Doi C, et al. Insulin resistance in patients with cancer: Relationships with tumor site, tumor stage, body-weight loss, acute-phase response, and energy expenditure. *Nutrition.* 2001;17:590–593.
11. Demark-Wahnefried W, Aziz NM, Rowland JH, et al. Riding the crest of the teachable moment: Promoting long-term health after the diagnosis of cancer. *J Clin Oncol.* 2005;23:5814–5830.
12. Hull MC, Morris CG, Pepine CJ, et al, Valvular dysfunction and carotid, subclavian, and coronary artery disease in survivors of Hodgkin lymphoma treated with radiation therapy. *JAMA.* 2003;290:2831–2837.
13. Schultz PN, Beck ML, Stava C, et al. Health profiles in 5836 long-term cancer survivors. *Int J Cancer.* 2003;104:488–495.
14. Ko CY, Maggard M, Livingston EH. Evaluating health utility in patients with melanoma, breast cancer, colon cancer, and lung cancer: A nationwide, population-based assessment. *J Surg Res.* 2003;114:1–5.
15. Hewitt M, Rowland JH, Yancik R. Cancer survivors in the United States: Age, health, and disability. *J Gerontol A Biol Sci Med Sci.* 2003;58:82–91.
16. Aziz NM. Cancer survivorship research: State of knowledge, challenges and opportunities. *Acta Oncol.* 2007;46:417–432.
17. Turk DC, Meichenbaum D. Adherence to self-care regimens: The patient's perspective. In: Sweet JJ, Rozensky RH, Tovian SM, eds. *Handbook of clinical psychology in medical settings.* New York: Plenum Press, 1991:249–266.
18. Kerns RD, Rosenberg R, Jamison RN, et al. Readiness to adopt a self-management approach to chronic pain: The Pain Stages of Change Questionnaire (PSOCQ). *Pain.* 1997;72:227–234.
19. Burns JW, Glenn B, Lofland K, et al. Stages of change in readiness to adopt a self-management approach to chronic pain: The moderating role of early-treatment stage progression in predicting outcome. *Pain.* 2005;115:322–331.
20. Turk DC, Swanson KS, Gatchel RJ. Predicting opioid misuse by chronic pain patients: A systematic review and literature synthesis. *Clin J Pain.* 2008;24:497–508.
21. Hurn J, Kneebone I, Cropley M. Goal setting as an outcome measure: A systematic review. *Clin Rehabil.* 2006;20:756–772.
22. Zaza C, Stolee P, Prkachin K. The application of goal attainment scaling in chronic pain settings. *J Pain Symptom Manage.* 1999;17:55–64.
23. Fisher K. Assessing clinically meaningful change following a programme for managing chronic pain. *Clin Rehabil.* 2008;22:252–259.
24. Engel GL. The need for a new medical model: A challenge for biomedicine. *Science.* 1977;196:129–136.
25. Hearn J, Higginson IJ. Do specialist palliative care teams improve outcomes for cancer patients? A systematic literature review. *Palliat Med.* 1998;12:317–332.
26. Franks PJ, Salisbury C, Bosanquet N, et al. The level of need for palliative care: A systematic review of the literature. *Palliat Med.* 2000;14:93–104.
27. Zech DF, Grond S, Lynch J, et al. Validation of World Health Organization Guidelines for cancer pain relief: A 10-year prospective study. *Pain.* 1995;63:65–76.
28. Linklater GT, Leng ME, Tiernan EJ, et al. Pain management services in palliative care: A national survey. *Palliat Med.* 2002;16:435–439.
29. Kay S, Husbands E, Antrobus JH, et al: Provision for advanced pain management techniques in adult palliative care: A national survey of anaesthetic pain specialists. *Palliat Med.* 2007;21:279–284.

SUMMARY: PAIN AND CANCER

Cancer is one of the medical conditions that patients fear most. In addition to anxiety about cancer as a potentially lethal disease, patient and family often believe that pain is an inevitable and untreatable consequence; these are major sources of distress. Controlling pain associated with cancer is a major health care problem. Lack of expertise by clinicians in assessing pain is an important cause of poor pain control. A stepwise approach to cancer pain assessment begins with a systemic clinical interview and ends with a clinically relevant diagnosis that outlines the mechanisms and contributing factors to the pain complaint. It involves determining the etiology of the pain and forecasting its future trajectory. It also involves determining the number of sites from which pain originates and the probable mechanisms involved. Assessment must include evaluation of the impact of pain on sleep, functional capability, activity level, and psychological well-being. In addition, the clinician must determine the nature, course, and impact of the cancer on the patient. A thorough evaluation will allow the clinician to obtain a basis for evaluating therapeutic intervention and determining the long-term goals of the patient and/or the patient's family.

Many health care professionals may become involved with the cancer pain patient at any one time. Successful pain management requires that the person or persons responsible for pain management adopt, or at least become familiar with, an interdisciplinary approach to care.

The goals of cancer therapy include cure, symptom palliation, psychological support, and research. Comprehensive cancer care encompasses a continuum that progresses from disease-oriented, curative, life-prolonging treatment through symptom oriented, supportive, and palliative care extending, for some patients, to terminal hospice care. Pain relief must be a priority in all stages of their disease for cancer patients. Pain is the most common symptom experienced by cancer patients and it requires aggressive treatment to maximize both quality and quantity of the patient's life.

Detailed assessment of pain and other quality-of-life concerns is the foundation for successful pain management in the cancer patient. Typically, the pain experience is multidimensional and treatment must address both the physical and emotional components. Failure to outline and diagnose the pain complaint will usually result in poor pain management. Interdisciplinary collaboration is essential for comprehensive care of the cancer patient. Disciplines and specialties involved in care commonly include pain management specialists, oncologists, surgeons, psychiatrists, psychologists, physical therapists, pharmacists, nurses, and social workers. Aggressive therapy of both cancer and pain are mutually beneficial and are best done by skilled, interdisciplinary teams.

Most patients can attain adequate symptomatic relief of cancer pain using appropriate oral pharmacotherapy. As more patients survive cancer and become long-term survivors, appropriate use of medications in this setting is essential. The concurrent use of adjunctive or specialized therapies is sometimes necessary, however, and referral for specialized surgical, anesthetic, or psychological intervention may benefit a significant number of patients. In addition, the growth of the home care industry has broadened the possibilities of extending all types of pain management strategies into the home.

The ideal clinician for management of pain in the cancer patient should be comfortable in assessing, diagnosing, and managing the complex issues that occur in this patient population. That person should be familiar with the patient's treatment environment and be aware of the many complex interactions that such treatment may have for the cancer patient in pain. Because of this potentially complex changing environment, the pain clinician should be comfortable with the many pharmacologic strategies available and be familiar with the appropriate interventional options. The rewards for successfully managing these patients are many, not least of which is the humanitarian component.

APPENDIX A ■ PAIN DISABILITY INDEX (PDI)

The rating scales below are intended to measure the degree to which several aspects of your life are presently disrupted due to chronic pain. In other words, we would like to know how much your pain is preventing you from doing what you would normally do, or from doing it as well as you normally would. Respond to each category by indicating the **overall** impact of pain in your life, not just when the pain is at its worst. For each of the 7 categories of life activity listed, please circle the number on the scale that describes the level of disability you typically experience. A score of 0 means no disability at all, and a score of 10 signifies that all of the activities in which you would normally be involved have been totally disrupted or prevented by your pain.

(1) Family/home responsibilities

This category refers to activities related to the home or family. It includes chores or duties performed around the house (eg, yard work) and errands or favors for other family members (eg, driving the children to school).

    0 1 2 3 4 5 6 7 8 9 10
    no   total
    disability   disability

(2) Recreation

This category includes hobbies, sports, and other similar leisure-time activities.

    0 1 2 3 4 5 6 7 8 9 10
    no   total
    disability   disability

(3) Social activity

This category refers to activities that involve participation with friends and acquaintances other than family members. It includes parties, theater, concerts, dining out, and other social functions.

    0 1 2 3 4 5 6 7 8 9 10
    no   total
    disability   disability

(4) Occupation

This category refers to activities that are a part of or directly related to one's job. This includes nonpaying jobs as well, such as that of a homemaker or volunteer worker.

    0 1 2 3 4 5 6 7 8 9 10
    no   total
    disability   disability

(5) Sexual behavior

This category refers to the frequency and quality of one's sex life.

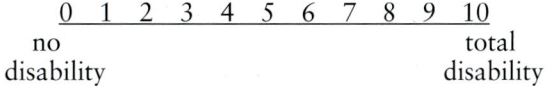

(6) Self-care

This category includes activities that involve personal maintenance and independent daily living (eg, taking a shower, driving, getting dressed, etc.).

<u>0   1   2   3   4   5   6   7   8   9   10</u>
no   total
disability   disability

(7) Life-support activity

This category refers to basic life-supporting behaviors such as eating, sleeping, and breathing.

<u>0   1   2   3   4   5   6   7   8   9   10</u>
no   total
disability   disability

APPENDIX B ■ FUNCTIONAL ASSESSMENT CANCER THERAPY – GENERAL (FACT-G)

Below is a list of statements that other people with your illness have said are important. By circling one (1) number per line, please indicate how true each statement has been for you during the past 7 days.

PHYSICAL WELL-BEING	Not at all	A little bit	Somewhat	Quite a bit	Very much
I have a lack of energy..................................	0	1	2	3	4
I have nausea...	0	1	2	3	4
Because of my physical condition, I have trouble meeting the needs of my family...	0	1	2	3	4
I have pain...	0	1	2	3	4
I am bothered by side effects of treatment...	0	1	2	3	4
I feel ill...	0	1	2	3	4
I am forced to spend time in bed.................	0	1	2	3	4

SCORE =

SOCIAL/FAMILY WELL-BEING	Not at all	A little bit	Somewhat	Quite a bit	Very much
I feel close to my friends.............................	0	1	2	3	4
I get emotional support from my family......	0	1	2	3	4
I get emotional support from my friends......	0	1	2	3	4
My family has accepted my illness................	0	1	2	3	4
I am satisfied with family communication about my illness..................	0	1	2	3	4
I feel close to my partner (or the person who is my main support)..................	0	1	2	3	4

Regardless of your current level of sexual activity, please answer the following question. If you prefer not to, please check this box ☐ and go to the next section.

I am satisfied with my sex life.......................	0	1	2	3	4

SCORE =

EMOTIONAL WELL-BEING	Not at all	A little bit	Somewhat	Quite a bit	Very much
I feel sad..	0	1	2	3	4
I am satisfied with how I am coping with my illness...	0	1	2	3	4
I am losing hope in the fight against my illness...	0	1	2	3	4
I feel nervous...	0	1	2	3	4
I worry about dying.....................................	0	1	2	3	4
I worry that my condition will get worse......	0	1	2	3	4

SCORE =

FUNCTIONAL WELL-BEING	Not at all	A little bit	Somewhat	Quite a bit	Very much
I am able to work (include work at home)	0	1	2	3	4
My work (include work at home) is fulfilling	0	1	2	3	4
I am able to enjoy life	0	1	2	3	4
I have accepted my illness	0	1	2	3	4
I am sleeping well	0	1	2	3	4
I am enjoying the things I usually do for fun	0	1	2	3	4
I am content with the quality of my life right now	0	1	2	3	4

SCORE =

RELATIONSHIP WITH DOCTOR	Not at all	A little bit	Somewhat	Quite a bit	Very much
I have confidence in my doctor(s)	0	1	2	3	4
My doctor is available to answer my questions	0	1	2	3	4
How much does your relationship with your doctor affect the quality of your life?	0	1	2	3	4

SCORE =

(Reprinted with permission from Cella D et al. The Functional Assessment of Cancer Therapy scale: development and validation of the general measure. *J Clin Oncol*, 1993;11(3):570–579. Copyright 1987, 1997 by David Cella, Ph.D.)

APPENDIX C ■ STRUCTURED OPIOID ASSESSMENT FOR PATIENTS WITH PAIN (SOAPP) - VERSION 1.0

Name:_____ Date:_____

The following are some questions given to all patients at the Pain Clinic who are on or being considered for opioids for pain management. Please answer each question as honestly as possible. This information is for our records and will remain confidential. Your answers alone will not determine your treatment but will help us provide the best medical care possible. Thank you.

	Never	Seldom	Sometimes	Often	Very Often
(1) How often do you feel that your pain is "out of control"?					
(2) How often do you have mood swings?					
(3) How often do you do things that you later regret?					
(4) How often has your family been supportive and encouraging?					
(5) How often have others told you that you have a bad temper?					
(6) Compared with other people, how often have you been in a car accident?					
(7) How often do you smoke a cigarette within an hour after you wake up?					
(8) How often have you felt a need for higher doses of medication to treat your pain?					
(9) How often do you take more medication than you are supposed to?					
(10) How often have any family members, including parents and grandparents, had a problem with alcohol or drugs?					

	Never	Seldom	Sometimes	Often	Very Often
(11) How often have any of your close friends had a problem with alcohol or drugs?					
(12) How often have others suggested that you have a drug or alcohol problem?					
(13) How often have you attended an AA or NA meeting?					
(14) How often have you had a problem getting along with the doctors who prescribed your medicines?					
(15) How often have you taken medication other than the way that it was prescribed?					
(16) How often have you been seen by a psychiatrist or mental health counselor?					
(17) How often have you been treated for an alcohol or drug problem?					
(18) How often have your medications been lost or stolen?					
(19) How often have others expressed concern over your use of medication?					
(20) How often have you felt a craving for medication?					
(21) How often has more than one doctor prescribed pain medication for you at the same time?					
(22) How often have you been asked to give a urine screen for substance abuse?					
(23) How often have you used illegal drugs (for example, marijuana, cocaine, etc.) in the past 5 years?					
(24) How often in your lifetime have you had legal problems or been arrested?					

Note: To score SOAPP, add the ratings of Questions 2, 7, 10, 11, 12, 13, 15, 17, 18, 19, 20, 22, 23, and 24. A score of 7 or higher is considered positive. (©2009 Inflexxion, Inc. Permission granted solely for use in published format by individual practitioners in clinical practice. No other uses or alterations are authorized or permitted by copyright holder. Permissions questions: PainEDU@inflexxion.com. The SOAPP was developed with a grant from the National Institutes of Health and an educational grant from Endo Pharmaceuticals.)

APPENDIX D ■ CURRENT OPIOID MISUSE MEASURE (COMM)

The following are some questions given to all patients at the Pain Clinic who are on or being considered for opioids for pain management. Please answer each question as honestly as possible. This information is for our records and will remain confidential. Keep in mind that we are only asking about **the past 30 days**. Thank you.

	Never	Seldom	Sometimes	Often	Very Often
(1) In the past 30 days, how often have you had trouble with thinking clearly or had memory problems?	O	O	O	O	O
(2) In the past 30 days, how often have people complained that you are not completing necessary tasks? (ie, doing things that need to be done, such as going to class, work or appointments)	O	O	O	O	O
(3) In the past 30 days, how often have you had to go to someone other than your prescribing physician to get sufficient pain relief from medications? (ie, another doctor, the emergency room, friends, street sources)	O	O	O	O	O
(4) In the past 30 days, how often have you taken your medications differently from how they are prescribed?	O	O	O	O	O
(5) In the past 30 days, how often have you seriously thought about hurting yourself?	O	O	O	O	O
(6) In the past 30 days, how much of your time was spent thinking about opioid medications (having enough, taking them, dosing schedule, etc.)?	O	O	O	O	O
(7) In the past 30 days, how often have you been in an argument?	O	O	O	O	O
(8) In the past 30 days, how often have you had trouble controlling your anger (eg, road rage, screaming, etc.)?	O	O	O	O	O
(9) In the past 30 days, how often have you needed to take pain medications belonging to someone else?	O	O	O	O	O

	Never	Seldom	Sometimes	Often	Very Often
(10) In the past 30 days, how often have you been worried about how you're handling your medications?	O	O	O	O	O
(11) In the past 30 days, how often have others been worried about how you're handling your medications?	O	O	O	O	O
(12) In the past 30 days, how often have you had to make an emergency phone call or show up at the clinic without an appointment?	O	O	O	O	O
(13) In the past 30 days, how often have you gotten angry with people?	O	O	O	O	O
(14) In the past 30 days, how often have you had to take more of your medication than prescribed?	O	O	O	O	O
(15) In the past 30 days, how often have you borrowed pain medication from someone else?	O	O	O	O	O
(16) In the past 30 days, how often have you used your pain medicine for symptoms other than for pain (eg, to help you sleep, improve your mood, or relieve stress)?	O	O	O	O	O
(17) In the past 30 days, how often have you had to visit the emergency room?	O	O	O	O	O

To score COMM, add the rating of all the questions. A score of 9 or higher is considered a positive.
(©2009 Inflexxion, Inc. Permission granted solely for use in published format by individual practitioners in clinical practice. No other uses or alterations are authorized or permitted by copyright holder. Permissions questions: PainEDU@inflexxion.com. The Current Opioid Misuse Measure was developed with a grant from the National Institutes of Health and an educational grant from Endo Pharmaceuticals.)

APPENDIX E ■ DRIVING INSTRUCTIONS FOR PATIENTS TAKING OPIOIDS

Opioid medications can cause side effects that impair your ability to drive. The final decision on whether you should drive while using opioid medications is a legal issue and should be addressed with your automobile insurance carrier. Out of concern for your safety and the safety of others, please observe the following guidelines:

- Do not drive for 4 to 5 days after beginning opioid treatment or after a change in opioid treatment, such as a dose increase.
- Do not drive if you ever feel sedated or cognitively impaired.
- Report sedation/unsteadiness/cognitive decline to our office as soon as possible.
- Under no circumstances should you use alcohol or illicit drugs, such as cannabis (marijuana), and drive.
- Avoid taking over-the-counter antihistamines, as contained in Tylenol PM and numerous cold and allergy medications.
- Do not make any changes in your medication regimen without consulting our office.

Patient Signature:_____ Date:_____

Practitioner Signature:_____ Date:_____

APPENDIX F ■ OPIOID AGREEMENT

Opioid analgesics (narcotics) are medications used to treat moderate to severe pain. The goal of the Oncology Pain Team is to control pain with few drug side effects and to improve quality of life. The Oncology Pain Team will monitor the effects of pain and treat that pain appropriately.

I, _____, understand that I need to follow the guidelines below to receive pain treatment with opioids by the _____.

1. I will take medications only at the dose and frequency prescribed.
2. I will take no additional opioid analgesics unless I talk to a care provider at _____.
3. No increases in pain medication will be made without prior approval from a _____ care provider.
4. I will ask for opioid analgesics for pain only from a _____ provider.
5. I will keep my scheduled appointments. If I need to cancel an appointment, I will give 24 hours prior notice.
6. I will not use illegal drugs or substances during treatment. I will consent to random drug screens if indicated or requested by a _____ provider.
7. I understand that opioid analgesic pain medications may be stopped if one of the following occurs:
   - The care provider feels that opioid analgesics are not helping to relieve my pain or my ability to function has not improved.
   - I repeatedly fail to follow care provider instructions on use of opioids.
   - I develop side effects that are of concern to the care providers.
   - I inappropriately obtain opioids from sources other than the _____.
8. I will telephone my request for renewal of medications 48 to 96 hours prior to needing them. The Oncology Pain Team reserves the right to specify refill notices for individual patients.
9. If the Oncology Pain Team choose to stop opioid analgesic medications, either these will be reduced over a safe period of time, or a referral will be made to an alternate care provider.
10. An important part of pain management may include non-drug therapies. If I do not follow through with all of the parts of this plan, I understand that the need for opioid therapy may be reevaluated.
11. I will protect my prescriptions and medications. If medications or prescriptions are stolen, it must be reported to the police and a case number given to _____ providers. Treatment with opioid analgesics will be reevaluated and may include discontinuation of care for recurrent losses.
12. When appropriate, I consent to allow the Oncology Pain Team to share information with other providers of my medical care.
13. If I have questions or concerns about my pain management, I will contact a _____ provider. During the week, a message may be left at [Contact Clinic Telephone #]. I understand that I may expect a response within 24 hours of leaving a message. If a call is urgent, I may phone the [CLINIC] at [Paging Operator #] and ask to have the Oncology Pain Service nurse paged. After 5:00 PM and on weekends the Oncology Pain Service team members may be reached by calling the [Paging Operator #] and asking to have the [Appropriate Personnel-Specify] paged.

Patient Signature:_____ Date:_____

Practitioner Signature:_____ Date:_____

APPENDIX G ■ CONSENT TO ASSUME RISKS FOR MEDICAL MARIJUANA

CONSENT TO ASSUME RISKS FOR MEDICAL MARIJUANA

I, __(PATIENT/MINOR PATIENT'S PARENT OR LEGAL GUARDIAN)__ am requesting permission for myself/patient to use medical marijuana under Washington's Medical Use of Marijuana Act (RCW Chapter 69.51 A), and in doing so, assume full responsibility for any and all risks of this action related to my/patient's current medical condition.

I have been informed by my/patient's physician as follows:

- Use of medical marijuana is of unknown benefit;

- Use of medical marijuana creates unknown risks;

- Use of medical marijuana may be harmful; and

- Medical marijuana is not government regulated by the Federal Food and Drug Admmistration for medicinal purposes and may contain unknown qualities of active ingredients and potentially contain contaminants and/or impurities.

- I understand that my/patient's physician may not be knowledgeable of all the associated risks involved in the use of medical marijuana.

- I know that there may be very little scientific information available about the usage of medical marijuana.

- I acknowledge that my/patient's physician has informed me/patient not to drive or operate heavy machinery or engage in potentially hazardous activities while using medical marijuana. I also understand that use of marijuana may affect my coordination and cognition. I assume full responsibility for any harm resulting to me/patient and/or other individuals as a result of my/patient's driving or engaging in potentially hazardous activities while under the influence of medical marijuana.

- I understand that there may be unanticipated side effects/symptoms as a result of this alternative therapy, and that it is my/patient's responsibility to let the physician know if any side effects/symptoms occur. If such side effects/symptoms occur, I understand that my/patient's physician may advise or direct that the use of medical marijuana be stopped.

- I understand that I/patient must be a Washington State resident to receive medical marijuana authorization, and I/patient have provided my physician with a current Washington driver's license or "identicard" card (issued by the Washington State Department of Licensing) to be photocopied and placed in my medical chart.

- I understand that the authorization for expires six months from today's date. I understand that it is my/patient's responsibility to see my/patient's physician to assess the possible continuance of medical marijuana use beyond expiration of the authorization.

- I hereby consent for a [CLINIC] physician or his/her designee, at his/her discretion, to affirm the signing of this authorization form.

- I hereby assume full responsibility for any or all risks of this action, and hereby release the [CLINIC] its employees, staff, and agents from any liability and for any consequences that may result by my action in voluntarily consenting to use of medical marijuana.

_____

Signature of Patient or Legal Representative   Date

_____

PLEASE PRINT – PATIENT OR LEGAL REPRESENTATIVE NAME

_____

If signed by Legal Representative – relationship to patient

_____

Signature of Physician or Medical Provider

Note: If the patient is less than 18 years of age, both the name of the patient and that of the patient's parent or legal guardian should be printed above and both the minor patient and his/her parent or legal guardian should sign the form.

(Reprinted with permission by University of Washington Medical Center.)

APPENDIX H ■ PHYSICIAN AUTHORIZATION FOR MEDICAL MARIJUANA

PHYSICIAN AUTHORIZATION FOR MEDICAL MARIJUANA

Patient Name:_____ Date of Birth:_____

If patient is less than 18 years of age – patient's parent or legal guardian's name:
_____

I am a physician licensed in the State of Washington. I am treating the above-named patient for a terminal illness or debilitating condition as defined in RCW 69.51A.010. According to Washington state law, the benefits of medical marijuana may include treating: nausea and vomiting from cancer chemotherapy; AIDS wasting syndrome; severe muscle spasms from multiple sclerosis or other spasticity disorders; glaucoma either acute or chronic; epilepsy or other seizure disorder; intractable pain which is unrelieved by standard medical treatments and medications; Crohn's disease; hepatitis C, and any other qualifying conditions which have been approved and adopted by the Washington State Medical Quality Assurance Commission.

I have advised the above-named patient and, if the patient is less than 18 years of age, the patient's parent or legal guardian, about the potential risks and benefits of the medical use of marijuana. I have assessed the above-named patient's medical history and medical condition. It is my medical opinion that the potential benefits of the medical use of marijuana would likely outweigh the health risks for this patient. Some risks of medical marijuana may include: possible long-term effects on the brain in the areas of memory; coordination and cognition; respiratory damage; possible lung cancer, and physical and psychological interdependence.

Consistent with the recommendations published in the Institute of Medicine Report, "Marijuana and Medicine: Assessing the Science Base" (1999), I affirm the following conditions are met:
- As appropriate, approved medications to treat the patient's symptoms have been prescribed and the medications have failed to provide the patient relief. This failure to provide relief has been documented in the patient's medical chart;
- The patient's symptoms can reasonably be expected to be relieved by rapid-onset cannabinoid drugs; and
- Such treatment (use of marijuana) is administered under medical supervision in a manner that allows for assessment of treatment effectiveness.

I have advised the above-named patient about the limited medical knowledge regarding the risks and benefits of marijuana usage, including: lack of conclusive scientific data regarding the health risks involved with medical marijuana usage; potential existence of impurities in the marijuana; unknown potency of marijuana; potential interactions with high-risk patient populations; potential interactions with existing psychiatric illness; potential interactions with current drug therapy; and potential unknown side effects resulting from medical marijuana usage.

I have cautioned this patient not to drive or engage in hazardous activities (such as operating machinery) while using medical marijuana.

This authorization form expires 6 months from today's date

_____

(Today's date)

I have completed the "Consent to Assume Risk for Medical Marijuana" Form, and both the patient/patient's authorized representative and I have signed it.

_____

Signature of Patient or Legal Representative   Date

_____

PLEASE PRINT – PATIENT OR LEGAL REPRESENTATIVE NAME

_____

If signed by Legal Representative – relationship to patient

_____

Signature of Physician or Medical Provider

(Reprinted with permission by University of Washington Medical Center.)

APPENDIX I ■ PITTSBURGH SLEEP QUALITY INDEX (PSQI)

The following questions relate to your usual sleep habits during **the past month** only. Your answers should indicate the most accurate reply for the majority of days and nights in the past month. Please answer **all** questions.

1. During the past month, when have you usually gone to bed at night?

   USUAL BED TIME_____

2. During the past month, how long (in minutes) has it usually taken you to fall asleep each night?

   NUMBER OF MINUTES_____

3. During the past month, when have you usually gotten up in the morning?

   USUAL GETTING UP TIME_____

4. During the past month, how many hours of actual sleep did you get at night? (This may be different than the number of hours you spend in bed.)

   HOURS OF SLEEP PER NIGHT_____

For each of the remaining questions, check the **one** best response. Please answer **all** questions.

5. During the past month, how often have you had trouble sleeping because you…

   (a) Cannot get to sleep within 30 minutes

   Not during the past month__   Less than once a week__   Once or twice a week__   Three or more times a week__

   (b) Wake up in the middle of the night or early morning

   Not during the past month__   Less than once a week__   Once or twice a week__   Three or more times a week__

   (c) Have to get up to use the bathroom

   Not during the past month__   Less than once a week__   Once or twice a week__   Three or more times a week__

   (d) Cannot breathe comfortably

   Not during the past month__   Less than once a week__   Once or twice a week__   Three or more times a week__

   (e) Cough or snore loudly

   Not during the past month__   Less than once a week__   Once or twice a week__   Three or more times a week__

   (f) Feel too cold

   Not during the past month__   Less than once a week__   Once or twice a week__   Three or more times a week__

   (g) Feel too hot

   Not during the past month__   Less than once a week__   Once or twice a week__   Three or more times a week__

   (h) Had bad dreams

   Not during the past month__   Less than once a week__   Once or twice a week__   Three or more times a week__

   (i) Have pain

   Not during the past month__   Less than once a week__   Once or twice a week__   Three or more times a week__

(j) Other reason(s), please describe_____
_____

How often during the past month have you had trouble sleeping because of this?

Not during the past month__ Less than once a week__ Once or twice a week__ Three or more times a week__

6. During the past month, how would you rate your sleep quality overall?

    Very good_____

    Fairly good_____

    Fairly bad_____

    Very bad_____

7. During the past month, how often have you taken medicine (prescribed or "over-the-counter") to help' you sleep?

Not during the past month__ Less than once a week__ Once or twice a week__ Three or more times a week__

8. During the past month, how often have you had trouble staying awake while driving, eating meals, or engaging in social activity?

Not during the past month__ Less than once a week__ Once or twice a week__ Three or more times a week__

9. During the past month, how much of a problem has it been for you to keep up enough enthusiasm to get things done?

    No problem at all_____

    Only a very slight problem_____

    Somewhat of a problem_____

    A very big problem_____

10. Do you have a bed partner or roommate?

    No bed partner or roommate_____

    Partner/roommate in other room_____

    Partner in same room, but not same bed_____

    Partner in same bed_____

If you have a roommate or bed partner, ask him/her how often in the past month you have had......

(a) Loud snoring

Not during the past month__ Less than once a week__ Once or twice a week__ Three or more times a week__

(b) Long pauses between breaths while asleep

Not during the past month__ Less than once a week__ Once or twice a week__ Three or more times a week__

(c) Legs twitching or jerking while you sleep

Not during the past month__ Less than once a week__ Once or twice a week__ Three or more times a week__

(d) Episodes of disorientation or confusion during sleep

Not during the past month__ Less than once a week__ Once or twice a week__ Three or more times a week__

(e) Other restlessness while you sleep; please describe_____
_____

Not during the past month__ Less than once a week__ Once or twice a week__ Three or more times a week__

Scoring Instructions for the Pittsburgh Sleep Quality Index

PSQI contains 19 self-rated questions and five questions rated by the bed partner or roommate (if one is available). Only self-rated questions are included in the scoring. The 19 self-rated items are combined to form seven "component" scores, each of which has a range of 0 to 3 points. In all cases, a score of "0" indicates no difficulty, while a score of "3" indicates severe difficulty. The seven component scores are then added to yield one "global" score with a range of 0 to 21 points, "0" indicating no difficulty and "21" indicating severe difficulties in all areas.

Component 1: Subjective sleep quality
Examine question #6, and assign scores as follows:

Response	Component 1 score
"Very good"	0
"Fairly good"	1
"Fairly bad"	2
"Very bad"	3

Component 1 score:___

Component 2: Sleep latency
1. Examine question #2, and assign scores as follows:

Response	Score
≤15 minutes	0
16–30 minutes	1
31–60 minutes	2
>60 minutes	3

Question #2 score:___

2. Examine question #5a, and assign scores as follows:

Response	Score
Not during the past month	0
Less than once a week	1
Once or twice a week	2
Three or more times a week	3

Question #5a score:___

3. Add #2 score and #.5a score

Sum of #2 and#5a:___

4. Assign component 2 score as follows:

Sum of #2 and#5a	Component 2 score
0	0
1–2	1
3–4	2
5–6	3

Component 2 score:___

Component 3: Sleep duration
Examine question #4, and assign scores as follows:

Response	Component 3 score
>7 hours	0
6–7 hours	1
5–6 hours	2
<5 hours	3

Component 3 score:___

Component 4: Habitual sleep efficiency
(1) Write the number of hours slept (question # 4) here: _____

(2) Calculate the number of hours spent in bed:
Getting up time (question # 3): _____
MINUS Bedtime (question #1): _____
EQUALS Number of hours spent in bed: _____

(3) Calculate habitual sleep efficiency as follows:
(# of hours slept/# of hours spent in bed) X 100 = Habitual sleep efficiency (%)
(_____/)_____ X 100 =_____%

(4) Assign component 4 score as follows:

Habitual sleep efficiency %	Component 4 score
>85%	0
75–84%	1
65–74%	2
<65%	3

Component 4 score:___

Component 5: Sleep disturbances
(1) Examine questions #5b-5j, and assign scores for each question as follows:

Response	Score
Not during the past month	0
Less than once a week	1
Once or twice a week	2
Three or more times a week	3

#5b score _____
c score _____
d score _____
e score _____
f score _____
g score _____
h score _____
i score _____
j score _____

(2) Add the scores for questions #5b-5j:

Sum of #5b-5j:_____

(3) Assign component 5 score as follows:

Sum of #5b-5i	Component 5 score
0	0
1–9	1
10–18	2
19–27	3

Component 5 score:___

Component 6: Use of sleeping medication
Examine question #7 and assign scores as follows:

Response	Component 6 score
Not during the past month	0
Less than once a week	1
Once or twice a week	2
Three or more times a week	3

Component 6 score: ___

Component 7: Daytime dysfunction
(1) Examine question #8, and assign scores as follows:

Response	Score
Never	0
Once or twice	1
Once or twice each week	2
Three or more times each week	3

Question #8 score:___

(2) Examine question #9, and assign scores as follows:

Response	Score
No problem at all	0
Only a very slight problem	1
Somewhat of a problem	2
A very big problem	3

Question #9 score: ___

(3) Add the scores for question #8 and #9:

Sum of #8 and #9: ___

(4) Assign component 7 score as follows:

Sum of #8 and #9	Component 7 score
0	0
1–2	1
3–4	2
5–6	3

Component 7 score: ___

Global PSQI Score
Add the seven component scores together:

Global PSQI Score:___

(Reprinted with permission from Busse D, Reynolds C, Monk T et al. The Pittsburgh Sleep Quality Index (PSQI): A new instrument for psychiatric research and practice, 1989; 28(2): 193–213. Copyright Sleep Medicine Institute, University of Pittsburgh, http://www.sleep.pitt.edu)

APPENDIX J ■ PATIENT HEALTH QUESTIONNAIRE-9 (PHQ-9)

Major depression is diagnosed if 5 or more of the 9 depressive symptom criteria have been present at least "more than half the days" in the past 2 weeks, and 1 of the symptoms is depressed mood or anhedonia. Other depression is diagnosed if 2, 3, or 4 depressive symptoms have been present at least "more than half the days" in the past 2 weeks, and 1 of the symptoms is depressed mood or anhedonia. One of the 9 symptom criteria ("thoughts that you would be better off dead or of hurting yourself in some way") counts if present at all, regardless of duration. As a severity measure, the PHQ-9 score can range from 0 to 27, since each of the 9 items can be scored from 0 (not at all) to 3 (nearly every day).

Name_____Date_____

Over the **last 2 weeks** how often have you been bothered by any of the following problems?

	Not at all	Several days	More than half the days	Nearly every day
1. Little interest or pleasure in doing things	0	1	2	3
2. Feeling down, depressed, or hopeless	0	1	2	3
3. Trouble falling or staying asleep, or sleeping too much	0	1	2	3
4. Feeling tired or having little energy	0	1	2	3
5. Poor appetite or overeating	0	1	2	3
6. Feeling bad about yourself, or that you are a failure or have let yourself or your family down	0	1	2	3
7. Trouble concentrating on things, such as reading the newspaper or watching television	0	1	2	3
8. Moving or speaking so slowly that other people could have noticed? Or the opposite—being so fidgety or restless that you have been moving around a lot more than more than usual	0	1	2	3
9. Thoughts that you would be better off dead or of hurting yourself in some way	0	1	2	3

(For office coding: Total Score =)

If you have checked off **any** problems, **how difficult** have these problems made it for you to do your work, take care of things at home, or get along with other people?

Not difficult at all ☐   Somewhat difficult ☐   Very difficult ☐   Extremely difficult ☐

(Developed by Drs. Robert L. Spitzer, Janet B.W. Williams, Kurt Kroenke and colleagues, with an educational grant from Pfizer Inc. Copyright 2005 Pfizer, Inc. All rights reserved. Reprinted with permission.)

APPENDIX K1 ■ TEMPLATE FOR INITIAL OUTPATIENT PAIN EVALUATION

HISTORY: Age: Date of Visit: Referral:

Tumor Diagnosis:

Chief Pain Complaint: Duration of Pain:_____

Chief Pain Complaint Descriptors: (4)

1) Onset:_____
2) Location:
3) Duration: ☐ continuous ☐ intermittent
4) Character:
   ☐ sharp ☐ burning ☐ aching ☐ dull ☐ heavy ☐ stabbing ☐ tender
   ☐ radiating ☐ shock-like ☐ unable to describe ☐ other:_____
5) Severity: average (0–10) _____ worst (0–10)_____ interval_____
   ☐ absent ☐ mild ☐ moderate ☐ moderate-severe ☐ Severe ☐ excruciating
   ☐ unable to describe
6) Aggravating factors:
   ☐ incident _____ ☐ other_____
7) Relieving Factors:
   ☐ rest ☐ position ☐ other_____
8) Associated Symptoms:
   ☐ numbness ☐ weakness ☐ insomnia ☐ none ☐ other_____
9) Functional activities: ☐ normal ☐ limited (specify) Performance Score (Karnofsky/ECOG) =

FACT-G: Physical = ; Social/Family = ; Emotional = ; Functional = ; Relationship with Doctor =
Pain Disability: Family/Home = /10; Recreation = /10; Social Activity = /10; Occupation = /10; Sexual behavior = /10; Self-Care = /10; Life Support Activity = /10.

Functional Goals:

Secondary Pain Complaint(s) + Descriptors:

PT.NO

NAME

DOB

ONCOLOGY PAIN CLINICS:

Initial Consultation

Tumor Treatment: Stage:_____ Date of Diagnosis:_____
Tumor Diagnosis:_____

1) Surgical:

2) Radiation:

3) Chemotherapy:

Known Tumor Location: (include mets)

Recent Diagnostic Tests: (include type/date)

Recent Laboratory Tests:

Clinical Status:
- ☐ known disease, palliative care
- ☐ known disease, surveillance
- ☐ known disease, treatment in progress
- ☐ no known disease, surveillance
- ☐ no known disease, treatment in progress
- ☐ no known disease, no surveillance

Medical Oncologist: Radiation Oncologist:

Other (include Primary Care Provider):

Describe long-term care plan (if known):

Current Medication Use:
- opioid: ☐ None   ☐ Duration of use:_____
  - Long-acting _____
  - Short-acting _____ Average/24 hr _____
    - Prior opioid use/problems ☐ no ☐ yes_____
    - Side Effects: _____
      _____
      _____

- anxiolytic: _____ ☐ Duration of use: _____
- antidepressant: _____ ☐ Duration of use: _____
- Other:

Known Allergies: ☐ no ☐ yes_____

Substance abuse:

☐ alcohol ☐ active N/Y describe_____
☐ opioid ☐ active N/Y describe_____
☐ recreationalv ☐ active N/Y describe_____
☐ other ☐ active N/Y describe_____

Substance Abuse Treatments: ☐ No ☐ Yes
History of Prescription Opioid Issues: ☐ No ☐ Yes
History of Opioid Diversion: ☐ No ☐ Yes
SOAPP Score (ver 1) =   **COMM Score** =

Past Medical History/Family History:

Personal/Family History addiction: ☐ No ☐ Yes

Psychosocial issues:

BDI Score = **Pittsburgh Sleep Quality Index:** Subjective Sleep Quality = ; Sleep Latency = ; Sleep Duration = ; Habitual Sleep Efficiency = ; Sleep Disturbance = ; Use of Sleeping medication = ; Daytime dysfunction = ; Global PSQI = /21.

Other issues:

Driving Consent addressed: ☐ no ☐ yes

Review of Systems: (10+; All other systems negative)

	Positive Findings No	Positive Findings Yes	Comments
Constitutional symptoms	☐	☐	
Eyes	☐	☐	
Ears, nose, throat	☐	☐	
CV	☐	☐	
Respiratory	☐	☐	
GI	☐	☐	
Genitourinary	☐	☐	
Musculoskeletal	☐	☐	
Skin	☐	☐	
Neurological	☐	☐	
Psychiatric	☐	☐	
Endocrine	☐	☐	
Hematologic/lymphatic	☐	☐	
Oncologic	☐	☐	

PHYSICAL EXAMINATION: (8 systems)

P__ BP__ RR__ SpO2____ Wt____ Temp____	Appears comfortable ☐ yes ☐ no Independent ADLs ☐ yes ☐ no Pupils:	Sedation (0–3) Confused ☐ yes ☐ no Speech clear ☐ yes ☐ no Affect
CVS/Respiratory:	Able to ambulate ☐ yes ☐ no Gait: ☐ normal ☐ antalgic	Oral intake: ☐ yes ☐ no Oral cavity:
Neurologic:		
Musculoskeletal:		
Other: (sketch affected area, if indicated): **Dermatologic (include surgical incisions)**		

IMPRESSION:

Pain:
   1) Intensity
   2) Etiology
   3) Source

Clinical Status:

Others:

MEDICAL DECISION-MAKING AND TREATMENT PLAN:

☐	Medication Management	Long Term Opioid Risks Explained: ☐ no ☐ yes
☐	Interventional Options	
☐	Further Investigations	
☐	Consultations Pending	
☐	Others (specify)	
☐	Toxicity Monitoring	☐ Opioid ☐ Others
☐	Counseling	>50% of time spent Time spent = ☐ 30 ☐ 45 ☐ 60

FOLLOW-UP:

☐	Telephone	
☐	Clinic Appointment	
☐	Management Primary Care MD	
☐	Other	
☐	Referral Home Infusion Services	

ADDITIONAL COMMENTS:

Dr._____, Attending, was present during interview, examined the patient, and was involved with decision making.

Date:_____   _____M.D./PA-C/Pharm-D/ARNP

APPENDIX K2 ■ TEMPLATE FOR OUTPATIENT PAIN CLINIC FOLLOW-UP VISITS

UPDATED HISTORY: Age: Date of Visit: Date of Last Evaluation:

Tumor Diagnosis:

Previous Pain Complaint: Duration of Pain:_____

Chief Pain Complaint Descriptors: (4)

1) New Complaint(s):   ☐ Yes   ☐ No
2) Location:
3) Duration: ☐ continuous   ☐ intermittent
4) Character:
   ☐ sharp ☐ burning ☐ aching ☐ dull ☐ heavy ☐ stabbing ☐ tender
   ☐ radiating ☐ shock-like ☐ unable to describe ☐ other:_____
5) Severity: average (0–10) _____   worst (0–10)_____   interval_____
6) Aggravating factors:
   ☐ incident _____   ☐ other_____
7) Relieving Factors:
   ☐ rest ☐ position ☐ other_____
8) Associated Symptoms:
   ☐ numbness ☐ weakness ☐ insomnia ☐ none ☐ other_____
9) Functional activities: ☐ normal   ☐ limited (specify)   Performance Score (Karnofsky/ECOG) =
10) Pain control adequate?:   ☐ Yes   ☐ No

FACT-G: Physical = ; Social/Family = ; Emotional = ; Functional = ; Relationship with Doctor =
Pain Disability: Family/Home = /10; Recreation = /10; Social Activity = /10; Occupation = /10; Sexual behavior = /10; Self-Care = /10; Life Support Activity = /10.

Functional Goals attained?   ☐ Yes   ☐ No

Secondary Pain Complaint(s) + Descriptors:

PT.NO

NAME

DOB

ONCOLOGY PAIN CLINICS:

Follow-Up Visit

Tumor Treatment Update (include most recent dates seen by Provider):

1) Surgical:

2) Radiation:

3) Chemotherapy:

Known Tumor Location: (include mets)

Recent Diagnostic Tests: (include results of tests ordered)

Recent Laboratory Tests:

Clinical Status:
- ☐ known disease, palliative care
- ☐ known disease, surveillance
- ☐ known disease, treatment in progress
- ☐ no known disease, surveillance
- ☐ no known disease, treatment in progress
- ☐ no known disease, no surveillance

<u>New Care Providerf(s):</u>

Current Medication Use:

Medication	Dose/Frequency	Average Daily Use	Dose Escalation

Recent Medication Issues:	
Prescription issues: ☐ Yes ☐ No Compliance: ☐ Yes ☐ No Benefit: ☐ Yes ☐ No	
COMM Score =	
Psychosocial issues:	
BDI Score = Pittsburgh Sleep Quality Index: Subjective Sleep Quality = ; Sleep Latency = ; Sleep Duration = ; Habitual Sleep Efficiency = ; Sleep Disturbance = ; Use of Sleeping medication = ; Daytime dysfunction = ; Global PSQI = /21.	
Other issues:	
Review of Systems: (10+; All other systems negative)	

	Positive Findings		Comments
	No	Yes	
Constitutional symptoms	☐	☐	
Eyes	☐	☐	
Ears, nose, throat	☐	☐	
CV	☐	☐	
Respiratory	☐	☐	
GI	☐	☐	
Genitourinary	☐	☐	
Musculoskeletal	☐	☐	
Skin	☐	☐	
Neurological	☐	☐	
Psychiatric	☐	☐	
Endocrine	☐	☐	
Hematologic/lymphatic	☐	☐	
Oncologic	☐	☐	

PHYSICAL EXAMINATION: (8 systems)

P__ BP__ RR__ SpO2_____ Wt_____ Temp_____	Appears comfortable ☐ yes ☐ no Independent ADLs ☐ yes ☐ no Pupils:	Sedation (0-3) Confused ☐ yes ☐ no Speech clear ☐ yes ☐ no Affect
CVS/Respiratory:	Able to ambulate ☐ yes ☐ no Gait: ☐ normal ☐ antalgic	Oral intake: ☐ yes ☐ no Oral cavity:

Neurologic:
Musculoskeletal:
Other: (sketch affected area, if indicated): **Dermatologic (include surgical incisions)**

IMPRESSION:

Pain: Complaint:
  1) Stability?
  2) New complaints?
 	
Disease Status:
  1) Stability?
  2) New issues?
 	
Medications:
  1) Appropriate?
  2) Compliance ?
  3) Toxicities ?
 	
Others:

MEDICAL DECISION-MAKING AND TREATMENT PLAN:

☐	Medication Management	
☐	Interventional Options	
☐	Further Investigations	
☐	Consultations Pending	
☐	Others (specify)	
☐	Toxicity Monitoring	☐ Opioid ☐ Others
☐	Counseling (reason)/Care coordination (method)	> 50% of time spent. Time spent = ☐15 ☐25 ☐40 ☐

FOLLOW-UP:

☐	Telephone	
☐	Clinic Appointment	
☐	Management Primary Care MD	
☐	Other	
☐	Referral Home Infusion Services	

ADDITIONAL COMMENTS:

Dr.____, Attending, was present during interview, examined the patient, and was involved with decision making.

Date:_____M.D./PA-C/Pharm-D/ARNP

APPENDIX L ■ PATIENT DISABILITY QUESTIONNAIRE (PDQ)

NAME:_____ ID#:_____ DATE:_____

Please read:
This questionnaire asks for your views about how your pain interferes with how you function in everyday activities at this time. This information will help you and your doctor know how you feel and how well you are able to do your daily tasks now.

Please answer every question by making an "X" along the line to show how much your pain problem affects you (from having no problems at all to having the most severe problems you can imagine).

BE SURE TO ANSWER ALL QUESTIONS.

1. Does your pain interfere with your normal work inside and outside the home?
   ]_____]_____]_____]_____]
   Work normally   Unable to work at all

2. Does your pain interfere with personal care (such as bathing, dressing, etc.)?
   ]_____]_____]_____]_____]
   Take care of myself   Need help with all
   completelymy   personal care

3. Does your pain interfere with your traveling?
   ]_____]_____]_____]_____]
   Travel anywhere I like   Cannot travel at all

4. Does your pain interfere with your ability to sit or stand?
   ]_____]_____]_____]_____]
   No problems   Cannot do at all

5. Does your pain interfere with your ability to lift overhead, grasp objects, or reach tor things?
   ]_____]_____]_____]_____]
   No problems   Cannot do at all

6. Does your pain interfere with your ability to bend, stoop, squat, or lift objects off the floor?
   ]_____]_____]_____]_____]
   No problems   Cannot do at all

7. Does your pain interfere with your ability to walk or run?
   ]_____]_____]_____]_____]
   No problems   Cannot do at all

8. Is your income less since your pain began?
   ]_____]_____]_____]_____]
   No decrease   No income at all

9. Do you have to take pain medication to control your pain?
   ]_____]_____]_____]_____]
   No pain medication   Taking pain medication
   needed   throughout the day

10. Does your pain force you to see doctors much more often than before your pain began?
]_____]_____]_____]_____]_____]
Never see doctors   See doctors weekly

11. Does your pain interfere with your ability to see the people who are important to you as much as you would like?
]_____]_____]_____]_____]_____]
No problems   Never see them

12. Does your pain interfere with recreational activities and hobbies that are important to you?
]_____]_____]_____]_____]_____]
No problems   Cannot do at all

13. Do you need the help of your family and friends to complete everyday tasks (including both work inside and outside the home) because of your pain?
]_____]_____]_____]_____]_____]
Never need help   Need help all the time

14. Do you now feel more depressed tense, or anxious than before your pain began?
]_____]_____]_____]_____]_____]
No depression/tension   Severe depression/tension

15. Are there emotional problems caused by your pain that interfere with your family, social, or work activities?
]_____]_____]_____]_____]_____]
No problems   Severe problems

Mild-moderate scores are 0–70; severe, 71–100; and extreme, 101–150.

APPENDIX M ■ NEUROPATHIC PAIN SCALE (NPS)

1. Please use the scale below to tell us how **intense** your pain is. Place an "X" through the number that best describes the intensity of your pain.

   No pain | 0 1 2 3 4 5 6 7 8 9 10 | The most **intense** pain sensation imaginable

2. Please use the scale below to tell us how **sharp** your pain feels. Words used to describe "sharp" feelings include "like a knife," "like a spike," "jabbing" or "like jolts."

   Not sharp | 0 1 2 3 4 5 6 7 8 9 10 | The most **sharp** sensation imaginable ("like a knife")

3. Please use the **scale** below to tell us how **hot** your pain feels. Words used to describe very hot pain include "burning" and "on fire."

   Not hot | 0 1 2 3 4 5 6 7 8 9 10 | The most **hot** sensation imaginable ("on fire")

4. Please use the scale below to tell us how **dull** your pain feels. Words used to describe very dull pain include "like a dull toothache," "dull pain," "aching" and "like a bruise."

   Not dull | 0 1 2 3 4 5 6 7 8 9 10 | The most **dull** sensation imaginable

5. Please use the scale below to tell us how **cold** your pain feels. Words used to describe very cold pain include "like ice" and "freezing."

   Not cold | 0 1 2 3 4 5 6 7 8 9 10 | The most **cold** sensation imaginable ("freezing")

6. Please use the scale below to tell us how **sensitive** your skin is to light touch or clothing. Words used to describe sensitive skin include "like sunburned skin" and "raw skin."

   Not sensitive | 0 1 2 3 4 5 6 7 8 9 10 | The most **sensitive** sensation imaginable ("raw skin")

7. Please use the scale below to tell us how **itchy** your pain feels. Words used to describe itchy pain include "like poison oak" and "like a mosquito bite."

   Not itchy | 0 1 2 3 4 5 6 7 8 9 10 | The most **itchy** sensation imaginable ("like poison oak")

8. Which of the following best describes the **time** quality of your pain? Please check only one answer.

    ( ) I feel a background pain <u>all of the time</u> **and** occasional flare-ups (break-through pain) <u>some of the time</u>.

    Describe the background pain:_____

    Describe the flare-up (break-through) pain:_____

    ( ) I feel a single type of pain <u>all the time</u>. Describe this pain:_____

    ( ) I feel a single type of pain only <u>sometimes</u>. Other times. I am pain free.

    Describe this occasional pain:_____

9. Now that you have told us the different physical aspects of your pain, the different types of sensations, we want you to tell us overall how **unpleasant** your pain is to you. Words used to describe very unpleasant pain include "miserable" and "intolerable." Remember, pain can have a low intensity, but still feel extremely unpleasant and some kinds of pain can have a high intensity but be very tolerable. With this scale, please tell us how **unpleasant** your pain feels.

    Not unpleasant | 0 | 1 | 2 | 3 | 4 | 5 | 6 | 7 | 8 | 9 | 10 | The most **unpleasant** sensation imaginable ("intolerable")

10. Lastly, we want you to give us an estimate of the severity of your <u>deep</u> versus <u>surface</u> pain. We want you to rate each location of pain separately. We realize that it can be difficult to make these estimates, and most likely it will be a "best guess," but please give us you best estimate.

    HOW INTENSE IS YOUR *DEEP* PAIN?

    No **deep** pain | 0 | 1 | 2 | 3 | 4 | 5 | 6 | 7 | 8 | 9 | 10 | The most **intense deep** pain sensation imaginable

    HOW INTENSE IS YOUR *SURFACE* PAIN?

    No **surface** pain | 0 | 1 | 2 | 3 | 4 | 5 | 6 | 7 | 8 | 9 | 10 | The most **intense surface** pain sensation imaginable

(Reprinted with permission from Galer B and Jensen M, Development and preliminary validation of a pain measure specific to neuropathic pain: the Neuropathic Pain Scale. *Neurology*, 1997. 48(2): 332–338.)

APPENDIX N ■ CAGE QUESTIONNAIRE

Post-test probability of alcohol dependence is 7%, 46%, 72%, 88%, and 98% with CAGE scores of 0, 1, 2, 3, and 4 respectively.

1. Have you ever felt you should Cut down on your drinking?
2. Have people Annoyed you by criticizing your drinking?
3. Have you ever felt bad or Guilty about your drinking?
4. Have you ever had a drink first thing in the morning to steady your nerves or get rid of a hangover (Eye-opener)?

(Reprinted with permission from Ewing J, Detecting alcoholism. The CAGE questionnaire. *JAMA*, 1984. 252(14):1905–1907. Copyright 1984 American Medical Association. All rights reserved.)

INDEX

Note: Page numbers followed by *f* and *t* indicate figures and tables, respectively.

A

Abdominal hollow organs, tumor infiltration of, 35
Abdominal pain
  colicky, 183–184
  true parietal, 87
Aβ fibers, in neuropathic pain, 90
Ablative procedures, for pain management, 154
  cordotomy, 278
  cryoablation, 257*f*, 312
  hormonal, for prostate cancer, 328
  neurolysis, 253–254
  neurosurgical, 248–253
  ovarian, 43
  thermal, 254–255, 254*f*
Abraxane, 324
Abscess, epidural, 291*f*
Abstinence syndrome, 176
Acetaminophen, 161–162
  in combination with
    hydrocodone, 206
    morphine, 165
    propoxyphene, 207
  drug interactions, 162
  hepatotoxicity, 161–162
  WHO recommendations for use, 156
N-Acetyl-para-amino-phenol (APAP). *See* Acetaminophen
Acetylsalicylic acid (ASA), 160. *See also* Aspirin
Acidosis, pain-inducing effect of, 17–18
Acid-sensing ion channels, 11, 18
Activities of daily living, assessment of, 121–122, 126*f*
Acupuncture, 324
Acute pain
  cancer treatment-related, 33*t*
  differentiated from chronic pain, 121
Addiction
  definition, 236
  recidivism in, 237
Adenocarcinoma
  cervical, 53
  colorectal, 49–50
  pancreatic, 58*f*
  prostate, 47
  pulmonary, 45
Adenoma
  colorectal, 50, 159
  pituitary, 65–66
Aδ fibers, in neuropathic pain, 90
Adjuvant drugs, 171–189
  analgesics, 175–184
    bone pain adjuvants, 182–183
    general purpose, 175–176
    musculoskeletal pain adjuvants, 176–177
    neuropathic pain adjuvants, 177–182
    visceral pain adjuvants, 183–184
  antiemetics, 171–173
  cannabinoids, 184–185
  ketamine, 185–186
  laxatives, 173–175
  memantine, 186
  psychotropic drugs, 184
  reasons for use of, 171
  WHO recommendations regarding, 155
Adrenocorticotrophic hormone (ACTH), 45, 47
Affective symptoms, cancer treatment-related, 24
After-sensations, as neuropathic pain symptom, 89
Agency for Health Care Policy and Research, 120
Agoraphobia, 317

Alcohol
  neurolysis agent, 253, 255–256
  drug interactions, 197, 232, 241–242
Alcohol abuse, 236, 240–242
  acetaminophen hepatotoxicity in, 161, 162
  adverse health effects, 240–241
  breast cancer risk factor, 42
  screening, 241
Alcohol misuse, 241
Alcohol withdrawal, untreated, 235
Alemtuzumab (Campath), 144
Alfentanil, hepatic metabolism of, 192
Alkaloids, opioid, 192
Allodynia, 89, 93
Alprazolam, 184, 317
Alvimopan, 174, 175
American Academy of Algology, 330
American Academy of Pain Management, 330
American Academy of Pain Medicine, 212, 329, 330
American Board of Anesthesiology, 330
American Board of Interventional Pain Practice, 330
American Board of Medical Specialties, 148, 329
American Board of Psychiatry and Neurology, 330
American Cancer Society, 148
American College of Radiology, 148
American College of Surgeons, 148
American Pain Society, 120, 132*t*, 330
American Society of Anesthesiologists, 120
American Society of Interventional Pain Practice, 330
5-Aminosalicylic acid, 161
Amitriptyline (Elavil), 315
  action mechanism, 179
  neuropathic pain treatment, 179, 181
Amputation
  central pain cause, 97
  palliative, 247
  phantom pain cause, 102
Amygdala, role in pain perception, 13, 14
Analgesic Ladder, 154–158, 155*t*, 156*f*, 195
Analgesics
  adjuvant
    bone pain adjuvants, 182–183
    definition, 175
    general purpose, 175–176
    musculoskeletal pain adjuvants, 176–177
    neuropathic pain adjuvants, 177–182
    visceral pain adjuvants, 183–184
  compliance/noncompliance in use of, 130–131
  nonopioid, 159–170. *See also* Acetaminophen; Acetylsalicylic acid (ASA); Nonsteroidal anti-inflammatory drugs (NSAIDs); Salicylates
    action mechanism of, 159
    serotonin syndrome risk factor, 217
Anastrazole, as pain cause, 108
Anemia, as fatigue cause, 27
Angiogenesis, 17
Angiogenesis inhibitors, as breast cancer treatment, 43
Anorexia nervosa, 28
Anterior cingulate cortex, role in pain perception, 13, 14
Antibiotics
  palliative therapy, 149–150
  serotonin syndrome risk factor, 217*t*
Anticholinergics, as visceral pain treatment, 183
Anticonvulsants
  neuropathic pain treatment, 177–178, 178–181
  serotonin syndrome risk factor, 217
  side effects, 178–179, 217
Antidepressants, 155, 314–316, 315*t*
  agoraphobia treatment, 317

insomnia treatment, 318, 320
neuropathic pain treatment, 177
panic disorder treatment, 317
serotonin syndrome risk factor, 217*t*
Antiemetics, 171–173, 172*t*, 173*t*, 184, 217*t*
Antifungal agents, 150
Antihistamines
  insomnia treatment, 319
  muscle relaxants, 176
Anti-Hu syndrome, 99–100
Antimetabolites, 143
Antimigraine drugs, as serotonin syndrome risk factor, 217*t*
Anxiety, 25
  treatment, 155, 316–317
Anxiolytics, 155, 184, 316–317
Apoplexy, pituitary, 66
Apoptosis, 89–90
  acidosis cause, 18
Appetite loss, depression-related, 25
Appetite stimulants, 185
Aprepitant, 171–173, 172*t*
Aripiprazole (Abilify), 239–240
Aromatase inhibitors
  arthralgia and myalgia cause, 18, 20, 43
  breast cancer treatment, 43
  pain cause, 39, 108
β-arrestin$_2$, 197, 221
Arthralgia/arthritis, 18, 19
Ascites, malignant, 149, 150, 150*t*
Asparaginase, as depression cause, 314*t*
Aspirin, 163
  absorption, 160
  action mechanism, 160
  adverse effects, 161
  antiplatelet activity, 160–161
  antipyretic activity, 160, 161
  cancer pain treatment, 154–155, 165
  contraindication in children, 161
Assessment
  cancer pain, 130
    intensity/severity, 32–33
    need for improvement in, 7
    systematic assessment, 120–125
  depression, 25
  neuropathic pain, 90
Astrocytomas, 66, 98, 98*f*
Ataxia, epidural spinal cord compression-related, 117
Autoimmune reactions, paraneoplastic syndrome cause, 99
Avinza, 197–198

B

Bacillus Calmette-Guerin, 144
Back pain
  bone metastases-related, 78, 79
  metastatic epidural spinal cord compression-related, 114, 115, 117–118
  pancreatic cancer-related, 59
  spinal cord tumor-related, 66
Baclofen
  intrathecal administration, 272–273
  muscle spasm treatment, 177
  neuropathic pain treatment, 182
Bariatric drugs, serotonin syndrome risk factor, 217*t*
Beck Depression Inventory (BDI), 26
Bed sores, 40
Benzodiazepine-receptor agonists, insomnia treatment, 318, 319–320

Benzodiazepines
  abuse, 320
  anxiety treatment, 316–317
  insomnia treatment, 318, 319–320
  pain treatment, 184
Benzodiazepine withdrawal, untreated, 235
Bevacizumab (Avastin), 50, 144
Bile duct cancer, 4t
Biliary obstruction, 149
Biliary tract cancer pain, 40
Bioinformatics, 220
Biologic response modifiers, 143–144
Biomarkers, cancer, 69–70
Biopsy, 147
Biotherapy, 143–144
Bisacodyl, 174
Bisphosphonates, 49, 182–183, 307
Black cohosh, 324
Bladder cancer
  5-year survival rate in, 2, 3
  metastatic to bone, 81
  mortality cause, 3, 4t
Bladder dysfunction
  cordotomy-related, 250
  spinal cord compression-related, 115, 117
Bladder spasms, 183
Blood vessels, tumor invasion, 35, 38, 87
Board certification, in pain medicine, 330
Bone cancer
  metastatic, 19
  sarcoma, 63, 64–65
Bone cancer pain, 41, 65
  acidosis, 18
Bone loss, radiographic assessment, 308
Bone marrow transplantation, 144, 145
Bone metastases, 76–85
  clinical consequences, 78–79
  clinical imaging, 76–77, 79–80
  differentiated from insufficiency fractures, 83
  fatigue cause, 26
  hematogenous spread, 77
  incidence, 80t
  molecular basis, 77, 78
  osteolytic, 76–77, 78
  osteosclerotic, 76, 77
  prevalence, 76, 76t
  prognosis, 80–81, 80t
  radiological appearance, 76–77
Bone metastases pain, 36–37
  characteristics, 77–78
  location, 120
  pathophysiology, 35
  prostate cancer-related, 48
  treatment, 182–183, 306–312, 307t
    adjuvant analgesics, 182–183
    algorithmic approach, 306, 306f
    chemotherapy, 307–309
    nonsteroidal anti-inflammatory drugs, 165
    percutaneous radiofrequency/cryoablation, 311–312
    radiation therapy, 309
    radiopharmaceuticals, 182
    vertebroplasty/kyphoplasty, 309–311, 312
Bone scans
  bone metastases, 81, 83–84f
  epidural spinal cord compression, 118
  sacral insufficiency fractures, 83
Bortezomib (Velcade), 63, 143
  peripheral neuropathy cause, 105t, 107–108
Botulinum toxin injections, muscle spasm treatment, 177
Bowel dysfunction
  opioids-induced, 173–175
  spinal cord compression-related, 115, 117
Bowel obstruction, 149
Brachial plexopathy
  radiation therapy-related, 103
  tumor infiltration-related, 37, 93–94, 93f, 95, 95t
Brachytherapy
  intracavitary, for cervical cancer, 55
  prostate cancer, 48–49, 139, 139f
Brain injury
  apoptosis, 89–90
  peripheral nerve injury-related, 89
Brain metastases, 68–69
Brain tumor pain, 34

Brain tumors, 65, 66
  imaging, 67
  mortality cause, 3, 4t
  nociceptive pain associated with, 97
  primary, 65–67
  treatment, 67
BRCA1/BRCA2 gene mutations, breast cancer risk factor, 42, 43, 69
Breakthrough pain, 36
  Analgesic Ladder treatment failure in, 158
  bone metastases-related, 78
  definition, 121
  during intrathecal therapy, 281
  opioid analgesics treatment, 198
  opioid rescue doses, 194–195
  oral transmucosal fentanyl citrate treatment, 195
Breast cancer, 42–44
  asymptomatic for pain, 19
  chemotherapy, 143
  diagnosis, 42–43
  estrogen receptor-positive, 43, 69
  5-year survival rate in, 3t
  fractures associated with, 76
  HER2-positive, 43, 69
  incidence, 3
  metastatic, 19
    cranial neuralgia cause, 90
    lumbosacral plexopathy cause, 95
    to bone, 76, 77f, 78–79, 81, 165, 307
    to brachial plexus, 93, 93f
    to brain, 34f, 68, 68f
    to chest wall, 93f
    to kidney, 34f
    to leptomeninges, 92f
    to spine, 256f
    vertebral, 117f
  mortality cause, 2, 3, 4t
  onset age, 2
  patient decision making in, 138
  recurrence, 327
  risk factors, 42
  treatment, 43–44
    abraxane, 324
    fatigue cause, 27
    surgical, 147
  tumor markers, 69, 69t, 70t
Breast cancer pain
  causes, 44, 44t
  incidence, 40
  location, 120
  prevalence, 19f
  severity, 19
  syndromes, 40
Breast conservation surgery, 147
  cellulitis cause, 150
Brief Fatigue Inventory, 27
Brief Pain Inventory, 7, 32, 121
"Brompton Cocktail," 195
Brownian movement, 280
Bupivacaine
  intrathecal administration, 272t, 279–281, 280f
    in combination with morphine, 281–283, 282t
  continuous intracisternal, 294–296
  high cervical, 294–296
  intracisternal, 295f
  microcapsule delivery, 325–326
  neurotoxicity, 283, 284
Buprenex, 206
Buprenorphine, 205–206, 234
  abuse, 236
  opioid-dependence treatment, 235–236
  transdermal, 206
Bupropion (Wellbutrin), 27, 315
  side effects, 315–316
"Burning" pain, 89
Buspirone, 317
Butorphnol, contraindication as cancer pain treatment, 210–211, 210t

C
Cachexia, 20
  lung cancer-related, 47
  primary or secondary, 28
  treatment, 28–29, 29f, 184
CAGE questionnaire, alcohol abuse diagnosis, 241
Calcitonin, bone pain treatment, 183
Calcium ion channels, 11

Camptothecins, 143
Cancer. See also specific types of cancer
  annual new cases, 130
  diagnosis, 138
  economic costs, 4
  incidence rates, 2, 3–4, 4f
  late sequelae, 328t
  mortality cause, 2–3
  survival rate, 211
Cancer Pain Relief (World Health Organization), 154, 256
Cancer-related pain. See also specific types of cancer pain
  adaptation to, 21–22
  causes, 18–20, 18t
  characteristics, 32–41
    cancer pain syndromes, 35–41
    chronicity, 32
    intensity and severity, 32–33, 120
    pathophysiology/mechanisms, 33–35
    patterns, 35
    syndromes, 36–41t
    timing and duration, 121
  differentiated from noncancer pain, 20
  emotional component, 21
  impact, 121
  intensity/severity, 18–19
    assessment, 32–33, 32t, 120
    predictive factors, 22
    relationship with cancer progression, 22
  management/treatment
    algorithmic approach, 133, 153, 153f
    approaches, 133t
    barriers, 7, 131
    celiac plexus block, 258–263
    comprehensive, 135–137
    individualized approach, 132–133
    interdisciplinary approach, 153
    medications, 153–158
    multimodality approach, 136f
    neuromodulatory treatments, 266–267
    neurosurgical procedures, 248–253
    pharmacological strategies, 154
    radiation therapy, 246
    strategy, 127f
    surgical interventions, 246–253
    symptom-directed, 246–269, 247t
    undertreatment, 7, 130, 131–132, 131t, 132t, 190
    WHO recommendations, 154
  modulating factors, 121
  most common cause, 78–79
  multiple syndromes, 19
  prevalence, 4–5, 5t, 18–19, 19t, 130
  process, 17–23
  psychological factors, 21–22
  radiation therapy-related, 142
  refractory, treatment, 185
  sensory component, 17
  tumor-related, differentiated from nontumor-related, 246
  underestimation, 32
Cancer-related pain syndromes, 35–41
Cancer risk, gender factors, 2
Cancer stem cells, 143
Cancer survivors
  fatigue, 26, 27–28
  of breast cancer, 42
  pain management, 327–329
  percentage of U.S. population, 327
  surveillance, 5
Cancer treatment. See also Chemotherapy; Radiation therapy
  cancer pain cause, 18, 19
  combined treatment, 138
  complementary and alternative medicine, 138–139
  continuum, 138–152
  interaction with cancer pain treatment, 136
  late sequelae, 328t
  neuropathic pain cause, 100–108
  primary, 138–152
  side effects, 24
    permanent, 138
    temporary, 138
  stages, 211
Candidiasis, 145, 150
CA19-1, 69

Cannabidiol, 185
Cannabinoids, 184-185. *See also* Marijuana
　analgesics, 185
　antiemetics, 184, 185
　antitumor cell activity, 184
　neuropathic pain treatment, 177, 178
　therapeutic effects, 238
Capsaicin
　action mechanism, 179
　neuropathic pain treatment, 177, 178, 179
Carbamazepine
　action mechanism, 179
　neuropathic pain treatment, 178, 179, 180, 182
Carboplatin, peripheral neuropathy cause, 105
Carcinoembryonic antigen (CEA), 50, 69*t*, 70, 70*t*
Carcinoid tumors, colorectal, 49–50
Carcinomatosis
　leptomeningeal, 38
　meningitis cause, 92*f*
　peritoneal, 87
Cardiovascular disease, in cancer survivors, 328
Cardiovascular risk, nonsteroidal anti-inflammatory drug-related, 164, 166–167
Carisoprodol (Soma), 176–177
Catechol-O-methyltransferase (COMT) enzyme gene, 221, 222
Catheters
　epidural externalized, 293
　　infection associated with, 291–292
　epidural percutaneous, 272, 274
　intracerebrovascular, 278
　intrathecal externalized, 289–292, 289*f*, 290*f*
　　infection associated with, 290–291
　　surgical implantation technique, 289
　intrathecal internalized, 276*f*, 292
　intrathecal percutaneous, 275–276
Cauda equina, compression, 305
Cavernous sinus syndrome, 90
Celecoxib, 165
　cardiotoxicity, 166, 167
Celiac plexus, anatomy and function, 258–259, 259*f*
Celiac plexus blocks, 258–263
　complications, 260–262
Cellulitis, of the breast, 150
Central nervous system
　neural injury adaptation in, 90
　role in pain perception and processing, 10–15, 21
　　descending pain modulatory system, 13–15
　　neuroanatomy of central pain processing, 12–13
　　nociceptive transmission, 10–12
　role in pain transmission, 18
Central nervous system tumors
　central pain cause, 97
　mortality cause, 67
　primary, 65–67
　radiosurgery treatment, 140–141
Central pain, 96–97
Central sensitization, 12
Cerebellar degeneration, 98
Cerebrospinal fluid
　drug distribution within, 270, 279–281, 281*t*
　dural puncture-related leakage, 146, 293–294
Cerebrospinal fluid analysis
　for leptomeningeal metastases evaluation, 92, 303
　in paraneoplastic neurological syndromes, 99
Certification, of pain medicine specialists, 330
Cervical cancer, 53–56
　5-year survival rate in, 2
　metastatic, 53–54, 53*f*, 54*f*, 55–56, 95
　staging, 54
　treatment, 54–55
Cervical cancer pain, 41, 56
Cervical cancer vaccine, 53, 144
Cervical flexion, 125
Cervical plexus, tumor infiltration, 92–93
Cervical spinal cord, astrocytomas, 98
Cervical spine
　as bone metastases site, 77–78
　in myogenic pain evaluation, 21
　range-of-motion assessment, 127
Cetuximab (Erbitux), 50, 144
C fibers, in neuropathic pain, 90
Chemotherapeutic agents. *See also specific chemotherapeutic agents*
　cytotoxicity, 143
　depression cause, 25, 314, 314*t*
　drug interactions, 178

emetogenicity, 171, 171*t*
myogenic pain cause, 20
peripheral neuropathy cause, 105*t*
Chemotherapy, 138, 142–146
　adjuvant, 143
　definition, 142–143
　multiple- *versus* single-agent, 143
　pain treatment, 143
　regional administration, 143
　side effects
　　fatigue, 26, 27
　　late sequelae, 328
　　nausea and vomiting, 171–173
　　oral mucositis, 144, 145
　　pain, 19, 33, 39, 97
　　peripheral neuropathy, 103–108
　systematic administration, 143
Chest wall, as metastases site, 258*f*
Chest wall pain
　lung cancer-related, 47
　metastatic breast cancer-related, 93*t*
Children, central nervous system cancer, 67
Chinese medicine, 145
Cholangiopancreatography, endoscopic retrograde (ERCP), 149
Choline magnesium trisalicylate, 160, 161, 163
Chondrosarcoma, 63, 64, 290*f*
Chordoma, 63, 63*f*, 66
Chronic pain, differentiated from acute pain, 121
Chronic pain disorders, mechanism, 15
Cingulotomy, 252
Cisplatin
　cervical cancer treatment, 55
　peripheral neuropathy cause, 105
Citalopram, 314
Clinical guidelines, for cancer treatment, 135
Clinical status, classification, 124*t*
Clinical trials, 136
Clodronate, 183
Clomipramine, 179
Clonazepam, 184, 317
Clonidine
　coadministration with opioid analgesics, 195
　neuraxial administration, 284–286
　　epidural, 285
　　intrathecal, 272*t*, 285–286
　use in detoxification, 235
Clotrimazole, 150
Cocaine abuse, 239–240, 242
Codeine
　bowel dysfunction cause, 175
　cancer pain treatment, 154–155
　metabolism, 206–207
Cognitive-behavioral therapy
　cancer survivors, 329
　depression, 318–319
　insomnia, 318–319
Cognitive function, modafinil-related improvement, 215
Cognitive impairment
　cancer treatment-related, 24
　opioid-related, 212, 213, 214–215
　radiation therapy-related, 141
Colon cancer
　5-year survival rate in, 2, 3, 3*t*
　metastatic, 261*f*
　mortality cause, 2, 3, 4*t*
　recurrence, 327
　surgical treatment, 147
Colon pain, 87
Colorectal cancer, 49–51
　aspirin-related prophylaxis, 159
　metastatic, 49, 50, 95, 297*f*
　prevalence, 19*t*
　recurrent, 51
　risk factors, 49
　treatment, 50–51
　tumor markers, 69*t*, 70
Colorectal cancer pain, 19, 40, 50
Combined treatment, for cancer, 138
Commission on Accreditation of Rehabilitation Facilities (CARF), 330
Complementary and alternative medicine (CAM), 138–139, 324
Complex regional pain syndromes, 38, 186, 266
Compliance, in prescription medication use, 130–131
Comprehensive cancer pain care, 135–137

Computed tomography (CT)
　bone metastases, 79, 80
　brain tumors, 67
　cervical cancer, 54
　lung cancer, 45–46
　sacral insufficiency fractures, 82, 84
　spinal metastases, 303
Constipation, opioid-related, 173–175, 194, 212, 213
　morphine-related, 274–275
Continuing education, in cancer pain management, 7
Controlled substances, guidelines for use, 131
Conus magus, 286
Conus medullaris lesions, 117
Coproxamol, 207
Cordotomy, 154, 250–251, 250*f*, 251*t*, 278
Corticosteroids
　adjuvant analgesics, 175
　antiemetic agents, 171–172, 173
　cachexia treatment, 28
　depression cause, 314*t*
　side effects, 16, 175, 314
Cotrimoxazole, 150
Cough medication, as serotonin syndrome risk factor, 217
Coumadin, interaction with acetaminophen, 162
Coxibs, 162–163
Cranial nerve palsies, 90
Cryoablation, of bone metastases, 312
Cryoneurolysis, 254
Cryproablation, 255, 257*f*
Curcumin, 167
Current Opioid Misuse Measure (COMM), 233
Cushing syndrome, 45
Cutaneous pain, 17, 20
Cyberknife Robotic Radiosurgery system, 140–141, 140*f*, 246
Cyclooxygenase-1 (COX-1)
　inhibition, 159
　　acetaminophen-related, 161
　　aspirin-related, 161
　　nonsteroidal anti-inflammatory drug-related, 159–160
　physiologic and pathophysiologic functions, 159, 159*t*, 160*f*
　prostaglandin biosynthesis effects, 159, 159*f*
Cyclooxygenase-2 (COX-2)
　inhibitors
　　antitumor activity, 163–164
　　bone cancer pain treatment, 165
　　cardiotoxicity, 166–167
　　prostaglandin biosynthesis effects, 159, 159*f*
　　selective, 163–164, 165
CYP3A4, in opioid metabolism, 192
CYP3A4 inducers, concomitant administration with methadone, 201
CYP2C19 enzyme system, impairment, 177
CYP2D6
　codeine metabolism, 206
　opioid metabolism, 192
　oxycodone metabolism, 198
CYP2D6 inhibitors, drug interactions, 317
CYP2E1, in acetaminophen metabolism, 162
CYP 450 enzyme system, 178, 201
Cyproterone, 49
Cystitis, 149
Cytarabine, 97, 108
Cytokines
　proinflammatory
　　bone metastases, 77, 78
　　cachexia, 28
　　interaction with opioids, 191
　therapeutic use, 144

D

Death
　cachexia-related, 28
　cancer patients' wish for, 314
Decision making, in cancer treatment, 4, 8, 138
Decompression, as spinal metastases treatment, 247
Deep brain stimulation, 267
Deep tissue pain, 17, 20
Delirium, hypoactive, 316
Depression, 24–26, 25*t*, 314–316, 314*t*
　detection and assessment, 25–26
　fatigue cause, 27
　treatment, 314–316, 318–319
Dermatomes, sensory examination, 125*f*

Descending pain modulatory system, 13–15, 14f
Desipramine (Norpamin), 179, 315
Detoxification, 234–235
Developing countries, cancer pain undertreatment, 190
Dexamethasone, 172, 173
 antiemetic agent, 171
 combination with bupivacaine, 325–326
Dextroamphetamine (Dexedrine), 316
Dextromethorphan, 179
Dextropropoxyphene, 207
 adverse effects, 211
 contraindication as cancer pain treatment, 210t
Dezocine, contraindication as cancer pain treatment, 210–211, 210t
Diagnosis
 cancer pain, 8–9
 components, 124f
 psychosocial effects, 4–5
 role in pain management, 127
Diagnostic and Statistical Manual of Mental Disorders (DSM), 24
Diagnostic procedures, as pain cause, 33
Diazepam
 abuse, 320
 muscle spasm treatment, 177
Diclofenac, 165, 167
Diclofenac sodium, 163
Dietary supplements
 cancer treatment, 138
 serotonin syndrome risk factor, 217t
Diffuse noxious inhibitory control (DNIC), 14–15
Diflunisal, 160, 163
Dihydrocodeine, 207
Dihydromorphine, 207
Diphenhydramine, 172t
 abuse, 320
Discharge, from medical care, 231–232, 232t
Divalproex sodium, 178
DNA damage, cancer treatment-related, 145
DNA synthesis, chemotherapy-related inhibition, 143
Docetaxel
 breast cancer treatment, 43
 peripheral neuropathy cause, 106–107
Docosahexaenoic acid (DHA), 29
Docusate, 175
Docusate sodium, 174
Dolasetron, as antiemetic agent, 171
Dorsal root acid-sensing ion channel (DRASIC), 18f
Dorsal root entry zone lesions (DREZ), 251–252
Dose dumping, 241–242
Double effect principle, 154
Doxepin, as oral mucositis pain treatment, 145
Doxorubicin, 143
 liposomal, 324
Drainage, therapeutic, 149
Driving ability, in patients using opioids, 214
Dronabinol (Marinol), 184
Drug abuse
 prescription drugs, 23, 233–236
 recidivism, 237
 serotonin syndrome cause, 217t
Drug Abuse Warning Network (DAWN), 232, 233, 234, 236–237
Drug control laws, implication for cancer management, 131
Drug delivery systems. See also Catheters
 nanotechnology-based, 324, 325–326
Drug Enforcement Agency (DEA), 238
Drug interactions. See also specific drugs
 among psychiatric drugs, 317
Drug response, genetic factors, 219–222
Duloxetine, as neuropathic pain treatment, 181–182
Duloxetine (Cymbalta), 315
Dural puncture
 cerebrospinal fluid leak cause, 293–294
 headache cause, 146
Dysesthesias, as neuropathic pain symptom, 89
Dysphoria, opioid-related, 212, 213, 215

E
Eastern Cooperative Oncology group, 122t
Eaton-Lambert syndrome, 45
Edema, cerebral, 34
Efferescence-type reactions, use in fentanyl adsorption, 205
Eicosapentaenoic acid (EPA), 28, 29

Elderly patients, methadone use, 202
Electrical stimulation, 249, 266–267
Embeda, 233
EMLA (lidocaine and prilocaine) cream, 176
Emotional component, of cancer pain, 21
Emotional factors, in pain perception, 13
Encapsulated organs, tumor involvement, 34
Encephalitis, limbic, 99
Encephalomyelitis, 98, 100
Encephalopathy, methadone use, 202
Endocannabinoid system, 184
Endocrine disorders, intrathecal opioid use-related, 275
End-of-life care, 5. See also Palliative care
 controlled sedation, 154
Endometrial cancer, recurrence, 327
Endothelins, 17, 18
Epidemiology, of cancer and cancer pain, 2–6
Epidermal growth factor, 17
Epidermoid tumors, 91
Epidural administration
 indications, 154
 opioids, 273–274
 percutaneous catheter use, 272
Epidural metastases, 296–297
 imaging, 303
Epidural space
 abscess, 291f
 anatomy and location of, 270, 270f, 271, 271f
 opioid movement from, 273
Epigastric pain, 58f, 260f
Epothilones, as breast cancer treatment, 43
Erlotinib (Tarceva), 143
Errors, diagnostic, 8–9
Escitalopram (Lexapro), 314, 315
Esophageal cancer, 51
 5-year survival rate, 2
 heartburn cause, 87
 mortality cause, 3, 4t
 prevalence, 19t
 recurrence, 327
 surgical treatment, 147
Esophageal cancer pain
 prevalence, 19
 severity, 19
Estazolam (ProSom), 319
 abuse, 320
Estradiol, as modulator of opioid effects, 191
Eszopiclone (Lunesta), 320
Etodolac, 163
Etoposide, as peripheral neuropathy cause, 105, 108
European Association for Palliative Care, opioid analgesia recommendations, 195
European Federation of Neurological Societies, report on painful polyneuropathy treatment, 181–182, 182t
European Organization for Research and Treatment of Cancer Quality of Life Questionnaire, 26, 123
Ewing sarcoma, 63–64
Exemestane, as pain cause, 108
Exercise, as cancer-related fatigue treatment, 27–28
Extramedullary metastases, 303
Extramedullary spinal tumors, 66

F
Face, squamous cell carcinoma, 91
Failed back syndrome, 276f
Fatigue
 cancer-related, 26–28, 27t
 cancer treatment-related, 24
 depression-related, 25
 radiation therapy-related, 141
Federation of State Medical Boards of the United States, 131
Femur
 bone metastases site, 79
 fractures, 308
Fentanyl, 203–205
 buccal, 205
 increased use, 232
 intrathecal, 272t, 274
 oral transmucosal, 204–205
 parenteral, 208–209
 transdermal (patch), 193, 194, 203–204
 iontophoretic, 204
Fentanyl citrate, oral transmucosal, 195

α-Fetoprotein, 69–70, 69t
Fiber, dietary, 175
Fiber bulking agents, 174
Fibromyalgia, 176
Fibrosarcoma, 63
Fibrosis, radiation therapy-related, 95, 103, 141, 142
Filgrastim, 144
Floxuridine, intrathecal administration, 143
Fluconazole, 150
Flunitrazepam, abuse, 320
5-Fluorouracil, cytotoxicity, 143
Fluoxetine (Prozac), 314, 315
Fluphenazine, 184
Flurazepam, abuse, 320
Flurbiprofen, 163
Fluvoxamine (Luvox), 314, 315
FOLFOX, 50
Fractures, pathologic, 76–77, 78
 clavicular, 101
 long-bone, prophylactic fixation, 308, 308t
 multiple myeloma-related, 63
 muscle wasting-related, 20
 radiation therapy-related, 142
 sacral insufficiency, 81–84, 82–83f
 thoracolumbar compression, 312f
 vertebral, 117
Functional Assessment of Cancer Therapy Fatigue Subscale, 27
Functional Assessment of Cancer Therapy-General (FACT-G), 27, 123
Functional limitations, in cancer survivors, 328
Funicular pain, 116

G
Gabapentin
 action mechanism, 179
 comparison with pregabalin, 180t
 as neuropathic pain treatment, 178, 179, 180, 181–182
Gait analysis, 127
Gait impairment, spinal cord compression-related, 114–115
Gamma-aminobutyric acid A receptors, in sleep disorders, 319–320
Gamma Knife, 141, 141f, 246, 253
Gamma probes, 147
Gastric pain, 87
Gastrointestinal stromal tumors (GISTs), 64–65, 143
Gastrointestinal tract, effects of opioids, 173, 174
Gemcitabane (Gemzar), 144
 cytotoxicity, 143
 pancreatic cancer treatment, 59
Gemtuzumab (Mylotarg), 144
Genetic factors, in drug response, 219–222
Genomics, of opioid use, 219–222
Germ cell tumors, tumor markers, 69t, 70
Gleason grading system, prostate cancer, 47
Glial cells, 97
Glial tumors, 66–67
Glioblastoma, 66, 67
Glioblastoma multiforme, 66f
Glioma, 65, 97, 316
Glossopharyngeal neuralgia, 90–91
Glycerin, as neurolysis agent, 256–257
Glycerol, as neurolysis agent, 253
Goal attainment scaling, 329
G protein-coupled receptor (GPCR) family, 191
Graft-versus-host disease, 145–146
Granisetron, as antiemetic agent, 171
Granuloma, intrathecal catheters-related, 275–276
Grief, 21
Growth factors
 in bone metastases, 77, 78
 hematopoietic, 108, 144
Guided imagery, 324
Gynecological cancer pain, 19, 19t
Gyrectomy, cortical, 252

H
Hallucinations, 214–215
Haloperidol, 172t
Headaches
 brain tumor-related, 65, 66
 leptomeningeal metastases-related, 92
 pituitary tumor-related, 65
 procedural puncture, 146

Head and neck cancer, 51–53
  metastatic, 52, 91
  sarcoma, 64
  squamous cell carcinoma, 144–145
  treatment, 52–53
Head and neck cancer pain
  intracerebroventricular opioid analgesia, 278–279
  prevalence, 19t
  severity, 19
Head and neck pain, post-cancer treatment, 20
Heartburn, 87
Helplessness, perceived, 21
Hematological cancers, varicella-zoster virus reactivation, 109
Hematopoietic agents, 27
Hematopoietic growth factors, 108, 144
Hemorrhage
  bone metastases-related, 35
  gastrointestinal, 163, 166
Hepatic artery, as chemotherapy infusion site, 143
Hepatitis B virus vaccine, 144
Hepatocellular carcinoma, 70, 144
Herbal remedies, 138, 217t, 324
Heroin addiction, 231
  methadone maintenance treatment, 234–235
Heroin withdrawal, 235
Herpes zoster virus, as neuralgia cause, 108–109, 109f
Histamine2-receptor antagonists, 163
Histiocytoma, fibrous, 63
Hodgkin disease, paraneoplastic neurological syndromes, 99
Home care, 323–324
Honda sign, of insufficiency fractures, 82
Hopelessness, 26, 314
Hormone replacement therapy, breast cancer risk factor, 3, 42
Horner syndrome, 90–91, 93
Hospital Anxiety and Depression Scale (HADS), 26
Hot flashes, 316
Human chorionic gonadotropin, 69t, 70t
Human immunodeficiency virus (HIV)-infected patients, illicit drug use, 238
Human papillomavirus vaccine, 53, 144
Humerus, fractures, 308
Hydrocodone, 194, 206
  abuse, 206, 232, 233
  side effects, 194
Hydromorphone, 200, 206
  as alternative to oral morphine, 195
  equianalgesic conversion, 219
  interaction with alcohol, 242
  intrathecal administration, 272t, 274
  myoclonus cause, 193
  postoperative pain treatment, 209
  subcutaneous administration, 210
Hydromorphone hydrochloride extended release capsules, 242
ortho-Hydroxybenzoic acid, 160
5-Hydroxytryptamine, as depressive and anxiety disorders treatment, 317
5-Hydroxytryptamine$_3$ receptor antagonists, 171, 172
Hyoscyamine, 172t
Hyperalgesia
  as neuropathic pain symptom, 89
  opioid-induced (OIH), 215–216
Hyperbaric oxygen therapy, 142
Hypercalcemia, of malignancy
  bone metastases-related, 78, 79
  lung cancer-related, 47
  treatment, 182–183
Hyperesthesia, brachial plexopathy-related, 93
Hyperpathia, as neuropathic pain symptom, 89
Hypnosis, 324
Hypnotics
  abuse, 320
  as insomnia treatment, 318, 319, 320
Hypogogic imagery, 212, 213
Hypophysectomy, 252–253
Hypothalamotomy, 252
Hypothalamus, role in pain perception, 14, 15

I
Ibandronate, 183
Ibritumomab tiuxetan (Zevalin), 144
Ibuprofen, 163
Illicit drug abuse, 231, 236

Imaging studies. See also Computed tomography (CT); Magnetic resonance imaging (MRI); Positron emission tomography (PET)
  for cancer assessment, 124
Imatinib (Gleevec), 64–65, 143
Imipramine, 179, 181
Imiquimod (Aldara), 144
Immune adjuvants, 144
Immune system
  components, 143
  opioid effects, 191
  response to cancer, 143–144
Immune therapy, 143–144, 144t
  prophylactic, 144
Immunization, passive, 144
Immunosuppression, opioid-related, 191–192
Incontinence, 96
Indomethacin, 165
Infection, intrathecal catheters-related, 290–292
Inflammatory bowel disease, salicylate treatment, 160, 161
Inflammatory cells, invasion of neoplastic cells, 17–18
Infusion pumps/systems
  ambulatory, 323
  intrathecal, 274
  neuraxial, 271
  programmable, 272
Infusion therapy, versus bolus injection, 276–277
Insomnia
  classification, 318, 318t
  pathogenesis, 319f
  treatment, 155, 317–321
Insufficiency fractures, sacral, 81–84
Insulin resistance, 327–328
Intercostal cryoablation, 257f
Intercostal nerve blocks, 325
Intercostal nerve injury, 91, 101–102
Interdisciplinary approach, to cancer treatment, 135–136
Interdisciplinary care team approach, to cancer pain treatment, 5f
Interferon therapy, 144
  depression cause, 314t
  peripheral neuropathy cause, 105, 108
Interleukins, 17, 144
International Association for the Study of Pain, 330
Intestine, radiation therapy-related injury, 142
Intracerebroventricular administration, of opioids, 278–279
Intracranial pressure, brain tumor-related elevation, 66
Intramedullary metastases, 303
Intramedullary spinal tumors, 66–67
Intrathecal administration
  advantages, 272
  bupivacaine, 279–281, 282t
    continuous intracisternal, 294–296
    high cervical, 294–296
  doses and concentration, 272t
  mechanism of drug distribution, 279–280
  of morphine, 279–281
  novel techniques, 294–296
  of opioids, 274
Intrathecal (subarachnoid) space, anatomy and location, 270, 270f, 271, 271f
Ion channels, in nociception, 10–11, 11f
Irinotecan, 50

J
Jaundice, pancreatic cancer-related, 58, 59
Joint pain, aromatase inhibitors-related, 18
Joints, steroids-related osteonecrosis, 19

K
Kadian, 197, 242
Karnofsky Performance Status, 81, 81t
Ketamine, 185–186
  neuraxial administration, 287–288
Ketoprofen, 163, 165
Ketorolac, 163, 165
Kidney cancer. See also Renal cell carcinoma
  metastatic to bone, 76
  as mortality cause, 3, 4t
Kidney cancer pain, pathophysiology, 34
Kyphoplasty, 309, 311, 311f

L
Laboratory studies, for cancer assessment, 124
Lactulose, 174
Lambert-Eaton syndrome, 98, 99
Laminectomy, 247, 251, 305
Lamotrigine, as neuropathic pain treatment, 178, 179, 180, 182
Laparoscopic surgery, 147
Laryngeal cancer, 51, 52
  metastatic, 35f
Laser ablation, 253–254
Laxatives, 173–175
Leiomyosarcoma, 63
  colorectal, 49–50
  metastatic to chest wall, 258f
Lenalidomide, 63
Leptomeningeal metastases, 90, 91–92, 303
Leptomeninges, anatomy, 270, 271
Letrozole, as pain cause, 108
Leucovorin, 50, 144
Leukemia
  chronic myelogenous, 143
  5-year survival rate, 2, 3, 3t
  leptomeningeal metastases, 91
  mortality cause, 4t
Leukemia pain, 41, 77
Leukoencephalopathy, methotrexate-related, 97
Levetiracetam, 80, 180–181
Levorphanol, 202–203
Lhermitte sign, 118
Lidocaine
  action mechanism, 179
  neurotoxicity, 283, 284
  topical, 176, 177, 178, 179
Lidocaine patch, 176
Life expectancy
  implication for neuraxial analgesia use, 293
  influence on treatment decisions, 136–137
Limb length discrepancy, radiation therapy-related, 142
Limb salvage, 247
Liposarcoma, 63
Liposomes, 324, 325
Lipoxygenase, 167
Liver cancer
  as mortality cause, 3, 4t
  recurrent, thermal ablation, 147–148
Liver cancer pain, 34, 40, 87
Liver disease patients, acetaminophen use, 161–162
Liver metastases, 50
Local anesthetic blocks, 154
Local anesthetics
  coadministration with opioid analgesics, 195
  intrathecal administration
    in combination with morphine, 281–283
  neurotoxicity, 283–284
  nanoparticle-based delivery, 325
Lorazepam, abuse, 320
Lorcet (hydrocodone), 206
Lortab (hydrocodone), 206
Low back pain, 176
Lower extremity
  nerve root examination, 125t
  radicular innervation patterns, 126
Lumbar spine
  metastases site, 247
  surgical instrumentation, 310f
Lumbosacral plexopathy
  radiation-related, 103, 104
  tumor infiltration/compression-related, 37, 94–96, 95t
Lumbosacral spine, as bone metastases site, 77–78
Lung cancer, 44–47
  depression associated with, 24
  5-year survival rate in, 3, 3t
  imaging, 45–46
  incidence, 3
  metastatic
    cranial neuralgia cause, 90
    to bone, 76–77, 81, 165
    to brachial plexus, 93
    to brain, 46
    to thoracic spine, 305
  mortality cause, 2, 3, 4, 45
  nonsmall cell, 45, 46
  Pancoast tumors, 45, 46, 46f, 47, 93
  paraneoplastic syndromes, 46–47

Lung cancer *(Continued)*
  pathologic fracture risk factor, 76–77
  prevalence, 19t
  small-cell, 45, 46–47
  treatment, 46
    surgical, 147
Lung cancer pain, 35, 40, 45f, 47
  location, 120
  prevalence, 19
  severity, 19
Lymphatics, tumor infiltration, 35
Lympho-hematologic cancer pain, 19, 19t
Lymphoma
  B-cell, as brachial plexopathy cause, 94f
  colorectal, 49–50
  metastatic, 91, 95
  monoclonal antibody therapy, 144
  as mortality cause, 4t
  5-year survival rate in, 2
Lymphoma pain, 41
Lyrica. *See* Pregabalin

M

Macrophages, of neoplasms, 17
Magnesium salts, 174
Magnetic resonance imaging (MRI)
  bone metastases, 79
  brain tumors, 67
  breast cancer, 43
  cervical cancer, 54
  epidural abscess, 291f
  epidural spinal cord compression, 118
  functional, for neuropathic pain syndrome evaluation, 90
  lung cancer, 45, 46
  sarcoma, 64
  sacral insufficiency fractures, 82–83, 83
  spinal metastases, 303
Magnetoencephalography (MEG), 90
Malnutrition, 28
Mammography, screening, 3
Mandible, radiation therapy-related injury, 142
Mandibular bone tumors, 91
Marijuana, medical use, 185, 238–239
  as cachexia treatment, 29
Mastectomy
  versus breast conservation surgery, 147
  neuropathic pain after, 100–101
  pain syndrome associated with, 39
  patient decision making regarding, 138
  phantom pain after, 102
McGill Pain Questionnaire, 120
Medical education, pain management component, 7
Medical history, 123
Medical model, application to cancer pain treatment, 133
Medtronic, 272
Megestrol, as cachexia treatment, 28–29
Melanoma
  5-year surival rate in, 3t
  metastatic, 81, 296f, 308f
Melatonin, 320
Melatonin-receptor agonists, as insomnia treatment, 318, 320–321
Memantine, 179, 186
Memorial Pain Assessment Card (MPAC), 121
Memorial Symptom Assessment Scale (MSAS), 124
Meninges, spinal, location, 271t
Meningioma, 66, 91
Meningitis, 92, 97
  carcinomatous, 92t
Meperidine, 194
  contraindication as cancer pain treatment, 210t
  hepatic metabolism, 192
  neuraxial administration, 274, 287
  side effects, 194
Meprobamate, 177
Mesalamine (5-ASA), 160
Mesothelioma, metastatic, 248f
Metabolic syndrome, in cancer survivors, 327–328
Metastases. *See also under specific types of cancer*
  as depression risk factor, 25
  number, 19
Metastatic disease, curable, 143
Metaxalone (Skelaxin), 177
Methadone, 233
  as cancer pain treatment, 200–202

cardiac safety recommendations, 201, 202, 202t
  intrathecal administration, 274
  as neuropathic pain treatment, 200
  pharmacokinetics, 200–201, 201t
  rotations, 218–219
  side effects, 194, 201, 202
Methadone maintenance treatment, for opioid addiction, 234–235
Methamphetamine abuse, 240, 242
Methotrexate, 97, 143
Methotrimeprazine, 184
N-Methyl-D-aspartate antagonists, 177, 178, 185, 186, 201, 202
Methylnaltrexone, 174–175
Methylphenidate (Ritalin), 27, 316
Methylprednisolone, as antiemetic agent, 171
Metoclopramide, 172t
Micelles, 325
Microglia, 90
Midazolam, neuraxial administration, 288–289
Middle cranial fossa syndrome, 90
Mind-body medicine, 324
Mirtrazapine (Remeron), 315, 316, 320
Misoprostol, 163
Misuse, of prescription medications, 130, 231t. *See also* Opioid abuse, factors contributing to, 231
Modafinil (Provigil), 27–28, 215, 316
Model Guidelines for the Use of Controlled Substances for the Treatment of Pain, 131
Molecular pain genetics, 220
Monoamine oxidase inhibitors, 217t, 320
Monoclonal antibody therapy, 144
Mononeuropathies, tumor-associated, 91
Morphine, 154–155, 195–298
  administration routes, 195, 196
  in combination with
    acetaminophen, 165
    bupivacaine, 281–283, 282t
    sequestered-release naltrexone, 233
  comparison with tramadol, 208
  dose titration, 195
  effect on driving ability, 214
  effect on tumor growth, 191–192
  efficacy of, genetic factors in, 221
  equianalgesic conversion, 219
  formulations, 195, 196–198
  hepatic metabolism, 192
  increased use, 232
  isolation, 190
  metabolites, 192–193
  neuraxial administration
    epidural administration, 273–274, 277–278
    infusion, *versus* bolus injection, 276–277
    intrathecal administration, 272–273, 274, 279–283
    technical issues related to, 293
  parenteral administration, 208–209
  as postoperative pain treatment, 209
  potency, 195, 232
  side effects, 194, 196, 274–275
  subcutaneous administration, 210
  tolerance to, 277
Morphine-3-glucuronide, 192–293, 209
Morphine-6-glucuronide, 192
Morphine IR, 194
Mortality rates, in cancer, 2–3, 3t, 4
Motor cortex stimulation, 267
Motor skills impairment, opioid-related, 214
M protein, as multiple myeloma marker, 61, 62
MS Contin, 196–197
Mucosa, serous, tumor infiltration, 35
Mucosal pain, treatment, 145
Mucositis, 20, 39, 144–145, 145t
Mucous membranes, necrosis of ulceration, 38
Multidisciplinary approach, to cancer treatment, 135–136
Multiple myeloma, 61–63
  chemotherapy, 143
  clinical and laboratory abnormalities, 62t
  fractures associated with, 76
  imaging, 62–63, 63
  metastatic to bone, 62, 63t, 76–77, 80
  osteosclerotic form, 99
Muscle, cachexia-related loss, 28
Muscle-related pain. *See* Myogenic pain
Muscle relaxants, 176–177

Muscle wasting, 20
Musculoskeletal pain, adjuvant analgesia treatment, 176–177
Myelofibrosis, radiation therapy-related, 141
Myelopathy
  methotrexate-related, 97
  radiation therapy-related, 39, 97, 102–103
Myelotomy, 154, 251
Myoclonus
  opioid-related, 212, 213
  parenteral opioid therapy-related, 209
  serotonin syndrome-related, 216
Myofascial pain, assessment, 125, 127
Myofascial pain syndrome, 20, 21, 176
Myogenic pain, 20–21
Myopathy, paraneoplastic necrotizing, 21

N

Nabilone (Cesamet), 184, 185
Nabumetone, 163
Nalbuphine, contraindication as cancer pain treatment, 210–211, 210t
Naloxone, 174, 190, 235–236
Naltrexone, 235
  sequestered-release, 233
Nanotechnology, 324–326, 325f
Naproxen, 163, 165, 167
Narcolepsy, 316
Nasal cavity cancer, 52
Nasopharyngeal cancer, 52
National Cancer Institute
  oral mucositis scoring criteria, 145, 145t
  Surgical Oncology Fellowship Program, 148
National Cancer Institute-designated cancer centers, 135
National Institutes of Health, statement on cancer symptom management, 24
National Survey on Drug Use and Health, 233
Nausea and vomiting
  antiemetic therapy, 171–173, 172t, 173t, 184, 217t
  complementary and alternative medicine therapies, 324
  morphine-related, 274–275
  nonsteroidal anti-inflammatory drug-related, 166
  opioid-related, 194, 212, 213
Neck dissection, 39, 52, 101
Neck pain, 176
Necropsy, 9
Necrosis
  aseptic, of bone, 39
  bone metastases-related, 35
  radiation therapy-related, 142
  tumor-induced, 35
Neostigmine, neuraxial administration, 286
Nephrostomy, percutaneous, 148
Nerve growth factor, 18
Nerve injury
  apoptosis cause, 89–90
  ectopic excitability cause, 89
  thoracotomy-related, 101–102
Nerve roots, examination, 124–125, 125t
Nerves, tumor infiltration, 17, 18, 34–35, 37–38
Nerve sheath tumor, 96
Neural degeneration, tumor-induced, 17
Neuralgia
  cranial, 90–91
  glossopharyngeal, 90–91
  postherpetic, 39, 108–109, 176, 177
  trigeminal, 91, 246
Neuraxial analgesia, 270–302, 294t
  alternative drugs, 284–289
  choice of drug delivery systems, 271–272
  choice of medication, 271t, 272–273
  definition, 270
  epidermal metastases and, 296–297
  indications, 271t
  limitations, 292–294
  opioids, 273–279
    adverse effects, 274–276
    bolus injection *versus*, 276–277
    epidural administration, 273–274
    failure rate, 273, 274, 277, 278
    intracerebroventricular administration, 278–279
    intrathecal administration, 274
    long-term efficacy, 277–278
  spinal canal occlusion and, 296–297
Neurectomy, peripheral, 249

Neurofibroma, 66
Neurokinin-1 receptor antagonists, 171, 172–173
Neurolysis
 chemical, 253
 intercostal, 258
 spinal, 255–258
 of splanchnic nerves, 262–263
 thermal, 253–254
Neuroma, acoustic, 91
Neuromodulatory treatment, for cancer pain, 266–267
Neuropathic pain, 98-113. See also Neuropathies
 brachial plexopathy-related, 93–94, 95
 cancer treatment-related, 100–108
 central pain, 96–97
 cervical plexopathy-related, 92–93
 characteristics of, 89
 cranial neuralgia-related, 90–91
 diagnosis, 177
 differentiated from nociceptive pain, 33–34
 herpes zoster neuralgia, 108–109
 leptomeningeal metastases-related, 91–92
 lumbosacral plexopathy-related, 94–96
 methadone treatment, 200
 mononeuropathy-related, 91
 multiple etiologies, 177
 paraneoplastic neurological syndromes-related, 98–100
 peripheral neuropathy-related, 97–98
 positive and negative symptoms, 89
 postherpetic neuralgia, 108–109
 prevalence in cancer patients, 17
 radicular, 91, 96
 sacrum/sacral nerve tumor infiltration-related, 96
 spinal, 96
 treatment
  adjuvant analgesics, 177–182, 178t, 179t
  memantine, 186
  tramadol, 208
Neuropathic Pain Scale (NPS), 90
Neuropathies
 axonal vasculitic, 97–98
 cancer treatment-related, 24
 cranial, 37
 motor paraneoplastic, 100
 peripheral, 37, 39, 97–98, 99t
  chemotherapy-induced (CIPN), 103–108, 106f, 107t, 177
  paraneoplastic, 100
 sensory, 100
 spinal, 37
Neurosurgical procedures, for cancer pain management, 248–253
Neurotonin. See Gabapentin
Neurotransmission, genetic variation in, 220–221
Neurotransmitters, release during nociceptor activation, 17
Neutrophils, of neoplasms, 17
Nociceptive pain
 differentiated from
  neuropathic pain, 33–34
  radicular pain, 96
 prevalence in cancer patients, 17
 somatic, 17
Nociceptive transmission, of pain, 10–12, 10f
Nociceptors, 10, 11, 11f, 18f
Nociceptor sensitization
 cancer-related, 17–18, 18f
 in myogenic pain, 20–21
Nociceptor stimulation, 33–34
Nonsteroidal anti-inflammatory drugs (NSAIDs), 162–167, 163t
 action mechanisms, 159
 antitumor activity, 163–164
 as bladder spasm treatment, 183
 as cancer pain treatment, 163, 164–166
 cardiotoxicity, 166–167
 as colorectal adenoma treatment, 159
 definition, 162
 side effects, 163, 166, 166t
 topical, 164
 WHO recommendations for use, 156
Norco (hydrocodone), 206
Nordextropropoxyphene, 207, 211
Nortriptyline, 179, 181, 315
Nuclear factor-κB, activation, 163
Nuclear factor-κ ligand (RANKL), 77, 78f

Nucleus cuneiformis, role in pain perception, 14, 15
Numerical Rating Scale, of pain severity, 32, 33
Nutritional supplements, as cachexia treatment, 28
Nystatin, 150

O
Obesity
 cancer risk factor, 327
  breast cancer, 42
  colorectal cancer, 49
 cancer treatment-related, 327
 in cancer survivors, 327–328
Obstruction, visceral, 38–39, 148–149
Obstructive sleep apnea, 316
Octreotide, 183–184
Oligodendroglioma, 67
Ommaya reservoir, 143, 278
Oncologists, surgical, 148
Onconeural antigens, 99
Ondansetron, 171, 172t
Ondine Cruse, 250
Opioid abuse, 231, 236–237
 deterrent technology, 232–233
Opioid addiction, 234–235
Opioid agonist-antagonists, action mechanism, 190
Opioid agonists
 action mechanism, 190
 partial, action mechanism, 190
Opioid analgesics, 190–230
 active metabolites, 192, 192t
 administration routes, 193
 cellular effects, 191
 in combination with nonsteroidal anti-inflammatory drugs, 165, 163, 165–166
 controlled-release (CR), 190
 definition, 190
 dosage, 193–194
  versus analgesic relationship, 216f
 dose titration, 211
 effect on driving ability, 214
 effect on motor skills, 214
 emetogenic effects, 173
 equianalgesic conversions, 219t
 extended-release (ER), 190
 as first-line therapy, 193
 gender-related response, 191
 immunomodulatory effects, 191–192
 implication for ablative neurosurgical procedures, 248–249
 improper use, 211–212
 interaction with alcohol, 241–242
 long-acting, 193
 long-term use, 211–212, 211t
 metabolism, 192
 neuraxial administration, 273–279
  adverse effects, 274–276
  bolus injection versus, 276–277
  bolus versus continuous administration, 276–277
  epidural administration, 273–274
  failure rate, 273, 274, 277, 278
  intracerebroventricular administration, 278–279
  intrathecal administration, 274
  long-term efficacy, 277–278
 as neuropathic pain treatment, 177, 178, 181–182
 not recommended for cancer pain management, 210–211, 210t
 oral and transdermal formulations, 194
 overview, 190–193
 parenteral administration, 154, 208–210
  intravenous, 208–209
  subcutaneous, 209–210
 problematic use, 327
 as rescue medication, 194
 rotation, 218–219, 218t
 selection, 193–195
 short-acting, 193
 side effects, 212–213, 212t
  bowel dysfunction, 173–175
  cognitive impairment, 214–215
  constipation, 173–175, 194, 212, 213
  gastrointestinal effects, 173, 173t, 174
  gender-related, 191
  hyperalgesia, 215–216
  prevention or minimization, 213
  treatment, 155, 213, 213t

 sustained-release (SR), 190
 tolerance, 130, 215–216, 277
 variability in response, 190–191
 WHO recommendations for use, 156–157
Opioid antagonists, as bowel dysfunction treatment, 174–175
Opioid contracts, 212
Opioid misuse, 237
Opioid poisonings, 236–237
Opioid receptors
 genetic encoding, 221–222
 location, 190
  central nervous system, 174
  gastrointestinal, 173–174
 types, 190, 191
Opioid resistance, 219–220
Opioids, definition, 190
Opium, alkaloids, 190
Oral cavity cancer, 2, 51, 52
Oramorph SR, 196–197
OraVescent technology, 205
Organ failure, methadone use, 202
Oropharyngeal cancer, 51, 52
Oropharyngeal cancer pain, 40
Orphenadrine, 176
Osmic acid, as chemical neurolysis agent, 253
Osmotics, 174
Osteonecrosis
 radiation therapy-related, 142
 steroids-related, 19
Osteoporosis, in cancer survivors, 328
Osteoproteregin, 77
Osteosarcoma, 63, 64
Outpatient oncology treatment, 130
Ovarian cancer, 56–58
 5-year survival rate, 3
 metastatic, 57f
 mortality cause, 3
 tumor markers, 69t, 70, 70t
Ovarian cancer pain, 41, 57–58, 88
Oxaliplatin, as peripheral neuropathy cause, 105
Oxaprozin, 163
Oxazepam, abuse, 320
Oxcarbazepine
 action mechanism, 179, 180
 as neuropathic pain treatment, 178
Oxycodone, 198–199
 abuse, 233, 234
 action mechanism, 179
 administration routes, 198–199
 as alternative to oral morphine, 195
 controlled release, 194
 immediate release, 194
 increased use, 232
 metabolism, 198
 as neuropathic pain treatment, 179, 182
 pharmacokinetics, 198
 side effects, 194
Oxycodone gelatin capsules, 233
OxyContin, 198, 199
 abuse, 234
Oxymorphone, 198, 199–200
 formulations, 194, 199–200
 side effects, 194

P
Paclitaxel acute pain syndrome, 107
Paclitaxel-induced arthralgia/myalgia syndrome, 20
Paclitaxel (Taxol)
 as myofascial pain syndrome cause, 20
 nanoparticle-containing, 324, 325
 as pain cause, 180
 as peripheral neuropathy cause, 106, 107
Pain: Its Mechanisms and Neurosurgical Control (White and Sweet), 248
Pain. See also Cancer-related pain; specific types of pain
 components, 22f
 definition, 10, 17
"Pain cocktail," methadone as component, 202
Pain Disability Index (PDI), 121
Pain Disability Questionnaire (PDQ), 121–122
Pain history, components, 120–122, 120t
Pain Management Index (PMI), 130
Pain matrix, 13, 13f, 90
Pain medicine, 329–330, 329t
Pain modulatory system, descending, 13–15

Pain perception, 10–16
  biologic factors, 42
  central nervous system, 13t
    descending pain modulatory system, 13–15, 14f
    neuroanatomy of central pain processing, 12–13
    nociceptive transmission, 10–12
    pain matrix, 13, 13f, 90
  emotional aspects, 13
  role in healing, 11
  variations, 190–191
Pain rating scales, 120
Pain specialists, 329–331
  role in palliative care, 330–331
Pain Stages of Change Questionnaire, 329
Pain syndromes
  cancer-related, 36–42t
  unrelated to cancer, 40t
Pain threshold, 33
Palliative care, 5
  antibiotics use, 149–150
  for bone metastases patients, 81
  cancer pain specialist's role, 330–331
  versus curative care, 135
  surgery as, 148
Palonosetron, as antiemetic agent, 171
Pamidronate, 183
Pancoast tumors, 45, 46, 46f, 47, 93
Pancreatic cancer, 58–59
  cachexia cause, 20
  chemotherapy, 143
  depression associated with, 24
  5-year survival rate, 3
  metastatic, 58, 58f, 59, 260f, 262f
  mortality cause, 3
  surgical resection, 147
Pancreatic cancer pain, 40, 58–59
  celiac plexus block treatment, 260, 262
  necrosis-related, 35
  syndromes, 59t
Panic disorder, 317
Panitumumab (Vectibix), 144
Panlor SS (dihydrocodeine), 207
Papanicolaou (Pap) smear, 53
Papaver bracteatum, 190
Papaver somniferum, 190
Paracentesis, 149
Paranasal sinus cancer, 52
Paraneoplastic syndromes
  definition, 98
  of lung cancer, 45, 46–47
  neurological, 98–100
    antibody markers, 99
  as pain cause, 40
Parathyroid hormone-related protein, 77, 78, 78f, 79
Parecoxib, cardiotoxicity, 166
Paresthesia
  brachial plexopathy-related, 93
  as neuropathic pain symptom, 89
  spinal cord tumor-related, 66
Paroxetine (Paxil), 27, 314, 315
Patient-controlled analgesia (PCA), 208
  home-based, 323–324
  intrathecal, 296
  for mucosal pain, 145
Patient Health Questionnaire (PHQ-9), 26
Patients, pain management training, 7
Pelvic pain
  localized, 120
  superior hypogastric plexus block treatment, 263–265
Pelvis
  as metastases site, 50f, 79, 95f
  radiation therapy-related injury, 83, 84, 142
  sarcoma, 257f
Pentazocine
  contraindication as pain treatment, 210–211, 210t
  hepatic metabolism, 192
Pentobarbital, abuse, 320
Performance Status Tables, 122
Perianal pain, 48, 257f
Periaqueductal gray area
  electrical stimulation, 267
  role in pain perception, 14, 15
Perineal pain, 87–88
Peripheral nerve(s), tumor infiltration, 34–35
Peripheral nerve injury, 89
Peripheral nerve sheath tumors, 63, 96f

Peripheral nerve stimulation, 266
Peripheral nerve tumors, radiation therapy-related, 39
Peripheral nervous system, 17
Peripheral neuroectodermal tumors, 64
Peripheral sensitization, 11, 12
Periventricular gray area, electrical stimulation, 267
pH, of tissue, tumor-related decrease, 17–18
Phantom pain, 89, 102, 186
Pharmacotherapy, for cancer pain. See also names of specific drugs for cancer pain, principles, 156–157, 157t
Pharyngeal cancer, 51
Phenol, as chemical neurolysis agent, 253, 255–257
Phenolics, of plants, 160
Phenytoin, 178
Physical examination, 124–127
Phytoestrogens, 324
Piroxicam, 163
Pittsburgh Sleep Quality Index, 318, 321
Pituitary gland tumors, 65–66
Placebo effect, in cancer pain treatment, 165
Plants, salicylic-like compounds, 160
Plasma cell disorders, 99
Platelet-derived growth factor, 17
Platinum chemotherapy agents, 143
  as peripheral neuropathy cause, 105
Pleural effusions, malignant, 149
Pleurodesis, 149
Plexopathy
  brachial, 93–94, 93f, 95, 95t
  cervical, 92–93
  drug-induced, 105t
  lumbosacral, 94–96, 95t
  radiation-related, 95t, 103, 104, 104t, 141
Pneumonitis, radiation-related, 141
POEMS syndrome, 62
Polymethyl methacrylate injections, in vertebroplasty, 309, 310
Polyneuropathies, 177
  painful, pharmacotherapy, 181–182
  paraneoplastic, 99–100
  sensorimotor, 99
Positron emission tomography (PET)
  bone metastases, 80
  brain injury, 90
  brain tumors, 67
  breast cancer, 42–43
  cervical cancer, 54
  epidural spinal cord compression, 118
  lung cancer, 45
Potassium ion channels, 10
Potassium ions, opioid receptor-mediated influx, 191
Pregabalin
  action mechanism, 179
  comparison with gabapentin, 180t
  as neuropathic pain treatment, 178, 179, 180, 181–182
Prescription medications, misuse, 130, 231
Prilocaine, topical application, 176
Procarbazine, 108, 314t
Prochlorperazine, 172t
Proctitis, radiation therapy-related, 141, 142
Profile of Mood States (POMS), Fatigue subscale, 27
Progestogens, as cachexia treatment, 28–29
Promathazine, 172t
Propoxyphene, 206, 207
Prostaglandin analogues, 163
Prostaglandin endoperoxide synthase, 159
Prostaglandins
  cyclooxgenase-mediated biosynthesis, 159
  role in angiogenesis and tumor growth, 17, 18
Prostanoids, 160
Prostate cancer, 47–49
  asymptomatic for pain, 19
  brachytherapy, 48–49, 139, 139f
  diagnosis, 47
  5-year survival rate in, 2, 3
  grading, 47
  hormone ablation therapy, 328
  hormone-refractory, 49
  incidence, 3
  metastatic
    to bone, 48f, 76, 77, 80f, 81, 120, 165
    as cranial neuralgia cause, 90
    as mortality cause, 4t
    prevalence, 19t
  treatment, 48–49

  tumor markers, 69t, 70t
Prostate cancer pain, 41, 47–48, 48t
  location, 120
  prevalence, 19, 19f
  severity, 19
Prostatectomy, radical, 49
Prostate-specific antigen (PSA), 47, 69t, 70t
Proteolytic enzymes, tumor-produced, 18
Proteomics, 220
Proton pump inhibitors, 163
Pruritus
  opioid-related, 212, 213
  radiation therapy-related, 141
Psychological assessment, of cancer patients, 122
Psychological factors, in cancer pain, 21–22
Psychological interventions, with cancer survivors, 329
Psychosocial assessment, of cancer patients, 122, 123t
Psychostimulants, 316
Psychotherapy, 314
Psychotropic drugs, 184
Purinergic receptor subtype X ion channels, 11

Q
QTc interval, methadone-related prolongation, 201
Quality improvement movement, 133
Quality of life
  assessment, 122–123, 122t
  of cancer survivors, 327
  as cancer treatment component, 135
  effect of cancer symptoms on, 24
  effect of symptom management on, 24
  fatigue-related decrease, 26, 27
  of head and neck cancer patients, 52–53
  radiation therapy-related decrease, 20
Quantum dots, 325
Quazepam, abuse, 320

R
Racial factors, in cancer survival, 2
Radiation therapy, 138, 139–142
  for bone metastases, 309
  brachytherapy, 139
  conformal, 139
  cranial, prophylactic, 46
  diseases commonly treated by, 139t
  for epidural spinal compression, 304–305
  external beam, 139–141
  hypofractionation, 139
  intensity-modulated, 139
  for metastatic spinal tumors, 303
  palliative, 139, 154, 246, 247
  for prostate cancer, 49
  radioimmunotherapy, 139
  side effects, 141–142
    acute and late effects, 20, 141t, 328
    brachial plexopathy, 95
    fatigue, 26, 27
    myelopathy, 102–102
    nausea and vomiting, 171–173
    oral mucositis, 144, 145
    pain, 20, 33, 39
    plexopathy, 95t, 103, 104, 104t, 141
  therapeutic, 246
  thoracic, as breast cancer risk factor, 42
  whole-brain, 68–69
Radicular innervation patterns, 126t
Radicular pain, 91, 96
  differentiated from nociceptive pain, 96
  epidural metastases-related, 115–116, 117
  leptomeningeal metastases-related, 92
  spinal cord tumors-related, 66, 67
Radiculopathies, 91
Radioactive tracers, 147
Radiofrequency ablation, 254–255, 254f
  of bone metastases, 311–312
  thermal, of liver tumors, 147–148
Radiofrequency cordotomy, 250–251
Radiofrequency cordotomyablation, 251t
Radioimmunotherapy, 139
Radiopharmaceuticals, as bone pain treatment, 182, 307
Radiosurgery, 139–141
  Cyberknife Robotic Radiosurgery system, 140–141, 140f, 246
  Gamma Knife, 141, 141f, 246, 253

spinal, 303–304, 304t
stereotactic
  pituitary, 253
  of spinal tumors, 303
Ramelteon (Rozerem), 320–321
  abuse, 320
Ramsay-Hunt syndrome, 109
Rectal cancer, 2, 3, 4t, 50f
Rectal pain, phantom, 102
Rectal spasms, 183
Referred pain
  epidural metastases-related, 116
  visceral, 87
Regional anesthesia, 154
Rehabilitation, of cancer survivors, 327
Remoxy, 233
Renal cell carcinoma
  biologic response modifier therapy, 144
  metastatic, 60–61, 60f, 76–77, 81
  recurrence, 327
Renal cell carcinoma pain, 61
Renal failure, opioid pharmacokinetics in, 192, 193, 193t
Research, in cancer survivorship, 328
Respiratory depression
  morphine-related, 196, 275
  opioid-related, 212, 213
Retroperitoneal lymph node dissection, 147
Retroperitoneal sarcoma, 64
Reye's syndrome, 161
Rhizotomy
  cranial, 249
  dorsal, 249–250
Rituximab (Rituxan), 144
Rizanidine, as muscle spasm treatment, 177
Robotic surgery, 147
Rofecoxib, cardiotoxicity, 166
Ropivacaine, neurotoxicity of, 283
Rostral ventromedial medulla, role in pain perception, 14, 15
Rotations, of opioid analgesics, 218–219, 218t

S

Sacral insufficiency fractures, 81–84, 82–83f
Sacral nerves, tumor infiltration, 96
Sacrum, tumor infiltration, 63f, 96f
Saddle blocks, intrathecal, 256–257
Salcatonin, 183
Salicin, 160, 161f
Salicylates, 160–162
Salicylate salts, 160, 161
Salicylic acid, structure, 161f
Salsalate, 161
Sarcoma
  of bone, 63, 64–65
  definition, 63
  metastatic, 64, 95, 105f, 165, 258f
  pelvic, 95
    epitheloid, 257f
  of skull base, 66
  soft-tissue, 63–64, 65
Sarcoma pain, 41
Sativex, 185
Scapular flip sign, 101
Schwannoma, 66
Sciatic notch, tumor invasion, 91
Scopolamine, 172t, 183
Screener and Opioid Assessment for Patients with Pain (SOAPP), 233
Sedation
  controlled, 154
  muscle relaxant-related, 176, 177
  opioid-related, 194, 212, 213
    minimization, 316
  palliative, 154
Selective serotonin reuptake inhibitors
  drug interactions, 317
  as hot flashes treatment, 316
  as insomnia cause, 320
  as serotonin syndrome cause, 217
  side effects, 314–315
Self-reports, of cancer pain severity, 32
Senna, 174
Sensitization
  central, 12
  peripheral, 11, 12
Sensory examinations, 124–125

Sensory testing, quantitative, 90
Serotonin-norepinephrine reuptake inhibitors, as neuropathic pain treatment, 178, 181–182
Serotonin syndrome, 216–217, 217f, 217t
Sertraline (Zoloft), 314, 315
Sexual dysfunction, intrathecal opioid use-related, 275
Shoulder syndrome, 101
Shunts, for ascites drainage, 149
Signal transduction, in pain
  genetic variation, 220–221
  pathways, 11, 11f, 12f
Skeleton, axial, as bone metastases site, 76. See also Bone metastases
Skull base, as metastases site, 79, 90, 91
Skull base tumors, 66
Sleep apnea, obstructive, 316
Sleep disturbances
  cancer treatment-related, 24
  as fatigue cause, 27
  treatment, 27, 316, 317–321
Sleep hygiene, 318–319, 318t
Small intestine pain, 87
Smoking, as lung cancer cause, 45
Social support, 314
Society of Surgical Oncology, 148
Sodium ion channels, 11
Sodium salicylate, 160
Soft tissues, tumor infiltration, 35, 63, 64–65
Somatization, 21
Somatostatin analogs, 183
Sorbitol, 174
Spasticity, treatment, 176–177
Specialized pain management, 327–331
Spheroidal Oral Drug Absorption System (SODAS), 197
Spinal canal
  drug administration. See Neuraxial analgesia
  occlusion, 296–927
Spinal cord
  signal transmission, 12f
  tumor infiltration, 35
Spinal cord compression
  acute, 118f
  bone metastases-related, 78
  metastatic epidural, 38, 79, 97, 114–119, 117t, 304–305, 305f
  pathophysiology, 106f
Spinal cord injury, as central pain cause, 97
Spinal cord metastases, radiation therapy, 246
Spinal cord stimulation, 266–267
Spinal cord tumors, 66–67, 98f
Spinal metastases, 303–305, 309t
  radiation therapy, 246
  radiosurgical treatment, 303–304
  surgical management, 247–248, 308
Spinal pain
  chronic, 96
  treatment, 186
Spinal tumors, as axial pain cause, 303
Spine, meninges, 270, 271
Spinocerebellar tract, compression, 115
Spinomesencephalic tract, 12
Spinoreticular (spinoparabrachial) tract, 12
Spinothalamic tract, 12, 18, 20
  compression, 115
  injury to, 97
Spinothalamic tractotomy, 252
Spiraea, 160
Splanchnic nerves, neurolysis, 262–263, 263f
Splenic cancer pain, 34
Squamous cell carcinoma
  cervical, 53f
  of face, 91
  of head and neck, 51f, 52, 91, 144–145
  laryngeal, 35f
  metastatic to spine, 257
  as perianal pain cause, 257f
  prostate, 47
  pulmonary, 45
Stem cells, cancer, 143
Stem cell transplants, hematopoietic, 143, 145–146
Stenting, as visceral obstruction treatment, 148–149
Steroids. See also Corticosteroids
  fracture risk factor, 312f
  pain cause, 39
  toxicity, 19, 176t
Stevens-Johnson syndrome, 178–179

Stomach cancer pain, 19, 19t
Stomach pain, 87
Stool softeners, 174, 175
Straight-leg raising test, 125
Stump pain, 102
Suboxone therapy, 206, 235–236. See also Buprenorphine
Substance abuse. See also Alcohol abuse; Drug abuse
  management, 236–237, 237t
  toxicology testing, 237–238
Substance Abuse and Mental Health Services Administration (SAMHSA), 233
Subutex. See Buprenorphine
Sufentanil
  intrathecal administration, 272t, 274
  parenteral administration, 208–209
  postoperative pain treatment, 209
Suffering, in cancer patients, 21, 22f
Suicidal ideation, hopelessness as risk factor, 26
Sulfasalazine, 160
Sulindac, 159, 163
Sulphasalazine, 161
Sunitinib (Sutent), 64–65
Superior hypogastric pelxus, anatomy, 263, 263f, 264f, 265f
Superior hypogastric plaxus block, 263–265
Suppositories, for constipation treatment, 174
Surgery, for cancer and cancer pain management, 138, 147–148, 246–253
  for metastatic lesions management, 247
  pain syndromes associated with, 20, 33, 39, 100–103
  palliative, 148
  positive surgical margins, 138
Surgical oncologists, 148
Survival rates, in cancer, 2, 2t, 3t, 130, 327
Sympathectomy, surgical, 249
Symptoms, cancer-related, 24
  assessment, 123–124
Symptoms burden, 24
Synalgos (dihydrocodeine), 207
Syncope, cranial neuralgia-related, 91
Syndrome of inappropriate secretion of antidiuretic hormone, 45, 47
Systemic lupus erythematosus, 143

T

Tactile sensory examination, 124–125
Tamoxifen, 43
  as depression cause, 314t
  drug interactions, 317
Taste, loss, 20
Taxanes
  breast cancer treatment, 43
  peripheral neuropathy cause, 106–107
Temazepam, abuse, 320
Tender points, 127
Tenesmoid pain, 183
Tetracaine, neurotoxicity, 283, 284
Tetrahydrocannabinol, 184, 185
  action mechanism, 179, 238
  neuropathic pain treatment, 179, 180
  psychoactive effects, 238
Thalamotomy, 252, 252t
Thalidomide, 63, 107
Thoracentesis, 149
Thoracic spine
  compression, 115
  metastases site, 115f, 247
Thoracotomy, pain syndromes associated with, 39, 101–102, 102t
Th2 cytokines, 143–144
Thymoma, paraneoplastic syndromes, 99
Thyroid cancer
  metastatic to bone, 76, 81
  tumor markers, 70
Tic douloureux, 91
Tizanidine hydrochloride (Zanaflex), 177
T-lymphocytes, of neoplasms, 17
Tolerance, to opioids, 130, 215–216
  to morphine, 277
  to neuraxial opioids, 273
Tonsils, squamous cell carcinoma, 51f
Topical analgesics, 145, 176, 177, 178
Topiramate, 178, 179
Topotecan, 143
Tositumomab (Bexxar), 144

Toxicology testing
  in chronic opioid therapy patients, 212
  for substance abuse, 237–238
Tractotomy
  spinothalamic, 252
  trigeminal, 251t
Training, in cancer pain management, 7
Tramadol, 207–208, 242
  action mechanism, 179
  neuropathic pain treatment, 177, 178, 179, 181–182
  side effects, 208
Transcutaneous skin stimulation, 266
Transforming growth factor, 17
Transient receptor potential (TRP) ion channels, 11
Trastuzumab (Herceptin), 144
Trazodone (Desyrel), 315, 316
Triazolam (Halcion), 319, 320
  abuse, 320
Tricyclic antidepressants
  insomnia cause, 320
  musculoskeletal pain treatment, 176
  neuropathic pain treatment, 178, 181–182
  side effects, 314
Trigeminal nerve tumors, 91
Trigger-point injections, 154
Trigger points, 20
Trophoblastic disease, tumor markers, 69t, 70t
Tropisetron, 171, 172
Tumor growth, 17
Tumor growth factor-β, in bone metastases, 77, 78
Tumor markers, 69–70, 69t
Tumor necrosis factor, 17
Tumor necrosis factor-α, therapeutic use, 144
Tyrosine kinase inhibitors, 143

U
Ultrasound, endoscopic, for celiac plexus block guidance, 262
Upper extremity
  in myogenic pain evaluation, 21
  nerve root examination, 125t
  radicular innervation patterns, 126

Upper motor neuron conditions, 176
Ureteral pain, 88
Urinary diversion, 148–149
Urinary tract cancer pain, 41
Urine toxicology testing
  in chronic opioid therapy patients, 212
  for substance abuse, 237–238
Uropathy, obstructive, 148–149
Uterine cancer, 2, 3
Uterine cancer pain, 41, 88

V
Valproate, 178, 179
Vanilloid receptor-1, 17, 18, 18f
Varicella-zoster virus infections, 108–109
Vascular endothelial growth factor, 17, 18f, 62, 77, 78
Vasculitides, as peripheral neuropathy cause, 97–98
Vasomotor symptoms, in postmenopausal women, 324
Venlafaxine (Effexor), 315t, 316
  action mechanism, 179
  insomnia cause, 320
  neuropathic pain treatment, 179, 181–182
Verbal rating scales, of pain severity, 32–33
Vertebrae, osteoporotic fractures, 309, 312
Vertebral bodies
  metastases site, 296f, 297f
  pathologic fractures, 117
  tumors, 115, 115f
Vertebral metastases, 35, 77–78, 79
  radiofrequency ablation, 255
  vertebroplasty, 310–311
Vertebral-venous plexus, role in bone metastases, 76
Vertebroplasty, 309–310, 309t, 311, 312f
Vicodin (hydrocodone), 206
Vicoprofen (hydrocodone), 206
Video-assisted thoracoscopic surgery (VATS), 102
Vinblastine, as depression cause, 314t
Vinca alkaloids, as peripheral neuropathy cause, 105, 107
Vincristine, adverse effects, 107, 314t

Vindesine, as peripheral neuropathy cause, 107
Vinorelbine, adverse effects, 107, 314t
Viscera, tumor infiltration and obstruction, 38–39, 86, 86t, 148–149
Visceral pain, 86–88
  adjuvant analgesic treatment, 183–184
  characteristics, 17
  description by site, 87
  mechanism, 86–87
  prevalence in cancer patients, 17
Visual Analog Scale, of pain severity, 32, 33, 33f, 121
Vomiting. See Nausea and vomiting

W
Wasting syndromes, 28
Weight loss, 25, 28
Well-being, factors affecting, 24–31
World Health Organization (WHO)
  Analgesic Ladder, 154–158, 155t, 156f, 195
  Cancer Unit, 131
  international cancer pain control efforts, 131
  nonopioid analgesia recommendations, 159, 165
  opioid analgesia recommendations, 196
  oral mucositis scoring criteria, 145, 145t
World Institute of Pain, 330

X
Xerostomia, 20, 142, 144–145
X-rays, of bone metastases, 79, 80

Z
Zaleplon (Sonata), 319, 320
ZerLo (dihydrocodeine), 207
Ziconotide, neuraxial administration, 272–273, 286–287
Zoledronate, 183
Zoledronic acid, 307
Zolpidem (Ambien), 319
  abuse, 320
Zopiclone, abuse, 320
Zydone, 206

CCS1209